THE ROUTLEDGE INTERNATIONAL HANDBOOK OF HEALTH PSYCHOLOGY

This state-of-the-art handbook provides authoritative, up to date coverage of health psychology topics, offering an excellent, in-depth view of the field. Leading experts provide essential insights into the discipline of health psychology, its roots, future directions, and the networks and organizations involved.

Structured into eight parts, the book starts with defining health psychology, including and providing an important historical overview. Subsequent sections examine theories and methodology, health behavior, interpersonal relations and health, chronic disease, and interventions. The concluding sections tackle the important areas of global health psychology and the future of health psychology. The editors and authors include leading experts in the field as well as early career researchers from over 20 countries across the world. Global representation was a key goal in selecting authors.

While familiar areas receive ample attention, this book strives to put the field of health psychology in context. As well as examining history, this book spotlights global issues and explicitly mentions future developments and opportunities. The role of health psychology in the COVID-19 pandemic is considered, and there is discussion more broadly on how health psychology can contribute to addressing societal challenges, including how to move forward sharing knowledge more firmly with policymakers.

This is an essential resource for scholars, PhD students and research masters students specializing in the field of health psychology.

Robbert Sanderman is Emeritus Professor of Health Psychology at the University Medical Center Groningen, the Netherlands. His research is focused on psychological and social adaptive processes in patients diagnosed with a chronic somatic disease (e.g., cancer, diabetes, heart failure, and COPD) and eHealth interventions. He supervised 70 PhD projects, co-edited several handbooks on chronic disease, and co-authored over 450 publications (articles, book chapters, and books). He has been on the boards of numerous societies in the field and is a Past President and Fellow of the European Health Psychology Society.

Karen Morgan is a Professor of Health Psychology at the Royal College of Surgeons in Ireland and is currently the President of the Royal College of Surgeons in Ireland and University College Dublin, Malaysia Campus. She has co(authored) over 100 international publications and book chapters, as well as 13 National Reports and policy briefs and is Co-editor in Chief of EHPS journal Health Psychology & Behavioral Medicine. She is a Past President and Fellow of the European Health Psychology Society who has taught health and organizational psychology in a number of countries across the world. Her research focuses on ageing, quality of life and population health, in particular the health of vulnerable populations. Based in Malaysia, she has a wide network of international multidisciplinary collaborators from fields as diverse as medicine to computer science and engineering.

ROUTLEDGE INTERNATIONAL HANDBOOKS

THE ROUTLEDGE HANDBOOK OF GREENING HIGH-DENSITY CITIES: CLIMATE, SOCIETY AND HEALTH
Edited by Peng Du, Kheir Al-Kodmany, and Mir M. Ali

THE ROUTLEDGE INTERNATIONAL HANDBOOK OF PERINATAL MENTAL HEALTH DISORDERS
Edited by Amy Wenzel

ROUTLEDGE HANDBOOK OF THE INFORMAL ECONOMY
Edited by Ceyhun Elgin

THE ROUTLEDGE HANDBOOK OF CHILD AND FAMILY SOCIAL WORK RESEARCHKNOWLEDGE-
Building, Application, and Impact
Edited by Elizabeth Fernandez, Penelope Welbourne, Bethany Lee and Joyce L. C. Ma

ROUTLEDGE HANDBOOK OF GENDER, CULTURE, AND DEVELOPMENT IN INDIA
Edited by N. B. Lekha and Pradeep Kumar M.

THE ROUTLEDGE INTERNATIONAL HANDBOOK OF VALUATION AND SOCIETY
Edited by Anne K. Krüger, Thorsten Peetz, and Hilmar Schäfer

THE ROUTLEDGE INTERNATIONAL HANDBOOK OF HEALTH PSYCHOLOGY: GLOBAL AND CONTEMPORARY ISSUES
Edited by Robbert Sanderman and Karen Morgan

THE ROUTLEDGE INTERNATIONAL HANDBOOK OF HEALTH PSYCHOLOGY

Global and Contemporary Issues

Edited by Robbert Sanderman and Karen Morgan

Routledge
Taylor & Francis Group
LONDON AND NEW YORK

Designed cover image: © smartboy10 via Getty Images

First published 2025
by Routledge
4 Park Square, Milton Park, Abingdon, Oxon OX14 4RN

and by Routledge
605 Third Avenue, New York, NY 10158

Routledge is an imprint of the Taylor & Francis Group, an informa business

Library of Congress Cataloging-in-Publication Data
Names: Sanderman, R. (Robbert), editor. | Morgan, Karen (Lecturer in psychology), editor.
Title: The Routledge international handbook of health psychology and behavior change / edited by Robbert Sanderman and Karen Morgan.
Description: Abingdon, Oxon ; New York, NY : Routledge, 2024. | Includes bibliographical references and index. |
Identifiers: LCCN 2024018460 (print) | LCCN 2024018461 (ebook) | ISBN 9781032330648 (hardback) | ISBN 9781032330662 (paperback) | ISBN 9781003318026 (ebook)
Subjects: LCSH: Clinical health psychology. | Sick--Psychology.
Classification: LCC R726.7 .R68 2024 (print) | LCC R726.7 (ebook) | DDC 616.001/9--dc23/eng/20240523
LC record available at https://lccn.loc.gov/2024018460
LC ebook record available at https://lccn.loc.gov/2024018461

ISBN: 978-1-032-33064-8 (hbk)
ISBN: 978-1-032-33066-2 (pbk)
ISBN: 978-1-003-31802-6 (ebk)

DOI: 10.4324/9781003318026

Typeset in Times New Roman
by SPi Technologies India Pvt Ltd (Straive)

CONTENTS

PREFACE

Every book starts somewhere, not just anywhere, but with an idea and an ambition. The idea for this book originated quite some years back. Prof. Ralf Schwarzer was talking with Routledge about an *International Handbook of Health Psychology*. He did have an impetus for a plan but indicated – at an EHPS (European Health Psychology Society) Conference – that he wanted to pass the project on to others. After consulting with Ralf and Lucy Kennedy (Routledge), we – Karen Morgan and Robbert Sanderman – agreed to take the project further.

The idea was there, but what was our ambition? Our ambition is to inspire readers with this book and help them reflect on the topics described. We wanted to create a book that would not just recount what we know but also what would be useful to record and pass on. This book takes in-depth approach to important topics and developments so that it will support readers, for example, when preparing new research, teaching, or learning about insights from subjects they are less familiar with. In choosing this approach of highlighting highly relevant issues we have explicitly chosen not to create an encyclopedia covering every inch of the field. In order to reach this ambition, we wrote a plan to divide the book into eight sections, each encompassing a certain theme and covering a selection of relevant associated issues. For each section, we described an outline with five possible chapters. To create what we had in mind, we proposed to work with section editors who would coordinate and ensure good balance across these five chapters, we asked these editors to lead the way by writing the first chapter of their section.

Although we had a wish list of authors, we left it to the section editors to flesh things out. Besides a good representation of women (not more than logical, but still good to mention explicitly, we thought), we asked to include (also) younger authors and people outside Europe and the USA. We had an aim to make this project as inclusive as possible and to make particular efforts to encourage contributions from countries where health psychology is in its infancy. Of course, we had to make the necessary choices. The field of health psychology is so extensive that it is impossible to summarize it in a book.

The sections in this book:

1 Defining Health Psychology
2 Theories and Methodology
3 Health Behavior
4 Interpersonal Relations and Health
5 Chronic Diseases
6 Interventions
7 Global Health Psychology
8 Current Challenges and Opportunities – The Future of Health Psychology

From the titles of the sections, it can be seen that, of course, the familiar areas receive ample attention (health behavior, chronic disease, interventions, and the like). With the design, we have tried not to stay too close to the substantive issues but to put the field in context. The choice was made to use oral history to look at how the area came into being and who was important in it and also to look at the global issues and explicitly mention future developments and opportunities. Certainly, the COVID-19 pandemic also had an impact in that respect. We have experienced and seen that health psychology can contribute to societal challenges, the pandemic being a good example. This also showed us how to step forward and share our knowledge more firmly with policymakers. Therefore, we hope this book demonstrates the area's strength and relevance in the service of societal challenges in health issues and behavior and beyond.

Thanks:

In a random order, we thank those who made the project possible. We want to thank the section editors; see also this book's list of section editors (the list is on page xv-xxxi). They have further punctuated the plans for the sections, improved these, sought authors for them, monitored and commented on the process, and commented in one or more rounds of reviews. It is not easy to manage such a project with 40 individual chapters, into which many authors put their heart and soul, and we are grateful to them for that. In doing so, we, of course, also mention the authors. Many authors contributed to this book, as so often happens, by putting a lot of time and energy into their contribution. We all know that academic life can be challenging, 'juggling' between teaching, research, writing applications, and – let's not forget – a family life. That so many again contributed to a project like this is highly commendable and speaks to the passion of so many researchers and experts in this area. However, we also certainly got the impression that many enjoyed doing so because the format provided gave a certain space and freedom to put a topic close to their hearts on the map.

Our heartfelt thanks also go to Lucy Kennedy of Routledge. Although the project got off to a somewhat slow start, and we suffered and faced delays in part due to the coronavirus period, she kept faith in the project and showed that by being patient at key moments. The help of Kiirtaara Aravindhan's tireless efforts made the task much easier. She supported us exceptionally well in organizing the project. Through countless online meetings and tons of emails and WhatsApp messages, we monitored content and progress and foucsed everyone on the finish line. Fortunately, we got there, and we hope you will enjoy reading as much as we enjoyed the process of editing this book.

Robbert Sanderman
Groningen, the Netherlands

Karen Morgan
Penang, Malaysia

LIST OF EDITORS AND SECTION EDITORS

Editors

Robbert Sanderman is emeritus professor of Health Psychology at the University Medical Center Groningen, The Netherlands. His research is focused on psychological and social adaptive processes in patients diagnosed with a chronic somatic disease (e.g., cancer, diabetes, heart failure, and COPD) and eHealth interventions. He supervised 70 PhD projects, co-edited several handbooks on chronic disease, and co-authored over 450 publications (articles, book chapters, and books). He has been on board of numerous societies in the field and is a Past President and Fellow of the European Health Psychology Society.

Karen Morgan is a Professor of Health Psychology at the Royal College of Surgeons in Ireland. She has co(authored) over 100 international publications and book chapters, as well as 13 National reports and policy briefs and is Co-editor in Chief of EHPS journal Health Psychology & Behavioral Medicine. She is a Past President and Fellow of the European Health Psychology Society who has taught health and organizational psychology in a number of countries across the world. Her research focuses on ageing, quality of life and population health, in particular the health of vulnerable populations. Based in Malaysia, she has a wide network of international multidisciplinary collaborators from fields as diverse as medicine to computer science and engineering.

Section Editors

Section 1: Defining Health Psychology

Angel Marie Chater is a Health Psychologist, Professor of Health Psychology and Behaviour Change (University of Bedfordshire/Centre for Behaviour Change, University College London (UCL)), and Co-director of the Policy Research Unit in Behavioural and Social Sciences. She has championed health psychology throughout her career through roles including UK National Delegate of the EHPS (2011–2018), Chair of the British Psychological Society's Division of Health Psychology (2019–2021), and Co-founder of the Behavioural Science and Public Health Network.

Felix Naughton is Professor of Health Psychology at the University of East Anglia and a Registered Health Psychologist. He leads a research program on the development and evaluation of digital interventions to promote and support health behavior change, particularly innovative technology-mediated approaches.

Section 2: Theories and Methodology

Lisa Marie Warner (Professor of Social Psychology, MSB Medical School Berlin) designs and tests theory-based behavior change programs in different behavioral domains (e.g., physical activity, healthy diet, medication adherence, volunteering) and populations (e.g., older/frail/multimorbid adults, health users) at the intersection of health, social, and lifespan psychology.

Rik Crutzen is Professor of Behaviour Change & Technology at the Department of Health Promotion, Care and Public Health Research Institute, Maastricht University in the Netherlands. Furthermore, he is a Honorary Professorial Fellow within the Melbourne School of Psychological Sciences, University of Melbourne, Australia. A central theme in his work is the systematic development, implementation, and evaluation of behaviour change interventions (i.e., using and developing the Intervention Mapping approach). He has a strong focus on methodological and theoretical progress.

Section 3: Health Behavior

Stephan U. Dombrowski is an Associate Professor at the University of New Brunswick, Canada. Stephan completed his PhD in health psychology at the University of Aberdeen in 2010. He held research posts at the University of Aberdeen, Newcastle University and the University of Stirling.

Gerard J. Molloy is Professor of Psychology at the University of Galway. Gerard completed his PhD in psychology at University of St. Andrews in 2004. He held research posts at the University of Aberdeen and UCL and was previously a Lecturer in Psychology at the University of Stirling

Section 4: Interpersonal Relations and Health

Mariët Hagedoorn is full Professor of Health Psychology at the Department of Health Sciences, University Medical Center Groningen, the Netherlands. She examines how individuals and their significant others adapt to chronic illness, and tests (dyadic) psychosocial (eHealth) interventions to improve their well-being.

Noa Vilchinsky, Associate Professor, serves as the Dean of the Division of Designated Programs and Director of the Psycho-Cardiology Research Lab at Bar Ilan University, Israel. Specializing in psycho-cardiology, coping with illness, caregiving, and patient dignity, her research explores individual, dyadic, and cultural dimensions.

Section 5: Chronic Diseases

Konstadina Griva is an Associate Professor of Health Psychology and Behavioural Medicine at Lee Kong Chian School of Medicine, Nanyang Technological University, Singapore. A Chartered Health Psychologist and honorary Fellow of EHPS, she has an established research record in health-related behavior change and chronic disease management with a particular focus on kidney disease and diabetes.

Stanton P. Newman ran the first Health Psychology MSc in the United Kingdom. He was Head of Psychiatry and Behavioural Science at University College London (UCL), Dean of Health Sciences, and Vice President and currently Professor of Behavioural Medicine, at City University of London. He has published over 350 papers and over 10 books

Section 6: Interventions

Barbara A. Mullan is Professor of Health Psychology at Curtin University. Her primary research interests and expertise lie in the use of social cognition models in predicting, changing, and improving health behaviors. She has held extensive leadership roles in academic societies, and has more than 230 peer-reviewed publications and 12,000+ citations.

Caitlin Liddelow is a Postdoctoral Research Fellow in the School of Psychology at the University of Wollongong and the President of the Australasian Society for Behavioural Health and Medicine (ASBHM). Caitlin is an expert in health behavior change, specifically in women's health, mental health, and sport

Section 7: Global Health Psychology

Bronwynè Coetzee is a Senior Lecturer and a Y1 rated (NRF) Researcher in the Department of Psychology at Stellenbosch University. Her research focuses on understanding and addressing psychosocial factors affecting treatment adherence among children, adolescents and adults living with chronic, infectious, and non-communicable disease in South Africa.

Rizwana Roomaney is a Research Psychologist and Associate Professor at the Department of Psychology at the Stellenbosch University in South Africa. She is a trained methodologist and works in the areas of reproductive health, women's health and online health-seeking behavior.

Lucie Byrne-Davis is a Professor of Health Psychology and a Health Psychologist at University of Manchester, United Kingdom. Working mainly with health partnerships across national borders, she studies and enables behavior change. Her work focuses on facilitating the development of a health workforce that delivers care and support prevention.

Section 8: Current Challenges and Opportunities – The Future of Health Psychology

Dominika Kwasnicka (PhD) is a Senior Research Fellow at University of Melbourne (Australia) and SWPS University (Poland). She is a behavioral scientist interested in health behavior change maintenance, innovative research methods, and applied health promotion interventions. She is a Co-founder of Open Digital Health (www.opendigitalhealth.org) and Lead Editor of Practical Health Psychology (www.practicalhealthpsychology.com).

Olga Perski is a Marie Skłodowska-Curie Postdoctoral Research Fellow at the University of California, San Diego (United States) and Tampere University (Finland). She is an interdisciplinary researcher working at the intersection of behavioral science and technology, with expertise in the development and evaluation of digital behavior change interventions

CONTRIBUTORS

Section 1

Julia Allan is Professor of Psychology at the University of Stirling, conducting research on the effortful control of health behavior and health professional stress and fatigue. She was Chair of the British Psychological Society Division of Health Psychology Scotland (2018–2020) and an EHPS Executive Committee member (2020–2024).

Vivi Antonopoulou works as a Senior Research Fellow for the NIHR Policy Research Unit in Behavioural Science, at UCL Centre for Behaviour Change, focusing on behavioral science theories and models and public health policies. Vivi is a Chartered Psychologist and Associate Fellow of the British Psychological Society (CPsychol AFBPsS).

Phoebe Brook-Rowland is a Researcher and PhD candidate based in the Institute for Sport and Physical Activity Research at the University of Bedfordshire. Her research focuses on increasing physical activity in people with long-term health conditions, specifically via training physical activity practitioners in effective behavior change.

Lucie Byrne-Davis is a Professor of Health Psychology and a Health Psychologist at University of Manchester, United Kingdom. Working mainly with health partnerships across national borders, she studies and enables behavior change. Her work focuses on facilitating the development of a health workforce that delivers care and support prevention.

Angel Marie Chater is a Health Psychologist, Professor of Health Psychology and Behaviour Change (University of Bedfordshire/Centre for Behaviour

Change, University College London (UCL)), and Co-director of the Policy Research Unit in Behavioural and Social Sciences. She has championed health psychology throughout her career through roles including UK National Delegate of the EHPS (2011–2018), Chair of the British Psychological Society's Division of Health Psychology (2019–2021), and Co-founder of the Behavioural Science and Public Health Network.

Hannah Family is Research Fellow in Behavioural and Qualitative Science at National Institute for Health and Care Research Collaboration (NIHR ARC) West and National Institute for Health Protection Research Unit in Behavioural Science and Evaluation (NIHR HPRU BSE) and conducts applied social research to support the development and evaluation of public health interventions, supporting projects in sexual health, substance misuse, medicines optimization and adherence.

Jo Hart is Professor of Health Professional Education, Health Psychologist, Head of Division of Medical Education, Deputy Head of School of Medical Sciences at University of Manchester, United Kingdom. Her research and practice focus on optimization of health professional education, leveraging behavior change theories and methods to improve practice nationally/internationally.

Lisa Hynes is a Health Psychologist with experience in the development, implementation and evaluation of health behavior change interventions focusing on self-management of long-term conditions such as type 1 diabetes and asthma. She currently works for a community-based charity that aims to promote the prevention of cardiovascular disease.

Elizabeth Jenkinson is a Health Psychologist, Associate Professor at the University of the West of England, Bristol, and currently National Training Director in Health Psychology and Workforce Redesign at NHS England. Her teaching, research and practice spans health psychology with a focus on enhancing NHS practice.

Lesley Lewis, a Registered Health Psychologist, leads the Behavioural Science Unit in Somerset Council's Public Health Team. With over a decade of experience in public health and behavior change, Lesley specializes in translating research into practice, applying behavioral science theories and techniques across a range of public health initiatives.

Marta Marques is an Assistant Professor at the NOVA National School of Public Health, Portugal (PhD Health Psychology, Leiden University). Her research interests are in applying behavior change theories to the design of health-related interventions and in advancing the methods for the development of the science of behavior change.

Daniel Masterson is an Assistant Professor in Social Psychology at Skövde University. With a background in health psychology, Daniel's research interest is within health communication, co-production, community-based action research, behavior change, workplace health, and healthy urban planning.

Karen Matvienko-Sikar is a Health Psychologist and Lecturer in the School of Public Health in University College Cork, Ireland. Her research focuses on maternal and child health, particular perinatal mental health and childhood obesity. Dr. Matvienko-Sikar is current chair of the Psychological Society of Ireland Division of Health Psychology.

Jenny McSharry is a Health Psychologist and Lecturer at the University of Galway. She leads a program of research that takes a systematic approach to behavior change to address health-care challenges. She has a particular interest in implementation science and promoting the uptake of research into practice.

Val Morrison's research has examined sociocognitive influences on illicit drug use and risk behavior, and the psychosocial influences on the impacts of physical illness or informal caregiving for 35 years. Working with multidisciplinary teams this research informs policy and practice. She also co-authors a leading European health psychology textbook.

Felix Naughton is Professor of Health Psychology at the University of East Anglia and a Registered Health Psychologist. He leads a research program on the development and evaluation of digital interventions to promote and support health behavior change, particularly innovative technology-mediated approaches.

Rachel Povey first worked in health psychology as a Research Assistant at the University of Kent in 1993. She was awarded her PhD from the University of Leeds in 1997. Rachel currently works as Associate Professor in Health Psychology at Staffordshire University where she co-directs the Professional Doctorate in Health Psychology.

Francis Quinn is an Academic Psychologist whose main interests are in health psychology, exercise psychology, applications of psychology to the fitness industry and mental well-being. He has also published on the history of health psychology. He is currently Lecturer in Psychology at the Robert Gordon University in Aberdeen, United Kingdom.

Karen Rodham is a health psychologist with academic and practice experience. She has worked in the UK National Health Service with people living with Complex Regional Pain Syndrome. She was Chair of the Division of Health Psychology (2015–2017). She specializes in helping people live well in spite of their chronic condition(s).

Jenny Scott is an academic and practicing Pharmacist with research and clinical interests in substance use and harm reduction. She works across multidisciplinary teams to improve the health of people who use drugs.

Vivien Swanson is a Professor of Health Psychology at the University of Stirling. Her research investigates determinants of maternal and infant health and well-being, including breastfeeding behavior. Professional interests also relate to training health psychologists and health psychology practice.

Section 2

Smita C. Banerjee is an Associate Attending Behavioral Scientist in the Department of Psychiatry and Behavioral Sciences at Memorial Sloan Kettering Cancer Center, New York, United States. Her research is in cancer prevention and control, with special emphasis on the role of communication between oncology care providers and patients.

Eva Asselmann is Professor of Differential and Personality Psychology at the HMU Health and Medical University in Potsdam, Germany. Her research focuses on personality development across the lifespan, the intersection of personality with mental and physical health, and targeted personality development, personality change interventions, health promotion, and prevention.

Shweta Chawak is Assistant Professor at Department of Humanities and Social Sciences at IIT Bombay, specializes in health and medical psychology, with a focus on health-care communication, diabetes management, and women's health. During her PhD, she developed a cancer communication intervention based on the Question Prompt List for Indian patients and their caregivers.

Mahati Chittem works as an Associate Professor of Health and Medical Psychology in the Department of Liberal Arts at the Indian Institute of Technology Hyderabad (IITH). Mahati conducts research in primarily two domains: (1) chronic disease management (specialized in psycho-oncology and endocrinology): focusing on communication skills, symptom identification and pathways to care, adherence, and end-of-life issues, and (2) health behaviors: examining the cultural underpinnings of engaging in dietary, exercise and safe sex behaviors.

Alexandra Lelia Dima is a Senior Researcher in Health Psychology. Her research focuses on person-centered care and patient empowerment. She has contributed to the development and validation of several patient-reported measures, statistical algorithms for estimating medication adherence from Real World Data, and interventions for adherence and self-management support in chronic conditions.

Christina M. Juchem is a Research Assistant and Teacher in differential and personality psychology. Her research focuses on how personality, health, and subjective well-being change and interact. As a behavioral science consultant, she has advised on health and talent development projects, and she facilitates mental health promotion workshops for adolescents.

Nicola O'Brien is a Health Psychologist and Associate Professor of Health Psychology at Northumbria University, United Kingdom. Her research includes developing innovative methods and evidence-based interventions to promote individual, population and global health, and well-being.

Ines Pfeffer is a Sport Scientist and does research in the field of Exercise Psychology. Her projects are about physical activity behavior and interventions to promote a physically active lifestyle. Since 2021, she has been Vice President and Treasurer of the German Association of Sport and Exercise Psychology.

Matsungshila Pongener, a PhD candidate at the Indian Institute of Technology Hyderabad, India, specializes in cervical cancer literacy, health behaviors, and preventive health in indigenous communities. Her research is published in international and national journals, and she contributes as a peer reviewer, contributing to the scholarly community in her field.

Lisa Marie Warner (Professor of Social Psychology, MSB Medical School Berlin) designs and tests theory-based behavior change programs in different behavioral domains (e.g., physical activity, healthy diet, medication adherence, volunteering) and populations (e.g., older/frail/multimorbid adults, ehealth users) at the intersection of health, social, and lifespan psychology.

Section 3

Julia Allan is Professor of Psychology at the University of Stirling, conducting research on the effortful control of health behavior and health professional stress and fatigue. She was Chair of the British Psychological Society Division of Health Psychology Scotland (2018–2020) and an EHPS Executive Committee member (2020–2024).

Amy L. Ahern is a Principal Research Associate and Program Leader in the MRC Epidemiology Unit at the University of Cambridge. Amy obtained a PhD in psychology from the University of Liverpool in 2008 and completed postdoctoral research at the University of Oxford (2008–2009) and MRC Human Nutrition Research Unit (2009–2016).

Stephan U. Dombrowski is an Associate Professor at the University of New Brunswick, Canada. Stephan completed his PhD in health psychology at the University of Aberdeen in 2010. He held research posts at the University of Aberdeen, Newcastle University and the University of Stirling.

Elizabeth H. Evans is Associate Professor of Psychology at Durham University. Elizabeth completed her PhD in psychology at Durham University in 2013. She previously held research posts and a lectureship at Newcastle University.

Lena Fleig is Professor of Health Psychology and Behavioral Medicine at the Medical School Berlin. Her research focuses on the role of goals and volitional processes in health behavior change, benefiting both healthy individuals and those with chronic diseases. She is currently an Associate Editor for Health Psychology and Behavioral Medicine.

Louise Foley is Postdoctoral Researcher at the School of Allied Health and Health Research Institute, University of Limerick, Ireland. Louise completed her PhD at University of Galway in 2022, researching medication adherence among people living with multiple long-term conditions.

Gerard J. Molloy is Professor of Psychology at the University of Galway. Gerard completed his PhD in psychology at University of St. Andrews in 2004. He held research posts at the University of Aberdeen and UCL and was previously a Lecturer in Psychology at the University of Stirling.

Theda Radtke is Professor of Health Psychology at the University of Wuppertal. Theda completed her PhD in psychology at the University of Zurich in 2011. She held research posts at the University of Zurich and Konstanz and was previously Professor in Health and Work Psychology at Witten/Herdecke University.

Milica Vasiljevic is an Associate Professor of Behavioural Science at Durham University. Milica obtained a PhD in Psychology from the University of Kent in 2012. She was a Senior Research Associate at the University of Cambridge Institute of Public Health prior to joining Durham University in 2018.

Section 4

Chiara Acquati, PhD, LMSW, FAOSW, is an Associate Professor in the Graduate College of Social Work at the University of Houston. Her research focuses on interpersonal processes that contribute to mental health, coping, and well-being related outcomes of cancer patients and partners, with an emphasis on intervention development and capacity building.

Arnstein Finset, PhD, is Professor Emeritus at Department of Behavioral Medicine, Faculty of Medicine, University of Oslo. He has published widely in health psychology in the last 25 years, with emphasis on clinical communication research. He has broad teaching experience in the fields of health psychology and communication skills training

Mariët Hagedoorn is full Professor of Health Psychology at the Department of Health Sciences, University Medical Center Groningen, the Netherlands. She examines how individuals and their significant others adapt to chronic illness, and tests (dyadic) psychosocial (eHealth) interventions to improve their well-being.

Val Morrison has examined sociocognitive influences on illicit drug use and risk behavior, and the psychosocial influences on the impacts of physical illness or informal caregiving for over 35 years. Working with multidisciplinary teams, this research informs policy and practice. She also co-authors a leading European health psychology textbook.

Nickola C. Overall is a Professor of Psychology at the University of Auckland, New Zealand. Nickola investigates how couples and families can best resolve conflict and support each other, including identifying the factors that influence these important relationship processes, such as biased perceptions, emotion regulation, and attachment insecurity.

Paula R. Pietromonaco is Professor Emerita at the Department of Psychological and Brain Sciences, University of Massachusetts, Amherst. Her research focuses on how romantic partners shape each other's physiological responses, behaviors, and perceptions; how individual differences (e.g., attachment insecurity) modulate these responses; and the link between these responses and downstream emotional and physical health.

Noa Vilchinsky, Associate Professor, serves as the Dean of the Division of Designated Programs and Director of the Psycho-Cardiology Research Lab at Bar Ilan University, Israel. Specializing in psycho-cardiology, coping with illness, caregiving, and patient dignity, her research explores individual, dyadic, and cultural dimensions.

Section 5

Yael Benyamini, PhD, is a Health Psychologist and a Professor at the Bob Shapell School of Social Work at the Tel Aviv University. She studies how people think about their health, focusing on self-regulation processes that affect psychological and physical outcomes in chronic diseases and around women's health issues.

Elizabeth Broadbent is a Professor of Health Psychology at the University of Auckland and Fellow of the Royal Society of New Zealand. Her research interests include patients' illness perceptions, psychoneuroimmunology, human-robot interaction, and embodied cognition. Her research develops empathetic robots and virtual humans for reducing stress and improving health.

Frederick H. F. Chan is a PhD candidate supervised by Associate Professor Konstadina Griva at Nanyang Technological University. Frederick's research interest lies in the area of symptom management and self-care behavior in chronic disease. Frederick's current research focuses on subjective cognitive complaints in end-stage renal disease patients receiving dialysis treatment.

Konstadina Griva is an Associate Professor of Health Psychology and Behavioural Medicine at Lee Kong Chian School of Medicine, Nanyang Technological University, Singapore. A Chartered Health Psychologist and honorary Fellow of EHPS, she has an established research record in health-related behavior change and chronic disease management with a particular focus on kidney disease and diabetes.

Evangelos C. Karademas is a Professor of Clinical Health Psychology at the Department of Psychology, University of Crete, Greece. He is an Honorary Fellow of the EHPS. His research interests include the role of stress in health, self-regulation, dyadic regulation and health, adaptation to chronic illness, and well-being.

Kate Loveys (PhD) is a Research Fellow at the University of Auckland School of Medicine in Auckland, New Zealand. Her research focuses on digital health, evidence syntheses, and guideline development. Dr Loveys is a consultant to the World Health Organization and serves in the International Telecommunication Union/World Health Organization Focus Group on Artificial Intelligence for Health.

Stanton P. Newman ran the first Health Psychology MSc in the United Kingdom. He was Head of Psychiatry and Behavioural Science at University College London (UCL), Dean of Health Sciences, and Vice President and currently Professor of Behavioural Medicine, at City University of London. He has published over 350 papers and over 10 books.

Rui She is a Research Assistant Professor at the Department of Rehabilitation Sciences, the Hong Kong Polytechnic University. She received her bachelor's degree in Medicine from Peking University and PhD in Public Health from the Chinese University of Hong Kong. Her research focuses on aging research related to multimorbidity and development of behavioral health promotion for patients with chronic diseases.

Section 6

Hayley Breare is a PhD candidate in the School of Population Health, Curtin University. She has a bachelor of psychology (honors). Her areas of research include health behavior change and the importance of training of health professionals in behavior change to improve patient care and outcomes.

Amelia J. Lake is a Behavioral Scientist and Postdoctoral Research Fellow at the Australian Centre for Behavioural Research in Diabetes. Amelia's research interests include evidence and theory-based approaches to health behavior change intervention development, and strategies to optimize intervention implementation and sustainability, particularly for populations with high unmet need.

Caitlin Liddelow is a Postdoctoral Research Fellow in the School of Psychology at the University of Wollongong and the President of the Australasian Society for Behavioural Health and Medicine (ASBHM). Caitlin is an expert in health behavior change, specifically in women's health, mental health, and sport.

Chloe Maxwell-Smith is a Lecturer at Curtin University. Her research is focused on psycho-oncology, cancer survivorship, chronic disease risk, remote interventions, and behavioral medicine. Dr. Maxwell-Smith teaches mixed methods research, supervises research students in health psychology, and is Deputy Chair of Curtin University's Behavioural Science and Health Research Group.

Matthew McDonald is a final year PhD candidate at Curtin University in Perth, Western Australia. His expertise lies broadly in trials and implementation science, particularly in relation to health behavioral interventions and health inequalities. His PhD is linked to the Aussie-Fans in Training Program, which uses Australian Rules Football as a 'hook' to engage men in a health behavior change intervention. McDonald is experienced in working on health behavior related projects both directly with communities in practice and in research, having previously held roles in Scotland working for the NHS and the University of Stirling respectively.

Matthew McLaughlin is a Physical Activity Researcher and Advocate. Dr. McLaughlin submitted his implementation science PhD thesis in November 2021 on the topic of scaling-up physical activity interventions. Dr. McLaughlin has taken leading roles in advocacy campaigns, including the "Eight Investments That Work for Physical Activity" and "Three Transport Priorities".

Rachel E. Menzies is a Clinical Psychologist and Postdoctoral Research fellow at the University of Sydney, where she completed her honors, master's, and doctoral degrees in psychology. She has published five books on the topic of existential issues and mental health.

Joanna C. Moullin is an Implementation Scientist, experienced in implementation theories, implementation research methodologies and measurement development. Dr. Moullin's research aims to investigate, expedite and increase the introduction and integration of evidence, programs and innovations into practice.

Barbara A. Mullan is Professor of Health Psychology at Curtin University. Her primary research interests and expertise lie in the use of social cognition models in predicting, changing, and improving health behaviors. She has held extensive leadership roles in academic societies, and has more than 230 peer-reviewed publications and 12,000+ citations.

Eleanor Quested's research focuses on the initiation and maintenance of health behaviors, particularly physical activity. Quested designs and implements theory-driven, evidence-based interventions that empower individuals to adopt healthy lifestyles and experience well-being. Quested has a particular interest in capitalizing on the appeal of sport to promote engagement in health behavior change.

Amelia J. Scott is a Clinical Psychologist and Research Fellow at Macquarie University, in Sydney, Australia. Her research specializes in adjustment to chronic disease and seeks to understand how to promote mental health and optimal functioning among people living with chronic diseases.

Hamsini Sivaramakrishnan is a PhD candidate within the Curtin School of Population Health at Curtin University. Her research focuses on the psychological and social aspects of sport participation among aging adults.

Jemma Todd is a Clinical Psychologist and Senior Lecturer in clinical and health psychology at the University of Sydney. Her research focuses on the interplay between physical and mental health, and how psychological factors contribute to chronic health conditions and health outcomes.

Amelia Williams is a Research Assistant at the Australian Centre for Behavioural Research in Diabetes, and provisional psychologist currently completing a master's in educational and developmental psychology. Amelia has contributed to various programs of research that have centered on experiences of living with a chronic condition and health behavior change.

Section 7

Benjamin Ambuehl researches the behavior of individuals and organizations. Currently researching cybersecurity, he has previously led research in water, sanitation, and hygiene (WaSH) in an international consortium. His interdisciplinary and mixed methods research focuses on behavior change for stewardship of shared resources, researching psychological ownership and systematic behavior change frameworks.

Richard Appiah leverages his training in clinical psychology and doctorate in health sciences, along with his expertise in positive psychology, to conduct research on community mental health. His primary focus is on developing and evaluating context-appropriate positive psychology interventions aimed at promoting mental health, building resilience, and increasing vocational productivity across various populations and contexts in sub-Saharan Africa.

Asma Bibi, a Human Rights Advocate and Program Manager at A. R. Brothers (Ltd.), Pakistan's first woman in alternative energy. With an MSc in health psychology, she has dedicated 12 years to various national and international non-governmental organizations, focusing on girls' education, gender-based violence, child marriage prevention, peace building, and mental health awareness. Through community projects like plantation drives and gender equality workshops, she actively promotes Sustainable Development Goals 3, 5, 13, and 16.

Lucie Byrne-Davis is a Professor of Health Psychology and a Health Psychologist at University of Manchester, United Kingdom. Working mainly with health partnerships across national borders, she studies and enables behavior change. Her work focuses on facilitating the development of a health workforce that delivers care and support prevention.

Bronwynè Coetzee is a Senior Lecturer and a Y1 rated (NRF) Researcher in the Department of Psychology at Stellenbosch University. Her research focuses on understanding and addressing psychosocial factors affecting treatment adherence among children, adolescents and adults living with chronic, infectious, and non-communicable disease in South Africa.

Darlina Hani Fadil Azim is a Clinical Psychologist, Lecturer, and Health Coach, and has a PhD in health psychology. Darlina's interests are in digital therapeutics, researching the efficacy of the internet and technology for improving the physical and mental well-being combining her expertise in clinical and health psychology.

Jo Hart is Professor of Health Professional Education, Health Psychologist, and Head of Division of Medical Education at University of Manchester, United Kingdom. Her research and practice focus on the optimization of health professional education, leveraging behavior change theories and methods to improve practice nationally and internationally.

Ashraf Kagee is Distinguished Professor of Psychology at Stellenbosch University, Co-director of the Alan J. Flisher Centre for Public Mental Health, and a member of the Academy of Science of South Africa. His research has focused on common mental disorders among persons living with HIV and the psychological and structural factors influencing adherence to antiretroviral therapy.

Irene A. Kretchy is an Associate Professor of Pharmacy Practice (Socio-behavioral) at University of Ghana. With a background in pharmacy and clinical psychology, she researches psychosocial factors in response to treatments, understanding and optimizing medication-related behaviors and patients' experiences of illness and treatment for chronic physical and mental illness.

Ifeanyichukwu Anthony Ogueji is a Health Systems Researcher. He has a bachelor's degree in psychology and a master's degree in clinical psychology from University of Ibadan. He has studied neonatal morbidity and mortality and quality improvement in the Nigerian health system. He has published qualitative and quantitative research in international journals.

Rizwana Roomaney is a Research Psychologist and Associate Professor at the Department of Psychology at the Stellenbosch University in South Africa. She is a trained methodologist and works in the areas of reproductive health, women's health and online health-seeking behavior.

Katherine Sorsdahl is the Co-director of the Alan J. Flisher Centre for Public Mental Health at the University of Cape Town. Over the last 20 years, her work has focused on improving access to and the quality of care for people living with mental health conditions, developing and adapting evidence-based mental health interventions for low- and middle-income country contexts, and integrating evidence-based mental health services into health systems with a focus on task sharing.

Enoch Teye-Kwadjo is a Senior Lecturer in Health Psychology and Psychometrics at the Department of Psychology, University of Ghana, and an Extraordinary Senior Lecturer at the Department of Industrial Psychology, Stellenbosch University. His research focuses on health behavior theory, psychometrics, HIV and sexual health, road traffic injury prevention, and mental health.

Vica Tomberge is dedicated to promoting global equal access to healthy living in occupational and family health. She earned her PhD from the University of Bern, focusing on health psychology and behavioral medicine. Previously, she worked in self-care, staff care, and stress-sensitive research methods in a women's rights organization.

Section 8

David K. Ahern, PhD is Director of the Digital Behavioral Health and Informatics Research Program in the Department of Psychiatry at the Brigham and Women's Hospital and Assistant Professor of Psychology at Harvard Medical School. The program focuses on investigating the role of emerging technologies in health care, leveraging informatics and data science.

Paquito Bernard (PhD) is Associate Professor at the University of Québec in Montréal (Canada) and Researcher at the University Institute of Mental Health in Montréal. His research activity focuses on the effects and mechanisms of physical activity on mental health, and the health behavior change for a better health and livable planet. His academic blog can be found at https://avuer.hypotheses.org/.

Guillaume Chevance is a Behavioral Scientist. His research focuses on developing behavior change interventions with the overall objective of helping people foster their efforts for climate change mitigation and adaptation.

Bradford W. Hesse, PhD, is a Psychologist with 40 years of experience in health psychology, human factors, and medical informatics. He served as Chief of the

National Cancer Institute's Health Communication and Informatics Research Branch from 2004 to 2018. He retired from federal service in 2019.

Dominika Kwasnicka (PhD) is a Senior Research Fellow at University of Melbourne (Australia) and SWPS University (Poland). She is a behavioral scientist interested in health behavior change maintenance, innovative research methods, and applied health promotion interventions. She is a Co-founder of Open Digital Health (www.opendigitalhealth.org) and Lead Editor of Practical Health Psychology (www.practicalhealthpsychology.com).

Jessica M. Lipschitz (PhD) is a Clinical Psychologist and Associate Director of the Digital Behavioural Health and Informatics Research Program at Brigham Women's Hospital. Her research focuses on implementation and optimization of digital behavioral health tools. Additionally, she has worked extensively with industry and the Veteran's Administration to create, evaluate, and implement mHealth solutions.

Olga Perski is a Marie Skłodowska-Curie Postdoctoral Research Fellow at the University of California, San Diego (United States) and Tampere University (Finland). She is an interdisciplinary researcher working at the intersection of behavioral science and technology, with expertise in the development and evaluation of digital behavior change interventions.

Robert A. C. Ruiter is Professor of Health and Social Psychology at Maastricht University, the Netherlands. His core research is within the systematic development, implementation, and evaluation of theory- and evidence-based behavior change interventions. He is co-author of "Intervention Mapping", a globally applied protocol for the planned design of behavior change interventions.

Catherine Sherrington is a Professor in the School of Public Health at the University of Sydney. Prof. Sherrington leads the Physical Activity, Ageing, and Disability Research Stream within the Institute for Musculoskeletal Health at Sydney Local Health District and has a background as a physiotherapist.

Gill A. ten Hoor is Associate Professor at Maastricht University (the Netherlands) and adjunct professor at the University of Texas at Houston. Gill is certified Intervention Mapping trainer and contributes to planned behavior change in various topics. One of his landmark publication is "Implementation Mapping", a protocol to develop implementation strategies.

Anne Tiedemann, PhD, is Professor of Physical Activity and Health in the Faculty of Medicine and Health, the University of Sydney. Anne has a professional background in exercise science. Her research develops scalable interventions that can enhance physical activity to promote health and prevent falls in middle to older age.

SECTION 1

Defining Health Psychology

1

HISTORY OF HEALTH PSYCHOLOGY

Angel Marie Chater, Francis Quinn, and Val Morrison

Introduction

This chapter gives an overview of the history of health psychology, covering the development of the discipline across a number of countries, including the United States of America (USA), Europe, the United Kingdom (UK), Japan, Africa, Canada, Australia and New Zealand. It takes a look at the key influences on its development, changes to job opportunities, discussions on the need for training models to accommodate standardised skill sets, core journals and books that were published to assist knowledge transfer of this new discipline, and how the growth in countries where health psychology is well-established such as the UK, differ from less developed countries. It includes extracts from interviews with 53 Health Psychologists (mainly trained in the UK) as part of the Royal Society–funded Oral History of Health Psychology (OHHP) in the UK Project (funded 2016–2018: Quinn & Chater; an overview in Quinn, Chater & Morrison, 2020), many of whom were involved in European and international developments. New oral testimony from this project, interviewed by the authors (Chater, Quinn & Morrison, 2019), is presented in this chapter for the first time, highlighted by the date on which people were interviewed as part of this historical work. The chapter concludes with practical tips to ensure that history continues to be able to be captured in the future on an international platform through good documentation at annual meetings and as part of professional network events, conferences, and peer-reviewed journals.

Health Psychology Beginnings: From the USA to Europe

In a novel about time travel, author Michael Crichton (1999, p. 85) writes, "*Professor Johnston often said that if you didn't know history, you didn't know anything. You were a leaf that didn't know it was part of a tree*". Historically, from

 DOI: 10.4324/9781003318026-2

the seeds of shared interest and passion, health psychology has produced some strong roots and an international family tree with many leaves. There are a number of significant roots to mention, captured in articles and books written by those who were there at the time, and transcripts from the OHHP Project. The first mention of health psychology is traced back to the early 1970s, influenced by scientists in the USA at a task force meeting with the American Psychological Association (APA) in 1973 (Johnston, Weinman, & Chater, 2011). The meeting agenda asked a question on how psychologists (who were mostly clinical) can support the maintenance of physical health, the management of those with physical health problems, and the effectiveness of health-care delivery. In the UK OHHP Project (Quinn, Chater & Morrison, 2020), which was the first of its kind for the health psychology discipline, Professor Marie Johnston recalls the task force and a conference the following year:

> *"Gerald Patterson was there, but in addition so was George Stone [...] George Stone is the editor of the first textbook in health psychology. And there's somebody else I need to mention, Philip Ley. So Phil Ley was in Liverpool. So you know there's all this research now on health professional behaviour? Well, Phil Ley way back then had a study, I think he called it non-compliance by doctors or something like that, showing that doctors didn't always do what they should do. But in addition he did experiments in which he experimentally altered leaflets and information given to patients in accord with cognitive theory. So he used primacy, he put the important message first, so that instead of telling people about their history, he would have doctors start off with "What I want you to do is this, and that is because..." and so he would reverse the order of the consultation.... So using primacy, the first message was what the person had to do. And he also did things where you reduced the complexity of leaflets. And all of those things had effects. So reducing the complexity of leaflets, he showed that you got more weight change in overweight women with his simple message than with a complex message. So Phil Ley, I think, is really important. Nobody knows about him nowadays. But the conference in 1974, George Stone was there and he basically laid out the agenda for health psychology [...]"*
>
> *"He showed where behaviour is important, behaviour is important in affecting your health, and behaviour was important everywhere in the healthcare system, in the decision to seek healthcare, the delivery of healthcare, in the design of policy, the design of health services. He had it all there. He had an amazing diagram which I'm sure must be published somewhere but I can't find it. And then he and Nancy Adler and somebody else, a third person, in 1979 published that book [Stone, Cohen & Adler, 1979] on health psychology".*
>
> *(Professor Marie Johnston, OHHP interview – 2 September 2016)*

The development of the discipline was led by the APA, which in 1978 created a member network in health psychology called Division 38. In an article written as part of an APA series on the development of their member networks and the '*Unification through Division*', Kenneth Wallston (1997) describes the development of Division 38 (Health Psychology). A history of shared passion and values of those with an interest in health psychology is told, with Steve Weiss coined the 'father of health psychology', acting as chair-elect to Joe Matarazzo, the first president of Division 38. In early 1978, Wallston (1997) reports that Matarazzo invited colleagues from experimental, clinical, and social psychology – namely, Joseph Brady, Richard Evans, Wilbert Fordyce, W. Doyle Gentry, David Glass, Irving Janis, Neal Miller, Gary Schwartz, Jerome E. Singer, and George Stone – to join him and Weiss to petition the APA Council to establish a new Division of Health Psychology. Over 600 members and fellows signed the petition, which was approved in August 1978. In his presidential address at the meeting of the APA in New York in September 1979, Matarazzo coined one of the most commonly cited definitions of health psychology, later published as:

> *"[Health psychology is] ... the aggregate of the specific educational, scientific, and professional contributions of the discipline of psychology to the promotion and maintenance of health, the prevention and treatment of illness, and the identification of etiologic and diagnostic correlates of health, illness, and related dysfunction".*
>
> *(Matarazzo, 1980, p. 815)*

Matarazzo (1980), in his article entitled "Behavioral Health and Behavioral Medicine: Frontiers for a New Health Psychology" published in the *American Psychologist*, goes on to write,

> *"I take no special pride of authorship in this beginning definition of health psychology, nor, for that matter, in the definition of behavioral health offered above. However, this beginning definition of health psychology is offered in the hope that it will stimulate further discussion among psychologists representing all areas of specialization within psychology, some of whom already are Charter members of the APA's recently formed Division of Health Psychology. As psychologists plow [plough] this field, sow a variety of seeds, and reap their harvests, the appellation health psychology will encompass as little or as much as such individuals wish of the domains in which psychology and medicine overlap. At the moment, health psychology seems a broader term than the more robust, and to many of us more familiar, term clinical psychology or than medical psychology, one of the subspecialties clinical psychology spawned three decades ago. However, if my reading of the history of the sociology of professions is correct, some of what is today called clinical and medical psychology will soon be labelled health psychology by some of the leaders in these fields, many of whom fortunately are part of the leadership of this new health psychology focus within American psychology."*
>
> *(Matarazzo, 1980, p. 815)*

Those who were working in the field of health psychology, without it formally having this title, began to feel that they belonged to a greater movement. Stone et al.'s (1979) book consolidated the identity that came with the use of the term 'health psychology', grouping experts together with a shared vision. Professor John Weinman recalls,

> *"This was the first time I had seen that [the term health psychology], yeah. It's a book that came out in 1979. And basically, this was a conference with a whole lot of Americans, who again, really, they were beginning to be aware of this discipline which they labelled health psychology, and they were the same group of people, really important group of people, went on to form the APA Section 38 or whatever they were. So, this was a great book, coping with stresses of illness, why people seek healthcare, looking at effects of cancer on people's lives, lots of psychology of clinical reasoning, which was very familiar with the sort of cognition stuff here, and so on. So, this, for me, really was a real eye-opener, which all of this, which is a disparate set of things, psychophysiology, cognition, various social psychology stuff, attributions, decision making and so on, that all of that could be part of a discipline. Where I saw myself as just teaching these various bits and pieces in a fairly piecemeal sort of way to medical students, then doing a bit of research here and there, and it all seemed a bit messy, compared with doing my PhD which was so narrow. And then all of a sudden somebody badged it all up and said "Hey, this is called health psychology." "Hey, I'm a health psychologist." So, it was great, it was really nice. I can remember having these conversations with Marie [Johnston], we were realising actually we were in a discipline, as it were. And then the thing in Holland really brought it together."*
>
> *(Professor John Weinman, OHHP interview – 24 October 2016)*

While health psychology was developing in America with the support of the APA, a meeting in the Netherlands was a pivotal point for the development of European health psychology. Professor Marie Johnston recalls,

> *"[...] we began to find other people, and a few things happened. So we met Stan Maes in the Netherlands. I don't know how we found Stan Maes, though. I think John Weinman may be able to tell you how we found him. [...] Stan Maes had a conference in 1986 in Tilburg. Because we were corresponding with Stan and working with him in a way that I can't quite remember. And we went to Tilburg, and that was how I met Howard Leventhal. [...] So in a way I moved on from Gerald Patterson. I'd collected Gerald Patterson and now I was collecting what I could get from Howard Leventhal. So we went to Tilburg, and we didn't quite establish EHPS [European Health Psychology Society] then, but we retrospectively think of that as the first EHPS meeting. And that was 1986 as well. But that was really important".*
>
> *(Professor Marie Johnston, OHHP interview – 2 September 2016)*

[Angel Chater: "*What made it important?*"]

"Because we were meeting people internationally who were caring about the same issues, and that we weren't a bunch of stupid isolates. John and I used to talk about we were developing this health psychology thing and was it a figment of our imagination? So we still joke about that. It may have been a figment of our imagination but we've managed to fool all these other people. […] Well, I think the world was ready for it. And we were just there worrying about it early because of the kind of jobs we had and what we were doing."

(Professor Marie Johnston, OHHP interview – 2 September 2016)

Stan Maes (1947–2018) has been described as a key figure in European health psychology (Johnston, 2018), being the first president of the EHPS, to be followed by Marie Johnston. In an article following his death, Johnston (2018) describes how Stan Maes connected those interested in health psychology from across Europe, to include Finland, Switzerland, Poland, Czechoslovakia, Italy, Germany, Belgium, Spain, the UK, and the Netherlands, facilitating an identity as European Health Psychologists and a shared focus for professional and scientific pursuits. In an interview with Professor John Weinman, he also recalls the meeting Stan organised in the Netherlands:

"Marie and I did a review together, a bit of an overview of the whole recovery from surgery bit between us, and we presented that at what turned out to be the very first ever European Health Psychology meeting. Which I think was in 1986 in Holland. Which is where we both met Stan Maes. … But also, at that meeting there was a very small group of people in Europe who were just beginning to find their way in what we would call health psychology, mid-'80s. I've jumped a bit so we might want to go back a bit. So there were I think only three of us in the UK, there was Marie, myself, and a guy called Tom Cox, who was very much a stress researcher. And then there were people from Germany, Belgium, and the Netherlands, I think. So, a very small group of Europeans just emerging, but we had about four or five big name American health psychologists came over. […] I don't know if I've got my book. Somebody wrote it up as a book, in the end. One of the big Americans there was Leventhal, so I spent a lot of time talking to Leventhal, really friendly with him, and he's been a bit of an inspiration and colleague ever since. The other person who I met there and who remained a really good friend in health psychology ever since was Ad Kaptein, Dutch guy. And he's part of that growing network of people."

(Professor John Weinman, OHHP interview – 24 October 2016)

[Angel Chater: "*So, a huge impact that conference must have had.*"]

"Yeah, and it was very small. And it was early … I was really beginning to expand the teaching I was doing for medical students to take in the stuff that Marie [Johnston] had drawn my attention to, some of the

psychophysiology, and then gradually talking about how patients cope with illness, impact of illness, issues like non-adherence. So, really got to be aware of all that behavioural side of illness. The symptom perception work was just coming out, there was a lot of very interesting work on symptom perception. So all of that was sort of bubbling up, I certainly wasn't calling it health psychology, because my course was called Psychology Applied to Medicine. Which was actually the title of my lectureship, I was a Lecturer of Psychology Applied to Medicine. And nobody was using the term. And then I think Marie or somebody drew my attention to that book." [referring to Stone et al., 1979]

(Professor John Weinman, OHHP interview – 24 October 2016)

Biomedical vs. Biopsychosocial Models of Health and Illness

From America to Europe and beyond in the 1970s–1980s, the development of health psychology was dominated by the application of psychology and behavioural medicine to physical health care, illness, preparation and recovery from surgery, and the health-care system (Quinn, Chater & Morrison, 2020). A key influence on this development was the need to understand human behaviour of those who were unwell or at risk of becoming ill and those who were treating them. The medical profession historically used a biomedical approach to treatment, with the aim to find the physiological root cause of a problem and treat it at the source via medical or surgical means. This approach aligned to the dualistic view of Descartes' (1596–1650), who proposed that the mind and the body are split into two domains: the mind seen as 'non-material' (i.e., not visible – such as a thought) and the body seen as 'material' (i.e., made of visible things such as organs) (see Chater & Cook, 2014 [Chapter 1]; Morrison & Bennett, 2006 [Chapter 12]). However, there came a realisation that treatment approaches needed to consider a wider view than what dualism could offer.

Engel (1977, 1980) challenged the biomedical view that disease occurred solely due to deviations from normative biological factors that can be measured. He proposed the Bio-Psycho-Social Model of Health and Illness (Engel, 1977, 1980), which offered an alternative view aligned to the concept of monism that suggested that the mind and the body are part of the same system or unit that can interact and work together (Chater & Cook, 2014). The model proposed interacting influences on health and illness from biological, psychological, and social factors, presented in Figure 1.1, adapted to represent the influences on health psychology. Job opportunities began widening to apply psychology and sociology to health and medicine. Clinical psychologists were being employed in medical departments, with the acknowledgement that there may be more to physical health and illness than biomedical factors. Psychology and sociology became of interest to those in charge of medical curriculums, broadening medical training and opportunities for psychologists to specialise in these areas. John Weinman explains,

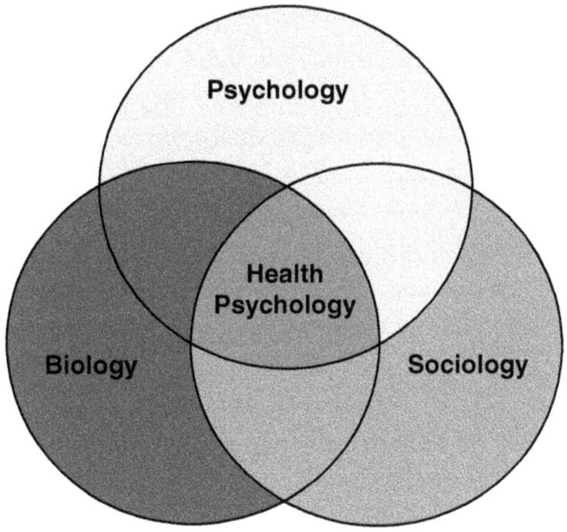

Figure 1.1 The Bio-Psycho-Social Model of Health and Illness (Engel, 1977, 1980). Adapted to include health psychology at the core.

> *"[...] I think they came to the conclusion that medical students needed to have a broader curriculum ... to have teaching in things like psychology and sociology and ethics and communication skills and so on [...] a few Medical schools offered these full-time lectureships [...] we could more or less develop our own curriculum [...] In these early days... we weren't even aware of health psychology back then but quite a number of the early people, like Marie and like that were based in medical schools. Chares Abraham I think was in Dundee ... Beth Alder... a lot of us were doing that, that's how we got exposed to more general medicine as opposed to the more mental health end or neurology and neuropsychology [...] there was this slow trickle of doctors coming across asking questions like "Well, you're a psychologist, can you tell me why it is that some of my patients that don't seem to be that ill, are coping so badly". [...] And these were doctors who could sort of see the bigger picture. [...] And so I started working with them."*
>
> *(Professor John Weinman, OHHP interview – 24 October 2016)*

The Bio-Psycho-Social Model later became a core component in the health psychology curriculum, and the history of Engel's work and the challenge to the medical model is well known. The application of this model to issues such as stress and pain was mentioned as being influential. Daryl O'Connor recalls,

> *"Of course there was the US mini revolution going on, which had started, I now know but didn't know then, in the early to mid-'80s. So you had the publication of Engel's work, and lots of people who have really started to challenge the medical model. So I think because certain key things started to happen where people were seeing that behaviour was important to health, but also that psychology could play an etiological role in predicting and changing*

and determining lots of illnesses and diseases, or at least there was some evidence of that happening. And actually I think one of the big areas that has actually moved that was stress. If you look back, stress is actually one of the most dominant areas of demonstrating the biopsychosocial model. And even pain, the work on pain, which is back in the '60s, the classic Melzack and Wall stuff which changed the way we think about pain. So I think there was movement from America, so you had the development of behavioural medicine and behavioural health, and then this biopsychosocial model starting to be talked about in the mid-'80s. And of course then the introduction of Division 38 of the APA. So I think those things, although I was not aware of them, to be honest, at the time, when I look back and see these things were pushing it forward. But certainly in Europe and in the UK it would be people like Marie Johnston, John Weinman who were then starting to really organise and develop this thing called health psychology."

(Professor Daryl O'Connor, OHHP interview – 12 December 2016)

International Development, Annual Meetings, and Member Networks

With the APA taking the lead on the development of the discipline of health psychology with Division 38, the European community followed swiftly. The meeting of experts in Tilburg in 1986, instigated by Stan Maes, brought together people with an interest in health psychology from many parts of Europe and the USA, signifying the beginnings of the EHPS. Over the years that followed, a team of like-minded individuals with a shared vision for health psychology worked together, and the EHPS became the society it is today, with Stan Maes as its first president (Johnston, 2018). Annual meetings continued in Trier (1988), Utrecht (1989), Oxford (1990), Lausanne (1991), and Leipzig (1992), and the proceedings from these meetings were published (Johnston, 2018). Alongside this, the group worked to develop the rules, articles, and legal status of the EHPS, with Marie Johnston taking over the presidency from Stan Maes in 1992 (Johnston, 2018). The year 2024 marks the 38th annual conference on the EHPS, bringing members (https://ehps.net/members/) and those with an interest in health psychology together annually from across the world.

In parallel to these developments were the beginnings of the British Psychological Society (BPS) Division of Health Psychology (DHP) in the UK. In August 1985, Marie Johnston and John Weinman wrote a letter to the *BPS Bulletin* (the precursor to *The Psychologist*) calling for a Health Psychology Section, which was granted in 1986 with Marie Johnston as the inaugural chair (Johnston, Weinman & Chater, 2011). The section had its first conference in Sussex in 1987, and the committee has hosted a meeting annually ever since. In 1993, the BPS Health Psychology Section became a Special Group, and in 1997, following the agreement of an established body of science and training routes, the BPS DHP was formed (Johnston, Weinman & Chater, 2011; Quinn, Chater

& Morrison, 2020). It wasn't long before the European and UK communities came together, and in 1990, the EHPS and the BPS Health Psychology Section hosted their first joint conference in Oxford, with more that followed with its successors, the most recent being the joint conference in Aberdeen in 2016.

From these early beginnings came further developments across the world. The Australian Psychological Society (APS) was a member of the BPS until 1966 and is now the major body representing the professional interests of psychologists in Australia. In late 1988, the society established a Working Party on Health Psychology, which recommended ways to develop the field in Australia. Many psychologists involved in this area were also members of the Australian Behaviour Modification Association, which was established in the late 1970s (Oldenburg & Owen, 1990). The College of Health Psychologists of the APS was established in 1997 (Martin et al., 2014). Australia is now one of the countries affiliated with the EHPS. Historical accounts of the developments in Japan (Takenaka, 2013) report the creation of the Japanese Association of Health Psychology (JAHP) in 1987.

A special issue of the *Journal of Health Psychology* in March 2018, entitled "Histor{y/ies} of Health Psycholog{y/ies}", edited by Ian Lubek and Michael Murray (2018), presents a series of articles on the development and expansion of health psychology in a number of other countries. These include France (Santiago-Delefosse & del Rio Carral 2018; Herzlich, 2018), Brazil (Spink, 2018), South Africa (Yen & Vaccarino, 2018), Ghana (de-Graft Aikins, 2018), Australia (Kippax, 2018), New Zealand (Chamberlain, Lyons & Stephens, 2018), the UK (Murray, 2018), the USA (Lubek et al., 2018), and Canada (Stam, Murray & Lubek, 2018). The journal editors (Lubek & Murray, 2018) recognise the journal's tradition in publishing with a critical health psychology lens, an important part of health psychology's history, and the influence of multidisciplinary origins, including psychoanalysis, behaviourism, behavioural medicine, cognitivism, social psychology, and anthropology. However, it is noted that several of the articles are autobiographical in nature, as opposed to narratives from a wider range of those present at the time. These articles are also not specifically about the development of professional networks but more often about the development of ideas, research methods, critical debate, and the science that we now call health psychology.

Similar to findings from the UK (Quinn, Chater & Morrison, 2020), initial scepticism towards this 'new discipline' and way of thinking was seen in France by some clinical psychologists (Santiago-Delefosse & del Rio Carral 2018). The 'fraught nexus' between academic research and political activism is described in the history of South Africa (Yen & Vaccarino, 2018), with the work related to health psychology deemed to be more appropriately termed 'psychology for health' and few people (2/12) interviewed identifying themselves as a 'Health Psychologist'. The HIV/AIDS pandemic is reported as an influential health focus in South Africa for those with psychological expertise, which mirrors reports from other countries, such as the UK OHHP (Quinn, Chater & Morrison, 2020), who describe psychology's response to the HIV/AIDS pandemic as an influencing part of the zeitgeist of its time. The narrative from Brazil (Spink, 2018) also reflects on the influence of the HIV/AIDS epidemic and its role in the history of psychology applied to health, as do the autobiographical accounts from France (Herzlich, 2018) and Australia (Kippax, 2018), who emphasise the influence of a multidisciplinary approach and the concept of 'social health' rather than health psychology. The emergence of health psychology in Ghana is reported to have begun with doctoral research by Ama de-Graft Aikins (2005), who studied social representations of diabetes in Ghana and was registered in the UK at the London School of Economics (de-Graft Aikins, 2018). However, the article concludes that there is currently no shared ideological vision of what health psychology in Ghana should be while acknowledging that there is a need for context-specific scientist-practitioner and scholar-activist models that engage in research as well as the development of evidence-based practice, interventions, and policies (de-Graft Aikins, 2018).

The development in New Zealand shines the light on the history of critical health psychology (Chamberlain, Lyons & Stephens, 2018), described as starting at the School of Psychology at Massey University. This account emphasises the importance of social justice and the application of knowledge for the benefit of society and the influences of behavioural, clinical, social, community, and medical psychology, alongside behavioural medicine, the sociology of medicine, psychosomatics, and psychoanalysis. In 1996, Kerry Chamberlain and John Spicer founded the New Zealand Health Psychology Society to provide a national and international identity for health psychology in New Zealand. Discussions between this newly formed society (Kerry Chamberlain and Glynn Owens) and the Australian Society for Behavioural Medicine (Christina Lee and Brian Oldenberg) were had in Brisbane in 2000 to plan a joint scientific meeting (conference). The outcomes of this meeting were to combine the two societies to create the Australasian Society for Behavioral Health and Medicine (ASBHM), which met annually from 2001, initially alternating conferences between Australia and New Zealand. However, as it developed, the ASBHM became more mainstream, and those who aligned with critical health psychology felt less at home. In 1999, Michael Murray convened the first International Conference on Critical and Qualitative Approaches to Health Psychology at Memorial University in St John's, Newfoundland, Canada, which met again two years later at Aston University, UK, leading to the development of the International Society of Critical Health Psychology.

Through these accounts, Lubek and Murray (2018) highlight the differing ways to collate historical narratives, from text analysis, bibliometric studies using citation counts, biographical interviews, case reports, archival research, to autobiographical accounts. Accessible (e.g., open access) documentation can assist in capturing the future history of health psychology as it continues to develop. Box 1.1 provides a current overview of health psychology 'in a nutshell', with many aspects discussed in greater detail later in this book.

Box 1.1 Health Psychology in a Nutshell

While there is no single definition, put simply, health psychology is the scientific study of health, illness, and the health-care system. The strength of health psychology lies in a core focus on evidence-based science, with expansive theoretical and methodological principles that can both be applied to and adapted by practice, drawing on the scientist-practitioner (Boulder) model. Health psychology draws from a range of paradigms, depending on the focus of investigation or application, and can be commended for its ability to be translational to the real world. Health psychology draws from the Bio-Psycho-Social Model of Health and Illness (Engel, 1977, 1980), using principles, frameworks, approaches, tools, and scientific evidence from a range of disciplines. Theories are used to explain how thoughts, feelings, and automatic processes, alongside the physical and social environment and physiological factors, influence behaviour and related outcomes (Chater, Whittaker, et al., 2020; Morrison & Bennett, 2022). Health psychology draws from a number of disciplines and areas, including other branches of psychology, such as clinical psychology, biology, medicine and behavioural medicine, medical anthropology, epidemiology, sociology, health economics, and public health. While health psychology covers an array of topics, a key focus is on the understanding of human behaviour and behaviour change. It seeks to address questions such as the following:

- What is the relationship between the mind and the body?
- How can mind and body interactions be measured?
- How are health and illness conceptualised and defined?
- How can health and well-being be maintained and optimised?
- What causes ill health?
- How are health and illness measured?
- How does illness impact those directly and indirectly affected?
- Who is responsible for maintaining health and treating illness?
- How should illness be treated?
- Who is responsible for treatment, and what might influence this?
- What is the role of psychology and psychologists in health and illness?
- How do biopsychosocial factors interact with health and illness?
- How can the health-care system be optimised to facilitate health and provide good care for those who are ill?
- What may influence health professional-patient/client interactions and behaviours?
- What are the key considerations for policy to enhance health, manage illness, and provide an effective health-care system?

The Beginnings of Health Psychology Journals and Textbooks

As professional member networks in health psychology developed, so too did ways to disseminate the most recent science, practice, and relevant activities. Those with an interest in health psychology from across the world began to create journals that specialised in the topic area. The first was *Health Psychology*, the official journal of the APA, launched in 1982, followed by *Psychology and Health* in 1987, officially affiliated to the EHPS. The *British Journal of Health Psychology* came a little later, in 1996, connected to the newly forming BPS DHP (Johnston, Weinman & Chater, 2011). John Weinman recalls the development of the European journal:

> *"That was about '85. And I talked about it and they [Harwood Academic] asked me to put forward an editorial board, so I got people like Marie [Johnston], Stan Maes, there was a guy in Miami, a guy called Ted Millon [Theodore Millon], various people around, because you had to be a bit international, they needed Americans on it. ... Don't think we had Leventhal on it early on. But it'd be interesting to look at that early editorial board, I can't remember all the people on it. Anyhow, it was that journal. The American Journal "Health Psychology" had started in about 1982, 1984, something like that, so that was around. So I wanted to call it the International Journal of Health Psychology. And I can remember arguing like crazy with somebody in the publishing company, and they were not that keen, and they wanted to call it Psychology and Health. And I can't remember why now. And I agreed to it, I thought "Well, that's okay, I don't mind, it's just a name." But I can remember one or two people, Stan Maes being one, who said "This is crazy, the discipline we're in is called health psychology, and if you change the name, the journal won't be linked in." Anyhow, I remember that being a bit of an issue. But it became Psychology and Health, An International Journal. Because they didn't want to call it an International Journal Of... because there's a million journals that are called that. So they wanted it a bit more punchy. Anyway, so I took charge of that and the first issue came out in 1986. And Marie [Johnston] had a really good paper in that on some psychosocial aspects of IVF or something. And then Mike Antoni, who is an eminent psychoimmunology researcher, had a really good paper in there. There were a few people on the editorial board who sort of got people to do papers. Anyway, that started, and it was a really interesting series of things that happened around the late 1970s, early 1980s. ... I said that I was going to only edit it for five years because I had a lot of work, and I think in the end I did six years and passed it on to Ad Kaptein."*
>
> *(Professor John Weinman, OHHP interview – 24 October 2016)*

Professor Theodore Millon (1928–2014), mentioned earlier, has been credited for his role in the development of health psychology and behavioural medicine (Antoni, 2015). Known for his work in personality theory, he edited an influential text published in 1975 entitled *Medical Behavioural Science* (Millon, 1975). Antoni (2015) recalls how his work was influencing the beginnings of health psychology prior to the development of the APA's Division 38. Like others at the time across Europe, Millon was tasked with developing a course for teaching medical students about the role of behavioural science in the practice of medicine in the USA. He published the *Handbook of Clinical Health Psychology* (Millon, Green, & Meagher, 1982) with the aim, in his words, to "*redefine this amorphous, but burgeoning field so as to place it squarely within the province of a broadly-based psychology – specifically, the emerging, substantive discipline of health psychology and the well-established and diverse technologies of clinical psychology*" (preface; Millon, Green & Meagher, 1982). The book included concepts such as 'health-care psychology' and historical and philosophical reflections on the emergence of clinical health psychology, where psychologists assume an active role in the management of the 'physically disordered'. Topics included psychological factors in bodily disease, injury, chronic illness, the role of stress and coping, and the clinical functions of the Health Psychologist. Through this text and the course, graduate students learned the unique role that clinical Health Psychologists play in various medical settings, from researchers to practitioners (Antoni, 2015). The handbook had a focus on training and clinical skills and embraced the Boulder (scientist-practitioner) Model, an approach adopted by the APA following the first conference for clinical psychology training, held in Boulder, Colorado, in 1949 (Frank, 1984).

Meetings between experts in health psychology and the need to present this 'new' discipline and its capabilities led to a number of influential textbooks. A pivotal book was the 1979 text led from the USA by George Stone and colleagues titled *Health Psychology: A Handbook: Theories, Applications, and Challenges of a Psychological Approach to the Health Care System*. Historical narratives earlier in this chapter refer to this as the first point the term 'health psychology' had been used in print. A later text in 1987 followed with a larger editorial team (Stone et al., 1987) titled *Health Psychology: A Discipline and a Profession*. A few years on in 1990, Sarafino published the text *Health Psychology Biopsychosocial Interactions* (1990), while in the UK, Paul Bennett, John Weinman, and Peter Spurgeon edited a book (1990) on *Current Developments in Health Psychology*.

There was an air of excitement in the introductions of these texts. Bishop (1994), in the book titled *Health Psychology: Integrating Mind and Body*, writes in the abstract, "*I have written this book as an invitation to the adventure that is health psychology*". International relationships were seen in texts such as the book *Health Psychology* (2004), edited by Ad Kaptein and John Weinman. Some influential texts were titled in relation to psychology applied to health as opposed to specifically health psychology, such as Marian Pitts and Keith Phillips's (1991) book *The Psychology of Health: An Introduction*, Beth Alder's (1995) *Psychology of Health: Applications of Psychology for Health Professionals*, and Paul Bennett and Simon Murphy's (1997) *Psychology and Health*.

Textbooks that have a number of editions still used today also began around this time. Shelly Taylor first published the textbook *Health Psychology* (1986), now on its 11th edition (Taylor & Stanton, 2020). Jane Ogden's first edition of the book *Health Psychology: A Textbook* was published in 1996, now on its seventh edition (2023). Paul Bennett wrote *Introduction to Clinical Health Psychology* (2000), and the first edition of Morrison and Bennett's *An Introduction to Health Psychology* was published in 2006, now in its fifth edition (2022). There are too many texts to mention in the development of health psychology resources; however, Murray (2014) has explored historical developments of the discipline through a study of the content of popular texts, offering insight into earlier work that has helped to shape the discipline. These texts and those that came after were important in the development of educational training routes, a topic covered in detail in Chapter 4, with the early history presented in Box 1.2.

Box 1.2 Health Psychology Training as a Route to Future Development

As health psychology became more established in terms of the research being conducted and published, there was a need to develop training courses to ensure a core educational foundation. There was recognition for the need for postgraduate training and the textbooks that developed alongside these professional training routes ensured that there was access to relevant knowledge.

> *"Might have been 1981, I think. And there was nothing that resembled health psychology in the curriculum at that point in time. Social psychology was of interest to me, Michael Billig was teaching there at that time. There was also a guy whose name I forget now who used to do stuff on psychiatric epidemiology, he was interested in things like migration and relationships to alcohol and mental wellbeing, things like that. So I was starting to think about those sorts of issues and how social phenomena might relate to health outcomes."*
>
> *(Professor Sheena Orbell, OHHP interview, 24 August 2018)*

> *"We were starting to talk about teaching MScs in Health Psychology [...] the conversation took place between Marie [Johnston] who was at the Royal Free, and Stan Newman who was at Middlesex, and we decided to create a University of London MSc in Health Psychology [...] It was the first one [1987/88]."*
>
> *(Professor John Weinman, OHHP interview – 24 October 2016)*

> *"Medical schools needed to start teaching social science, so it became part of the GMC curriculum, and so they all appointed a health psychologist in the medical schools, so that's why John [Weinman] was appointed at Guy's and Marie [Johnston] was appointed at the Royal Free, Jane [Wardle] was doing the teaching at King's."*
>
> *(Professor Jane Ogden, OOHP interview – 28 November 2016)*

"John Weinman, Stan Newman and I developed one of the first Masters courses in Health Psychology as a London University degree taught through three medical schools. It started in 1988."

(Professor Marie Johnston, OHHP interview – 2 September 2016)

Education and training in health psychology have continued to develop, and in some countries (e.g., the UK) lead to formalised registration to practise as a Health Psychologist. However, there are many countries without access to such training and/or lack national professional representation, such as that provided by the APA or BPS in America and the UK. Training routes can assist the professionalisation of a discipline and ensure that core competencies are connected to evidence-based curriculum. This in turn can assist in the development of career pathways and job opportunities. This is a topic to be discussed in further detail in Chapter 4. Historically, this was something that those who were present at the time were aware of and championed to develop to provide future opportunities within a health-care setting and later to align with public health, where many were already working in relation to health and illness and health promotion.

"At that time [late '80s] there were Masters in Health Psychology, but you wouldn't have called them training courses, they weren't training people for a job, there was no recognition within the NHS that health psychologists existed [...] there was absolutely no clinical skills in there at all."

(Professor Paul Bennett, OHHP interview – 19 October 2016)

"And so we had real chicken and egg situations around the training. We need health psychologists but we haven't got any training. So the training came along, so how do you recruit people into that? We have to persuade them that there's a career route."

(Professor Chris Armitage, OHHP interview – 21 of November 2016)

"Around the same time [early 2000s] there was a group set up to look at the development of public health competencies and see how they matched with the training of health psychology. And we had meetings with the Faculty of Public Health."

(Professor Tony Cassidy, OHHP interview – 8 of July 2016)

"We went out of our way to incorporate some elements of the public health curriculum into the MSc curriculum so we could meet their [UK Faculty of Public Health] demands. What actually happened was that they pulled out of that agreement [...] remnants of that decision still present in the curriculum now."

(Professor Mark Forshaw, OHHP interview – 15 November 2016)

Conclusion

Capturing the history of the development of a discipline relies on existing documentation and people's recollections. It is worth noting that some of the people mentioned in the history of health psychology in this chapter are no longer alive. Useful historical data has been captured by text analysis of previous manuscripts, documentation of meetings, autobiographical reflections, and those offering remembrance. While there remains no universal definition of health psychology, historical accounts show the influence of champions in the field, connected by a shared passion for the scientific application of theory, biopsychosocial principles, and evidence-based approaches to the understanding and intervention of health, illness, and the health-care system. Annual and professional meetings and events should ensure good minute-taking and documentation to enable the future history of health psychology to continue to be captured. Journal editors should utilise their editorial space to further contribute to the developing narrative of health psychology, as these can provide important reflections of the current landscape of the science and practice, and will become the historical archives of the future. There are many aspects not discussed in this chapter, such as the historical development of theoretical models and frameworks; the relationship with other disciplines as health psychology became a discipline in its own right; the professionalisation through member networks, training and registration; and the challenges and opportunities ahead. These will all be discussed in the next few chapters in this section. As the discipline continues to blossom, those within it have the responsibility to share the narrative of the history that came before them and to nurture and mentor the future generation and champions of health psychology.

Acknowledgements

This chapter includes material that was funded by the Royal Society (UK – grant no. RG150648), interviewed by the authors. Thanks go to all those who were interviewed in the OHHP in the UK project and to Professor Tony Cassidy, who assisted in the initial phase of the project.

Further Reading

Johnston, M., Weinman, J., & Chater, A. (2011a). A quarter century of health psychology. *The Psychologist*, *24*(12), 890–902.

Lubek, I., & Murray, M. (2018a). Doing histor {y/ies} of health psycholog {y/ies}. *Journal of Health Psychology*, *23*(3), 361–371. https://doi.org/10.1177/1359105317753627

Quinn, F., Chater, A., & Morrison, V. (2020a). An oral history of UK Health Psychology. *British Journal of Health Psychology*, *25*(3), 502–518. https://doi.org/10.1111/bjhp.12418

Matarazzo, J. D. (1980a). Behavioral health and behavioral medicine: Frontiers for a new health psychology. *American Psychologist*, *35*(9), 807–817. https://doi.org/10.1037/0003-066X.35.9.807

References

Alder, B. (1995). *Psychology of health: Applications of psychology for health professionals*. The Netherlands: Harwood Academic Publishers.

Antoni, M. H. (2015). Effects of Theodore Millon's teaching, mentorship, theory, and scientific contributions on health psychology and behavioral medicine research and practice. *Journal of Personality Assessment*, *97*(6), 550–562.

Bennett, P. (2000). *Introduction to clinical health psychology*. London: McGraw-Hill Education.

Bennett, P., & Murphy, S. (1997). *Psychology and health promotion*. London: Open University Press.

Bennett, P., Weinman, J., & Spurgeon, P. (Eds.). (1990). *Current developments in health psychology*. The Netherlands: Psychology Press.

Bishop, G. D. (1994). Health psychology: Integrating mind and body. Allyn & Bacon.

Chamberlain, K., Lyons, A. C., & Stephens, C. (2018). Critical health psychology in New Zealand: Developments, directions and reflections. *Journal of Health Psychology*, *23*(3), 457–471. https://doi.org/10.1177/1359105317734871

Chater, A., & Cook, E. (2014). *Psychology express: Health psychology*. Harlow: Pearson.

Chater, A., Quinn, F. & Morrison, V. with Chair: Hart, J; Discussants: Johnston, M. & Weinman, J. (2019). *An oral history of Health Psychology*. Structured Discussion. BPS Division of Health Psychology Annual Conference (Manchester, July 2019).

Chater, A., Whittaker, E., Lewis, L., Arden, M. A., Byrne-Davis, L., Chadwick, P., Drury, J., Epton, T., Hart, J., Kamal, A., McBride, E., O'Connor, D., Shorter, G., Swanson, V. & Armitage, C., (2020). Health psychology, behavioural science, and Covid-19 disease prevention. *Health Psychology Update*, *29*(SI), 3–9.

Crichton, M. (1999). *Timeline*. Alfred A. Knopf.

De-Graft Aikins, A (2005) Healer-shopping in Africa: New evidence from rural-urban qualitative study of Ghanaian diabetes experiences. *British Medical Journal*, *331*, 737. https://doi.org/10.1136/bmj.331.7519.737

De-Graft Aikins, A. (2018). Health psychology in Ghana: A review of the multidisciplinary origins of a young sub-field and its future prospects. *Journal of Health Psychology*, *23*(3), 425–441. https://doi.org/10.1177/1359105317752805

Engel, G. L. (1977). The need for a new medical model: A challenge for biomedicine. *Science*, *196*, 129–135.

Engel, G. L. (1980). The clinical application of the biopsychosocial model. *American Journal of Psychiatry*, *137*, 535–544.

Frank, G., (1984). The Boulder Model: History, rationale, and critique. *Professional Psychology: Research and Practice*, *15*(3), 417–435. https://doi.org/10.1037/0735-7028.15.3.417

Herzlich, C. (2018). A journey in the field of health: From social psychology to multidisciplinarity. *Journal of Health Psychology*, *23*(3), 386–396. https://doi.org/10.1177/1359105317709474

Johnston, M. (2018). Stan Maes: The founder of European health psychology. *Psychology & Health*, *33*(11), 1317–1320.

Johnston, M., Weinman, J. & Chater, A. (2011). A quarter century of health psychology. *The Psychologist*, *24*(12), 890–902.

Kippax, S. (2018). A journey to HIV prevention research: From social psychology to social health via multidisciplinarity. *Journal of Health Psychology*, *23*(3), 442–456. https://doi.org/10.1177/1359105317707529

Lubek, I., Ghabrial, M., Ennis, N., Crann, S., Jenkins, A., Green, M., Badali, J., Salmon, W., Moodley, J., Sulima, E., & Yen, J. (2018). Notes on the development of health psychology and behavioral medicine in the United States. *Journal of Health Psychology*, *23*(3), 492–505. https://doi.org/10.1177/1359105318755156

Lubek, I., & Murray, M. (2018). Doing histor {y/ies} of health psycholog {y/ies}. *Journal of Health Psychology, 23*(3), 361–371. https://doi.org/10.1177/1359105317753627
Matarazzo, J. D. (1980). Behavioral health and behavioral medicine: Frontiers for a new health psychology. *American Psychologist, 35*(9), 807–817. https://doi.org/10.1037/0003-066X.35.9.807
Martin, P. R., Cairns, R., Lindner, H., Milgrom, J., Morrissey, S., & Ricciardelli, L. A. (2014). The training crisis in health psychology in Australia. *Australian Psychologist, 49*(2), 86–95.
Millon, T. (Ed.). (1975). *Medical behavioral science*. Philadelphia, PA: W. B. Saunders.
Millon, T., Green, C., & Meagher, R. (Eds.). (1982). *Handbook of clinical health psychology*. New York, NY: Plenum Press.
Morrison, V., & Bennett, P. (2006). *An introduction to health psychology*. Harlow: Pearson Education.
Morrison, V., & Bennett, P. (2022). *An introduction to health psychology* (5th Ed.). Harlow: Pearson Education.
Murray, M. (2014). Social history of health psychology: Context and textbooks. *Health Psychology Review, 8*(2), 215–237. https://doi.org/10.1080/17437199.2012.701058
Murray, M. (2018). The pre-history of health psychology in the United Kingdom: From natural science and psychoanalysis to social science, social cognition and beyond. *Journal of Health Psychology, 23*(3), 472–491. https://doi.org/10.1177/1359105317705879
Ogden, J. (1996). *Health Psychology: A textbook*. London: McGraw Hill.
Ogden, J. (2023). *Health Psychology: A textbook* (7th Ed.). London: McGraw Hill.
Oldenburg, B., & Owen, N. (1990). Health psychology in Australia. *Psychology and Health, 4*(1), 73–81.
Pitts, M., & Phillips, K. (Eds.). (1991). *The psychology of health: An introduction*. London: Taylor & Francis.
Quinn, F., Chater, A & Morrison, V. (2020). An oral history of UK Health Psychology. *British Journal of Health Psychology, 25*(3), 502–518. https://doi.org/10.1111/bjhp.12418
Santiago-Delefosse, M., & del Rio Carral, M. (2018). The rapid expansion of (mainstream) health psychology in France: Historical foundations. *Journal of Health Psychology, 23*(3), 372–385. https://doi.org/10.1177/1359105317714484
Sarafino, E. (1990). *Health psychology biopsychosocial interactions*. New York: Wiley.
Spink, M. J. P. (2018). Interlaced strands: Health psychology in Brazil from an autobiographic perspective. *Journal of Health Psychology, 23*(3), 397–407. https://doi.org/10.1177/1359105317738259
Stam, H. J., Murray, M., & Lubek, I. (2018). Health psychology in autobiography: Three Canadian critical narratives. *Journal of Health Psychology, 23*(3), 506–523. https://doi.org/10.1177/1359105318755409
Stone, G. C., Weiss, S. M., Matarazzo, J. D., Miller, N. E., Rodin, J., Belar, C. D., Follick, M. J. & Singer, J. E. (Eds.). (1987). *Health psychology: A discipline and a profession*. Chicago: University of Chicago Press.
Stone, G. C., Adler, N. E. & Cohen, F. (1979). *Health psychology: A handbook: Theories, applications, and challenges of a psychological approach to the health care system*. San Francisco: Jossey-Bass.
Takenaka, K. (2013). Introductory remarks on the fifth term as president of the JAHP. The Japanese Association of Health Psychology. Accessed 27-05-24 https://kenkoshinri.jp/english/message.html
Taylor, S. E. (1986). *Health Psychology*. California, LA: Random House.
Taylor, S. E., & Stanton, A. L. (2020). *Health psychology* (11th Ed.). California, LA: McGraw-Hill.

Wallston, K. A. (1997). A history of Division 38 (Health Psychology): Healthy, wealthy, and Weiss. In D. A. Dewsbury (Ed.), *Unification through division: Histories of the divisions of the American Psychological Association* (Vol. 2, pp. 239–267). American Psychological Association. https://doi.org/10.1037/10234-009
Yen, J., & Vaccarino, O. (2018). 'Health psychology' or 'psychology for health'? A history of psychologists' engagement with health in South Africa. *Journal of Health Psychology*, *23*(3), 408–424. https://doi.org/10.1177/1359105317708201

2

HEALTH PSYCHOLOGY THEORIES AND MODELS OF BEHAVIOUR

Phoebe Brook-Rowland, Felix Naughton, Vivi Antonopoulou, Marta Marques, and Angel Marie Chater

Introduction

Theories, models, and their application are a crucial part of the development and growth of health psychology. This chapter contextualises health psychology in its foundations of the biopsychosocial model and discusses, non-exhaustively, key theories, models, and concepts used in the field relating to behaviour. The development of theories and models over the decades will be presented, showcasing the movement from cognitive to socio-cognitive, self-regulation to whole systems approaches, and where they are applied, to include individuals, populations, environments, behaviours, and conditions. This chapter will help to situate health psychology in the health and social care system, and critically discuss its contribution to science, education, policy, and practice.

Theoretical Underpinnings

One of the strengths of health psychology is the theoretical foundations that it is based on, with theories developing over time. Theory has been described *as "a set of concepts and/or statements which specify how phenomena relate to each other, providing an organizing description of a system that accounts for what is known, and explains and predicts phenomena*" (Davis, Campbell, Hildon, Hobbs, & Michie, 2015, p. 327). Theoretical models and frameworks allow for the assessment of hypothesised assumptions related to influences on behaviour and what needs to be considered when trying to achieve desired outcomes. A theory may identify (1) factors influencing a phenomenon (e.g., why some people engage in recommended physical activity levels whilst others do not), (2) the relationship between these factors (e.g., whether this behaviour is related to interacting levels of knowledge, ability, confidence, risk perception, attitudes, beliefs about outcomes, influence of other people, the physical environment, and so on), and, in

DOI: 10.4324/9781003318026-3

some cases, (3) the conditions under which these relationships occur (e.g., whether the behaviour changes in different conditions or when there is a national focus on activity, such as the Olympic Games). Understanding interlinking factors in relation to behaviour, its influences, and outcomes can assist in the maintenance of health and flourishing, the prevention and treatment of illness, and the optimisation of the health-care system and the experiences of those within it.

Whilst early behavioural theories and approaches focused mainly on the importance of providing access to information about threats of a disease or illness (e.g., fear appraisal models), research rapidly showed that the complexity of human behaviour required the development of more complex theories and models that could capture a variety of factors associated with behaviours. Theoretical models have greatly influenced the direction of health behaviour research and are often used in the development, delivery, and evaluation of behaviour change interventions. If we only consider theories explaining behaviour and behaviour change, there are at least 83 theories identified (Davis et al., 2015; Michie, West et al., 2014) and recently represented in an open-access database using an ontology-based modelling system (Hale et al., 2020; https://theory-database.appspot.com/). These theories vary considerably in their scope, specificity, and types of phenomena they aim to explain (e.g., motivation, cognitions), but there is also overlap between them (for example, self-efficacy is a construct addressed in more than one theory). In this chapter, we provide an overview of the most impactful and/or widely used theories in health psychology.

Health Belief Model

One of the oldest theories taught in health psychology linked to human cognition is the Health Belief Model (HBM), proposed by Rosenstock (1966) and further developed by Becker, Haefner, and Maiman (1977). The updated HBM, which added the construct of self-efficacy (Figure 2.1, from Chater and Cook 2014), suggests that behaviour is a result of the following beliefs and evaluations:

- **Susceptibility** to illness (e.g., "*My chances of getting diabetes are high*")
- **Severity** of the illness (e.g., "*Diabetes is a serious illness*")
- **Costs** vs. **benefits** involved in carrying out behaviour (e.g., "*The benefits of knowing whether I am at risk of diabetes outweigh the uncomfortableness of the assessment procedure*") and perceived self-efficacy (e.g., "*I am confident that I can attend an assessment procedure*")
- **Cues to action** (added by Becker & Maiman in 1975) (e.g., "*I have been feeling more tired than usual; perhaps something is wrong*")
- **Health motivation** (added by Becker et al. in 1977) (e.g., "*I want to be healthy*")

Demographics (age, gender, ethnicity) are also seen as influencing factors within the HBM, along with socio-psychological (personality, religion, social economic status) and educational (knowledge about disease, prior contact with disease) influences. However, the HBM fails to include intentions to perform behaviour, social factors, and a measure of coping appraisal.

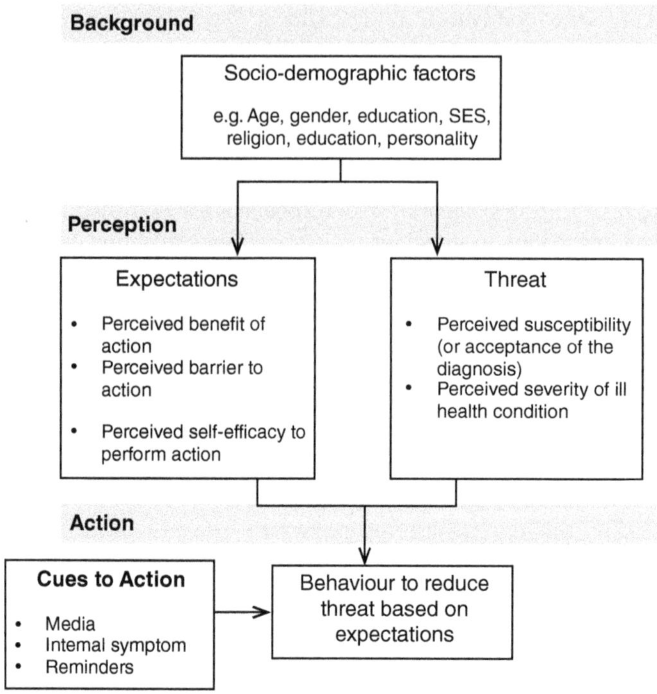

Figure 2.1 The HBM.

Source: Based on Rosenstock (1966, 2005); Becker and Maiman (1975); Becker et al. (1977).

HBM – Research and Application

The HBM has been widely used to predict a range of health behaviours. In a systematic review of COVID-19 vaccine hesitancy (Limbu et al., 2022), of 30,242 participants included, perceived barriers (positively) and perceived benefits (inversely) were commonly associated with vaccine hesitancy. Furthermore, perceived susceptibility, cues to action, perceived severity, and self-efficacy (not included in the original HBM) were inversely associated with vaccine hesitancy. However, additional social constructs, which were measured though missing from the HBM, were also found to be influential, such as placing value in government, public health, and health-care experts' cues to action. Though the review identified numerous influencing factors (e.g., gender, education, age, geographical location, income, race and ethnicity, religion, and political leaning), there is no explanation of underlying mechanisms of change provided and no indication of how to target them, for example, through behaviour change techniques.

Whilst evidence of the predictive utility of the HBM exists, the model has been described as weak in its ability to explain behaviour and being 'static', with no distinction between the motivational (cognitive) and volitional (planning) stages of behaviour change (Conner & Norman, 1995).

Health Locus of Control

Theoretical development was a focal point of research in the early decades, with many having their origins in the social learning tradition which focuses on expectancies, incentives, and reinforcement. Rotter (1954) introduced the concept of 'locus of control', which, based on a theory of incentives and rewards, postulated that if a behaviour has an incentive (i.e., a healthier body) or is reinforced (i.e., makes you feel good), you are more likely to want to engage in it. A distinction was made between an internal and an external locus of control:

- **Internal locus of control**: Individuals are more likely to believe that outcomes (i.e., their health) are a consequence of their own efforts
- **External locus of control**: Individuals are more likely to believe that outcomes are determined by factors beyond their control.

Rotter's theory was developed further by Wallston, Wallston, and DeVellis (1978), who created the Multidimensional Health Locus of Control (MHLC) Scale, measuring health expectancy beliefs along three dimensions: *internal*, *powerful others*, and *chance*.

- **Internal** – the belief that health is under your own influence: "*I am directly responsible for my health*".
- **Powerful others** – the belief that your health is determined by powerful others (i.e., health professionals): "*I can only do what my doctor tells me to do*".
- **Chance** – the belief that your health is uncontrollable and is in fact in the hands of fate or destiny: "*Whether I am well or not is a matter of luck or fate*".

Health Locus of Control – Research and Application

Research on health locus of control (HLOC) shows it to be a relatively weak theoretical model. A meta-analysis of global health appraisal, specific health behaviours, and health locus of control (Cheng et al., 2016) showed all HLOC domains had a weak correlation (r's = −.07 to .10) with specific health behaviours. Somewhat stronger correlations were found between HLOC and global health appraisals (mental quality of life and physical quality of life) (r's = −.16 to .21). This is in line with previous research which indicated HLOC could explain an average of <10% variance of specific health behaviours (Wallston, 1992).

Investigating intentional and non-intentional medication adherence in 188 primary care patients in Germany, Gerland and Prell (2021) found overall HLOC scores did not correlate with overall medication adherence. When looking at individual constructs, internal HLOC was associated with non-adherence, and external HLOC (powerful others and chance) was associated with better adherence, however the variance explained by these factors was low. Furthermore, it was reported that high depression scores had negative effects on both intentional and unintentional adherence, which suggests the impact of emotion should also be considered when trying to explain health behaviour. Additionally, Gerland and Prell (2021) note that whilst HLOC can be considered a trait, self-efficacy is state-related; therefore, an individual may believe they have a certain level of control over their health generally but may have differing beliefs over specific health behaviours and in different contexts.

In summary, although the HLOC can correlate with global health appraisals, its utility with specific health behaviours is inconsistent, and thought needs to be given to additional, sometimes underpinning constructs, such as self-efficacy and emotion.

Social Cognitive Theory

The social learning tradition moves the focus from merely cognition to one that considers the role of social influences on cognition and behaviour (Conner & Norman, 2015). Social Cognitive Theory (SCT: Bandura, 1982) evolved from this as a theory of human motivation based on three types of expectancies (Chater & Cook, 2014; Conner & Norman, 2005):

- **Situation-outcome expectancies**: Beliefs about what outcome will occur without personal action, such as susceptibility to a health threat (e.g., "*My eating behaviour may lead to diabetes*")
- **Action-outcome expectancies**: Beliefs that outcomes occur as a result of personal action (e.g., "*Changing my consumption of high fat, sugar, and salt will lead to a reduced risk of diabetes*")
- **Perceived self-efficacy**: Beliefs about the capability to perform a specific action required to reach a desired outcome (e.g., "*I can change my consumption of high fat, sugar, and salt to reduce my risk of diabetes*")

It has been argued (Schwarzer, 1992) that there is a clear causal ordering among these three expectancies, with the assumption that situation-outcome expectancies influence behaviour by the impact they have on action-outcome expectancies. This could, for example, be related to risk perception (situation-outcome expectancy), which makes you feel susceptible to an illness, and consequently motivates you to consider changing behaviour to reduce the risk. This is thought to be a precursor to an evaluation of action-outcome expectancies, e.g., how the behaviour could reduce the risk, and perceived self-efficacy, e.g., the confidence to make the change in behaviour to reduce the risk.

The updated SCT considers outcome expectations (physical, social, self-evaluative), self-efficacy, socio-structural factors (facilitators and impediments), and goals to influence behaviour (Bandura, 2004). At a more granular level, this includes knowledge, task self-efficacy, self-efficacy to overcome barriers, self-regulation, outcome expectations, outcome values, observational learning (modelling), emotional adaptation, environment, and situational perception (Luszczynska & Schwarzer, 2005). This means that the expansive theory can be used with varying levels of precision, with researchers favouring different levels of detail.

Social Cognitive Theory – Research and Application

In a quasi-experimental study to improve self-care behaviours in patients with type 2 diabetes, Ghoreishi et al. (2019) used a survey to identify which SCT constructs predicted self-care behaviours. This information was then used to design a tailored education intervention of six 45-minute sessions across 30 days targeting the constructs of emotional adaptation, self-efficacy to overcome barriers, and self-regulation. Pre- and post-between-group testing showed the educational intervention successfully increased scores in these domains and increased self-care behaviours. This demonstrates the benefit of specifically tailoring interventions to target influential psychological constructs.

Self-Efficacy

Though perceived self-efficacy is included in SCT, Self-Efficacy Theory (SET) (Bandura, 1977) preceded SCT, and self-efficacy later became the focus of extensive research, suggesting that self-efficacy was one of the most important cognitive constructs to explain adoption and persistence in a given behaviour (Bandura, 1992). SET proposes that the likelihood of behavioural engagement depends on an individual's confidence that the behaviour is under their control and can be successfully performed (Bandura, 1992; Schwarzer, 1992). Self-efficacy can be developed via past success (mastery), vicarious learning, and persuasion, alongside physiological and emotional states (Bandura, 1977, 1997). When a person believes that they can do something (e.g., with evidence from past experience, watching others, or through others having faith in their ability), they are more likely to try and be committed to this intention and behaviour. Evidence has shown that those with high self-efficacy beliefs pursue more challenging and ambitious goals (Luszczynska, Scholz, & Schwarzer, 2005), picture themselves succeeding, and are strongly related to better health, higher achievement, and more social interaction (Schwarzer, 2014).

Self-Efficacy – Research and Application

Self-efficacy is commonly reported as a strong predictor for behavioural intentions and health behaviours, whether measured alone or as part of a wider theory such as SCT. It has been associated with many health behaviours, such as smoking cessation (Gallus et al., 2023), safe sexual behaviours (Torregosa & Patricio, 2022), self-management of chronic diseases (Chen et al., 2023), and physical activity (Garland et al., 2021). However, some have argued that at least part of self-efficacy measures' ability to predict behaviour is because it is often indirectly measuring other constructs, such as intentions, outcome expectancies, and external challenges (Kirsch, 1995; Klassen & Klassen, 2018; Williams & Rhodes, 2016).

Theory of Reasoned Action and Theory of Planned Behaviour

One of the best-known theories in health psychology is the Theory of Planned Behaviour (TPB: Ajzen, 1985), an extension of the Theory of Reasoned Action (TRA: Fishbein & Ajzen, 1975). These social-cognition models see individual behaviour in a social context. Initially, the TRA hypothesised that intentions to perform a behaviour are influenced by attitudes and subjective norms. The TPB expanded this theory by adding perceived behavioural control (PBC), a construct similar to self-efficacy (see Figure 2.2 from Chater & Cook, 2014). This updated theory postulates that behaviour can be directly predicted by intentions and perceived behavioural control, and intentions in turn are predicted by attitudes, subjective norms, and perceived behavioural control:

- **Attitude** – underpinned by ***'behavioural beliefs'*** (the likelihood of an outcome occurring as a result of performing a behaviour) and ***'outcome evaluation'*** (the evaluation of that outcome)
- **Subjective norms** – underpinned by ***'normative beliefs'*** (the perception of how significant others, e.g., parents, friends, would view the behaviour) and ***'motivation to comply'*** with these significant others
- **Perceived behavioural control** – belief in the ability to perform the behaviour linked to ***'internal'*** (knowledge, skills, emotions) and ***'external'*** (opportunities, dependence on others, resource barriers) ***control factors***
- **Intention** – the conscious decision to perform a behaviour, reflecting a person's motivation to exert effort into trying
- **Behaviour** – the action, broken down to (a) the action/behaviour, (b) performed on or towards a target, (c) in a context, (d) at a time or occasion (e.g., (a) swallows, (b) medicine, (c) in the kitchen, (d) at 8 a.m. every morning with a cup of tea)

Theory of Planned Behaviour – Research and Application

The TPB has been applied to a variety of health behaviours. Whilst its predictive validity has been found to be fairly consistent, it explains only modest variance in behaviour. A systematic review of 237 prospective statistical tests found that the TPB accounted for approximately 19% of variability in health behaviour, with intention being the strongest predictor, as posited by the theory (McEachan, Conner, Taylor, & Lawton, 2011).

Wollast et al.'s (2021) TPB study of COVID-19 behaviours (handwashing and limiting social contact) in a sample of 4,804 participants in Belgium and France found increased positive attitudes, social norms, perceived behavioural control and intentions were associated with higher adherence to the health behaviours in both countries. The model accounted for 33% and 35% of variation in *intention* to perform handwashing and limiting social contact respectively, leading the authors to suggest further investigation into additional concepts such as cooperation, resilience and emotion were warranted. Additionally, the model was only able to account for 10% and 5% of variance in reported *behaviour*. This is

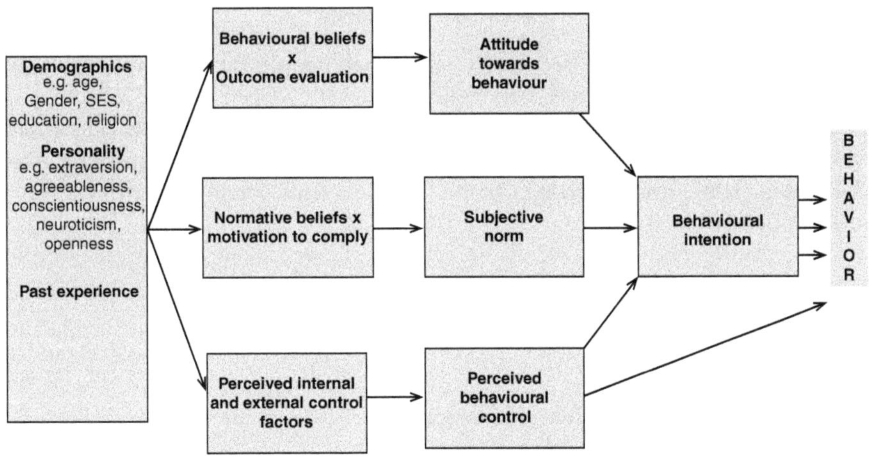

Figure 2.2 TPB.

Source: *From intentions to action: A theory of planned behaviour*. In J. Kuhl & J. Beckham (Eds.), Action control: From cognitions to behaviors, New York: Springer (Ajzen I. 1985) pp. 11–39, with kind permission from Springer Science and Business Media. Copyright © 1985, Springer-Verlag Berlin Heidelberg.

indicative of the 'intention-behaviour gap' (Rhodes & de Bruijn, 2013; Sniehotta et al., 2005), again suggesting additional constructs are required to improve the prediction of behaviour.

Meta-analyses of physical activity in adults with physical disabilities found social norms to have a non-significant effect on intention (Sur et al., 2022), and to be weakly correlated in general adult populations (Schüz et al., 2017). Noting subjective norms as an area for improvement in the TPB and the importance of social identity, Willis et al. (2020) found that adding measures of group identification and behavioural group importance predicted attitudes and norms, and therefore intentions towards binge drinking in 246 Australian university students. This suggests, although not accounted for in the TPB, understanding whether individuals associate a behaviour with their social identity may be integral to understanding behavioural engagement. Furthermore, executive function tasks such as behavioural regulation and decision processes have been found to partially account for the translation from intention to behaviour in binge drinking among students (Mullan et al., 2011a).

Despite the TPB having shaped psychological theorising for health-related preventive behaviours, it has also been heavily criticised for excluding affective and unconscious influences on behaviour (Sniehotta et al., 2014). To address such criticisms, new components have been added to the model to increase its predictive value. Myers and Goodwin (2012) noted a substantial improvement in the TPB's predictive value with the addition of anticipated regret. Additionally, factors such as past behaviour and knowledge were also found to be useful predictors of intention and behaviour in previous research on swine flu vaccination (Gallagher & Povey, 2006).

Unrealistic Optimism

Unrealistic optimism (Weinstein, 1982) theorised people are often not motivated to protect their health because they believe "*It won't happen to me*", reflecting an inaccurate or 'unrealistically optimistic' perception of their risk. The potentially egocentric and selective perception of risk has been termed **'optimistic bias'** (Weinstein, 1987) and is thought to be linked to four cognitive factors (Chater and Cook, 2014, p. 31):

1) Lack of personal experience with the problem
2) The belief that the problem is preventable by individual action
3) The belief that if the problem has not yet appeared, it will not appear in the future
4) The belief that the problem is infrequent

Unrealistic Optimism – Research and Application

A study of 373 adults collected ratings of perceived risks and benefits of different medical scenarios (Hanoch et al., 2019). Unlike previous studies, the authors included a range of uncommon and common conditions, provided information and probabilities of the risks (treatment failure or side effects) and benefits (successful treatment, reduction in symptoms), and took a measure of participant's numeracy skills (as this was thought to be important for risk perception). The results showed participants were still optimistic about their chances of avoiding the risk, though they were less optimistic about receiving the benefits. These findings are important, as patients must give consent to medical interventions but may still not be consenting to an accurate perception of risk. Therefore, it is important for future research to understand how unrealistic optimism can be challenged.

Protection Motivation Theory

Many health campaigns, particularly in the early days of health psychology, aim to induce feelings of risk or threat. However, evidence from the HBM and unrealistic optimism have shown that feelings of susceptibility and severity only explain a small amount of the variance in health behaviours. SCT and TPB help us to understand behaviour a little more, focusing on expectancies, and the social context in which behaviour is or is not performed. The Protection Motivation Theory (PMT: Rogers, 1975) combines elements from these other theories (see Figure 2.3) and suggests that behaviour is a result of two cognitive factors:

- **Threat appraisal** – made up of both perceived ***'severity'*** of illness and ***'vulnerability'*** to it (which leads to fear arousal)
- **Coping appraisal** – a function of both ***'response efficacy'*** (similar to an outcome expectancy) and ***'self-efficacy'*** beliefs, leading to an evaluation of ***'response costs'***.

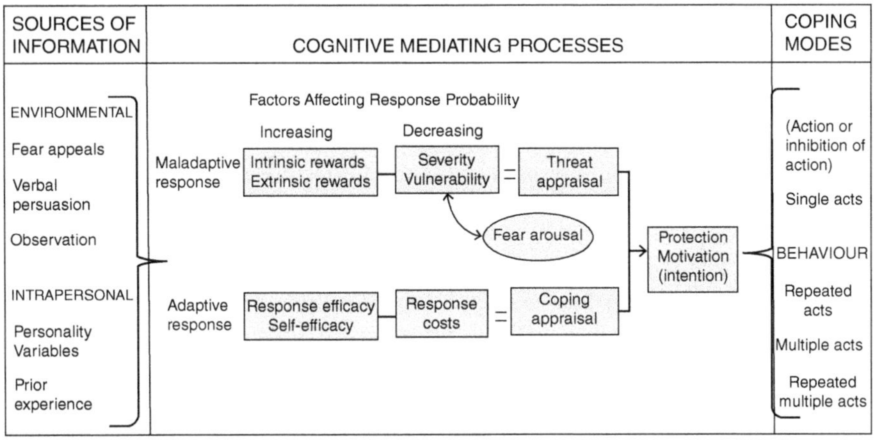

Figure 2.3 PMT.

Source: A protection motivation theory of fear appeals and attitude change, Rogers, R. W., *Journal of Psychology*, 1975, Taylor & Francis Ltd, reprinted by permission of the publisher (Taylor & Francis Ltd, http://www.tandf.co.uk/journals).

These appraisals are thought to lead to an **intention** (protection motivation), which then leads to **behaviour**. Chater and Cook (2014; p. 30) highlight that **behaviour** is more likely to occur if a person holds the following beliefs:

a) They are vulnerable to disease ("*My chances of getting bowel cancer are high*": **'*vulnerability*'**)
b) The disease will have severe consequences ("*Bowel cancer is a serious illness*": **'*severity*'**)
c) They believe a change in behaviour will reduce risk/improve outcomes ("*Eating more fruit and vegetables will reduce my risk of getting bowel cancer*": **'*response efficacy*'**)
d) They believe that they are capable of engaging in the behaviour ("*I am confident I am able to eat more fruit and vegetables*": **'*self-efficacy*'**)
e) They have a high intention towards the behaviour ("*I will definitely eat more fruit and vegetables*": **'*intention*'**)

Protection Motivation Theory – Research and Application

Findings from meta-analyses examining the use of the PMT (Floyd, Prentice-Dunn, & Rogers, 2000; Milne, Sheeran, & Orbell, 2000) show that components of coping appraisal (response efficacy and self-efficacy) are stronger predictors of the protection motivation (intention) than components of threat appraisals (perceived vulnerability and severity). A protective motivation theory skills-based sexual health programme attempting to increase condom use intentions in

American Indian adolescents was found to be unsuccessful in changing boys' condom use intentions but successful in girls (Rosenstock et al., 2020). Though all PMT constructs were measured, the change in girls was significantly mediated primarily by condom use self-efficacy and secondarily by response efficacy. This suggests, in this instance, that self-efficacy is the most influential feature from PMT for girls for condom use intention and that for boys, this intention may be better addressed via a different model, perhaps one that provides a greater understanding of 'response cost'.

Although PMT includes threat appraisals, the utility of appealing or augmenting individuals' fear has been questioned. A meta-analysis (Witte & Allen, 2000) has indicated that whilst fear appeals may increase levels of susceptibility and severity, if self-efficacy is not simultaneously enhanced, it may lead to health messaging resistance and denial of a health threat. A more recent meta-analysis (Tannenbaum et al., 2015) has concluded fear appeals are effective without identifying instances of undesirable outcomes. Though the authors highlight that effectiveness was improved via the inclusion of a self or response efficacy statement, fear appeals without efficacy statements were still effective. However, this meta-analysis has since been challenged (Kok et al., 2018) due to its methodology, such as the inclusion of attitudes, intentions, and behaviours as outcome measures rather than looking at behavioural change in isolation. This led Kok et al. (2018) to question whether the data truly supports fear appeals as an effective means of changing behaviour.

During COVID-19, concern was raised over the use of fear appeals and the potential negative mental health effects for an already vulnerable population (Chater et al., 2023; Demirtaş-Madran, 2021; Dong & Zheng, 2020). Heffner et al. (2021) found both fear and prosocial messaging equally influenced COVID-19 disease prevention behaviours; however, prosocial messaging effectiveness was more dependent on creating a greater emotional response. It is argued that although fear appeals may be used as more of a blunt instrument, targeting other psychological constructs may reduce potential negative spillover effects (Demirtaş-Madran, 2021).

Theoretical Domains Framework

With the intention of making psychological theory more accessible, a panel of behaviour change experts used consensus tasks to consolidate 128 theoretical constructs from 33 psychological theories into 12 domains, creating the original Theoretical Domains Framework (TDF) (Michie et al., 2005). Theory consolidation saw domains such as 'Beliefs about capabilities', which denotes the extent to which an individual feels capable of enacting a particular behaviour, drawing together SET (Bandura, 1977), 'perceived self-efficacy' from SCT (Bandura, 1986) and the HBM (Rosenstock, 1974), and 'perceived behavioural control' from the TPB (Ajzen, 1985, 1991).

Through a subsequent TDF validation study, Cane et al. (2012) used 112 theoretical constructs (after removing duplicates) to identify 14 theoretical domains, which encompass 84 psychological constructs, now commonly referred to as the

TDF – namely, (1) Knowledge, (2) Skills, (3) Social/Professional Role and Identity, (4) Beliefs about Capabilities, (5) Optimism, (6) Beliefs about Consequences, (7) Reinforcement, (8) Intentions, (9) Goals, (10) Memory, Attention and Decision Processes, (11) Environmental Context and Resources, (12) Social Influences, (13) Emotions, and (14) Behavioural Regulation.

Theoretical Domains Framework – Research and Application

The TDF has been used both qualitatively and quantitatively to explain a number of different health behaviours. Using semi-structured interviews, it has been used to understand prescribing behaviour (Chater, Williams & Courtenay, 2019; Courtenay et al., 2019; Spillane et al., 2021), sitting behaviour (Brierley et al., 2021; Ojo et al., 2019a,b), and COVID-19 prevention behaviours (Chater, Brook-Rowland, et al., 2023). Using survey design, it has been used to understand antimicrobial stewardship behaviours (Chater, Family, et al., 2022). It has also been used in systematic reviews and evidence synthesis, for example, to identify influences on uptake and engagement with health and well-being smartphone apps (Szinay et al., 2020) and for coding prescribing behaviour (Chater, Family et al., 2020).

The Behaviour Change Wheel and COM-B Model of Behaviour Change

The Behaviour Change Wheel (BCW) (Michie et al., 2011, 2014) provides a framework to identify influences on behaviour and their mechanisms of action, and to systematically match these influences to behaviour change intervention strategies (Michie et al., 2014; West et al., 2019). Developed from the consolidation of 19 behaviour change frameworks (Michie et al., 2011), the BCW offers a whole-system approach to intervention design, delivery, and evaluation, going beyond traditional theories in health psychology where the end point is often predicting behaviour.

Whilst creating the BCW, Michie et al. (2011) created an integrated model compromising the minimum factors necessary to enact a behaviour – the Capability, Opportunity, Motivation – Behaviour (COM-B) Model of Behaviour Change. The COM-B model is an integrative approach intended for practical application via understanding biopsychosocial influences on behaviour, highlighting an individual's capability, both physical (such as skills, strength, or stamina) and psychological (such as knowledge or ample mental resources); their opportunity, both social (norms) and physical (environmental contexts and resources); and their motivation, both reflective (influenced by beliefs such as confidence and intention) and automatic (influenced by emotion or habit).

To assist in its use to develop behaviour change interventions, the TDF has been mapped (Cane et al., 2012; Michie et al., 2014) to the COM-B model at the hub of the BCW (Michie et al., 2011). In this mapping, the TDF domain 'skills' features both physical and psychological capability, which has been visually depicted to include 'physical skills' and 'cognitive and interpersonal skills' by Chater et al. (2022) in Figure 2.4.

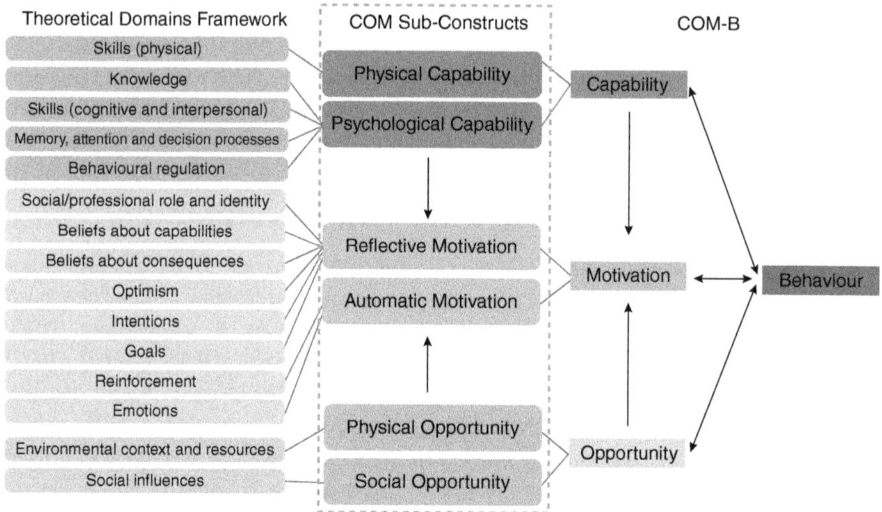

Figure 2.4 The TDF mapped to the sub-constructs of the COM-B model (from Chater et al., 2022).

COM-B – Research and Application

There is growing research evidence that the COM-B model, often used with the TDF, forms an integral 'behavioural diagnosis' for behaviour change interventions to be based upon, featured in Stage 1 of the BCW. A study (Carstairs et al., 2020) of health-care professional's barriers to connecting patients with community-based physical activity opportunities revealed that 'awareness of opportunities' (Psychological Capability – Knowledge), 'time' (Physical Opportunity – Environmental context and resources), and 'perceived patient engagement' (Reflective Motivation – Beliefs about consequences) were important areas for future interventions to consider. This enabled recommendations such as creating resource solutions via an intermediary person who could have the time and awareness to increase patient engagement in physical activity options.

Dual Processing and Heuristics

The assumption that humans are governed by rational and conscious decision-making is a significant limitation of many of the theoretical models and constructs discussed so far.

Thinking Fast and Slow: System 1 and System 2

Since the 1970s, psychologists have proposed that cognition and reasoning are determined by two separate, though often interacting, systems, referred to as 'dual-process' models. They broadly adhere to two types of processes: one as automatic, unconscious, quick to activate but usually slow to change (often referred to as system 1; Stanovich, 1999) and a second as reflective, conscious, slow to activate but potentially quick to change (system 2) (Kahneman, 2011). Dual-process models have been increasing in popularity in health psychology and have been applied to health-related decision-making and behaviour. As with other types of models, there are numerous dual-process theories. Some have categorised these models into groups based on how individuals are conceptualised within the models (Houlihan, 2018) or on attributes of the cognitive systems they describe (Evans, 2008).

Houlihan (2018) categorises health-related dual-process models as either treating individuals as irrational actors (e.g., Elaboration Likelihood Model of Persuasion; Petty and Cacioppo, 1986), as social actors (e.g., Social Identity Theory; Tajfel and Turner, 1979), as actors in a physical environment (e.g., COM-B model; Michie et al., 2011) or as self-regulated actors (e.g., Control Theory; Carver & Scheier, 1982). Houlihan proposes a general purpose dual-process model of health-related behaviour where external cues (e.g., social and physical) interact with internal cues (e.g., heuristics, beliefs, affect) through self-regulatory factors (e.g., habit, feedback processes) and act on behaviour via unconscious and propositional reasoning. However, Evans (2008) challenges whether the different dual-process models can be integrated into a generic model and considers this overly simplistic. Evans categorises dual-process models into those with attributes of consciousness (vs. unconsciousness), evolution (evolutionarily old vs. new), functional characteristics (associative vs. rules-based), and individual differences (universal vs. heritable). They add that thinking of system 1 as one single and universal system is problematic, as is thinking about system 2 as the conscious mind, and suggests that system 2 is likely a mixture of automatic (e.g., working memory) and reflective processes. Even though Houlihan and Evans come from different areas of psychology, the almost zero overlap between the dual-process models identified in their respective reviews, with only one overlapping model out of 34 identified across the two papers, highlights a broader discrepancy regarding how dual processes are conceptualised.

The consideration of automatic and unconscious processes for understanding behaviour expands our ability to predict it within a broader context of determinants. For example, Hamilton et al. (2020) found that drinking behaviour among students is more determined by unconscious and automatic processes than intentional ones. Similarly, a review found young people with overweight or obesity had greater deficits in conscious regulation-related processing, with their eating and weight-related behaviours governed more by automatic processes, compared to those classified within a 'healthy' weight (Kemps et al., 2020). System 1/automatic processes are likely to be more important in determining some behaviours more than others. For example, the Typology of Interventions in Proximal Physical Micro-Environments (TIPPME) is largely focused on system 1 type processes and is focused on the selection, purchase, and consumption of food, alcohol, and tobacco (Hollands et al., 2017). Medication adherence is also another area strongly driven by unintentional habit-based processes (Horne et al., 2013). Evidence from smoking cessation medication adherence intervention trials indicates that those focused on practicalities (e.g., capabilities, resources, levels of support or skills), aligning with system 1 determinants, show larger effect sizes compared to those based on perceptions (e.g., beliefs, cognitions, concerns, and preferences), aligned with system 2 determinants (Hollands et al., 2019). These align with the perceptions and practicalities approach (PAPA: Horne et al., 2019) often used to explain medication adherence.

Stage Models of Behaviour

Most causal theories and models in health psychology specify that key behavioural determinants, such as motivation, affect behaviour linearly, i.e., the stronger the determinant, the greater its influence on behaviour will be. These are referred to as continuum theories/models. Stage models, on the other hand, specify that individuals pass through a sequence of discrete stages, typically starting at inaction and ending at behavioural maintenance. Transitions between these phases are due to step changes in the staging construct, e.g., motivation, which in turn is affected by different factors or a combination of factors for each stage transition (Sutton, 2015).

Transtheoretical Model

The Transtheoretical Model (TTM) is one of the best-known examples of a stage model. It conceptualises behaviour change as the progression through six 'Stages of Change': precontemplation, contemplation, preparation, action, maintenance, and termination, and accounts for relapse. These stages are considered in relation to three dimensions: processes of change, decisional balance, and self-efficacy (Prochaska & DiClemente, 1982). However, it has been noted that many interventions are developed without appropriate consideration of all the dimensions (Hutchison et al., 2009), and efforts have been made to encourage researchers to utilise all elements of the theory (Romain, Caudroit, et al., 2018). Though Stages of Change constructs are helpful in establishing to what extent an individual is 'ready to change', it does not allow for exploration as to reasons why or provide tailored recommendations as to how to facilitate moving through the process. Additionally, as TTM is routed in individual motivation, it does not widely consider external factors. Furthermore, critiques of the model highlight weaknesses in the arbitrary staging process, need for people's intentions to be stable for stages to be meaningful, and underplaying the role of associative learning and habits (i.e., system 1 influences) on behaviour and behaviour change (West, 2005). Studies have also not consistently supported a key tenet of the model, that stage-matched interventions are more effective than stage-mismatched interventions (Schüz et al., 2007; de Vet et al., 2008).

Transtheoretical Model – Research and Application

A recent study of post-menopausal women found an educational intervention based on TTM to be successful in moving women out of the precontemplation stage and saw increases in self-reported physical activity (PA) in comparison to the control group (Masoudy et al., 2022). It is noteworthy that the educational intervention also included participation in three walking groups; therefore, it is possible that having the opportunity to participate in walking groups was what increased PA scores and moved women out of precontemplation. This could be identified if the study was repeated, including a walking group only, as well as the education group and control. Conversely, de Freitas et al.'s (2020) study split a group of women in a weight management programme and provided half with monthly behaviour change counselling based on the TTM. The intervention specified which process of change was used to target each stage of change. The TTM counselling group reported better adherence to weight management which addressed four behaviours; however, there was no between-group difference for PA. This is counter to a recent review which found that TTM interventions which target self-efficacy and processes of change were twice as likely to increase PA than those that did not (Romain et al., 2018). de Freitas et al. (2020) proposed that this was because both groups had access to exercise classes, suggesting this was an issue of opportunity and targeting psychological constructs was not additionally necessary.

The Health Action Process Approach

The Health Action Process Approach (HAPA) Model is one of the few theoretical approaches developed within health psychology (Schwarzer, 1992; Schwarzer & Luszczynska, 2008). It is considered both an integrative and a hybrid model. Integrative because it integrates constructs from different social cognitive and action theories, and hybrid as it can be used as a stage (pre-intenders, intenders, and actors) or continuous model. HAPA is a social cognitive model that distinguishes between motivational and volitional or post-motivational processes (see Figure 2.5):

- **Motivational processes**: include (a) ***risk perception*** (perceived severity and susceptibility to a health threat), (b) ***outcome expectancies*** (potential emotional, social, or physical outcomes resulting from performing the behaviour), c) ***action self-efficacy*** (confidence in ability to perform the behaviour also referred to as task self-efficacy), and (d) ***intention*** to perform a behaviour which is hpyothesised to be influenced by the first three determinants
- **Volitional processes**: comprise (a) ***planning***, i.e., the specification of the implementation of the behaviour made up of – action planning (e.g., when, how, where, and with whom the person will do the behaviour) and coping planning (identification of potential barriers and how to deal with them); (b) ***coping self-efficacy*** (confidence in ability to maintain the behaviour, even if certain barriers occur); (c) ***recovery self-efficacy*** (confidence in ability to re-engage in the target behaviour after a relapse); and (d) ***action control*** (conscious processes needed for the maintenance of behaviour such as self-monitoring, self-regulation efforts). Action and coping planning are considered to mediate the intention-behaviour relationship.

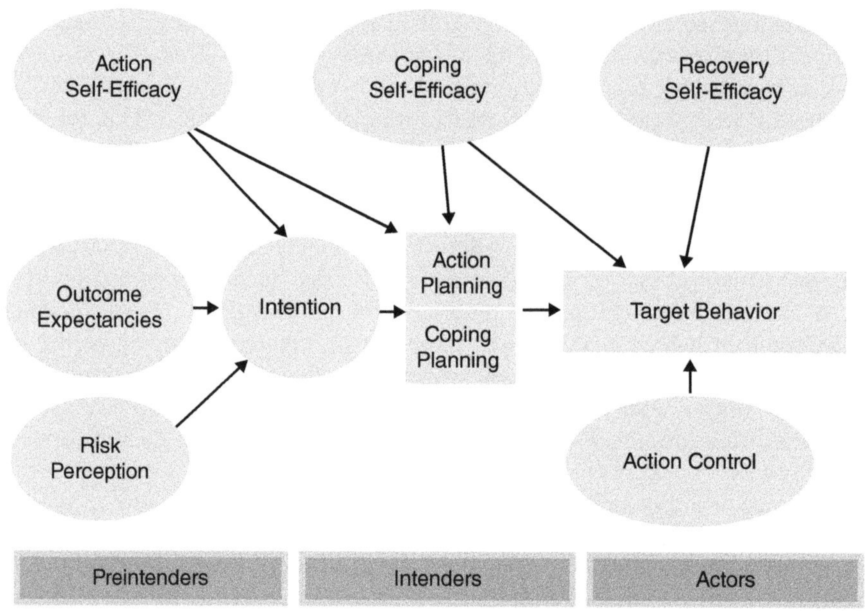

Figure 2.5 HAPA.

Source: Self-efficacy: Thought control of action, Washington, DC: Hemisphere Publishing Corporation (Schwarzer, R. 1992), republished with permission of Informa plc., permission conveyed through Copyright Clearance Center, Inc.

The Health Action Process Approach – Research and Application

There is an increasing body of research investigating the relationships between HAPA constructs in multiple health behaviours. A meta-analysis (Zhang et al., 2019) examined the HAPA model assumptions in 95 studies across health behaviours. Correlations between HAPA constructs were found to be positive with small to medium effect sizes, with the exception of risk perception and recovery self-efficacy. Action self-efficacy had the largest effects on health behaviour through intentions and maintenance self-efficacy. Further, past behaviour attenuated the intention-behaviour relationship.

The HAPA model has been used to underpin a range of health behaviour change interventions, providing a useful and solid theoretical basis in which all constructs can be linked with specific behaviour change techniques, and the relationships between constructs can inform the design of an intervention (e.g., Lippke, Schwarzer, Ziegelmann, Scholz, & Schüz, 2010; Gellert et al., 2014).

Misalignment of 'Between-Person' and 'Within-Person' Differences in Theoretical Designs

A major critique of much of the evidence underpinning theories and models in health psychology is that it is based on between-person rather than within-person data. At best, this means findings from between-person analyses will hide any individual variation, and at worst, it means identified relationships are misrepresented or incorrect for many individuals (Johnston & Johnston, 2013).

As an example, Innauen et al. (2016) looked at the association between intention and unhealthy snack eating using a longitudinal diary (five measures per day for seven days). When they aggregated all intention scores across the time points together to see how well they predicted aggregated unhealthy snack eating, there was a small non-significant association. However, using the same data, they undertook a within-person analysis looking at whether intention at a specific time point predicted snack eating over the next three hours. They found a strong significant association, showing that, at the individual level, the higher the intention to not eat unhealthy snacks, the lower the subsequent snacking behaviour. This discrepancy between the between- and within-person findings is described by two connected phenomena: Simpson's paradox, where fundamentally different relationships can be found when accounting for a higher level of clustering, i.e., looking at within-person data rather than data aggregated at the person level, and an ecological fallacy, where inferences from groups are inappropriately applied to individuals (Fisher et al., 2018).

A related issue is that individuals differ from one another and even themselves when examined over time, often due to changes in context. For example, Hojjatinia et al. (2021) found that digital messages promoting PA had an overall positive average effect on their sample of increasing objectively measured PA. However, the average effect hid a detrimental effect for some individuals when within-person analyses were undertaken, with one-third of participants modelled to actually reduce their PA after receiving the messages. Furthermore, for some individuals, the same messages had a positive effect on activity when received on a weekend but a neutral or negative effect on a weekday. Similar inter- and intra-individual differences have been observed across a range of phenomena.

To validly apply theories to individuals, they need to be tested on individuals using within-person methodologies. If within-person findings correspond with between-person (aggregated) findings, then relationships can be considered ergodic, and an ecological fallacy will be avoided. However, based on the limited within-person investigations to date, individuals often seem to vary in what determines their behaviour, somewhat contrary to predictions made by theories and the between-person data supporting them (e.g., Kwasnicka et al., 2017; Perski et al., 2019). Under such conditions, within-person methodologies, including N-of-1 (single case designs), would be preferable to between-person ones when testing the relationships between theory-derived constructs.

Shift towards Ecological and Whole Systems Models

A final note on the recent emphasis on ecological models in the field of health psychology. Health behaviour theories provide systematic ways to comprehend and predict why individuals engage in certain health-related actions. Whole systems approaches involve a more holistic understanding of the complex interplay between individuals and their environments. Social ecological models (SEMs) for health behaviour extend beyond individual factors to encompass the influence of social, environmental, and policy contexts in shaping individuals' health-related decisions and actions. These models depict dynamic relationships among individuals, groups, and their environments and recognise the role of social and economic factors in creating and sustaining health disparities (Baron et al., 2014). By emphasising the interplay of the social determinants of health across multiple levels, SEMs can help researchers and practitioners identify points of intervention at different levels for effective health promotion and behaviour change initiatives (Sallis et al., 2015; Mehtälä et al., 2014).

Conclusion

This chapter has demonstrated the strong theoretical foundations within health psychology, with emphasis on core theories, models, and approaches related to health behaviours and health outcomes. Furthermore, methodological complexities of understanding and improving health at both an individual and population level have been highlighted. Continuing efforts to address gaps and create theories, models, and approaches which are accessible to researchers and practitioners whilst maintaining sufficient depth have been discussed. The chapter has presented a recent move towards a consolidation of theories combined with more holistic whole systems approaches to maintain and improve health and health services.

Further Reading

Cane, J., O'Connor, D., & Michie, S. (2012). Validation of the theoretical domains framework for use in behaviour change and implementation research. *Implementation Science*, *7*(1), 37. https://doi.org/10.1186/1748-5908-7-37

Chater, A. M., & Cook, E. (2014). *Psychology express: Health psychology*. Pearson.

Conner, M., & Norman, P. (2015). *Predicting and changing health behaviour: Research and practice with social cognition models*. McGraw-Hill Education (UK).

Michie, S., Johnston, M., Abraham, C., Lawton, R., Parker, D., & Walker, A. (2005). Making psychological theory useful for implementing evidence based practice: A consensus approach. *Quality & Safety in Health Care*, *14*(1), 26–33. https://doi.org/10.1136/qshc.2004.011155

References

Ajzen, I. (1985). *From intentions to action: A theory of planned behaviour*. In J. Kuhl & J. Beckham (Eds.), *Action control: from cognitions to behaviors* (pp. 11–39). New York: Springer.

Ajzen, I. (1991). The theory of planned behavior. *Organizational Behavior and Human Decision Processes*, *50*(2), 179–211.

Bandura, A. (1977). Self-efficacy: Toward a unifying theory of behavioural change. *Psychological Review*, *28*(2), 191–215.

Bandura, A. (1982). Self-efficacy mechanism in human agency. *American Psychologist*, *37*, 122–147.

Bandura, A. (1986). *Social foundations of thought and action*. Englewood Cliffs, NJ, (23–28).
Bandura, A. (1992). Self-efficacy mechanism in psychobiologic functioning. In R. Schwarzer (Ed.), *Self-efficacy: Thought control of action*. Washington, DC: Hemisphere.
Bandura, A. (1997). *Self-efficacy: The exercise of control*. New York, NY: W.H. Freeman and Co.
Bandura, A. (2004). Health promotion by social cognitive means. *Health Education & Behavior*, *31*(2), 143–164. https://doi.org/10.1177/1090198104263660
Baron, S. L., Beard, S., Davis, L. K., Delp, L., Forst, L., Kidd-Taylor, A., ... Welch, L. S. (2014). Promoting integrated approaches to reducing health inequities among low-income workers: Applying a social ecological framework. *American Journal of Industrial Medicine*, *57*(5), 539–556. https://doi.org/10.1002/ajim.22174
Becker, M. H., Haefner, D. P., & Maiman, L. A. (1977). The Health Belief Model in the prediction of dietary compliance: A field experiment. *Journal of Health & Social Behavior*, *18*, 348–366.
Becker, M. H., & Maiman, L. A. (1975). Sociobehavioral determinants of compliance with health and medical care recommendations. *Medical Care*, *13*(1), 10–24.
Brierley, M. L., Smith, L. R., Bailey, D. P., Every, S. A., Staines, T. A., & Chater, A. M. (2021). Perceived influences on reducing prolonged sitting in police staff: a qualitative investigation using the Theoretical Domains Framework and COM-B model. *BMC Public Health*, *21*(1): 2126. https://doi.org/10.1186/s12889-021-12019-6
Cane, J., O'Connor, D., & Michie, S. (2012). Validation of the theoretical domains framework for use in behaviour change and implementation research. *Implementation Science*, *7*(1), 37. https://doi.org/10.1186/1748-5908-7-37
Carstairs, S. A., Rogowsky, R. H., Cunningham, K. B., Sullivan, F., & Ozakinci, G. (2020). Connecting primary care patients to community-based physical activity: A qualitative study of health professional and patient views. *BJGP Open*, *4*(3). https://doi.org/10.3399/bjgpopen20X101100
Carver, C. S. & Scheier, M. F. (1982). Control theory: A useful conceptual framework for personality–social, clinical, and health psychology. *Psychological Bulletin*, *92*(1), 111.
Chater, A. M., Brook-Rowland, P., Tolani, F., Christopher, E., Hart, J., Byrne-Davis, L. M. T., Moffat, A., Shorter, G. W., Epton, T., Kamal, A., O'Connor, D. B., Whittaker, E., Lewis, L. J. M., McBride, E., Swanson, V., & Arden, M. A. (2023). Understanding a constellation of eight COVID-19 disease prevention behaviours using the COM-B model and the theoretical domains framework: A qualitative study using the behaviour change wheel. *Frontiers in Public Health*, *11*, 1130875. https://doi.org/10.3389/fpubh.2023.1130875
Chater, A. M., & Cook, E. (2014). *Psychology express: Health psychology*. Pearson.
Chater, A. M., Family, H., Abraao, L. M., Burnett, E., Castro-Sanchez, E., Du Toit, B., Gallagher, R., Gotterson, F., Manias, E., Mcewen, J., Figueiredo, R. M., Nathan, M., Olans, R., Padoveze, M. C., & Courtenay, M. (2022). Influences on nurses' engagement in antimicrobial stewardship behaviours: A multi-country survey using the Theoretical Domains Framework. *Journal of Hospital Infection*, *129*, 171–180. https://doi.org/10.1016/j.jhin.2022.07.010
Chater, A., Family, H., Lim, R., & Courtenay, M (2020). Influences on antibiotic prescribing by non-medical prescribers for respiratory tract infections: A systematic review using the Theoretical Domains Framework. *Journal of Antimicrobial Chemotherapy*, *75*(12), 3458–3470. https://doi.org/10.1093/jac/dkaa335
Chater, A., Williams, J., & Courtenay, M. (2019). The prescribing needs of community practitioner nurse prescribers: A qualitative investigation using the Theoretical Domains Framework and COM-B. *Journal of Advanced Nursing*, *75*(11), 2952–2968. https://doi.org/10.1111/jan.14170

Chen, J., Tian, Y., Yin, M., Lin, W., Tuersun, Y., Li, L., Yang, J., Wu, F., Kan, Y., Li, X., Gan, Y., Sun, X., Wu, Y., & He, F. (2023). Relationship between self-efficacy and adherence to self-management and medication among patients with chronic diseases in China: A multicentre cross-sectional study. *Journal of Psychosomatic Research*, *164*, 111105. https://doi.org/10.1016/j.jpsychores.2022.111105

Cheng, C., Cheung, M. W.-L., & Lo, B. C. Y. (2016). Relationship of health locus of control with specific health behaviours and global health appraisal: A meta-analysis and effects of moderators. *Health Psychology Review*, *10*(4), 460–477. https://doi.org/10.1080/17437199.2016.1219672

Conner, M., & Norman, P. (1995). *Predicting health behaviour*. Buckingham: Open University Press.

Conner, M., & Norman, P. (2005). *Predicting health behaviour* (2nd Edn.). Buckingham: Open University Press.

Conner, M., & Norman, P. (2015). *Predicting and changing health behaviour: Research and practice with social cognition models*. McGraw-Hill education (UK).

Courtenay, M., Rowbotham, S., Lim, R., Peters, S., Yates, K., & Chater, A. (2019). Examining influences on antibiotic prescribing by nurse and pharmacist prescribers: A qualitative study using the Theoretical Domains Framework and COM-B. *BMJ Open*, *9*(6): e029177. https://doi.org/10.1136/bmjopen-2019-029177

Davis, R., Campbell, R., Hildon, Z., Hobbs, L., & Michie, S. (2015). Theories of behaviour and behaviour change across the social and behavioural sciences: A scoping review. *Health Psychology Review*, *9*(3), 323.44. https://doi.org/10.1080/17437199.2014.941722

de Freitas, P. P., de Menezes, M. C., Dos Santos, L. C., Pimenta, A. M., Ferreira, A. V. M., & Lopes, A. C. S. (2020). The transtheoretical model is an effective weight management intervention: a randomized controlled trial. *BMC Public Health*, 20, 1–12.

Demirtaş-Madran, H. A. (2021). Accepting restrictions and compliance with recommended preventive behaviors for COVID-19: A discussion based on the key approaches and current research on fear appeals. *Frontiers in Psychology*, *12*. https://www.frontiersin.org/articles/10.3389/fpsyg.2021.558437

De Vet, E., De Nooijer, J., De Vries, N. K., & Brug, J. (2008). Testing the transtheoretical model for fruit intake: comparing web-based tailored stage-matched and stage-mismatched feedback. *Health Education Research*, *23*(2), 218–227.

Dong, M., & Zheng, J. (2020). Letter to the editor: Headline stress disorder caused by Netnews during the outbreak of COVID-19. *Health Expectations: An International Journal of Public Participation in Health Care and Health Policy*, *23*(2), 259–260. https://doi.org/10.1111/hex.13055

Evans, J. S. B. (2008). Dual-processing accounts of reasoning, judgment, and social cognition. *Annual Review of Psychology*, *59*, 255–278.

Fishbein, M., & Ajzen, I. (1975). *Belief, attitude, intention and behavior: An introduction to theory and research*. Reading, MA: Addison-Wesley.

Fisher, A. J., Medaglia, J. D., & Jeronimus, B. F. (2018). Lack of group-to-individual generalizability is a threat to human subjects research. *Proceedings of the National Academy of Sciences*, *115*(27), E6106–E6115.

Floyd, D. L., Prentice-Dunn, S. & Rogers, R. W. (2000). A meta-analysis of protection motivation theory. *Journal of Applied Social Psychology*, *30*, 407–429.

Gallagher, S., & Povey, R. (2006). Determinants of older adults' intentions to vaccinate against influenza: A theoretical application. *Journal of Public Health*, *28*(2), 139–144.

Gallus, S., Cresci, C., Rigamonti, V., Lugo, A., Bagnardi, V., Fanucchi, T., Cirone, D., Ciaccheri, A., & Cardellicchio, S. (2023). Self-efficacy in predicting smoking cessation: A prospective study in Italy. *Tobacco Prevention & Cessation*, *9*, 15. https://doi.org/10.18332/tpc/162942

Garland, M., Wilbur, J., Fogg, L., Halloway, S., Braun, L., & Miller, A. (2021). Self-efficacy, outcome expectations, group social support, and adherence to physical activity in African American Women. *Nursing Research, 70*(4), 239–247. https://doi.org/10.1097/NNR.0000000000000516
Gellert, P., Krupka, S., Ziegelmann, J. P., Knoll, N., & Schwarzer, R. (2014). An age-tailored intervention sustains physical activity changes in older adults: A randomized controlled trial. *International Journal of Behavioral Medicine*. https://doi.org/10.1007/s12529-013-9330-1
Gerland, H.-M. E., & Prell, T. (2021). Association between the health locus of control and medication adherence: An observational, cross-sectional study in primary care. *Frontiers in Medicine, 8*. https://www.frontiersin.org/articles/10.3389/fmed.2021.705202
Ghoreishi, M.-S., Vahedian-Shahroodi, M., Jafari, A., & Tehranid, H. (2019). Self-care behaviors in patients with type 2 diabetes: Education intervention base on social cognitive theory. *Diabetes & Metabolic Syndrome: Clinical Research & Reviews, 13*(3), 2049–2056. https://doi.org/10.1016/j.dsx.2019.04.045
Hale, J., Hastings, J., West, R., Lefevre, C. E., Direito, A., Connell Bohlen, L., Godinho, C., Anderson, N., Zink, S., Goarke, H., and Michie, S. (2020) An ontology-based modelling system (OBMS) for representing behaviour change theories applied to 76 theories [version 1; peer review: awaiting peer review]
Hamilton, K., Gibbs, I., Keech, J. J., & Hagger, M. S. (2020). Reasoned and implicit processes in heavy episodic drinking: An integrated dual-process model. *British Journal of Health Psychology, 25*(1), 189–209.
Hanoch, Y., Rolison, J., & Freund, A. M. (2019). Reaping the benefits and avoiding the risks: Unrealistic optimism in the health domain. *Risk Analysis, 39*(4), 792–804. https://doi.org/10.1111/risa.13204
Heffner, J., Vives, M.-L., & FeldmanHall, O. (2021). Emotional responses to prosocial messages increase willingness to self-isolate during the COVID-19 pandemic. *Personality and Individual Differences, 170*, 110420. https://doi.org/10.1016/j.paid.2020.110420
Hollands, G. J., Bignardi, G., Johnston, M., Kelly, M. P., Ogilvie, D., Petticrew, M., Prestwich, A., Shemilt, I., Sutton, S., & Marteau, T. M. (2017). The TIPPME intervention typology for changing environments to change behaviour. *Nature Human Behaviour, 1*(8), 1–9.
Hollands, G. J., Naughton, F., Farley, A., Lindson, N., & Aveyard, P. (2019). Interventions to increase adherence to medications for tobacco dependence. *Cochrane Database of Systematic Reviews, 8*, CD009164.
Hojjatinia, S., Hojjatinia, S., Lagoa, C. M., Brunke-Reese, D., & Conroy, D. E. (2021). Person-specific dose-finding for a digital messaging intervention to promote physical activity. *Health Psychology, 40*(8), 502–512. https://doi.org/10.1037/hea0001117
Horne, R., Chapman, S. C., Parham, R., Freemantle, N., Forbes, A., & Cooper, V. (2013). Understanding patients' adherence-related beliefs about medicines prescribed for long-term conditions: A meta-analytic review of the Necessity-Concerns Framework. *PloS one, 8*(12), e80633. https://doi.org/10.1371/journal.pone.0080633
Horne, R., Cooper, V., Wileman, V., & Chan, A. (2019). Supporting adherence to medicines for long-term conditions. *European Psychologist, 24*, 1.
Houlihan, S. (2018). Dual-process models of health-related behaviour and cognition: A review of theory. *Public Health, 156*, 52–59.
Hutchison, A. J., Breckon, J. D., & Johnston, L. H. (2009). Physical activity behavior change interventions based on the transtheoretical model: A systematic review. *Health Education & Behavior*, 36(5), 829–845.
Inauen, J., Shrout, P. E., Bolger, N., Stadler, G., & Scholz, U. (2016). Mind the gap? An intensive longitudinal study of between-person and within-person intention-behavior relations. *Annals of Behavioral Medicine, 50*(4), 516–522.

Kahneman D. (2011) *Thinking, Fast and Slow*. Penguin books Ltd.
Kemps, E., Goossens, L., Petersen, J., Verbeken, S., Vervoort, L., & Braet, C. (2020). Evidence for enhancing childhood obesity treatment from a dual-process perspective: A systematic literature review. *Clinical Psychology Review*, *77*, 101840.
Kirsch, I. (1995). *Self-efficacy and outcome expectancies: A concluding commentary*. In Self-efficacy, adaptation, and adjustment: Theory, research, and application (pp. 331–345). Boston, MA: Springer US.
Klassen, R. M., & Klassen, J. R. L. (2018). Self-efficacy beliefs of medical students: A critical review. *Perspectives on Medical Education*, *7*(2), 76–82. https://doi.org/10.1007/s40037-018-0411-3
Kok, G., Peters, G.-J. Y., Kessels, L. T. E., ten Hoor, G. A., & Ruiter, R. A. C. (2018). Ignoring theory and misinterpreting evidence: The false belief in fear appeals. *Health Psychology Review*, *12*(2), 111–125. https://doi.org/10.1080/17437199.2017.1415767
Kwasnicka, D., Dombrowski, S. U., White, M., & Sniehotta, F. F. (2017). N-of-1 study of weight loss maintenance assessing predictors of physical activity, adherence to weight loss plan and weight change. *Psychology & Health*, *32*(6), 686–708.
Johnston, D. W., & Johnston, M. (2013). Useful theories should apply to individuals [Editorial]. *British Journal of Health Psychology*, *18*(3), 469–473. https://doi.org/10.1111/bjhp.12049
Limbu, Y. B., Gautam, R. K., & Pham, L. (2022). The health belief model applied to COVID-19 vaccine hesitancy: A systematic review. *Vaccines*, *10*(6), Article 6. https://doi.org/10.3390/vaccines10060973
Lippke, S., Schwarzer, R., Ziegelmann, J. P., Scholz, U., & Schüz, B. (2010). Testing stage-specific effects of a stage-matched intervention: A randomized controlled trial targeting physical exercise and its predictors. *Health Education & Behavior*, *37*, 533–546. https://doi.org/10.1177/1090198109359386.
Luszczynska, A., Scholz, U., & Schwarzer, R. (2005). The general self-efficacy scale: Multicultural validation studies. *The Journal of Psychology*, *139*(5), 439–457.
Luszczynska, A., & Schwarzer, R. (2005). Social cognitive theory. In M. Conner & P. Norman (Eds.), *Predicting health behaviour* (2nd Ed.). Berkshire: Open University Press.
Masoudy, G., Dehghani, A. S., Ansari, H., Abbasi, M. H., Bagheri, H. & Shahraki, J. (2022). Promoting the Physical Activity in Postmenopausal Women. Trans-Theoretical Model-based intervention. *Research in Health and Medical Sciences*, 1(2). https://jrhms.thums.ac.ir/article-1-39-en.pdf
McEachan, R., Conner, M., Taylor, N. J., & Lawton, R. (2011). Prospective prediction of health-related behaviours with the Theory of Planned Behaviour: A meta-analysis. *Health Psychology Review*, *5*(2), 97–144.
Mehtälä, M. A. K., Sääkslahti, A. K., Inkinen, M. E., & Poskiparta, M. E. H. (2014). A socio-ecological approach to physical activity interventions in childcare: A systematic review. *International Journal of Behavioral Nutrition and Physical Activity*, *11*(1), 1–12.
Michie, S., Atkins, L., & West, R. (2014). *The Behaviour Change Wheel Book: A Guide To Designing Interventions*. Silverback Publishing. http://www.behaviourchangewheel.com/
Michie, S., Johnston, M., Abraham, C., Lawton, R., Parker, D., Walker, A., et al. (2005). Making psychological theory useful for implementing evidence based practice: A consensus approach. *Quality & Safety in Health Care*, *14*(1), 26–33. https://doi.org/10.1136/qshc.2004.011155
Michie, S., van Stralen, M. M., & West, R. (2011). The behaviour change wheel: A new method for characterising and designing behaviour change interventions. *Implementation Science*, *6*(1), 42. https://doi.org/10.1186/1748-5908-6-42
Michie, S., West, R., Campbell, R., Brown, J., & Gainforth, H.L. (2014). *ABC of Behaviour Change Theories*. Surrey: Silverback Publishing.

Milne, S., Sheeran, P., & Orbell, S. (2000). Prediction and intervention in health-related behaviour: A meta-analytic review of Protection Motivation Theory. *Journal of Applied Social Psychology*, *30*, 106–143.
Myers, L. B., & Goodwin, R. (2012). Using a theoretical framework to determine adults' intention to vaccinate against pandemic swine flu in priority groups in the UK. *Public Health*, *126*, S53–S56.
Ojo, S. O., Bailey, D. P., Brierley, M. L., Hewson, D. J., & Chater, A. M. (2019a). Breaking barriers: Using the behavior change wheel to develop a tailored intervention to overcome workplace inhibitors to breaking up sitting time. *BMC Public Health*, *19*(1), 1–17.
Ojo, S. O., Bailey, D. P., Hewson, D. J., & Chater, A. M. (2019b). Perceived barriers and facilitators to breaking up sitting time among desk-based office workers: A qualitative investigation using the TDF and COM-B. *International Journal of Environmental Research and Public Health*, *16*(16), 2903.
Perski, O., Naughton, F., Garnett, C., Blandford, A., Beard, E., West, R., & Michie, S. (2019). Do daily fluctuations in psychological and app-related variables predict engagement with an alcohol reduction app? A series of N-Of-1 studies. *JMIR mHealth and uHealth*, *7*(10), e14098.
Petty, R., & Cacioppo, J. (1986). The elaboration likelihood model of persuasion. In L. Berkowitz (Ed.), *Advances in experimental social psychology* (Vol. 19). New York: Academic Press.
Prochaska, J. O., & DiClemente, C. C. (1982). Transtheoretical therapy: Toward a more integrative model of change. *Psychotherapy: Theory, Research & Practice*, *19*(3), 276.
Rhodes, R., & de Bruijn, G.-J. (2013). How big is the physical activity intention-behaviour gap? A meta-analysis using the action control framework. *British Journal of Health Psychology*, *18*, 296–309. https://doi.org/10.1111/bjhp.12032
Rogers, R. W. (1975). A protection motivation theory of fear appeals and attitude change. *Journal of Psychology*, *91*, 93–114.
Romain, A. J., Caudroit, J., Hokayem, M., & Bernard, P. (2018). Is there something beyond stages of change in the transtheoretical model? The state of art for physical activity. *Canadian Journal of Behavioural Science*/Revue canadienne des sciences du comportement, 50(1), 42.
Rosenstock, I. M. (1966). Why people use health services. *Milbank Memorial Fund Quarterly*, *44*, 94–124.
Rosenstock, I. M. (1974). The health belief model and preventive health behavior. *Health Education Monographs*, *2*(4), 354–386.
Rosenstock, I. M. (2005). Why people use health services. *The Milbank Quarterly*, *83*(4), 1–32.
Rosenstock, S., Chambers, R., Lee, A., Goklish, N., Larzelere, F., & Tingey, L. (2020). Self-efficacy and response-efficacy: Critical components of sexual and reproductive health interventions targeting condom use intention among American Indian adolescents. *AIDS Care*, *32*(3), 379–385. https://doi.org/10.1080/09540121.2019.1695726
Rotter, J. B. (1954). *Social learning and clinical psychology*. New York: Prentice-Hill.
Sallis, J. F., Owen, N., & Fisher, E. (2015). Ecological models of health behavior. *Health Behavior: Theory, Research, and Practice*, *5*(43–64).
Schwarzer, R. (1992). *Self-efficacy: thought control of action*. Washington, DC: US: Hemisphere Publishing Corporation.
Schwarzer, R., & Luszczynska, A. (2008). How to overcome health-compromising behaviors: The health action process approach. *European Psychologist*, *13*(2), 141–151.
Schwarzer, R. (2014). *Self-efficacy: Thought control of action*. Taylor & Francis.
Schüz, B., Li, A. S.-W., Hardinge, A., McEachan, R. R. C., & Conner, M. (2017). Socioeconomic status as a moderator between social cognitions and physical activity:

Systematic review and meta-analysis based on the Theory of Planned Behavior. *Psychology of Sport and Exercise*, *30*, 186–195. https://doi.org/10.1016/j.psychsport.2017.03.004

Schüz, B., Sniehotta, F. F., & Schwarzer, R. (2007). Stage-specific effects of an action control intervention on dental flossing. *Health Education Research*, *22*(3), 332–341.

Sniehotta, F. F., Presseau, J., & Araújo-Soares, V. (2014). Time to retire the theory of planned behaviour. *Health Psychology Review*, *8*(1), 1–7. https://doi.org/10.1080/17437199.2013.869710

Sniehotta, F. F., Scholz, U., & Schwarzer, R. (2005). Bridging the intention–behaviour gap: Planning, self-efficacy, and action control in the adoption and maintenance of physical exercise. *Psychology & Health*, *20*(2), 143–160. https://doi.org/10.1080/08870440512331317670

Spillane, D., Courtenay, M., Chater, A., Family, H., Whitaker, A., & Acton, J. H. (2021). Factors influencing the prescribing behaviour of independent prescriber optometrists: a qualitative study using the Theoretical Domains Framework. *Ophthalmic and Physiological Optics*, *41*(2), 301–315. https://doi.org/10.1111/opo.12782

Stanovich, K. E. (1999). *Who is rational?: Studies of individual differences in reasoning*. Mahwah, NJ: Elrbaum, Psychology Press.

Sur, M. H., Jung, J., & Shapiro, D. R. (2022). Theory of planned behavior to promote physical activity of adults with physical disabilities: Meta-analytic structural equation modeling. *Disability and Health Journal*, *15*(1), 101199. https://doi.org/10.1016/j.dhjo.2021.101199

Sutton, S. (2015). Stage theories. In M. Conner & P. Norman (Eds.), *Predicting and changing health behaviour* (3rd ed., pp. 279–320), McGraw-Hill.

Szinay, D., Jones, A., Chadborn, T., Brown, J., & Naughton, F. (2020). Influences on the uptake of and engagement with health and well–being smartphone apps: Systematic review. *Journal of Medical Internet Research*, *22*(5), e17572.

Tajfel, H., Turner, J. C., Austin, W. G., & Worchel, S. (1979). An integrative theory of intergroup conflict. *Organizational Identity: A Reader*, *56*(65), 9780203505984-16.

Tannenbaum, M. B., Hepler, J., Zimmerman, R. S., Saul, L., Jacobs, S., Wilson, K., & Albarracín, D. (2015). Appealing to fear: A meta-analysis of fear appeal effectiveness and theories. *Psychological Bulletin*, *141*(6), 1178–1204. https://doi.org/10.1037/a0039729

Torregosa, M., & Patricio, O. (2022). The mediating role of sexual self-efficacy on protected sex. *Journal of Primary Care & Community Health*, *13*, 21501319221129934. https://doi.org/10.1177/21501319221129934

Wallston, K. (1992). Hocus-pocus, the focus isn't strictly on locus: Rotter's social learning theory modified for health. *Cognitive Therapy and Research*, *16*(2), 183–199.

Wallston, K. A., Wallston, B. S., & DeVellis, R. (1978). Development of multidimensional health locus of control (MHLC) scales. *Health Education Monographs*, *6*, 160–170.

Weinstein, N. (1987). Unrealistic optimism about illness susceptibility: Conclusion from a community-wide sample. *Journal of Behavioural Medicine*, *10*, 481–500.

Weinstein, N. D. (1982). Unrealistic optimism about susceptibility to health problems. *Journal of Behavioural Medicine*, *5*, 441–460.

West, R. (2005). Time for a change: Putting the Transtheoretical (Stages of Change) Model to rest. *Addiction*, *100*(8), 1036–1039. https://doi.org/10.1111/j.1360-0443.2005.01139.x.

West, R., Michie, S., Atkins, L. et al. (2019). *Achieving behaviour change: A guide for local government and partners*. London: Public Health England.

Williams, D. M., & Rhodes, R. E. (2016). The confounded self-efficacy construct: Conceptual analysis and recommendations for future research. *Health Psychology Review*, *10*(2), 113–128. https://doi.org/10.1080/17437199.2014.941998

Willis, L., Lee, E., Reynolds, K. J., & Klik, K. A. (2020). The theory of planned behavior and the social identity approach: A new look at group processes and social norms in the context of student binge drinking. *Europe's Journal of Psychology*, *16*(3), 357–383. https://doi.org/10.5964/ejop.v16i3.1900

Witte, K., & Allen, M. (2000). A meta-analysis of fear appeals: Implications for effective public health campaigns. *Health Education & Behavior*, *27*(5), 591–615.

Wollast, R., Schmitz, M., Bigot, A., & Luminet, O. (2021). The Theory of Planned Behavior during the COVID-19 pandemic: A comparison of health behaviors between Belgian and French residents. *PLOS ONE*, *16*(11), e0258320. https://doi.org/10.1371/journal.pone.0258320

Zhang, C. Q., Zhang, R., Schwarzer, R., & Hagger, M. S. (2019). A meta-analysis of the health action process approach. *Health Psychology*, *38*(7), 623. https://doi.org/10.1037/hea0000728

3

HEALTH PSYCHOLOGY'S ROLE WITHIN THE BIOPSYCHOSOCIAL SCIENCES

Karen Rodham, Lesley Lewis, Daniel Masterson, Rachel Povey, Angel Marie Chater, Jenny Scott, and Hannah Family

Introduction

This chapter focuses on understanding health psychology in the wider system. The main aim is to show the interdisciplinary reach of health psychology and to highlight the importance of interconnectivity and collaborative working. Initially, synergies and differences between health psychology and other practitioner psychology branches will be discussed. The chapter will then focus outwards on the connection of health psychology with the biopsychosocial sciences. A particular focus will be made on behavioural, social, and medical sciences. The chapter will conclude with a discussion on the role health psychology plays and could play in multi-, inter-, and transdisciplinary teams.

Health Psychology and Other Branches of the Psychology Family

In a special edition of the *Journal of Health Psychology*, the focus was on the social, cultural, and political contextual factors that have impacted the development of health psychology (Lubek & Murray, 2018). Murray (2018, p. 472) notes, "*Psychological theory and practice are not constructed in isolation from the social world but rather are shaped by it*". Authors from around the world (e.g., de-Graft Aikins, 2018; Herzlich, 2018; Spink, 2018; Stam, Murray & Lubek, 2018; Yen & Vaccarino, 2018) shared their experiences and viewpoints. A clear example of the cultural and political impact was shared by Santiago-Delefosse and Carral (2018), who clearly show how health psychology was shaped by and forged from clashes between and within theoretical, practice-based, and cultural approaches and standpoints. Stam et al. (2018: p. 507) suggest that health psychology is not a '*single coherent discipline*'. Herzlich (2018:

DOI: 10.4324/9781003318026-4

p. 386), sharing her French perspective, states, "*[H]ealth psychology is a newer sub-discipline whose research methodologies, theories, and practices were borrowed from diverse areas of psychology*". Similar accounts were shared in the oral history of United Kingdom (UK) health psychology published by Quinn, Chater, and Morrison (2020). Common to this collection of narratives was the multidisciplinarity, not just of the origins but also of the current and potential future of the profession.

With this in mind, we offer some context for our chapter exploring health psychology in the wider system. Whilst we draw from a range of Health Psychologists' work, spanning different countries and areas of focus, we are mindful that all the authors of this chapter were trained in the UK, and although some have experience working in other countries, our main health psychology experience is inevitably shaped by the context in which we have trained and worked. We include some UK background that we see as being particularly important for the context to the focus of this chapter on the reach of health psychology.

Chapter 1 highlighted that formal recognition of health psychology in the UK began in the mid-1980s when a British Psychological Society (BPS) Health Psychology Section was created. In the 1990s, the section became a BPS Special Group and was working towards 'Division' status. In order to be recognised as a BPS Division, suitable competencies and training routes had to be developed and then approved by a vote of representatives from all the existing BPS Divisions. Quinn et al. (2020) note that at that time, the Division of Clinical Psychology (DCP) opposed the inclusion of one-to-one clinical work by Health Psychologists. A compromise was reached whereby training for Health Psychologists would focus on professional skills, consultancy, teaching/training, and research as core competencies, with behaviour change as an optional competency (Quinn et al. 2020). The compromise was approved, and the Special Group became the BPS Division of Health Psychology (DHP) in 1997. Over time, the competencies have been refined, and currently, psychological interventions are now included as core elements. Behaviour change (now encompassed by the term 'psychological interventions') is no longer an option but is at the heart of what Health Psychologists do, whether that be research or practice.

There are two things to note here. First, the decision to oppose rather than welcome the proposed clinically based practice of a new psychology specialism. Second, the word 'division' to denote the different psychology specialisms. Indeed, the UK is not the only country to adopt the term 'division'. The health psychology section of the American Psychological Association (APA) is known as Division 38, established in 1978 (France, 2013). For this chapter, we have chosen to use the word 'family' as an umbrella term to describe the different domains of the psychology profession. The *Oxford English Dictionary* defines family as a group of allied genera of animals or plants. Looking up 'genus', we see that the definition extends to "a group having common structural characteristics distinct from those of all other groups, and usually containing several species". This perhaps sums up the family of psychology ... we complete an approved undergraduate degree, so we have the same common structural characteristics. We then go on to specialise and become different 'species' with the same common structural foundations.

Unfortunately (in our opinion), as a profession in the UK, the term 'division' has been historically used to denote the different specialisms. Returning to the dictionary, the word 'division' is associated with being divided. It could be argued that our decision as a psychology profession to call specialisms 'divisions' has had unintended consequences which obstruct recognition of the commonality between the different psychology family members. Instead of celebrating the complementary nature of our respective specialisms, noticing the similarities and identifying the ways in which the services we offer can be enhanced by working together, we can sometimes feel as though we are in competition with one another. When this happens, barriers and protective behaviours (for example, blocking the proposal that a new specialism practices clinically) can increase the distance. This is a shame because if we look at the competencies across the divisions, there are more similarities than differences. By way of example, Rodham put together a symposium for the BPS Annual Conference 2017. The symposium was designed to bring together representatives from both health psychology and sport and exercise psychology with a view to exploring similarities and differences in approach. Prior to the symposium, two case studies were designed. Each was shared with one Health Psychologist (Angel Chater/Vincent Deary) and one sport and exercise psychologist (Sarah Edmunds/Mikel Mellick), who were asked to prepare a presentation for the conference where they would outline their approach to the case and share their formulation for a behaviour change intervention (Rodham et al., 2017). The purpose of this symposium was to explore the common ground between health and sport and exercise psychology, and to look for opportunities to integrate evidence-based practice from the two perspectives. The symposium was written up by Catherine Loveday (2017), who concluded, "*[G]iven that none of the speakers were given anything other than the details of their case study and had no idea what each other might say, there was striking consistency between their approaches. [...] There was an overwhelming consensus in the room that working together is something health and sports psychologists should do more*". The symposium was in effect a small intervention – a way of bridging the gap, overcoming preconceptions between divisions, and recognising that we had more in common than might be indicated by the word 'division'.

Perhaps the divided nature of UK psychology combined with the multidisciplinary origins of health psychology is why Health Psychologists are often connected with disciplines from outside the psychology family. Indeed, in the afterword of Forshaw and Sheffield's (2013: p. 222) edited collection *Health Psychology in Action*, they note that Health Psychologists are "*genuine multidisciplinarians, part of a wider community of academic and health professionals of all kinds, working together to find things out and change lives for the better*". This interconnectedness is, in our view, embedded in the research and practice of health psychology.

Health Psychology and the Behavioural, Social, and Medical Sciences

Having noted earlier, the challenge of collaborating within the psychology family, stepping outside psychology and into other disciplines brings further challenges. Jacob (2008: p. 177) noted: "*scientific knowledge is divided among many disciplines, each with its own vocabulary, methods, and concepts. Disciplines create boundaries. They have become so disparate that it is sometimes difficult for members of one discipline to communicate with members of another*". Jacob (2008: p. 178) also notes, "*No single discipline can deal with all the complexity of a social phenomenon*". Now more than ever, there is a need for collaboration. Indeed, Lubek and Murray (2018: p. 367) issued what could be seen as a call to arms for health psychology when they noted,

> *The new global challenges of mass migration, climate change and population ageing are ones with serious health implications that demand health psychology more than ever to connect with sociopolitical psychology and with other disciplines, professions and organizations if it is to make a serious contribution to health for all in the 21st century.*

Connecting and collaborating with other disciplines in a way that exchanges, interactions, and cooperation move beyond disciplinary lines is therefore important. Patricia Rosenfeld (1992) outlined three ways in which relations between disciplines could be characterised. Neal et al. (2013) summarised the processes thus:

Multidisciplinarity: different disciplines work separately to address the same problem from their perspective.
Interdisciplinarity: different disciplines work together to address a problem but still use their own discipline's perspectives.
Transdisciplinarity: different disciplines work together to address a problem by developing new theories or methodologies that merge their unique disciplinary perspectives.

Multidisciplinarity keeps disciplines separate; each contributes its knowledge irrespective of what the other is doing. Interdisciplinary working allows for some sharing of knowledge. Although disciplines use their own perspectives, they are "*more likely to become aware of the conceptual frameworks and theoretical bases of the disciplines with whom they are collaborating*" (Rosenfeld, 1992: p. 1354). Transdisciplinary working enables disciplines to join forces and build on their distinct traditions and in doing so build new models and new ways of working that combine the strengths of the different disciplines.

The next section of the chapter focuses on the contribution health psychology has made to the behavioural, social, and medical sciences. Inevitably in one chapter, we cannot possibly share the breadth and depth of the focus of health psychology. Instead, we have chosen to share examples that we think give an indication of the reach, impact, and connectivity of health psychology. We provide case studies drawn from the authors' practice and research experiences to show in greater depth how Health Psychologists and health psychology have worked with other professions to overcome the challenges inherent in collaboration in behavioural, social, and medical sciences.

Behavioural Sciences

Strangely, although much is written about behavioural science, an agreed definition of 'behavioural science' is lacking. It seems writers tend to assume that readers (a) already understand what behavioural science is and (b) know which disciplines are considered to contribute to the behavioural sciences. The online *Encyclopaedia Britannica* (2023) states that any discipline dealing with human actions is a behavioural science. Fulton (2021: p. 3) defines behavioural science as the "science of human behaviour and decision-making". In other words, the focus is on understanding why we behave the way we do and how we might change this. It is also about understanding the things that drive our decisions, choices and habits. Fasolo (2016), writing on a blog for the London School of Economics (LSE), sees behavioural science being the "*science of understanding, predicting and influencing how people behave*". McBride et al. (2021; p. 5) define behavioural science as "*an umbrella term for a selection of disciplines (such as health psychology) that study human behaviour*". They go on to elaborate that "*behavioural scientists often aim to understand behaviours related to health and what can predict and change behaviour in individuals, communities, populations, and systems*".

The term 'behavioural science' is often used in conjunction (and sometimes interchangeably) with 'social science'. For example, the phrase '*behavioural and social sciences*' is commonly used. Indeed, in their strategy guidance document titled 'Improving People's Health: Applying Behavioural and Social Sciences' Public Health England (2018: p. 25) note,

> *It is sometimes difficult to say which discipline is responsible for a particular approach or framework, so our classification is necessarily somewhat imprecise.*

We suggest that one way of distinguishing between behavioural and social sciences is that behavioural sciences focus more on behaviour, whereas social sciences focus more on what people say they do, think, believe, and/or intend to do in (or not) a social system. In other words, social sciences focus more on cognitions, intentions, narratives, and beliefs. Psychology, and more specifically health psychology, could indeed fall into both the behavioural and social sciences.

Davis et al. (2014) highlighted the key role that human behaviour plays in many of the leading causes of death. They note that even small behavioural changes can translate into large effects on population outcomes. In our introduction to this chapter, we highlighted that behaviour change is at the heart of health psychology. As such, it is not surprising to learn that health psychology has made strong contributions to behavioural science. For example, health psychology can be used to identify target behaviours for change, highlight biopsychosocial factors that may influence selected target behaviours, and identify intervention strategies, behaviour change techniques, and ways to effectively deliver them to develop and evaluate health-behaviour interventions.

Most recently, Health Psychologists have been turning their attention to the COVID-19 pandemic. In the UK, Schüz and colleagues (2021) set out to identify the factors that predicted COVID-19 protection intentions and behaviours. Specifically, they wanted to see whether health cognitions, perceived susceptibility, and (bio)socio-structural factors (sex, age, ethnicity, and area-level deprivation) influenced the associations. Their findings suggested that intervention components that aim at increasing intentions might not benefit people who come from more disadvantaged backgrounds, with lower autonomy, and may inadvertently increase health inequalities. Suggestions were made as to how interventions could be better tailored to help people from disadvantaged backgrounds translate their intentions into behaviour. In contrast, Zhang et al. (2022) in the Netherlands focused on the process of habit formation with respect to the protective behaviours of physical distancing and hand washing. Their participants generally had strong intentions to adhere to the preventive behaviours and reported that their behaviours had become more automatic over time. The increase in habit strength was more evident for physical distancing than hand washing. Of course, the context to our behaviours plays an important role, and although increased hand washing was strongly recommended, physical distancing became a new social norm that was more strictly enforced than the act of handwashing, which was more often performed in private.

As the previous examples demonstrate, health psychology was able to play an important role during COVID-19. This is in part due to its already strong links with public health. Vinck et al. (2004: p. 6), writing about health psychology's contribution to public health (a discipline which draws heavily from behavioural science), use a wonderful word – 'armamentarium' –when describing the set of 'diagnostic instruments, tests, and assessment tools' that psychology brings to a collaboration. The case study in Box 3.1 highlights the contribution health psychology made to an important public health issue: increasing the uptake of the flu vaccine.

Box 3.1 The Contribution of Health Psychology to Public Health

Public health and health psychology are arguably a perfect match. The golden thread tying these two disciplines together is behaviour change; public health aims to monitor and change the public's (as well as professionals') behaviour to improve and protect population health, whilst a core part of health psychology is to understand what influences, and how to change behaviours that can influence health and the health-care system. With health psychology specialising in behaviour change, public health national and local teams are increasingly interested in this profession, alongside the wider behavioural sciences.

This case study focuses on the work of a UK local council's public health team. This team has invested in a Behavioural Science Unit led by a Health Psychologist (Lesley Lewis during the examples in this case study). The unit acts as a consultancy unit, utilising and applying knowledge and skills of the core competencies in health psychology to public health programmes. This has covered a wide range of public health areas, such as childhood immunisations, hypertension, active travel, smoking cessation, and sexual health, to name a few.

Uptake of the flu vaccine is one such public health programme aimed at protecting vulnerable populations from getting seriously ill and potentially dying from the virus. One particular target population to increase uptake of the flu vaccine is health and social care workers, a common priority group across the UK. The Behavioural Science Unit contributed health psychology knowledge and skills to a project targeting this population group.

Firstly, a literature review was conducted to understand the barriers and facilitators to uptake of the flu vaccine in this population group. This found population-specific insights such as health and social care workers believing they have a strong immune system due to working in health care and being exposed to infection.

Secondly, these insights, along with others, were mapped to the capability, opportunity, motivation – behaviour (COM-B) model of behaviour change (Michie, van Stralen, & West, 2011), identifying influencing factors related to capability, opportunity, and motivation; after which behaviour change techniques (BCTs: Michie et al., 2013) were selected to make recommendations on core messages to include in a communication campaign.

These recommendations were captured within a 'messaging matrix' which detailed relevant insight, the COM-B construct it related to, and the BCTs to target it. The BCTs were interpreted in relation to the insight to make it as easy as possible to understand and apply them to the development of campaign messages.

Notably, this ensured that behaviour change theories and techniques were used within this campaign – an approach which has been used across other public health programmes. This highlights the opportunity health psychology has in contributing not only to individual-level interventions but also to population-level interventions and the valuable use of primary and secondary research skills to inform the development of such interventions.

Another example of intervention development to increase uptake of the flu vaccine was the development and evaluation of flu vaccine email invitations to increase uptake within local authority staff (Lewis & Dunn, 2022). This involved creating three different email invitations applying BCTs in different ways to evaluate which was the most effective email for wider rollout. The results indicated that the emails using health psychology and other behavioural science considerations had greater uptake, demonstrating the value of behaviour change, research design, and evaluation skills.

Although this emphasises just one area that health psychology has contributed to in public health, there are numerous opportunities and examples. Both the public health and health psychology workforce have their own unique set of skills to improve and protect health amongst individuals, communities, and populations and, working together, can achieve shared outcomes. Using the core competencies of health psychology, this discipline can contribute to the ultimate goal of public health: to reduce health inequalities and improve population health.

Social Sciences

Whilst behavioural science focuses on trying to understand behaviour and what influences how we behave, social scientists focus on human society and social relationships and how these influence the world around us. The Academy of Social Sciences (2023) on its website defines social science as being,

> *the study of people: as individuals, communities and societies; their behaviours and interactions with each other and with their built, technological and natural environments.*

As noted in the introduction to this chapter, when health psychology was establishing itself, the practitioners leading the development of the new profession drew from other disciplines. In the UK context, Theresa Marteau is quoted as saying,

> *The psychology I was drawing upon were social psychologists like Lazarus and Folkman, looking at coping.*
>
> *(Quinn et al., 2020: p. 508)*

Mark Conner and Paul Norman (2005) note that a large body of research has focused on exploring the role that social cognitive factors might play in predicting health behaviour. The types of behaviour explored have been extremely varied and include health-enhancing behaviours (e.g., exercising, eating healthily), health protective behaviours (such as health screening and vaccinations), and health-harming behaviours (smoking, excessive alcohol consumption). Researchers developed models to explain how cognitive factors might influence social behaviours. These became known as social cognitive models. Indeed, Rory O'Connor noted,

> *I think in the 1990s we were so fixated on the social cognitive models. Now, I think that was really important in some ways because it led to an enhanced understanding of the determinants of health behaviour.*
>
> *(Quinn et al., 2020: p. 512)*

There is a rich history of social sciences being inter-weaved with the developing field of health psychology. Indeed, in her keynote at the 2022 European Health Psychology Society (EHPS) conference, Professor Urte Scholz (2022) noted that health-related behaviours usually happen in a social context. As such, there is a need to move away from the temptation to focus on how an individual's thoughts and beliefs might influence their behaviour and instead explore the influence of the social context.

One issue that really highlights the interconnectedness of health psychology and social science is obesity. There are concerns across the globe about obesity and increasing recognition that solving the problem will require more than individual behaviour change, though this will be an important component. In terms of social context, there are growing inequalities in terms of access to food and an increasing understanding of how our food consumption might be impacting the environment in the short and long term. This combination of factors provides an opportunity for Health Psychologists to contribute to the solutions from a biopsychosocial stance. For example, Sproesser et al. (2022) explored the extent of traditional and modern eating behaviours of older Indian adults in Gujarat. They gained insight into whether eating behaviour might be changing and the potential impact that could have on well-being, cultural identity, health, nutrient intake, and availability of food groups. Similarly, in Finland, Erkkola et al. (2022) investigated the influence of socio-demographic characteristics on food motives. Grocery purchase data with individual attributes on nearly 30,000 consenting loyalty card holders were analysed. They found that the most important resources for choosing more sustainable food profiles were education and stage of family life, whilst also highlighting that low income was not a barrier to a more sustainable purchase profile. This kind of work provides Health Psychologists with opportunities to collaborate with other professions and contribute expertise that helps to address the problems facing societies.

As noted earlier in this section, social science includes the study of built environments. One area where health psychology can have a role to play is town planning. The case study in Box 3.2 highlights the skills and expertise health psychology can bring to professions that perhaps may not have previously considered its contribution. Perhaps after reading the case study, you may consider that if town planners and developers reimagined their approach and embraced the idea of Health Impact Assessments, they could one day be included in the umbrella term 'allied health professional'.

Medical Sciences

The biopsychosocial model (Engel, 1977) moved our understanding of health and illness away from a biomedical model towards one that recognised the importance not just of life context but as a result of "*interacting mechanism at the cellular, tissue, organismic, interpersonal and environmental level as essential components of the whole system*" (Fava & Sonina, 2017, p. 258). Indeed, Engel (1977) noted,

Box 3.2 The Contribution of Health Psychology to Town Planning

Where we live, work, and play has a profound impact on our health and well-being. Our surrounding environment offers both potential and limits our choices for an active life. Interventions which seek to promote a conducive environment for health require consideration of the complex systems which shape the wider environment. This case study summarises action research undertaken to embed health considerations into urban planning, provides key reflections, and identifies why Health Psychologists are ideally suited for this area of work.

The National Planning Policy Framework (2012, most recently updated in 2021) in the UK called for planning decisions to enable and support a healthy life (e.g., layouts that encourage walking and cycling, safe and accessible green infrastructure). In response, local authorities developed policies requiring Health Impact Assessments to be undertaken on large-scale developments (e.g., more than 200 houses).

In this case study, the local authority, in negotiation with academic partners, recruited a Health Psychologist in training (Dr Daniel Masterson, with supervision and support from Professor Chris Gidlow, Professor Karen Rodham, and Dr Rachel Povey) to help them better understand why Health Impact Assessments were not being consistently applied. The Health Psychologist in training was tasked with

1. gaining insight into the barriers and challenges that prevented planning officers and architects from applying Health Impact Assessments, and
2. collating and providing evidence to better demonstrate the need to include health matters in local policy.

The Health Psychologist in training interviewed planning officers and architects, as well as observed and participated in the planning process. The outcomes of this work showed that planners and architects perceived health to be a result of individual choice and, as such, was not considered to be an integral part of the planning process. This meant that the new policy requiring Health Impact Assessments was viewed as an administrative process that was completed at the end of the planning process in order to comply with the new policy. A lack of understanding of the rationale for the Health Impact Assessments meant that planners and architects viewed them as a 'tick-box exercise' that needed to be done in order for a planning application to be approved. Indeed, discussions with architects identified that by the time a Health Impact Assessment was undertaken, much of the design had already been costed and justified. Any suggested changes at this late stage as a consequence of a Health Impact Assessment were likely to be both small and resisted. If not due to cost, then due to time constraints. In the context of a demand for housing and development, especially in areas with lower income, any 'bolt-on' considerations that were perceived to hinder developments were easily removed.

The work showed that in order for Health Impact Assessments to be applied consistently and to make a positive difference to population health, there needed to be increased capability within the planning department, which could then offer guidance in the earliest possible stages of development, such as during pre-planning applications. Such a change would increase the likelihood that health considerations would be embedded in planning applications, which in turn would allow for swifter Health Impact Assessments to be undertaken. More recently, an update to the UK National Planning Policy Framework (2021: p. 39) has called for local planning authorities to make appropriate use of "workshops to engage the local community, design advice and review arrangements, and assessment frameworks such as Building for a Healthy Life" (Birkbeck et al., 2020) all of which, if implemented will ensure health becomes part of the planning process, instead of a last-minute addition, or indeed, deduction.

The skills required for these activities are an understanding of how the environment impacts an individual's health, interpretation of epidemiological data to identify evidence to justify guidance, facilitating workshops, research, and consultancy skills. These are skills embedded within health psychology training. Health Psychologists are trained in communication and research skills which can be used to facilitate dialogue with those who can make a difference. Health Psychologists are also trained in understanding the importance of behaviour for implementing interventions. Breaking down problems in behavioural terms and exploring solutions with those most affected are also skills which a Health Psychologist is well prepared for and can help guide these consultations to ensure they go beyond a tick-box exercise and have meaningful outcomes which benefit the community in which these developments are built. This case study, and many others like it, shows the impact of embedding the knowledge and skills acquired during training and has led to further job opportunities for those trained in health psychology.

> *The boundaries between health and disease, between well and sick, are far from clear and never will be clear, for they are diffused by cultural, social, and psychological considerations. The traditional biomedical view, that biological indices are the ultimate criteria defining disease, leads to the present paradox that some people with positive laboratory findings are told that they are in need of treatment when in fact they are feeling quite well, while others feeling sick are assured that they are well, that is, they have no "disease". A biopsychosocial model which includes the patient as well as the illness would encompass both circumstances.*
>
> *(Engel, 1977: pp. 132–133)*

In including the patient, Engel was opening up space for a new approach for health and illness. He recognised that there are more influences on health and illness than those encompassed by the term 'biomedical'. Health psychology, with its multidisciplinary origins and focus on behavioural interventions, was growing around the same time Engel shared his model. The similarities are clear in a quote from Val Morrison in the UK health psychology oral history (Quinn et al., 2020):

> *People with drink and drug problems were either criminalised or they had a disease that had to be treated. What we [psychology] were trying to say was "yes, but there are social, contextual, emotional factors, beliefs and expectation factors that are influencing these behaviours". It is easy to frame it now, but we were bringing a psychosocial model to the biomedical model of drug use. And I didn't know about health psychology. I was an addictions researcher.*
>
> *(Quinn et al., 2020: p. 508)*

Health Psychologists as we have noted have expertise in behaviour and behaviour change. Sharing this knowledge and expertise with medical science professionals has created opportunities for collaborations that make a difference on a wide range of fronts. In this next section of the chapter, we focus on stress, suicide, and antibiotic use.

Stress can affect health directly and indirectly, and the "*cumulative science linking stress to negative health outcome is vast*" (O'Connor et al., 2021: p. 663). Stress, its impact on health and how it is experienced and coped with, has long been a focus of Health Psychologists. Cheetham-Blake et al. (2019) explored children's experiences of stress and coping. The children were interviewed with their mothers or fathers, which allowed for a deeper understanding of child and parent perspectives on stress. Round et al. (2022) focused on UK teachers, whom they described as a group particularly prone to suffering from burnout. The researchers invited a group of teachers and a group of non-teachers to employ a positive writing intervention for 20 minutes per day for 3 consecutive days. Although they did not note any special benefits for the teacher group specifically, there were benefits across both groups. They suggest that positive expressive writing reduces anxiety and enhances aspects of job satisfaction. As such, it may be a useful technique for enhancing job satisfaction in full-time workers.

In Australia, Murphy et al. (2022) wanted to learn more about the stresses and concerns experienced by people who had survived a spontaneous artery dissection (SCAD). A SCAD happens when a coronary vessel develops a blood clot within the arterial wall which bulges inwards, obstructing blood flow and causes what laypeople would call a heart attack. Thirty SCAD survivors took part in focus groups and shared their experiences with the research team. The findings were clear. There was an urgent need for psychosocial support and better information for this group that could complement and enhance the medical treatment offered to this population.

Suicide is a global health issue. Understanding the process that a person moves through as they consider and then engage in suicidal behaviour is important if we are to design appropriate and effective interventions. O'Connor and Kirtley (2018) developed a model to explain how people might move from having suicidal thoughts to behavioural enactment. In parallel, research exploring the impact of bereavement by suicide is also important. Cerel et al. (2016) argue for a reconceptualisation of who is impacted after bereavement by suicide, suggesting the impact is more diffuse and not restricted to loved ones or family members. With this in mind, Sandford et al. (2022) note that little attention had been paid to the impact of bereavement by client suicide on mental health practitioners working in primary care. They interviewed seven practitioners who had experienced the death by suicide of one of their patients. Whilst recognising the limitations of their study, the findings led to clear suggestions, including how best to prepare practitioners for the possibility of a patient dying by suicide, how to mitigate a potential sense of guilt, and how to overcome barriers to recovery following this experience. Further health psychology research highlights how simple behaviours such as physical activity and talking to others could benefit health professionals such as doctors after the death of a patient (Williams et al., 2021). These insights can assist both those seeking to design and improve interventions as well as those who are coping with the impact of suicide.

Antibiotics and the problem of antimicrobial resistance (AMR) have extremely serious implications if they are not resolved, and they are issues which cause health professionals considerable stress. Flowers (2018: p. 198) argues, "*Imaginative, innovative and interdisciplinary interventions are needed to reduce the drivers of antimicrobial resistance across the coming decades*". He makes it clear that we need to overcome the challenges of working with professionals from other disciplines so that we can work effectively together. Thorpe et al. (2021) note that people often ask for antibiotics even if they are clinically inappropriate for the presenting symptoms. It can be challenging for general practitioners (family doctors) to refuse to prescribe and to maintain a positive relationship with their patients (van der Zande et al., 2019). Indeed, antimicrobial stewardship (AMS), ensuring that patients only receive antibiotics when clinically appropriate, is not just an important role; it is also a behaviour.

Health psychology and nursing researchers have collaborated to explore the role, challenges, barriers, and experiences of antimicrobial stewards (e.g., Courtenay & Chater, 2021) in order that we can better prepare our health professionals to manage the delicate balance between patients perceived needs and what is clinically sound. The prescribing of antibiotics is not just a concern for health professionals but is also something that both vets and farmers must consider. As such, Health Psychologists have also explored the experiences of UK veterinarians and farmers and showed that although they seemed motivated to be antimicrobial stewards, they felt challenged by the day-to-day reality of their jobs (Golding et al., 2019). Training has been found to be an influential factor in AMS (Chater et al., 2022, 2020), and there is a call for further training in communication skills and behaviour change to meet a competency framework (Courtenay & Chater, 2021). The rise in antibiotic resistance is a very serious threat to public health globally, and there is a clear need to ensure that the public and health professionals are better educated about responsible antibiotic use.

From antibiotics to pharmacy-based research is not a great leap. The case study in Box 3.3 shares a pharmacist's experience of collaborating with Health Psychologists and incorporating health psychology models into their research.

Box 3.3 The Contribution of Health Psychology to Community Pharmacy-Based Research

This case study reports research funded by the UK Medical Research Council (MRC) Public Health Intervention Development programme, which combines health psychology with pharmacy practice. The research idea came from the practice experience of a pharmacist (Jenny Scott) and was led by a psychologist who teaches and researches health psychology in pharmacy settings (Hannah Family). Co-investigators had particular expertise in intervention design and behaviour change theory (a Health Psychologist – Angel Chater) and sociology of drug use (a social scientist – Joanne Neale). In this case study, the pharmacist reflects on how this interaction between health psychology, sociology, and pharmacy practice was essential and fruitful in the conduct and output of the project.

The Background

Women who use drugs like heroin often experience an absence of periods (menstruation). Fertility, and consequently periods, often return when the woman begins opioid substitution therapy (OST) such as methadone or buprenorphine. The woman could be at risk of an unplanned pregnancy if she had not received advice on this point and had not been supported to use contraception to manage her pregnancy possibilities. Anecdotally, the pharmacist involved in this collaboration knew that this issue was not often discussed when OST was prescribed. When OST is begun, in line with UK guidelines, it is usually given under daily supervised consumption by a community (retail) pharmacist. The team identified an opportunity for a pregnancy planning and management advice intervention to be delivered by the community pharmacist to women at the start of OST. The study aimed to find out what women in receipt of OST and pharmacists thought about this idea, and if acceptable, what the intervention might need to comprise. To do this, the team interviewed 40 women in receipt of OST and 20 community pharmacists.

Health Psychology Involvement

Traditionally, pharmacy practice research has been accused of lacking rigour and not being theoretically informed. Intervention development approaches have arisen out of practices which failed to take account of the needs, attitudes, and views of key actors. The team wanted to use an approach that would help them understand what the potential recipients and providers of the intervention thought about the following:

a Whether pharmacists felt they could deliver the intervention, what support and training they needed to do so, how they would offer and provide the intervention, and the factors that impacted their motivation to provide it (Al Husein et al., 2021).
b Whether the idea was acceptable to women receiving OST, and if it was, how they would want the intervention to be offered and delivered, what they would want it to contain, and the key issues that they felt the pharmacists needed to understand. The team also talked to women about their experiences, contraception preferences, and factors that helped, hindered, and motivated them to use contraception when they needed it (Neale et al., 2021)

The project used the Behaviour Change Wheel (BCW: Michie et al., 2011), expanded with the Theoretical Domains Framework (TDF: Cane et al., 2012) to identify the barriers and facilitators to pharmacists providing contraception advice and for women accessing and using contraception when receiving opiate substitution treatment. By using a well-established approach like the BCW and TDF, which bring together theories and frameworks of behaviour change, the team was able to conduct a transparent and rigorous approach to planning and developing our intervention by linking the factors that determine and influence behaviour through intervention options. The strength given to the project from the health psychology component cannot be understated. It enabled us to think from the perspective of the deliverers and recipients, to think through and evidence each component. Although the BCW is designed to be applied broadly, had the team been from only a pharmacy background, we would not have come to understand our participants with the depth and clarity that the health psychology lens brought.

Summary and Implications

In this chapter, we have offered a brief insight into the interconnectedness of health psychology. We have described its multidisciplinary beginnings to its current incarnation as a profession with significant expertise in behaviour change. We have shown health psychology to be a profession which reaches out to professionals in behavioural, social, and medical sciences. We have also highlighted through our examples the importance of moving away from multidisciplinary research (where different disciplines work separately on a problem), towards interdisciplinary research (where different disciplines work together on a problem but still use their own disciplinary perspectives), or even better, towards transdisciplinary research (where different disciplines work together to address a problem and in so doing, combine their strengths, knowledge, and perspectives to form new theories and approaches). We conclude our chapter by sharing some suggestions for research, practice, and global implications.

Research Implications

We have shown that much health psychology research is conducted in an interdisciplinary manner, where researchers from different disciplines work together to address a problem but still work from their own disciplinary perspectives. Given the hugely important health and climate issues we face, moving towards Rosenfeld's (1992) transdisciplinary model, where true collaboration and merging of theories and perspectives begin to take place, seems important. How we do this against what can feel like an increasingly indecent jostling for recognition of being 'world-leading' is something we ought to be putting our collective minds towards. Now is no time for ego, it is a time to put ego aside and collectively focus on the bigger picture.

Practice Implications

Practice is about more than designing and delivering psychological interventions. We have shown that practice is, and should be, about sharing expertise and knowing how best to collaborate with different professions. For us, a clear practice implication arising from this is the need to train Health Psychologists about working collaboratively across disciplines and silos, and in particular about how to develop communication skills and an air of curiosity that opens up discussion and advances scientific application. We ought to be training the next generation of Health Psychologists about Rosenfeld's (1992) three types of collaboration and be encouraging them to consider how they might aim for transdisciplinarity.

Global Implications

It would be neglectful of us in a chapter all about interconnectedness not to focus on the bigger global picture. One of the most important issues facing our world at present is that of climate change and our current age of the Anthropocene. The Anthropocene age is characterised by biophysical changes happening in our environment as a consequence of human actions. Health psychology, with its behaviour change expertise has much to offer in a joint effort to address this. Bernard (2019: p. 198), in a call to action when reflecting on the role of health psychology in the age of Anthropocene, notes that health psychology should "*collaborate with other scientific communities from anthropology, sociology, implementation sciences, behavioral medicine, neurosciences and ecology*" to address such global issues.

Conclusion

This chapter has highlighted the interconnectedness of health psychology with a number of disciplines which share a similar agenda. We suggest that the multidisciplinary influences that originally led to the development of health psychology as a discipline have ensured that interconnectivity and collaborative working are embedded at the heart of health psychology. This ability to collaborate is needed more now than ever before. We are hopeful that our profession, with its strengths in behaviour change and interconnectivity, can be part of the solution to the pressing global health and climate problems facing us.

Further Reading

Davis, R., Campbell, R., Hildon, Z., Hobbs, L. & Michie, S. (2014). Theories of behaviour and behaviour change across the social and behavioural sciences: A scoping review. *Health Psychology Review*, *9*(3), 323–344.

Engel, G.L. (1977). The need for a new medical model: A challenge for biomedicine. *Science*, *196*, 129–136.

McBride, E., Hart, J., O'Connor, D., Shorter, G., Arden, M.A., Armitage, C. J., Epton, T., Byrne-Davis, L., Chadwick, P., Drury, J., Kamal, A., Lewis, L., Swanson, V., Whittaker, E. & Chater, A. (2021). *Behavioural science investment needed to mitigate long-term health impacts of COVID-19*. Leicester: British Psychological Society.

Public Health England (2018). *Improving people's health: Applying behavioural and social sciences to improve population health and well-being in England*. London: Public Health England.

References

Academy of Social Sciences website: https://acss.org.uk/what-is-social-science/ [Accessed on 14th June 2023].

Al Husein, N., Scott, J., Neale, J., Chater, A., & Family, H. E. (2021). Community pharmacists' views on providing a reproductive health service to women receiving opioid substitution treatment: A qualitative study using the TDF and COM-B. *Exploratory Research in Clinical and Social Pharmacy*, *4*, 100071. https://www.sciencedirect.com/science/article/pii/S2667276621000718

Bernard, P. (2019). Health psychology at the age of Anthropocene. *Health Psychology and Behavioral Medicine*, *7*(1), 193–201.

Birkbeck, D., Kruczkowski, S., Jones, P., Singleton, D. & McGlynn, S. (2020). *Building for a Healthy Life: A Design Toolkit for neighbourhoods, streets, homes, and public spaces*. Available at: https://www.udg.org.uk/publications/othermanuals/building-healthy-life. [Accessed 18 January 2023].

Cane, J., O'Connor, D. & Michie, S. (2012). Validation of the theoretical domains framework for use in behaviour change and implementation research. *Implementation Science*, *7*(37). https://doi.org/10.1186/1748-5908-7-37

Cerel, J., Maple, M., van de Venne, J., Moore, M., Flaherty, C. & Brown, M. (2016). Exposure to suicide in the community: Prevalence and correlates in one U.S. State. *Public Health Reports*, *131*(1), 100–107.

Chater, A.M., Family, H., Abraao, L.M., Burnett, E., Castro-Sanchez, E., Du Toit, B., Gallagher, R., Gotterson, F., Manias, E., McEwen, J., Figueiredo, R.M., Nathan, M., Olans, R., Padoveze, M.C. & Courtenay, M. (2022). Influences on nurses' engagement in antimicrobial stewardship behaviours: A multi-country survey using the Theoretical

Domains Framework. *Journal of Hospital Infection, 129*, 171–180. https://doi.org/10.1016/j.jhin.2022.07.010

Chater, A., Family, H., Lim, R. & Courtenay, M. (2020). Influences on antibiotic prescribing by non-medical prescribers for respiratory tract infections: A systematic review using the Theoretical Domains Framework. *Journal of Antimicrobial Chemotherapy, 75*(12), 3458–3470. https://doi.org/10.1093/jac/dkaa335

Cheetham-Blake, T.J., Family, H.E. & Turner-Cobb, J.M., 2019. 'Every day I worry about something': A qualitative exploration of children's experiences of stress and coping. *British Journal of Health Psychology, 24*(4), 931–952.

Conner, M. & Norman. P. (2005). Predicting Health Behaviour: A special Cognition Approach in M. Conner & P. Normal (Eds.), *Predicting Health Behaviour*. 2nd edition. Maidenhead. Open University Press.

Courtenay. M. & Chater, A. (2021). Antimicrobial stewardship: A competency framework to support the role of nurses. *Primary Health Care, 31*(2), 36–42. 10.7748/phc.2021/e1709.

Davis, R., Campbell, R., Hildon, Z., Hobbs, L. & Michie, S. (2014). Theories of behaviour and behaviour change across the social and behavioural sciences: A scoping review. *Health Psychology Review, 9*(3), 323–344.

De-Graft Aikins, A. (2018). Health psychology in Ghana: A review of the multidisciplinary origins of a young sub-field and its future prospects. *Journal of Health Psychology, 23*(3), 425–441.

Encyclopaedia Britannica [accessed 16th January 2023] https://www.britannica.com/science/behavioral-science

Engel, G.L. (1977). The need for a new medical model: A challenge for biomedicine. *Science, 196*, 129–136.

Erkkola, M., Kinnunenm S.M., Vepsäläinen, H.R., Meinilä, J.M., Uusitalo, L., Konttinen, H., Saarijärvi, H., Fogelhorn, M. & Nevalainen, J. (2022). A slow road from meat dominance to more sustainable diets: An analysis of purchase preferences among Finnish loyalty-card holders. *PLOS Sustainability and Transformation, 1*(6), e0000015.

Fasolo, B. (2016) What is Behavioural Science at the LSE? https://blogs.lse.ac.uk/behaviouralscience/2016/05/24/what-is-behavioural-science-at-the-lse/ [Accessed 16th January 2023].

Fava, G.A. & Sonina, N. (2017). From the lesson of George Engel to current knowledge: The Biopsychosocial Model 40 years later. *Psychotherapy and Psychosomatics, 86*, 257–259.

Flowers, P. (2018). Antimicrobial resistance: A biopsychosocial problem requiring innovative interdisciplinary and imaginative interventions. *Journal of Infection Prevention, 19*(4), 195–199.

Forshaw, M. & Sheffield, D. (Eds.). (2013). *Health Psychology in Action*. Chichester: Wiley Blackwell.

France, C. (2013). *American Psychological Association Division 38 (Health Psychology)*. In: Gellman, M.D., Turner, J.R. (Eds.), *Encyclopedia of Behavioral Medicine*. New York, NY: Springer. https://doi.org/10.1007/978-1-4419-1005-9_1358

Fulton, E. (2021). An introduction to behavioural science. Published by Public Health England and the Behavioural Science and Public Health Network. https://global-uploads.webflow.com/63236652b830869ac6463e34/6332f062bf0b714650ea4253_1-An-Introduction-to-Behavioural-Science-Dr-Emmie-Fulton-BSPHN-Summer-2021.pdf [Accessed 14th June 2023].

Golding, S. E., Ogden, J. & Higgins, H.M. (2019). Shared goals, different barriers: A qualitative study of UK veterinarians' and farmers' beliefs about Antimicrobial resistance and stewardship. *Frontiers in Veterinary Science, 6*, 132. 10.3389/fvets.2019.00132

Herzlich, C. (2018). A journey in the field of health: From social psychology to multidisciplinarity. *Journal of Health Psychology, 23*(3), 386–396.

Jacob, S. (2008). Cross-Disciplinarization: A new talisman for evaluation? *American Journal of Evaluation, 29*(2), 175–194.

Lewis, L. J. M. & Dunn, O. (2022). *Evaluation of a behaviourally-informed email to increase flu vaccination uptake in local authority employees*. https://www.bsphn.org.uk/publication/evaluation-of-a-behaviourally-informed-email-to-increase-flu-vaccination-uptake-in-local-authority-employees [Accessed 25th January 2023].

Loveday, C. (2017). Working together to get off the medical merry go round, *The Psychologist*, June 5, 2017. British Psychological Society, London. https://www.bps.org.uk/psychologist/working-together-get-medical-merry-go-round [Accessed 25th January 2023].

Lubek, I. & Murray, M. (2018). Doing Histor{y/ies} of Health Psycholog{y/ies}. *Journal of Health Psychology, 23*(3), 361–371

McBride, E., Hart, J., O'Connor, D., Shorter, G., Arden, M.A., Armitage, C. J., Epton, T., Byrne-Davis, L., Chadwick, P., Drury, J., Kamal, A., Lewis, L., Swanson, V., Whittaker, E. & Chater, A. (2021). *Behavioural science investment needed to mitigate long-term health impacts of COVID-19*. Leicester: British Psychological Society.

Michie, S., Richardson, M., Johnston, M., Abraham, C., Francis, J., Hardeman, W., Eccles, M. P., Cane, J., & Wood, C.E. (2013). The behavior change technique taxonomy (v1) of 93 hierarchically clustered techniques: Building an international consensus for the reporting of behavior change interventions. *Annals of Behavioral Medicine, 46*(1), 81–95. https://doi.org/10.1007/s12160-013-9486-6.

Michie, S., van Stralen, M., & West, R. (2011). The behaviour change wheel: A new method for characterising and designing behaviour change interventions. *Implementation Science, 23*(6), 42, https://doi.org/10.1186/1748-5908-6-42

Murphy, B.M., Rogerson, M.C., Hesselson, S., Iismaa, S.E., Graham, R.M. & Jackson, A. (2022). Psychosocial impacts of spontaneous coronary artery dissection: A qualitative study. *PLoS ONE, 17*(9): e0273978.

Murray, M. (2018). The pre-history of health psychology in the United Kingdom: From natural science and psychoanalysis to social science, social cognition and beyond. *Journal of Health Psychology, 23*(3), 472–491.

National Planning Policy Framework (2021). Published by the Ministry of Housing Communities and Local Government. https://www.gov.uk/government/publications/national-planning-policy-framework--2 [Accessed 18 January 2023].

Neal, J.W., Janulis, P. & Collins, C. (2013). Is community psychology "too insular"? A network analysis of journal citations. *Journal of Community Psychology, 41*(5), 549–564.

Neale, J., Werthern, H., Alhusein, N., Chater, A., Scott, J. & Family, H. (2021). Contraceptive choice and power amongst women receiving opioid replacement therapy: Qualitative study. *Drugs: Education, Prevention & Policy*, 1–12. https://doi.org/10.1080/09687637.2021.1954599

O'Connor, D.B., Thayer, J.F. & Vedhara, K. (2021). Stress and Health: A review of psychobiological processes. *Annual Review of Psychology, 72*, 663–688.

O'Connor, R.C. & Kirtley, O.J. (2018). The integrated motivational-volitional model of suicidal behaviour. *Philosophical Transactions of the Royal Society B, 373*, 20170268–20170268

Public Health England (2018). *Improving people's health: Applying behavioural and social sciences to improve population health and wellbeing in England*. London: Public Health England.

Quinn, F. Chater, A. & Morrison, V. (2020). An oral history of health psychology in the UK. *British Journal of Health Psychology, 25*(3), 502–518.

Rodham, K. Chater, A., Edmunds, S., Mellick, M. Deary, V. & Smith, M. (2017). *Wellbeing: Converging approaches from Health and Sport and Exercise Psychology, Symposium. British Psychological Society Annual Conference*, Brighton, 3–5 May.

Round, E., Wetherell, M., Elsey, V. & Smith, M. (2022). Positive expressive writing as a tool for alleviating burnout and enhancing wellbeing in teachers and other full-time workers. *Cogent Psychology*, *9*(1), 2060628, https://doi.org/10.1080/23311908.2022.2060628

Rosenfeld, P. (1992). The potential of transdisciplinary research for sustaining and extending linkages between the health and social sciences. *Social Science and Medicine*, *35*(11), 1343–1357.

Sandford, D.M., Kirtley, O.J., Thwaites, R. & O'Connor, R.C. (2022). Exploring the impact on primary care mental health practitioners of the death of a patient by suicide: An IPA Study. *Psychology and Psychotherapy Theory, Research and Practice*, (Early online publication). https://doi.org/10.1111/papt.12426

Santiago-Delefosse, M. & Carral, M.D.R. (2018). The rapid expansion of (mainstream) health psychology in France: Historical foundations. *Journal of Health Psychology*, *23*(3), 372–385.

Scholz, U. (2022). Better together? The role of others in health behaviour change. *Keynote speaker at European Health Psychology Society conference 2022*. https://2022.ehps.net/speakers/ [Accessed 3rd February 2023].

Schüz, B., Conner, M., Wilding, S., Alhawtan, R., Prestwich, A. & Norman, P. (2021). Do socio-structural factors moderate the effects of health cognitions on CPVID-19 protection behaviours? *Social Science & Medicine*, *285*, 114261.

Spink, M.J.P. (2018). Interlaced strands: Health psychology in Brazil from an autobiographic perspective. *Journal of Health Psychology*, *23*(3), 397–407.

Sproesser, G., Bhangaokar, R., Ruby, M.B., Fischler C., Rozin, P., Schupp, H.T. & Renner, B. (2022). Traditional and modern eating in older adults: A comparison between an urban and rural sample from Gujarat, Western India. *Health Psychology and Behavioral Medicine*, *10*(1), 816–836.

Stam, H.J., Murray, M. & Lubek, I. (2018). Health psychology in autobiography: Three Canadian critical narratives. *Journal of Health Psychology*, *23*(3), 506–523.

Thorpe, A., Sirota, M., Orbell, S. & Juanchich, M. (2021). Effect of information on reducing inappropriate expectations and requests for antibiotics. *British Journal of Psychology*, *112*, 804–827.

Van der Zande, M.M., Dembinsky, M., Aresi, G. & van Staa, T.P. (2019). General practitioners' accounts of negotiating antibiotic prescribing decisions with patients: A qualitative study on what influences antibiotic prescribing in low, medium, and high prescribing practices. *BMC Family Practice*, *20*, 172. https://doi.org/10.1186/s12875-019-1065-x

Vinck, J., Oldenburg, B. & Von Lengerke, T. (2004). Editorial: Health Psychology and Public Heath – Bridging the gap. *Journal of Health Psychology*, *9*(1), 5–12.

Williams, J., Shorter, G. W., Howlett, N., Zakrzewski-Fruer, J., & Chater, A. M. (2021). Can physical activity support grief outcomes in individuals who have been bereaved? A systematic review. *Sports Medicine Open*, *7*(1), 1–17. https://doi.org/10.1186/s40798-021-00311-z

Yen, J. & Vaccarino, O. (2018). 'Health psychology' or 'psychology for health'? A history of psychologists' engagement with health in South Africa. *Journal of Health Psychology*, *23*(3), 408–424.

Zhang, C., Adriaanse, M.A., Potgieter, R., Tummers, L., de Wit, J., Broersen, J., de Bruin, M. & Aarts, H. (2022). Habit formation of preventive behaviours during the COVID-19 pandemic: A longitudinal study of physical distancing and hand washing. *BMC Public Health*, *22*, 1588.

4
PROFESSIONALISATION OF HEALTH PSYCHOLOGY

Karen Matvienko-Sikar, Julia Allan, Lisa Hynes, Jenny McSharry, Marta Marques, Vivien Swanson, and Angel Marie Chater

Introduction

The route to the professionalisation of health psychology has had many roads. For those working within health psychology, and for others with an interest in it, professional events, publications, and training assist the advancement of the science and its translation into policy and practice. Professional networks can also strengthen the identity of health psychology, offering a home to those with an interest in the area. This chapter will discuss professional meetings, events, conferences, and networks of health psychology, alongside networks wider than health psychology that have evolved to facilitate interdisciplinary and transdisciplinary working and professionalisation. Key publications, including journals and newsletters, will be evaluated with an international lens on dissemination of health psychology. Training from professional societies and networks in relation to accredited routes in the field and continuing professional development (CPD) will further be discussed, and links to more formalised practice-based organisations such as the Health and Care Professions Council (HCPC) in the United Kingdom (UK) will be explored. The chapter will conclude with a discussion on the challenges to the professionalisation of health psychology, accompanied by potential solutions and examples of successes to date.

Developing a Professional Discipline

The development of health psychology as a professional discipline was led by those with a shared passion for creating a home for those from different branches of psychology, such as clinical, social, and experimental psychology, who were applying their science and practice to areas related to health and medicine. Chapter 1 discussed how the American Psychological Association (APA) was at

DOI: 10.4324/9781003318026-5

the forefront of these developments and coined the term 'health psychology' (Matarazzo, 1980; Wallston, 1997). This was followed in the mid-80s by developments in Europe, the UK, and Japan described by Johnston (2018), Quinn et al. (2020), and Takenaka (2013), respectively.

Health Psychology Annual Meetings and Conferences

The historical accounts of health psychology often began with a scientific meeting and/or academic conference. These were usually attended by those with an interest in psychology applied to health and medicine. A series of academic meetings (discussed in Chapter 1) that became pivotal to the development of health psychology as a discipline, both in the United States of America (USA) and across Europe, brought together people passionate about the topic to share their ideas and work.

Academic conferences, also termed scientific meetings, conventions, or congress, serve many purposes. They provide a platform for researchers and (more recently) practitioners to present their most recent findings, methodological approaches, and/or theoretical ideas. Conferences are usually organised by a group of researchers who may or may not be part of a member network. They often have an agenda with a shared vision or purpose. Many larger gatherings will have a scientific committee that will ensure the academic quality of the content being presented and the invitation of keynote speakers, ensuring that work presented is at the cutting edge of science and/or practice.

The definition of health psychology, offered by the APA's first Division 38 (Health Psychology) president, Joseph Matarazzo (1980), during an opening address, is still used today, showing the significance of such academic events in the development of the discipline. Health psychology conferences have changed in stature and focus over the years, from small gatherings of people keen to develop a community of practice to large international conferences facilitated by more fluid transport opportunities globally (e.g., cheaper airfare) and hybrid (in-person and online) options. The content of such meetings has shifted from a focus on behavioural medicine, understanding psychology's role in health and illness and experimental designs, to the development of theories to predict behaviour and health outcomes, through to intervention development, behaviour change, and translational transdisciplinary working, advancing science, policy, and practice. This, in turn, has changed the outward-facing scope, focus, and goal of health psychology as a discipline, and a single accepted definition of the field does not exist. The British Psychological Society (BPS), a member network in the UK, defines the goal of health psychology as

> *to study the psychological processes underlying health, illness and health care, and to apply these findings to the promotion and maintenance of health, the analysis and improvement of the healthcare system and health policy formation, the prevention of illness and disability, and the enhancement of outcomes for those who are ill or disabled.*
>
> *(https://www.bps.org.uk/member-networks/division-health-psychology)*

Communities of Practice and Identity

From annual meetings and conferences came the development of more formalised communities of practice and learned societies that provide a forum and platform for bringing those with an interest in health psychology together. There are a number of communities of practice across the globe. The formation of the APA Division 38 occurred in 1978. This was quickly followed by the European Health Psychology Society (EHPS), developed in 1986. The roots of the UK BPS Division of Health Psychology (DHP) began alongside the EHPS, starting as a Health Psychology Section in 1986 and becoming a division and branch member network of the BPS in 1997.

With a wide international membership, the EHPS is one of the most diverse communities of practice and representation of health psychology. Many of the counties included in the EHPS have a National Delegate who represents the interests of health psychology from their country to the EHPS Executive Committee. In 2023, the EHPS had 33 National Delegates representing health psychology in Australia, Belgium, Brazil, Bulgaria, Costa Rica, Croatia, Cyprus, Czech Republic, Denmark, Germany, Greece, Hungary, Ireland, Israel, Italy, Japan, Latvia, Luxembourg, Malta, North Macedonia, Poland, Portugal, Romania, Slovakia, Slovenia, South Africa, Spain, Sweden, Switzerland, the Netherlands, Ukraine, the UK, and the USA.

There are pockets of historical evidence of the development of health psychology member networks in other countries internationally, such as the Japanese Association of Health Psychology (JAHP) founded in 1987 (Takenaka, 2013) and the establishment of the College of Health Psychologists of the Australian Psychological Society (APS) in 1997 (Martin et al., 2014). However, there is little written on the global development of health psychology other than that written in Chapter 1 of this book. This is a topic worthy of future academic investment.

Many of the aforementioned professional groups are members of the European Federation of Professional Psychologists Associations (EFPPA). David Marks led a Taskforce on Health Psychology, convened in 1992 by EFPPA (Marks et al., 1998), which set out the nature and scope of health psychology and what it may look like in the future. The Taskforce highlighted the training needs and desired objectives to develop a professional workforce in health psychology that could be used across Europe. Implications for practice and policy were considered in relation to medical advancement and societal change, alongside ethical and legal regulation. Yet to date, there is no internationally accepted training programme. This is another area worthy of investment.

Over the years, more targeted communities of practice have developed to facilitate the interaction between health psychology and aligned disciplines such as public health. The Health Psychology and Public Health Network (HPPHN), which began in the UK, is an example of such a grouping, described in more detail in Box 4.1.

Other groupings formed when there was a call for health psychology support during the COVID-19 pandemic. The Health Psychology Exchange (HPX)

Box 4.1 Development of a Health Psychology and Public Health Network

The HPPHN began with a desire to bring the fields of public health and health psychology together. Leading its development were key champions who held seats in relevant learned society committees: the Faculty of Public Health (Jim McManus) and the BPS DHP (Angel Chater), alongside those working within local authority and academia (see Chater & McManus, 2016). It was developed to be a community of practice, to bring those with shared interests together through events, an annual conference, a website with shared materials, on social media, and via a regular newsletter and podcast. You can listen to more about its development here: Real World Behavioural Science Podcast: #19 https://open.spotify.com/episode/5cJq2Zn7YKOHwx0k6iEWIB?go=1&sp_cid=cdd4870fa2e5cdc3a37a47848f6abafc&utm_source=embed_player_p&utm_medium=desktop&nd=1.

Since its inception, the HPPHN, now the Behavioural Science and Public Health Network (BSPHN, 2021), has benefited from the close relationships created by those working in health psychology and public health. The HPPHN was re-branded to become the BSPHN in June 2018 following a survey and vote by members to widen the remit of the network and identity. This was supported with income from the then Public Health England, to create a community of practice to bring professionals together and was publicly launched in September 2018. The change in name moved from health psychology *in* public health to a wider remit of behavioural science *and* public health to promote the two-way interaction of knowledge exchange. While this change of name received some criticism in removing the term 'health psychology' from the title, it benefited from enabling health psychology principles to reach a wider audience, maximising its impact.

The BSPHN is a forum and community of practice for professionals interested in all domains of public health and health psychology wishing to develop an understanding of health and well-being from a behavioural, social, and psychological perspective. The core mission of the BSPHN is to share best practices and maximise opportunities and insights from a multidisciplinary approach. Those who engage with the BSPHN have a variety of backgrounds and specialist areas, and include behavioural scientists, Health Psychologists, behavioural economists, social scientists, public health consultants and practitioners, and those working and training in these areas. The network now offers CPD events, workshops, and an annual conference; a website with access to a range of resources, including past events, recorded interviews with top experts, and a BSPHN publication; inclusion in a contact directory; and social media connections. It hosts the Behavioural and Social Science Strategy, "*[I]mproving people's health: applying behavioural and social sciences to improve population health and wellbeing in England*" produced by Public Health England (2018) that promotes training in and the use of health psychology in a public health setting. More details can be found here: www.bsphn.org.uk.

represents an example of the rapid mobilisation of knowledge and resources that is possible when an organised, well-developed network is in place. The HPX was formed to support the health, social care, and public health systems in the UK during the COVID-19 pandemic (Health Psychology Exchange, 2020). Over 150 health psychology professionals, including trainees, formed a collective to translate relevant evidence to guide policy and decision-makers, and inform, produce, deliver, and evaluate psychological and behavioural interventions across a variety of settings (Health Psychology Exchange, 2021). The collective used an Open Science Framework (OSF: Health Psychology Resources for COVID-19: https://osf.io/q5n3d/) to facilitate resource sharing, formed sub-groups to organise skills and address needs, and established partnerships with organisations such as city councils and charities (Armstrong et al., 2021; Chater et al., 2020; Health Psychology Exchange, 2021). This approach enabled the group, which was operating on a voluntary basis, to deliver a wide range of projects at speed, including an alcohol awareness campaign during lockdown and psychological support for staff across a range of health settings (Armstrong et al., 2021; Brady et al., 2021). It further assisted a national COVID-19 Behavioural Science and Disease Prevention Taskforce (BSDPT), convened by the BPS, to develop a series of public health roadmaps, COVID-19 guidance documents, and rapid reviews of the literature (Chater, Shorter et al., 2021). This work aimed to support research, policy, and practice at speed and led to the development of the Template for Rapid Iterative Consensus of Experts, which the team named TRICE (Chater, Shorter et al., 2021).

Health Psychology Journals

Any scientific community needs outlets to disseminate research evidence, extend methodological approaches, present and discuss theoretical ideas, and provide space for opinion pieces to advance knowledge and practice. The *Scimago Journal* and Country Rank website (https://www.scimagojr.com/journalsearch.php?q=health+psychology) lists 15 journals with 'health psychology' in the title. These can be found in Table 4.1, alongside their journal metrics as of January 2024. Of these, six are published from the USA, five from the UK, with the others from Germany, Poland, Switzerland, and Spain.

The journal metrics offer an evaluation of reach and significance, which is important to many academic assessments, such as the UK Research Excellence Framework (REF: https://www.ref.ac.uk/). The top five journals with the highest impact factors (IF) are *Applied Psychology: Health and Well-Being* (IF = 9.9), followed by *Health Psychology Review* (IF = 9.8), *International Journal of Clinical and Health Psychology* (IF = 8.8), the *British Journal of Health Psychology* (IF = 8.8), and the *Journal of Occupational Health Psychology* (IF = 5.1). There are other journal metrics that show reach and significance, such as the h-index, which accounts for the number of papers (h) published in a journal that have been cited at least 'h' times. The journal with the highest h-index is the APA journal *Health Psychology* (h-index = 182), which has an IF of 4.2. This is followed

Table 4.1 International health psychology journal details and metrics in 2024

Journal Name	*Country of Publication*	*Publisher/Affiliation*	*Impact Factor*	*Five-Year Impact Factor*	*Quartile*	*h-Index*	*SJR-Ranking*
Applied Psychology: Health and Well-Being	USA	Wiley-Blackwell/ International Association of Applied Psychology	9.9	-	Q1	43	2.05
British Journal of Health Psychology	USA	Wiley-Blackwell/BPS	7.9	8.1	Q1	98	2.37
European Journal of Health Psychology	Germany	Hogrefe-Verlag GmbH and Co. KG	2.1	2.7	Q2	18	0.51
European Journal of Investigation in Health, Psychology and Education	Switzerland	MDPI AG	3.2	3.5	Q3	18	0.54
Health Psychology	USA	APA	4.2	4.9	Q1	182	1.4
Health Psychology and Behavioral Medicine	UK	Taylor and Francis Ltd./ EHPS	2.7	3.2	Q1	12	0.77
Health Psychology Open	USA	SAGE Publications Inc.	2.9	3.4	Q2	25	0.78
Health Psychology Report	Poland	Termedia Publishing House Ltd.	2.16	-	Q3	10	0.45
Health Psychology Research	USA	Open Medical Publishing	2.51	-	Q2	8	0.5

(*Continued*)

Table 4.1 (Continued)

Journal Name	*Country of Publication*	*Publisher/Affiliation*	*Impact Factor*	*Five-Year Impact Factor*	*Quartile*	*h-Index*	*SJR-Ranking*
Health Psychology Review	UK	Routledge/EHPS	9.8	9.8	Q1	66	3.1
International Journal of Clinical and Health Psychology	Spain	Elsevier BV	8.8	-	Q1	51	2.32
Journal of Health Psychology	UK	SAGE Publications Ltd	3.2	3.1	Q2	98	0.91
Journal of Occupational Health Psychology	USA	Educational Publishing Foundation/APA	5.1	11.7	Q1	140	2.48
Psychology and Health	UK	Routledge/EHPS	3.3	4.0	Q1	101	1.03
Psychology, Health, and Medicine	UK	Routledge	3.8	3.5	Q2	73	0.94

by the *International Journal of Occupational Health Psychology* (h-index = 140), *Psychology and Health* (h-index = 101; IF = 3.3), the *British Journal of Health Psychology* (h-index = 98) and the *Journal of Health Psychology* (h-index = 98; IF = 3.2).

While it is useful to know the journals specific to health psychology, often, academics in the field publish in journals related to a disease area or topic such as the *International Journal of Obesity* or *BMC Public Health*. There are also journals that are linked to member networks that do not feature traditional metrics, such as the *Health Psychology Update* (HPU) from the BPS DHP and the publication from the BSPHN (https://www.bsphn.org.uk/collection/behavioural-science-and-public-health). Journals and member network publications are important in the professionalisation of a discipline, giving those with a shared interest the opportunity to share ideas and research findings while also adding to the group identity within the topic area. Publishing both within the discipline in health psychology–specific journals and across other disciplines, such as subject specific, ensures that those working in the area are up to date with key issues and science while also sharing the science with others who could assist in its translation.

Training Pathways as a Route to Professionalisation

Another key method of establishing health psychology as a reputable and valuable professional discipline is the development of formal training pathways and standards. Formal training pathways raise the profile of the discipline by promoting career pathways and ensuring consistency and quality within the discipline by providing a structured route to qualification. Training pathways also promote awareness of the value of the profession in different health-care contexts. Training standards and regulatory oversight provide the public and employers with information about the remit and scope of health psychology and with assurances about the quality and competence of Health Psychologists in practice.

As a relatively young psychological discipline, health psychology's training pathways are less concretely established internationally than those in larger, more established areas of psychological practice, such as clinical psychology. However, this is changing, with training programmes and pathways developing around the world in response to increased interest from students and increased demand for scientists and practitioners with the skills required to tackle pressing societal problems such as obesity, ageing populations, and infectious disease pandemics.

At present, health psychology training in many countries, including, but not limited to, Costa Rica, Croatia, Cyprus, Denmark, Israel, Japan, Luxembourg, and Slovakia, is typically conducted as part of training within a related or broader topic area such as clinical, medical, applied, or general psychology (McSharry et al., 2017). While this carries some advantages, for example, providing students with a broader, interdisciplinary perspective on the topics studied and recognising the real-world overlap between disciplines, it also limits the development and recognition of the value of professional health psychology as a distinct field with unique areas of focus and expertise. Health Psychologists need to be able to understand and change psychological and behavioural processes in the context of health, illness, and health care through research, education, training, and psychological intervention; to train and upskill other health and social care professionals; and to support health and wellness maintenance and the management of health conditions effectively. These competencies form a substantial part of health psychology professional training curricula, distinguishing health psychology from other areas of applied psychology (Chater, Rockliffe et al., 2021; Michie, Abraham & Johnston, 2007).

In a survey of National Delegates representing 27 countries as part of the EHPS, 6 (Germany, Japan, Lithuania, Sweden, Turkey, and the UK) reported that their country had health psychology–specific programmes at the undergraduate (BSc, BA) level (McSharry et al., 2017). Health psychology training is more commonly (16/27 countries surveyed) found at the postgraduate (MSc) level and reported in many countries (including, but not limited to, Australia, Bulgaria, Ireland, the Netherlands, Malta, Poland, Spain, and the UK (McSharry et al., 2017), alongside the USA). However, few nations legally regulate the practice of Health Psychologists after qualification. The European Federation of Psychologists Associations (EFPA) provides psychologists across Europe with EuroPsy certification, entitling them to practice as a psychologist, but this is for general psychological practice per se, and there is not currently an option to achieve EuroPsy certification in health psychology specifically. One of the few countries to register Practitioner Health Psychologists as a distinct professional group is the UK through the HCPC.

The oral history of health psychology in the UK word Project (Quinn et al., 2020) and the APA Taskforce (Wallston, 1997) highlighted calls for training to develop health psychology as a profession. In case studies published by the EHPS (McSharry et al., 2017) and BPS (Chater, Rockliffe et al., 2021), there is a clear pathway to health psychology practice in the UK via the HCPC, harmonised with BPS training. On this route, trainees must usually complete a BPS-accredited undergraduate psychology degree (usually 3 years full-time, equating to 360 UK credits/180 ECTS: European Credit Transfer and Accumulation System points), which offers the BPS Graduate Basis for Chartership (GBC). This is followed by a BPS-accredited MSc in Health Psychology (180 UK credits at M-level/90 ECTS points) for one year full-time (or part-time equivalent), which would provide the Stage 1 Qualification in Health Psychology. Those 'in-training' would then undergo two years of supervised practice (for 37.5/40 hours per week; 46 weeks per year or part-time equivalent) at the doctoral level via a university or independent route known as 'Stage 2' (see Chater, Rockliffe, et al., 2021, for more detail). Health psychology trainees must show competency in the key areas of generic professional practice, research, teaching/training, consultancy, and psychological interventions/behaviour change (see Box 4.2 for more detail). Once in receipt of GBC, Stage 1 and Stage 2 health psychology training, trainees are eligible to apply

Box 4.2 Health Psychology Training in the UK

In the UK, all psychology training standards, pathways, and qualifications are overseen and accredited by a single national body, the BPS. Once qualified, individuals must register with a national regulatory body, the HCPC, in order to practice and legally call themselves a 'Health Psychologist'.

Those pursuing a career in health psychology in the UK must first complete an undergraduate degree in psychology which may or may not include specific modules on health psychology. They must then complete two further stages of post-graduate training: 'Stage 1', a 1-year (or equivalent) master's programme which covers the core knowledge base of health psychology, and 'Stage 2', doctoral-level training focused on translating the knowledge acquired during Stage 1 into the skills needed for research, training, and practice.

The exact content of Stage 1 programmes varies from provider to provider, often reflecting the research and practice strengths of the staff delivering the programme. However, all programmes must cover the same nine curriculum areas:

1 Research and research methods
2 Contexts and perspectives in health psychology
3 Physiological and psychosomatic disease processes
4 Client groups and other stakeholders
5 Health-related behaviours and cognitions
6 Interventions/applications of health psychology
7 Health-care and professional settings
8 Measurement issues
9 Professional issues

This approach allows some flexibility to training providers while ensuring that all Stage 1 trainees graduate with comparable knowledge and skills in health psychology methods, theory and interventions.

Stage 2 involves training in health psychology professional practice. This can take the form of a full or part-time university course (which confers a professional doctorate qualification) or a doctoral-level, 'independent-route' qualification in health psychology (QHP) where trainees register with the BPS and engage in supervised practice by a supervisor registered on the Register of Applied Practice Psychology Supervisors (RAPPS) for at least two years full-time equivalent. During this period of supervised practice, trainees must produce a portfolio demonstrating work that evidences competencies in five core areas:

1 Generic professional practice
2 Psychological interventions

3 Research
4 Consultancy
5 Teaching and training

The requirements to achieve each competency are substantial, with clear learning outcomes that should be mapped to a plan of training (see the Stage 2 handbook for more detail https://cms.bps.org.uk/sites/default/files/2022-07/QHP%20Candidate%20Handbook.pdf). For example, within 'psychological interventions', trainees must design, deliver, and evaluate interventions based on psychological theory to groups, communities, or populations and individuals, accruing direct and observed client contact. Similarly, within the area 'research', trainees must plan, implement, analyse, and disseminate both a systematic review and an empirical research project.

Upon successful completion of Stage 2, trainees become fully qualified and are eligible to register with the HCPC, the UK body responsible for the regulation of allied health and care professions, including practitioner psychologists, physiotherapists, radiographers, dietitians, and paramedics. It is only at this point that the protected title 'Health Psychologist' can be legally used. Up until this point, trainees can use the terms 'Health Psychologist in Training' or 'Trainee Health Psychologist' (see Chater, Rockliffe, et al., 2021 for more details).

Trainees who do not wish to practice clinically and prefer to pursue an academic or research career can choose to complete a PhD instead of a 'Stage 2' qualification. If the PhD is completed within the area of health psychology, those completing it become eligible for full membership of the BPS DHP but cannot register with the HCPC or practice using the title 'Health Psychologist' unless they have completed Stage 2 before, after, or alongside their PhD.

for full membership of the BPS DHP, which also provides chartered status. Practitioner psychologists in the UK are regulated by the HCPC, and therefore, this training must also meet the Standards of Proficiency (SoPs) needed to register with the HCPC, as this is a legal requirement to be able to practice and legally use the term 'Health Psychologist'. While those in practice must be registered, academics, including researchers and teachers in the area of health psychology, are not required to be registered; however, they are therefore not eligible to call themselves a 'Health Psychologist' unless registered with the HCPC. Those who have studied abroad or do not have these qualifications or pre-requisites are also limited in their ability to register and practice in the UK. This can cause an unfortunate divide between 'academics' and 'practitioners', and those trained in the UK and international counterparts.

Clinical health psychology is recognised as a '*specialty, subspecialty, or proficiency in professional psychology*' within the APA (2014, 2022), but health psychology as a stand-alone is not. Clinical health psychology is described by the APA as "*a professionally recognized specialty that investigates and implements clinical services across diverse populations and settings to promote health and well-being and to prevent, treat and manage illness and disability*" (APA, 2022). To practice clinically as a Health Psychologist in the USA, students must complete an undergraduate (bachelor's), postgraduate (master's), and doctor of psychology (PsyD) or doctor of philosophy (PhD) degree. At the master's level, accredited courses require students to complete at least 2,000 hours of clinical experience through a practicum or internship. At least 1,000 hours of supervised experience in clinical settings are required as part of PsyD and PhD programmes, in addition to an internship which includes up to 2,000 hours of clinical placement (Smith-Kimble, 2022). The majority of people working in health psychology in the USA begin their training in clinical, counselling, or school psychology. Requirements for licensure vary between states of America, for example, in terms of level of qualification required (e.g., some states allow people to practice as a psychologist with a master's degree) and number of hours of supervised training. Licensure is only required for Health Psychologists who plan to practice clinically or who require it for their position, and some people working in academic settings may not be licenced (Smith-Kimble, 2022).

In New Zealand, Health Psychologists can attain a similar professional degree qualification to the UK, allowing them to register with the New Zealand Psychologists Board. In 2018, the University of Auckland was the only New Zealand University offering such a qualification through an MSc in Health Psychology, followed by a clinically focused postgraduate diploma (Chamberlain, Lyons & Stephens, 2018).

Formal training pathways contribute greatly towards the professionalisation of health psychology, strengthening recognition of health psychology as a discipline that adds value to applied research and practice in the domains of health, illness, and health care. To further improve career pathways and opportunities for health psychology researchers and practitioners, and to build the international health psychology workforce, it is important that those already working in the field continue to build and improve dedicated training pathways for psychology graduates. The lack of an international curriculum and mobility of qualifications must be considered as a priority to continue to strengthen the international recognition of health psychology as a profession. Furthermore, there is an urgent need to invest in funded training opportunities to enable fair access to training across the potential workforce, ensuring the qualification has equity, diversity, and is inclusive to all who wish to train in the area. There have been a series of calls to action to create funded training pathways in health psychology (Bull et al., 2020; Chater & Hart, 2019; McBride et al., 2021; Chater, Rockliffe, et al., 2021), and the National Health Service Education for Scotland (NES) has led the way (see Box 4.3), with the National Health Service for England (NHSE) following suit.

Box 4.3 Embedding health psychology training in a National Health Service (NHS)

Arguably, the most innovative and impactful development in health psychology training worldwide has been the development and implementation of Scotland's NES Trainee Health Psychology Programme.

The NES programme was launched in 2008 and was the first training programme in the world to offer health psychology trainees the opportunity to complete their training while employed full time within a national health-care system (Swanson, 2017). This was a hugely innovative step, involving collaboration between the Scottish government (which recognised the benefits of expanding the health psychology workforce), NHS Education for Scotland (which carries a remit to support and develop training for the NHS and the wider health and social care sector), the BPS (which oversee psychology-specific training in the UK), the heads of psychological services and directors of public health in the different Scottish health boards (who host and part fund trainees to work on projects of strategic importance or which address local health-care development needs).

How Does the Programme Work in Practice?

Programme leads at NES identify broad priority areas of current relevance to national health improvement policy and practice (e.g., long-term conditions, obesity, early years) and invite health boards in an annual recruitment round to submit bids to host trainees to work on specific projects within these strategic target areas. Leads from public health and psychological services in each health board are invited to collaborate in identifying local services which might benefit from health psychology input. This may include, for example, a health board submitting a bid indicating that they want to host a trainee in the area of obesity and propose that the trainee works with them to develop a weight management service for a particular target group and behaviour change training for staff to better support the delivery of this weight management service.

Submitted bids are evaluated and those selected are advertised nationally as fully funded 'Health Psychologist in Training' posts. These posts are graded at the same level as trainee clinical psychologists to achieve professional parity. Graduates with GBC with the BPS, holding an accredited MSc in Health Psychology are eligible for the posts and apply centrally to NES. Candidates are shortlisted, interviewed, and allocated to available posts through a central process. Those who are successful are jointly funded full time by the hosting health board and NES, who also contribute qualification and supervision fees. Appointed trainees are provided with an NHS line manager to supervise their day-to-day work, a clinical supervisor to supervise their intervention work, an academic supervisor to supervise their research work, and a BPS-approved course tutor/ coordinating supervisor from NES who provides support and oversight in the development of their training portfolio. This team-based approach to supervision means that trainees have access to a broad range of specialist input and guidance and ensures that their work takes account of current practices and developments in the health service, professional training regulations, and up-to-date scientific evidence. It also encourages collaboration between health-care providers and academic partners for mutual benefit. In addition to supervision, trainees have access to a central NES-provided curriculum which supports the acquisition of skills in areas such as systematic reviewing, publication, assessment and formulation, behaviour change, and the delivery of teaching and training. NES also encourages networking and mutual peer-based support for trainees. On completion of the training, the portfolio of competence is examined by the BPS for the award of its QHP, which confers eligibility for HCPC registration.

What Areas Do Trainees Work In?

The NES training model is one designed to achieve mutual benefits: trainees benefit from practice-based experience, being embedded within multidisciplinary teams within the health-care system, and health boards benefit from gaining an employee with the psychological knowledge and skills to conduct specialised work in areas of strategic importance. Trainee work is focused on areas related to national and local health improvement targets. Projects completed by trainees to date have involved working with client groups across the lifespan, and health and social care staff. They have spanned a diverse array of topic areas, including diabetes prevention, child healthy weight, alcohol interventions, weight management, behaviour change training for health professionals, health coaching in primary care, public health support in community pharmacies, psychological well-being in health-care staff, breastfeeding, falls prevention, dementia care, oral health, and cancer screening.

A Success Story

To date, the NES training programme has been hugely successful, with all Scottish mainland health boards choosing to participate in the scheme and more than 50 trainees undertaking training since the programme's inception. The programme contributes directly to the health improvement agenda at a national level, and trainees have produced an impressive number of outputs in terms of reports, academic papers, awards, presentations, and assets for health boards, such as new services, interventions, and evaluative tools. This has illustrated to health boards the added value of health psychology in the development and improvement of interventions, services, care pathways, and policies. A further notable feature of the scheme is that it has produced an active network of current and previous trainees across Scotland

and beyond, who are well integrated with each other but also with their professional body, the health-care service, and the higher education sector. This has raised the profile of health psychology nationally as a profession and introduced 'psychological mindedness' to diverse areas of service provision.

By including the development of training for health professionals within the required competencies, trainees on the NES programme can directly impact the quality of health care delivered, for example, by delivering training which increases the implementation of evidence-based practice, increases guideline compliance, or increases the ability to support behaviour change in patients. Finally, the programme is directly contributing to efforts to increase the professional workforce in health psychology; many NES-funded trainee Health Psychologists remain working in the health service after qualification while others move into academia or specialist areas of practice.

The programme is not free from challenges. It is, as with all government-funded initiatives, dependent on continued funding and, therefore, somewhat vulnerable to economic fluctuations or policy changes. Also, when compared with training programmes in applied psychology specialties such as clinical psychology, it is modest in scale: the NES programme currently supports an average of four fully funded training posts each year. This means that the calibre of trainees is consistently excellent as entry into the programme is highly competitive but also that there are many more high-quality applicants each year than can be supported.

As an innovative and extremely successful training model, the NES programme provides a useful blueprint for other countries looking to develop formal training pathways in health psychology. In recent years, the Scottish model has been used as the basis for the development of a comparable fully funded training programme in England, launched in 2022 (described in more detail in Chapter 5), and it is hoped that similar programmes can be established across the globe.

Challenges to Professionalisation of the Discipline and Ways to Self-Correct

Despite their benefits, professional health psychology networks and societies can experience a number of challenges linked to issues around the awareness and identity of health psychology and Health Psychologists, and in opportunities for funded training, professional roles, and career pathways.

Moreover, at their outset, establishing a society, network, or special interest group in health psychology is not without challenges tied to garnering support, potentially politicised landscapes, and recognition of health psychology as a stand-alone discipline of importance (Coetzee et al., 2023). For instance, the establishment of the APA Division 38 in 1978 is described as requiring its founding members to "*garner enough clout*" in the form of established and respected psychologist signatories to ensure the political support required to establish the division in the APA (Wallston, 1997). The oral history of health psychology in the UK identified contentions with more established disciplines, such as clinical psychology, and the importance of champions and an open dialogue to navigate such controversies (Quinn et al., 2020).

Evidence from areas in which health psychology is currently emerging as a stand-alone discipline, such as Jamaica (Marks et al., 2022), also speaks to the need for targeted advocacy to raise awareness about health psychology, which typically requires multiple advocates and champions and may not always be successful. This is echoed in experiences of attempts to establish a health psychology society in South Africa, where despite calls for a greater focus on health psychology in 2006, a previously established health psychology society no longer exists (Coetzee et al., 2023). However, a health psychology special interest group (SIG) in the Psychological Society of South Africa (PsySSA) has more recently been established and represents a move towards re-establishing the role of a health psychology network for members to share, collaborate, and contribute to improved health outcomes.

Similarly, as noted earlier, there are numerous 'success stories' of established national (e.g., BPS DHP) and international (e.g., EHPS) societies that can be looked to in guiding establishment of successful member networks. It is important to note that the development of any society, network, or SIG requires the input and efforts of individuals, which can pose challenges to the set-up and longevity of these formations. This is because those involved in establishing and running these groups tend to also be health psychology researchers, academics, and/or practitioners for whom involvement in health psychology societies, networks, and SIGs is often done in a volunteer capacity, in addition to the 'day job'. It is clear from examples of established societies and groups that the contribution of motivated individuals is central to such developments and moving the discipline forward. Thus, providing professional 'space' and time, and building capacity in individuals to contribute to the development and governance of such societies and networks is important.

One clear challenge faced by established societies and networks is tied to perceptions of the identity of health psychology at both the level of individual Health Psychologists and in society, education, policy, and practice more generally. There are multiple descriptions and definitions of health psychology, with no consistent international consensus on *what* health psychology is, *who* Health Psychologists are, and what they *do* (Hamilton et al., 2017; Marks et al., 2022). Even when taking the view that, at its core, health psychology involves biological, psychological, and social factors and behaviours related to health outcomes, this broad remit can lead to differences in perceptions of what health psychology is. Similarly, variability in the terminology used to describe or delineate the work and identity of Health Psychologists can arise due to blurred disciplinary boundaries and the varied settings in which Health Psychologists work (Hamilton et al., 2017; Plass et al., 2017). Examples of varied terminology include Health Psychologists being called clinical or medical psychologists in some settings and regions (Hamilton et al., 2017), and, more recently, behavioural scientists (see Chapter 3 & 5). Such differences in perceptions and variability in terminology can impact individuals' professional identity in terms of perceived cohesiveness and self-recognition of fit with the term 'health psychology'. This in turn can influence perceived relevance, usefulness, and appropriateness of health psychology societies and networks, and, ultimately, their membership and survival.

While challenges around identity are seen internationally, there are numerous examples of large and synergistic societies where Health Psychologists have found a professional 'home'. The APA Division 38, BPS DHP, EHPS, and the Psychological Society of Ireland (PSI) Division of Health Psychology are good examples of this. Despite the existence of such successful societies or disciplinary 'homes', it remains important to consider how health psychology and Health Psychologists can address issues around identity that impact engagement with professional societies and networks. For instance, there is a clear and necessary need for standardisation of the term 'health psychology' and the recognised remit of Health Psychologists internationally. Such standardisation would help address ambiguity in the disciplinary boundaries that define health psychology, as well as the identities of Health Psychologists in diverse roles (Thielke, Thompson, & Stuart, 2011). Similarly, as has been previously suggested (Byrne et al., 2017; Plass et al., 2017), there is a need for a standardised framework of health psychology competencies and skills, as well as funded training (Chater & Hart, 2019; McSharry et al., 2017). The UK case studies provide a good example of how standardised competencies and skills can be taught while retaining flexibility in training needs and approaches

Such standardisation of competencies and skills can contribute to addressing a further challenge of health psychology networks and societies, which relates to advocating for professional career pathways for Health Psychologists nationally and internationally. For instance, having standardised health psychology competencies and skills can enhance recognition of the importance and unique identity of health psychology (Plass et al., 2017). It would also enhance mobility for Health Psychologists who are currently limited by the broad range of definitions, terminology, and roles ascribed to Health Psychologists in different countries (Berndt et al., 2017; Plass et al., 2017). In addition, standardisation of skills and competencies could feed into regulations and requirements for the registration of Health Psychologists in practitioner posts, as such requirements currently vary (Berndt et al., 2017; Hamilton et al., 2017). This alone would not solve challenges in facilitating secure career pathways for Health Psychologists nationally and/or internationally, however, because in many instances, there are relatively few formally recognised professional opportunities and roles for Health Psychologists.

There is clearly work to be done, and at present much of that work is being led by national health psychology societies that advocate for professional training and practitioner posts. At this national level, health psychology societies can face challenges in terms of legal recognition of the term 'Health Psychologist' and funding. For instance, in the survey of EHPS National Delegates (Hamilton et al., 2017), in only 7 of 27 countries was the professional title 'Health Psychologist' legally protected. As such, societies need to work with regulatory systems and bodies to advocate for recognition of health psychology registration and practitioner posts. There are, however, positive examples of where professional training models and health service posts have been successfully developed, such as that of the NES training in Scotland and in the UK training models and practitioner posts that have been developed and are recognised (Moss, 2013). Across the globe in New Zealand, there is a professional health psychology degree qualification, which enables Health Psychologists to register with the New Zealand Psychologists Board under a general scope of practice (Chamberlain et al., 2018).

Rising to Meet the Challenges

Despite the challenges described in this chapter, health psychology networks and societies demonstrate a strong capacity to rise to meet these and other challenges. For instance, through the existence of networks and societies, Health Psychologists can work together to address societal and research-related challenges. For instance, the annual EHPS Synergy Expert meeting, which takes place as part of the EHPS annual conference, prepares papers and viewpoints on topics from research integrity and open science (Kwasnicka et al., 2021), through to the application of health psychology and behavioural science to policy and practice (Marques & Chater, 2022) and is able to pool expertise and enthusiasm together with a shared passion for promoting the professionalisation, application, and translation of the discipline.

The ability of Health Psychologists to come together and respond quickly to address a significant public challenge was clearly seen in the development of the Health Psychology Exchange (HPX) during the COVID-19 pandemic. The HPX represents an example of the rapid mobilisation of knowledge and resources that is possible when an organised, well-developed network is in place. The collective, with over 150 health psychology professionals and trainees, contributed to the translation of relevant evidence to inform policy and practice using open science principles. The existence of established networks and societies facilitated the rapid development of this initiative, providing the springboard for Health Psychologists to come together and work towards common goals.

Conclusion

It is clear that the discipline of health psychology has made real progress, with established networks, scientific meetings, professional journals, accredited training, and established career paths, although issues remain. As we reflect on our current position and focus on the question of professionalisation in the current context, it appears to be time to look outward, beyond the focus of the development of our shared professional networks. The purpose of professionalisation of health psychology is to realise the potential of the field through implementation of the science. Awareness and growth of the workforce, alongside registration of

Health Psychologists, regardless of their role or work setting, is crucial to this. Looking outwards now from a relatively well-developed, very well-organised, and influential core, the real challenge that faces the future of health psychology is the formal recognition of professional definitions, areas of scientific expertise, boundaries, curriculum, training, and career pathways. This speaks to the ongoing and well-documented issues of regulation, funding for education and training, employment issues, continuous professional development, supervision, and recognition of health psychology qualifications in different countries. It's now time to '*garner enough clout*' to internationalise the professionalisation of health psychology, uniting 'divisions' across the world to work together as a family.

Further Reading

Byrne, M., Gethin, N., & Swanson, V. (2017). Health Psychology Practice in Europe: Taking Stock and Moving Forward Together. *The European Health Psychologist, 19*(2), 314–320.

Chater, A. M., Shorter, G. W., Swanson, V., Kamal, A., Epton, T., Arden, M. A., Hart, J., Byrne-Davis, L., Drury, J., Whittaker, E., Lewis, L., McBride, E., Chadwick, P., O'Connor, D. B. & Armitage, C. J. (2021). Template for Rapid Iterative Consensus of Experts (TRICE). *International Journal of Environmental Research and Public Health, 18*(19), 10255. https://doi.org/10.3390/ijerph181910255

McSharry, J., Chater, A. M., Lučanin, J. D., Höfer, S., Paschali, A., & Warner, L. (2017). Health psychology education and training in countries represented in the EHPS. *European Health Psychologist, 19*(6), 375–381.

Plass, A. M., Gruszczynska, E., Andersson, S. I., & Kassianos, A. P. (2017). Health psychology practice in Europe and other countries represented in EHPS: A first step to moving forward together. *The European Health Psychologist, 19*(6), 367–374.

References

American Psychological Association. (2014) Pursuing a career in health psychology. Retrieved: https://www.apa.org/education-career/guide/subfields/health/education-training.pdf

American Psychological Association. (2022) Retrieved: https://www.apa.org/ed/graduate/specialize/health

Armstrong, S., Watson, D., Byrne, J., Howells, L., Byrne-Davis, L., Bull, E. & Brady, R. (2021). Supporting organisations to improve the psychological wellbeing of their staff during COVID-19 pandemic: Case studies. *The European Health Psychologist, 21*(1), 736–744.

Behavioural Science and Public Health Network: BSPHN (2021). Real World Behavioural Science Podcast, March 2021: #19 BSPHN Committee Leads. Retrieved: https://open.spotify.com/episode/5cJq2Zn7YKOHwx0k6iEWIB?go=1&sp_cid=cdd4870fa2e5cdc3a37a47848f6abafc&utm_source=embed_player_p&utm_medium=desktop&nd=1 [accessed 27-02-2024].

Berndt, N., Höfer, S., Kolesnikova, J., & Vilchinsky, N. (2017). Legal regulation of Health Psychology as a profession. *The European Health Psychologist, 19*(6), 390–394.

Brady, R., Bull, E., Armstrong, S., Watson, D., Lavallée, J., Cross, A., Howells, L., Byrne-Davis, L., Hart, J. & Chater, A. (2021). Translating the guidance on promoting front-line healthcare worker psychological wellbeing during COVID-19 pandemic: Psychological Needs Assessment Tool. *European Health Psychologist, 22*(1), 745–756.

Bull, E., Newman, K., Cassidy, T., Anderson, N. & Chater, A. (2020). Reflecting on the Stage 2 Health Psychology independent training route: A survey of trainee and graduate experiences of employability. *Health Psychology Update, 29*(2), 19–30.

5

FUTURE DIRECTIONS FOR THE DISCIPLINE OF HEALTH PSYCHOLOGY

Angel Marie Chater, Lucie Byrne-Davis, Elizabeth Jenkinson, and Jo Hart

Introduction

For the profession of health psychology to continuously evolve, we need to consider our history, roots, and core philosophy. We further need to embrace teachable moments, critically evaluate where we may have missed opportunities to contribute or lead and identify how we can overcome historical challenges for the discipline and profession. In doing so, we can strategically consider where we are heading and how we can work together to achieve great things. This chapter will consider the previous four chapters in this section, and offer a strategic vision of the future direction of health psychology. This will include a global view of the growth of the discipline, linking to research and the paradigms that are drawn upon, education, policy and practice. The relevance of health psychology to achieving national and international goals will be highlighted, and the need for wider funded opportunities, placements, mentoring, career pathways, and connections with stakeholders, employers, and policy will be discussed. The chapter will set the scene for future sections of the book that will discuss these issues in more detail. This chapter will end with a call to action to unite the global 'divisions' of health psychology, connecting countries to a central family tree, reducing structural barriers and silos, and optimising opportunities wherever they may lie.

Health Psychology: Its Roots, Branches, Core Strengths and Paradigms

The health psychology family tree has its foundations rooted in traditional psychology, defined in brief as the scientific study of the human mind and behaviour. Health psychology is one of the most exciting and rapidly growing branches of psychology. As a discipline that falls under the remit of the behavioural and social sciences (as described in Bunten, Constable, Chater, McManus &

 DOI: 10.4324/9781003318026-6

Chadborn, 2017; Chater, 2019; Chater, Whittaker et al., 2020; McBride et al., 2021; Public Health England, 2018), health psychology's core strengths lie in its use of the Bio-Psycho-Social Model (Engel, 1977, 1980) of health and illness, and an interdisciplinary scientist-practitioner approach (Chater, Whittaker et al., 2020). This enables the discipline to be truly holistic and evidence-based in its focus on maintaining health; preventing, treating, and coping with illness; and advancing the health-care system, taking into account biological, psychological, and social factors.

Health psychology as a discipline has developed and evolved partly in response to working with professionals from other fields, such as clinical psychology, medicine, public health, pharmacy, and biomedical science, to help understand behaviour to optimise health, reduce ill health and premature death, and enhance health-care systems (Chater, Whittaker, et al., 2020; Quinn, Chater & Morrison, 2020). Training in health psychology covers many disciplines that deal with human actions and sit under the auspices of the behavioural and social sciences, including psychology, sociology, anthropology, epidemiology, biology, economics, and political science (Chater, Whittaker, et al., 2020; McBride et al., 2021). This interdisciplinary perspective provides those trained in health psychology with the capability to develop and use complex theoretical, methodological, and analytical approaches to understand, predict, and change behaviour. Health psychology theories explain how thoughts, feelings, and automatic processes, alongside the environment and physiological factors, influence behaviour. Research methods are used from across the spectrum of qualitative, quantitative, experimental, and mixed methods approaches.

Health psychology draws from across the scientific paradigms. It can use a Postpositivist (and Positivist) paradigm drawing from a deterministic philosophy that tests assumptions through observation or measurement, most commonly aligned with quantitative research methods. However, it may also take an Interpretivist/Constructivist paradigm, more commonly associated with qualitative or mixed research methods, influenced by the philosophy of Phenomenology and the investigation of experiences and consciousness. More recently, there is growing evidence of health psychology drawing from a Pragmatic paradigm (Chater, Schulz, et al., 2022), where the researcher is not committed to any one system of philosophy or reality but instead focuses on using the most suitable research methods to address real-world research problems, which lies central to the approach. Whilst this stance can be criticised as having no philosophical loyalty, Pragmatism provides the underlying philosophical framework for mixed methods research (Tashakkori & Teddlie, 2003) and can be valuable in a real-world setting. Given its social science and political influences, health psychology is also well attuned to a person-centred approach, and the issues of equality, diversity, and inclusion (EDI). Creswell (2003) describes a Transformative paradigm that ensures the issues of social justice and factors that influence people from marginalised and underserved groups are given proper consideration. Mixed methods are again often used here, but with greater focus on a more complete presentation of the social world, through multiple perspectives, using culturally competent strategies. This is an area worthy of advancement for health psychology and all future scientific endeavours. Drawing on this eclectic set of scientific paradigms, and taking the holistic, interdisciplinary approach common to health psychology, provides the ability to develop truly transdisciplinary solutions to global problems, reaching new knowledge that one core discipline or philosophical stance alone, or many professionals working in cross-discipline silos would be unable to reach. The very fact that health psychology is built on knowledge and skills from a multitude of disciplines, taught through its core curriculum, allows it to be at the forefront of transdisciplinary science and practice.

Whilst there is evidence of the use of vast research methods, as a scientific discipline and profession, health psychology is still relatively young. Chapter 1 saw that it became a subdiscipline of psychology through the American Psychological Association (APA) in 1978, termed Division 38, and the term 'health psychology' was first coined in a textbook by Stone et al. (1979). Although, it is likely to have existed under another name before this time, as recognised by several historical accounts (Chater & Cook, 2014; Johnston, Weinman & Chater, 2011; Quinn, Chater & Morrison, 2020). Its agility to develop and use science to inform and address real-world health and societal problems on a global platform has given it an important seat at the table of scientific and applied professions. Those who work within the field are often seen as entrepreneurial, creating opportunities to advance scientific contributions and career prospects (Quinn, Chater & Morrison, 2020). However, there is still a long way to go to fully describe health psychology as 'mainstream'. Pioneers in health psychology have made one thing very clear: if we want people to know what health psychology is, we need to tell them (Quinn, Chater & Morrison, 2020).

Opportunities, Challenges, and Teachable Moments

Upon reflection of the development of health psychology as a discipline, it is important to ask whether we have missed a trick or two in voicing what health psychology is and what it can offer. This was certainly a focal point and view shared in the Oral History of Health Psychology (OHHP) Project described in Chapter 1 (Quinn, Chater & Morrison, 2020). Whilst health psychology internationally has seen great growth, there are also areas to reflect upon, critique, and correct. We have undoubtedly been too cautious in voicing the potential benefits of the application of our science to policy and practice. This is exacerbated by the lack of shared end-to-end examples of best practices, which clearly articulate the value of health psychology to those who may wish to commission or use it. This is an area for growth as we move forward as a discipline, creating impact case studies that can tangibly evidence its value.

COVID-19, whilst a global threat, created an opportunistic teachable moment on the value of the application of health psychology and its ability to generate evidence at speed (Arden, Byrne-Davis et al., 2020; Chater, Whittaker et al., 2020; Chater et al., 2021). Similar to the HIV epidemic of the 1980s, which was described as a zeitgeist for the health psychology movement in the OHHP Project (Quinn, Chater & Morrison, 2020), COVID-19 gave an opportunity for the world to see how health psychology could assist in a pandemic response when so much early on was unknown about the virus at hand.

Early in the pandemic, and throughout the course of time, the use of psychology by government and public health professionals varied, and '*following the science*' was influenced by political and economic decisions. A tongue-in-cheek article commissioned by *The Psychologist* prior to the onset of the pandemic on future outlooks of psychology (Chater, 2020) warned of the risk of psychology becoming '*a thing of the past*'. As the COVID-19 pandemic first hit the media, the article painted the picture of a robotic mechanical government unaware of psychology and behavioural science, making uninformed decisions based on habit (*what they've always done*) rather than theory or evidence, to the detriment of society. Chater (2020) highlighted the danger of a government who '*don't know what they don't know*' in a call to action to create a more psychologically informed society. She wrote:

> "*The answer … Psychology. From top-down to bottom-up, we need to be psychologically-informed. But people outside of psychology don't know what they don't know. We need a psychologically-informed society. One led by a functional psychologically-informed government that invests in training and career opportunities to see psychological professionals as important as doctors and nurses within a multidisciplinary team. To help inform policy and practice, training and service development. The leading causes of illness and death in society today can be supported by psychology. That may be through direct psychological support, to enhance mental wellness. Or through the psychological understanding and intervention with a multitude of detrimental behaviours, engagement with the health care system and professional communication. We are the voice of psychology and we need to shout louder than ever before, with gravitas*"
>
> *(p. 71 Chater, 2020)*

The ironic reality of the need for psychologically informed decision-making shone brightly in the months that followed its publication as the COVID-19 pandemic progressed. Whilst there is still a long way to go, this created an opportunity to call for and support the use of health psychology and behavioural science in government, policymaking, education, and practice at international, national, and local levels. Research confirmed that whilst people were keen to use health psychology and behavioural science within public health and health-care settings, further knowledge and skill development is needed to build capacity, alongside investment and 'buy-in' from senior leadership (Byrne-Davis et al., 2022; Chater et al., 2023; Moffat et al., 2022). In 2021, a call to action produced by the British Psychological Society (BPS, 2020) COVID-19 Behavioural Science and Disease Prevention Taskforce (McBride et al., 2021; Chater et al., 2022) was sent to policymakers in central and local governments, alongside commissioners and other key stakeholders, globally (such as the World Health Organisation), highlighting the need for investment in the use of health psychology and behavioural science, including better access to training and career pathways. Interest grew rapidly in how to employ those with a health psychology skill set.

In 2020, many countries began to mobilise health psychology expertise (Karekla et al., 2021), and journal editors highlighted the importance of health psychology during this time, calling for research contributions (Arden & Chilcot, 2020; Kazak, 2020). To ensure that health psychology was available and could be accessed by those who may benefit from it during this time, there was a need to collectivise our science, pool resources, develop mentoring, offer leadership, and amplify the voice of health psychology globally. In the United Kingdom (UK), the BPS created a COVID-19 Core Co-ordinating Group, overseeing a number of workstreams to mobilise a psychologically informed response to the pandemic. The BPS COVID-19 Behavioural Science and Disease Prevention (BSDP) Taskforce was one of these working groups. This was a cross-psychology workstream, most closely aligned to the BPS Division of Health Psychology (DHP, 2020; the UK national members' network for health psychology, chaired at the time by Professor Angel Chater). As a collective, the BSDP Taskforce aimed to build capacity to use, or at the very least consider, behavioural science, and specifically health psychology, in the prevention of infection and disease management during COVID-19. The taskforce developed a strategy to engage policymakers, practitioners, communicators, and the public in the complexity of human behaviour and behaviour change, highlighting the things that they "*may not know they don't know*". It included a core membership of 15 experts and offered ways to overcome common pitfalls in the translation of evidence to policy and public health recommendations to real-world practice. The team was guided by a forum of professionals working within a public health setting and communications with local and national government, alongside members from the World Health Organisation (WHO), all requesting behavioural insight and guidance, which was produced for a range of behaviours including hand hygiene (Byrne-Davis et al., 2020), physical distancing (Hart et al., 2021), self-isolation (Arden, Armitage, Lewis, et al., 2020), vaccination uptake (Epton, Lawes-Wickwar et al., 2020), public health messaging (Epton, Ghio et al., 2020), and using the track and trace mobile phone app (Arden, Armitage, Byrne-Davis, et al., 2020), alongside behaviours that may have been impacted by the pandemic such as physical activity (Chater, Abdin, Dryden et al., 2020), sitting (Chater, Abdin, Dryden et al., 2020), eating behaviour (Whittaker et al., 2020), smoking (Knowles et al., 2020), alcohol consumption (Shorter et al., 2020), sleep hygiene (Jenkinson et al., 2020), medication adherence (Coppin et al., 2022), opioid substitution treatment adherence (Family et al., 2022), and accessing appropriate health care (Lewis et al., 2022).

The taskforce developed the Template for Rapid Iterative Consensus of Experts (TRICE; Chater et al., 2021) and, using this methodology, produced over 20 guidance documents that can be considered as 'roadmaps' to using health psychology and behavioural science to optimise performance of a range of disease prevention behaviours. These roadmaps are evidence-based and theoretically driven and used a template for development based on the Behaviour Change Wheel (BCW: Michie et al., 2011, 2014) and the initial behavioural science guidance (Chater, Arden, Armitage et al., 2020) whereby a problem was identified, and a target behaviour to address the problem was selected and specified. A behavioural diagnosis using a COM-B analysis was then presented, based on research evidence and theoretical mapping of the influences related to Capability (e.g., knowledge, skills, memory, attention, decision processes, behavioural regulation), Opportunity (e.g., environmental context and resources, social influences), and Motivation (e.g., identity, beliefs about capabilities, beliefs about consequences, optimism, intention, goals, emotions, reinforcement) on Behaviour, ensuring that all of the domains from the Theoretical Domains Framework (TDF: Cane et al., 2012) were present. Intervention strategies, specifically the nine intervention types (namely, education, persuasion, incentivisation, coercion, training, enablement, modelling, environmental restructuring, and restrictions) and seven policy options (namely, guidelines, environmental/social planning, communication/marketing, legislation, service provision, regulation, and fiscal measures) of the BCW were recommended, and relevant literature and signposting were provided. All guidance documents were disseminated widely and have been used by a number of public health agencies in their COVID-19 response (see Chater et al., 2021; Chater, Whittakar, et al., 2020). The taskforce was forward-focused and connected with public health colleagues to identify areas of concern that would benefit from behavioural insight. It highlighted the importance of considering EDI in all decision-making and intervention development activities, highlighting that whilst we may all be in the same storm, we are not all in the same boat (Chater, Whittaker, et al., 2020). A focal point in their initial guidance (Chater, Arden, Armitage, et al., 2020) and throughout the work of the taskforce was the need to recognise factors that influence different populations, emphasising that this should be at the forefront of policy decision-making and public health campaigns at all times.

Health Psychology Communities of Practice

There are a number of communities of practice globally. One of the most diverse with global membership and representation is the European Health Psychology Society (EHPS), which in 2024 included 33 National Delegates representing health psychology in Australia, Belgium, Brazil, Bulgaria, Costa Rica, Croatia, Cyprus, Czech Republic, Denmark, Germany, Greece, Hungary, Ireland, Israel, Italy, Japan, Latvia, Luxembourg, Malta, North Macedonia, Poland, Portugal, Romania, Slovakia, Slovenia, South Africa, Spain, Sweden, Switzerland, the Netherlands, Ukraine, the UK, and the United States of America. Countries also have their own member networks and communities of practice, such as those discussed in Chapter 4, many of which are members of the European Federation of Psychologists' Associations (EFPA: https://www.efpa.eu/), which has 37 members.

Communities of practice have also emerged due to need. The Health Psychology Exchange (HPX) was a natural development in the early days of the COVID-19 pandemic that became a collective community of practice, mainly based in the UK but with contributions from across the globe. The UK already had strong connections across the four nations (England, Northern Ireland, Scotland, and Wales) and internationally through the national and European bodies representing health psychology (namely DHP, the EHPS, and EFPA). When COVID-19 became apparent in the UK in March 2020, Professor Lucie Byrne-Davis (who at the time was the future Chair of DHP), Professor Jo Hart (who at the time was the past Chair of DHP), and Professor Angel Chater (who at the time was Chair of DHP) developed this collective that brought over 155 people together. The HPX was a safe space for those with an interest or expertise in health psychology to collectivise and exchange information and mentorship through an open science framework (OSF: https://osf.io/q5n3d/) and regular online meetings. With a 'hive mind' approach, the HPX offered a crowd-sourced bank of resources, rapid reviews for evidence synthesis, scientific advancement, and academic expertise to those who requested it whilst also providing the health psychology community with a spirit of collegiality, informal mentoring, and consultancy opportunities (Armstrong et al., 2020). Over time, however, the activities during the acute stages of the COVID-19 pandemic began to dwindle due to the voluntary nature of the response and the lack of structural support and financial recompense for time allocated to the work of those within the grouping (Chater et al., 2021). Whilst the HPX still exists in spirit, it no longer meets as a collective, though the communities of practice (e.g., in public health) that developed out of it are still thriving, and academic connections still remain strong.

Developments such as the BSDP Taskforce and HPX were happening in other countries across the world too. In August 2022, the EHPS convened a synergy meeting of global experts who had led similar developments in other countries across the world titled "Behavioural Science and Public Health: Enhancing Impact through Policy and Practice during COVID-19 and Beyond". In a two-day meeting, international experts shared their contributions with case studies provided by Marta Marques (Portugal), Marijn de Bruin (Netherlands), Angel Chater (UK), Oliver Luminet (Belgium), and Molly Byrne (Ireland). A guide on how to write policy briefings was also presented by Vivi Antonopoulou, who is based in the UK National Institute for Health Research (NIHR) Policy Research Unit (PRU) in Behavioural Science (Antonopoulou et al., 2021), recently re-funded as the PRU in Behavioural and Social Sciences (https://behscipru.nihr.ac.uk/). The aim of this EHPS synergy meeting was to generate consensus on how those with expertise in health psychology across the world can work together within a policy environment and with key stakeholders in a more connected community of practice (Special Interest Group) hosted by the EHPS. The EHPS has created similar groups, such as the EHPS-UN Committee, developed to be formally associated with the United Nations (UN) and which has been granted special consultative status in the UN Economic and Social Council (ECOSOC).

Considerations should be given as to how to sustain such agile networks of experts for future rapid responses to global emergencies and how we can maintain a global health psychology community, sharing best practices from generation to generation.

Building Capacity: Education, Training, and Fair Access for Funding and Employment

Attempts have been made to map education and training opportunities globally to create a standardised level of training with shared core competencies (McSharry et al., 2017). We are yet to have an agreed global core curriculum in health psychology with the ability for those trained in one country to easily mobilise and work in another. In a report based on 27 countries from the EHPS (McSharry et al., 2017), it was found that 43/599 (7%) universities offer health psychology programmes at undergraduate level, and 87/474 (18%) universities offer master's level programmes in health psychology. In a survey of the National Delegates representing these countries, all except one agreed that there is a need for a shared and global consensus on a core curriculum in health psychology (McSharry et al., 2017). The lack of a shared curriculum hampers Health Psychologists wishing to register their skills and work globally, alongside limiting the diversity and career development of those in the field. This is an area for future development.

Two significant achievements of moving the discipline of health psychology forward with funded training are the success of the Scotland Stage 2 training route (Swanson, 2017: described in Chapter 4) and the development of the Health Education England (now called National Health Service (NHS) England) funded Stage 2 route, described in Box 5.1. It is essential for the survival of the discipline of health psychology going forward to retain accreditation-level

Box 5.1 Applying a Health Psychology Approach to Workforce Redesign

In 2022, Health Education England (HEE), now called NHS England (NHSE), launched a new programme to explore the contribution and impact of applying a health psychology approach to workforce transformation and redesign. Closely following the successful Scottish model (Swanson, 2017) and calls to action for a funded health psychology training model (Chater, 2017; Chater & Hart, 2019). Professor Lucie Byrne-Davis, Professor Jo Hart, and Professor Angel Chater worked closely with colleagues at NHSE, in particular Lucy Renwick and Kirstie Baxter, alongside Dr Adrian Whittington, National Lead for Psychological Professions, NHS England, to secure funding for a health psychology trainee (BPS Stage 2 Independent Route) in each of the seven NHSE regions. The team created a steering group, inviting Dr Liz Jenkinson to lead the development of the programme as the

National Training Director (Jenkinson, 2022), working closely with NHSE, regions, and the BPS. As a team, the steering group has been driving this programme forward in collaboration with stakeholders in seven NHS Trusts across England and a team of experienced Health Psychologist co-ordinating supervisors – namely, Dr Eleanor Bull, Dr Debbie Smith, and Professor Karen Rodham, alongside Dr Elizabeth Jenkinson and Professor Angel Chater, who each supervise one or two trainees.

This initiative was timely, and the foundations had been laid by decades of championing for funded training in the discipline (Quinn, Chater & Morrison, 2020), a call to action for funded Stage 2 training in health psychology (Chater & Hart, 2019) and the Teams Together Programme, also funded by HEE, that had supported clinical teams to implement new models of care (Bull, Byrne-Davis, et al., 2019; Bull, Hart, et al., 2019). Health psychology is recognised, valued, and included as one of the 12 psychological professions of the Psychological Professions Network (PPN: https://ppn.nhs.uk/resources/careers-map), and this initiative is a trailblazing investment. During this pilot programme, health psychology trainees will lead and deliver projects and shared learning within a two-year, fixed-term post to support the NHS in England in achieving its workforce transformation and redesign goals. They will support the development of an NHS workforce that is responsive to changes in health care by enhancing the way the NHS recruits, retains, deploys, develops, and supports the workforce to meet the growing and changing needs of local populations whilst ensuring high-quality care for patients. Behaviour change approaches, particularly the use of the BCW and COM-B model (Michie et al., 2011), are an integral part of this work, building the capacity of others within relevant organisations and systems to ensure that they are equipped and able to respond in an agile way to the new and revised models of care required in the recovery, restoration, and improvement of services.

This work is informed by research, drawing from the strength of the scientist-practitioner model of health psychology, whilst also developing and conducting research whilst in post where findings can be used within the system that the trainee is based, increasing the evidence-base and impact of health psychology in a real-world setting.

Champions of health psychology, with commissioning power, are widening the opportunities to train and employ Health Psychologists and those with training in the field to work within integrated health-care systems, in education and training, and in clinical practice. Scaling this initiative up in other areas and other countries is an area for future development.

standards of proficiency and extend funded training in the area. There can often become blurred lines between health psychology and behavioural science, and whilst there are exciting developments in both areas, there is also cause for concern with unrecognised credentials in roles that require core competencies. As a discipline, whilst we hold strength in the ability to train others to use our scientific and theoretical approaches, this should not be diluted to the point where the application by others lacks fidelity or regulation of specialised knowledge and skills. There is a need for global investment, not just in workforce redesign to train others to use health psychology but also growth in the number of those qualified in health psychology who are employed to embed their skills within organisations, systems, and workstreams.

Interest in how to fund health psychology trainees and employ a Health Psychologist has been growing, with some examples provided in Chapter 3. This has been of particular interest since the COVID-19 pandemic and the development of the Health Psychology in Public Health Network (HPPHN), now called the Behavioural Science and Public Health Network (BSPHN: discussed in Chapter 4; Chater, 2019). Yet there is still some misunderstanding of the varied roles those with health psychology expertise can perform. To support the promotion of health psychology careers, a series of 64 individual career case studies has been published (Chater, Rockliffe, Newman & Bull, 2021), featuring Health Psychologists in training, through to those in their early to mid-careers and those in senior roles. The call for the use of (Chater, Arden, Armitage, et al., 2020) and investment in (McBride et al., 2021) behavioural science and, in particular, health psychology followed requests for support in recruitment. To facilitate this, a recruitment pack was published (Bull, Dale & Chater, 2021), which includes modifiable job descriptions and person specifications to enable organisations to recruit Health Psychologists and/or Health Psychologists in training. It is currently unknown how many trainees and those qualified in health psychology there are globally. This is another area for future investigation to measure the workforce capacity and needs in terms of training posts or increased employment and leadership opportunities. It is important to get this balance right, country by country, to ensure there are stable progressions in education, training, supervision, and employability, and that one is not saturated over the other (e.g., more trainees than roles or supervisors, or more roles than those qualified to apply).

Equally, the characteristics and needs of our existing health psychology workforce are poorly understood. Whilst our discipline has shown clear application to challenging issues impacting EDI in health care and public health settings, we have yet to substantively target barriers to EDI in our profession. Professional societies and member networks for health psychology have an important role to play here, to address barriers to training and careers in health psychology on the one side and, on the other, to ensure health psychology as a discipline is considering and working in areas of EDI, where it could make an impact. This should be embedded within all directions of the future of health psychology.

The Value of Mentoring

There is a strong tradition of mentoring in health psychology, recognised in the development of the Chairs' Mentoring Award through the BPS DHP (2021) in the UK, first awarded to Professor Marie Johnston (see Box 5.2), and through

Box 5.2 The DHP's Chair's Mentoring Award – 2021

In 2020, the BPS's DHP launched the Chair's Mentoring Award. This was inspired by the unexpected death and loss to psychology of Professor Marcia Worrell in April 2020, who was the then DHP Chair's (Professor Angel Chater) former PhD supervisor and one of her esteemed mentors. The award recognises the importance of mentoring and gives people an opportunity to thank their mentors for the impact that they have had on them whilst they are still able to do so.

The first award winner was a familiar name to global health psychology, Professor Marie Johnston. Nominees gave permission for their words to be shared, and the following are just a few presented at the 2021 Annual General Meeting (Chater, presenting at the DHP AGM, 2021) that speak volumes to the value of mentoring.

> "Marie is not a mentor to just passively lean on. Her support is demanding – it is offered in a way that challenges you. As her mentee, you are always developing – always becoming better at whatever is in your best interest to be better at. Uniquely, Marie's mentoring is selfless and without ego."
>
> *(Professor Diane Dixon)*

> "Whilst working with her, I was able to see how she navigated through differences of opinion whilst sticking to her principles, and as a result I still sometimes have a "little Marie on my shoulder" who helps me see how best to approach a sticky situation, and how to work out what I and others need. When the little Marie on my shoulder can't see the way forward, the real Marie can – I am always impressed that she never answers the question I have, but reformulates the problem much more clearly and we answer that together."
>
> *(Professor Jo Hart)*

> "From the first time I met Marie, I was struck by how Marie took an interest in everyone she spoke to, encouraging us all to value Health Psychology and consider how we might contribute to this important discipline in the future.... I consider her to be my "guardian angel" – and I know I am one of many who think of her like this."
>
> *(Professor Molly Byrne)*

> "A key way in which Marie influenced my personal growth was in giving me confidence in myself."
>
> *(Dr Rachael Powell)*

> "Finally, as a woman, Marie is an inspiration – she is a role model herself of course but also a fierce advocate for other women and not afraid to be "difficult", to advocate for women and to call out the unconscious bias facing women in science. She has certainly helped me reframe my view of situations, how I define "success" and how I advocate for others (and myself). Everyone should have a Marie!"
>
> *(Dr Barbara Farquharson)*

the EHPS mentoring programme, named after Ari Haukkala, launched in 2023 (EHPS, 2023). This tradition has created a legacy of 'paying it forward', growing the discipline from generation to generation as described in the oral history of UK health psychology (Quinn, Chater & Morrison, 2020). Like the wording imprinted on the outer edge of the British £2 coin, health psychology is '*standing on the shoulders of giants*', a phrase used by Professor Susan Michie in her oral history interview with Angel Chater in 2016: "*Standing on the shoulders of giants, that's what we're all doing. We're standing on each other's shoulders. And thank goodness for those shoulders that have come before…*" (Professor Susan Michie, from Chater, Quinn & Morrison, 2019). Many in health psychology have dedicated valuable time to mentoring alongside championing opportunities in health psychology. Susan went on to say "*I remember when I became president elect of the EHPS, Marie [Johnston] saying "The first thing you need to do is think about legacy. Ensure that the right people are in place to pass the baton on to*" (Professor Susan Michie, from Chater, Quinn & Morrison, 2019). Professor Theresa Marteau affirms the importance of mentoring, stating "*[I]t's a really good way of asking the kinds of questions that you've asked but to be asking them of somebody that you admire… to learn this very qualitative way about 'how's it done'*" (Professor Theresa Marteau, from Chater, Quinn & Morrison, 2019).

However, mentoring specifically is not something traditionally taught in the health psychology curriculum, and it deserves further focus. More needs to be done to develop mentoring skills alongside supervision, leadership, and management. These skills, in addition to mentoring opportunities, relationships, and protected time to engage in such activities, are important for the strategic development and succession planning of a discipline; however, they are often neglected in both training programmes and within employment settings. Investment should be made in each country nationally and collectively as a global learned community to support the future direction of health psychology and the new generations ready to drive the discipline forward. Time for mentoring and leadership should be embedded into routine contracts, for both mentors and mentees, and supported through professional societies and member networks. Without this investment, successful health psychology departments and research centres may deteriorate and falter as leaders pass on, and with them, historical, scientific knowledge and practice will be lost. That being said, in the words of Professor Falko Sniehotta, "*I think we have an outstanding number of big mentors who have a huge influence in the career of other people*" (Professor Falko Sniehotta, from Chater, Quinn & Morrison, 2019), and as a discipline, our foundations are strong. The challenge for future health psychology is to maintain strong foundations to assist the discipline to flourish and grow.

Improving Health Psychology Impact

The impact of health psychology research and practice on global challenges can be assessed in many ways. One example is the Research Excellence Framework (REF: https://www.ref.ac.uk), which offers a helpful system to record research impact at UK higher institutions. Research outputs, impact, and environment are rated in terms of their originality, significance, and rigour in a number of Units of Assessment (UoAs), with the gold standard being classed as 'world-leading' receiving 4*, followed by 'internationally excellent' described as 3*. The two most recent REF assessment periods collated detail on research outputs, impact, and the research environment across six to seven years, presented in 2014 and 2021. When searching the REF Impact Case Study databases for the term 'health psychology', the term appeared 45 times in REF2014 and 48 times in REF2021. Focusing on the most recent REF2021, of the 48 case studies that mention health psychology, 13 specifically and directly mentioned that the case study was informed by health psychology as a discipline. The most common reason the term health psychology was used in the case studies was due to the journals that research evidence underpinning the impact was published in, with 30 case studies publishing in health psychology journals. Journals used to disseminate research included in the REF Impact Case Studies were the *Journal of Health Psychology*, the *British Journal of Health Psychology*, *Health Psychology*, the *Journal of Occupational Health Psychology*, *Health Psychology Review*, and the *International Journal of Clinical and Health Psychology*. These peer-review vehicles for dissemination clearly play a crucial role in promoting the health psychology discipline for which journal editors should be congratulated. In terms of the staff who were included in the REF2021 impact case study submissions, 14 case studies included staff that used the phrase 'health psychology' in their job titles. It should be noted, however, that several staff who are aligned and well-known in the field of health psychology did not name the discipline in their job description. This could be an easy win for future REF submissions (the next is REF2029) to ensure that health psychology is mentioned and therefore credited more widely.

The case studies presented in REF2021 included a broad scope of topic areas, such as those related to public health and safety, changing sedentary behaviour and physical activity, dietary behaviour, reducing alcohol-related harm, medication use, and promoting the health and well-being of those with long-term conditions such as cardiovascular disease, obesity, cystic fibrosis, allergies, tinnitus, Crohn's disease, dementia, cancer, and mental health concerns, such as depression, anxiety, and stress, including dental anxiety. They also included advancements in theoretical, methodological, and analytical approaches, including the BCW (Michie et al., 2011) and Interpretative Phenomenological Analysis (IPA: Smith, 2004).

Whilst these case studies showcase an excellent example of areas where health psychology has contributed to world-leading and internationally excellent impact, there are almost certainly more examples globally. As a discipline we need to get better at specifying and promoting the disciplinary roots of our work. Occupational psychology promote that they invented the tea break (BPS: https://www.youtube.com/watch?v=WYpBHLSS3lw) based on research that highlighted occupational risk without adequate breaks. These examples for health psychology will be helpful in showing the value of our discipline to commissioners, employers, colleagues, clients, current/prospective students, and the general population. Moving forward, a global database where health psychology professionals can share their impact would enable better sharing of best practices and create a stronger outward-facing message of the power of health psychology for global, societal, and health challenges.

Future Direction and Closing Thoughts

This chapter presents some key strengths of health psychology as a discipline and as a family that offers a valued identity and sense of belonging. As a profession, we are entrepreneurs who seek out opportunities and solutions through transdisciplinary approaches. It is essential that we continue to grow as a discipline together, uniting divisions globally to become stronger as a whole system and international community/family. Sharing best practices and promoting health psychology's impact whilst at the same time reducing scientific and professional silos will enable swifter developments with more secure and funded training opportunities and career prospects. Mentoring and succession planning will ensure historical knowledge is not lost, providing investment in leadership and development. The future of health psychology globally is exciting, with everything to play for. Lessons learned from the past 50 years can assist in the strategic development of the pathway forward. This section has set the scene of health psychology's past, present and future, and the importance of the advancement of the discipline. The world is our oyster.

Further Reading

Arden, M., Byrne-Davis, L., Chater, A., Hart, J., McBride, E. & Chilcot, J. (2020a). The vital role of health psychology in the response to Covid-19. *British Journal of Health Psychology*, *25*(4), 831–838. https://doi.org/10.1111/bjhp.12484

Bull, E. R., Hart, J. K., Swift, J., Baxter, K., McLauchlan, N., Joseph, S., & Byrne-Davis, L. M. (2019a). An organisational participatory research study of the feasibility of the behaviour change wheel to support clinical teams implementing new models of care. *BMC Health Services Research*, *19*(1), 1–12.

Chater, A. & Hart, J. (2019). Building capacity in behavioural science and public health using the stage 2 training route: Ideas for the development of a funded model. *Behavioural Science and Public Health*, *1*(1), 40–42.

Moffat, A., Cook, E. J., & Chater, A. M. (2022a). Examining the influences on the use of behavioural science within UK local authority public health: Qualitative thematic analysis and deductive mapping to the COM-B model and Theoretical Domains Framework. *Frontiers in Public Health*, *3742*.

References

Antonopoulou, V., McGee, O., Sniehotta, F., Lorencatto, F., Meyer, C., O'Donnell, A., Lecouturier, J., Kelly, M. P. & Michie, S. (2021). Research engagement with policy makers: a practical guide to writing policy briefs. Behavioural Science Policy Research Unit (PRU). *OSF Preprints*: https://osf.io/m25qp/

Arden, M. A., Armitage, C. J., Byrne-Davis, L., Hart, J., O'Connor, D. B., Chadwick, P., Drury J., Lewis, L., McBride, E., Perriard-Abdoh, S., Shorter, G. W., Swanson V., Thompson, S., Whittaker, E. & Chater, A. (2020). *Behavioural science and success of the proposed UK digital contact tracing application for Covid-19*. London: British Psychological Society.

Arden, M. A., Armitage, C. Lewis, L., Whittaker, E., Hart, J., O'Connor, D., Chadwick, P., Drury, J., Swanson, V., Byrne-Davis, L., McBride, E., Perriard-Abdoh, S., Shorter, G. Epton, T., Kamal, A. & Chater, A. (2020). *Encouraging self-isolation to prevent the spread of COVID-19*. Leicester: British Psychological Society.

Arden, M., Byrne-Davis, L., Chater, A., Hart, J., McBride, E. & Chilcot, J. (2020). The vital role of health psychology in the response to Covid-19. *British Journal of Health Psychology*, *25*(4), 831–838. https://doi.org/10.1111/bjhp.12484

Arden, M. A., & Chilcot, J. (2020). Health psychology and the coronavirus (COVID-19) global pandemic: A call for research. *British Journal of Health Psychology*, *25*(2), 231.

Armstrong, S., Watson, D., Byrne, J. & Howells, L. M. (2020). Teaching, training, consultancy and practice: Summaries of work relating to health psychology and Covid-19. *Health Psychology Update*, *29*, 28–29.

British Psychological Society (2020). *Being a psychologist*. Retrieved from https://www.youtube.com/watch?v=WYpBHLSS3lw

Bull, E., Dale, H., & Chater, A. (2021). *Employing trainee and qualified practitioner health psychologists: A resource pack for recruiters*. Leicester: British Psychological Society. https://cms.bps.org.uk/sites/default/files/2022-05/DHP%20job%20advertising%20resource%20pack%20%283%29.pdf

Bull, E. R., Byrne-Davis, L. M. T., Swift, J., Baxter, K., McLauchlan, N., & Hart, J. K. (2019). Exploring what teams perceive by 'culture' when implementing new models of care. *International Journal for Quality in Health Care*, *31*(6), 492–494.

Bull, E. R., Hart, J. K., Swift, J., Baxter, K., McLauchlan, N., Joseph, S., & Byrne-Davis, L. M. (2019). An organisational participatory research study of the feasibility of the behaviour change wheel to support clinical teams implementing new models of care. *BMC Health Services Research*, *19*(1), 1–12.

Bunten, A., Constable, M., Chater, A., McManus, J., & Chadborn, T. (2017). *The Role of Behavioural Sciences in Public Health. Public Health England*. Retrieved from https://www.academia.edu/32699468/The_Role_of_Behavioural_Sciences_in_Public_Health_A_Quick_Guide

Byrne-Davis, L., Chater, A., Arden, M., Armitage, C., Chadwick, P., Drury, J., Epton, T., Hart, J., Kamal, A., Lewis, L., McBride, E., O'Connor, D., Perriard-Abdoh, S., Shorter, S., Swanson, V., Whittaker, E., Kilpatrick, C. & Storr, J. (2020). *Encouraging hand hygiene in the community*. Leicester: British Psychological Society.

Byrne-Davis, L. M. T., Turner, R. R., Amatya, S., Ashton, C., Bull, E. R., Chater, A. M., Lewis, L. J. M., Shorter, G. W., Whittaker, E. & Hart, J. K. (2022). Using behavioural science in public health settings during the COVID-19 pandemic: The experience of public health practitioners and behavioural scientists. *Acta Psychologica*, *224*, 103527, ISSN 0001-6918, https://doi.org/10.1016/j.actpsy.2022.103527

Cane, J., O'Connor, D., & Michie, S. (2012). Validation of the theoretical domains framework for use in behaviour change and implementation research. *Implementation Science*, *7*, 1–17.

Chater, A. (2017). Building capacity in the workforce: How can we best use education and training to benefit public health? *Health Psychology and Public Health*, *1*(2), 2–3.

Chater, A. (2019). From Health psychology to behavioural science: Using a multidisciplinary approach to benefit public health and wellbeing. *Behavioural Science and Public Health*, *1*(1), 2–3.

Chater, A. (2020). Psychology a thing of the past? Prof-bots or a psychologically informed future? You decide. *The Psychologist*, *33*, 70–71. https://www.bps.org.uk/psychologist/psychology-thing-past

Chater, A., Arden, M., Armitage, C., Byrne-Davis, L., Chadwick, P., Drury, J., Hart, J., Lewis, L., McBride, E., Perriard-Abdoh, S., Thompson, S., Whittaker, E. & O'Connor, D. (2020). *Behavioural science and disease prevention: Psychological guidance*. Leicester: British Psychological Society.

Chater, A., Abdin, S., Dryden, J., Lewis, L., Shorter, G., Lewis, L., Hart, J., Armitage, C., Epton, T., Byrne-Davis, L., Arden, M. A., Chadwick, P., Kamal, A., Drury, J., McBride, E., O'Connor, D., Swanson, V., Thompson, S., Whittaker, E., Howlett, N. (2020). *COVID-19 Public Health Road Map: Sedentary Behaviour*. Leicester: British Psychological Society.

Chater, A. M., Brook-Rowland, P., Tolani, F., Christopher, E., Hart, J., Byrne-Davis, L. M. T., Moffat, A. Shorter, G., Epton, T., Kamal, A., O'Connor, D. B., Whittaker, E., Lewis, L. J. M., McBride, E., Swanson, V., & Arden, M. A. (2023). Understanding a constellation of eight COVID-19 disease prevention behaviours using the COM-B model and the Theoretical Domains Framework: A qualitative study using the Behaviour Change Wheel. *Frontiers in Public Health*, *11*, https://doi.org/10.3389/fpubh.2023.1130875

Chater, A., & Cook, E. (2014). *Psychology express: Health psychology*. Harlow: Pearson.

Chater, A. & Hart, J. (2019). Building capacity in behavioural science and public health using the stage 2 training route: Ideas for the development of a funded model. *Behavioural Science and Public Health*, *1*(1), 40–42.

Chater, A., Quinn, F. & Morrison, V. with Chair: Hart, J; Discussants: Johnston, M. & Weinman, J. (2019). *An oral history of health psychology. Structured Discussion. BPS Division of Health Psychology Annual Conference* (Manchester, July 2019).

Chater, A., Rockliffe, L., Newman, K. & Bull, K. (2021). *Health psychology career case studies*. Leicester: British Psychological Society https://www.bps.org.uk/sites/www.bps.org.uk/files/Member%20Networks/Divisions/DHP/DHP%20case%20studies-28Apr%202021.pdf

Chater, A. M., Schulz, J., Jones, A., Burke, A., Carr, S., Kukucska, D., Troop, N., Trivedi, D. & Howlett, N. (2022). Outcome evaluation of Active Herts: A community-based physical activity programme for inactive adults at risk of cardiovascular disease and/or low mental wellbeing. *Frontiers in Public Health*. *10*, 903109. https://doi.org/10.3389/fpubh.2022.903109

Chater, A. M., Shorter, G. W., Swanson, V., Kamal, A., Epton, T., Arden, M. A., Hart, J., Byrne-Davis, L., Drury, J., Whittaker, E., Lewis, L., McBride, E., Chadwick, P., O'Connor, D. B. & Armitage, C. J. (2021). Template for Rapid Iterative Consensus of Experts (TRICE). *International Journal of Environmental Research and Public Health*, *18*(19), 10255. https://doi.org/10.3390/ijerph181910255

Chater, A., Whittaker, E., Lewis, L., Arden, M. A., Byrne-Davis, L., Chadwick, P., Drury, J., Epton, T., Hart, J., Kamal, A., McBride, E., O'Connor, D., Shorter, G., Swanson, V. & Armitage, C., (2020). Health psychology, behavioural science, and Covid-19 disease prevention. *Health Psychology Update*, *29*(SI), 3–9.

Coppin, S., Family, H., Chapman, S., Howlett, H., Shorter, G. W., Lewis, L., Hart, J., Epton, T., Whittaker, E., O'Connor, D. B., Swanson, V., Armitage, C. J., Kamal, A., Byrne-Davis, L., Drury, J., McBride, E., Arden, M. A., Chadwick, P., & Chater, A. M. (2022). *Covid-19 public health road map: Medication adherence*. Leicester: British Psychological Society.

Creswell, J. W. (2003). *Research design: Qualitative, quantitative, and mixed methods approaches* (2nd ed.). Thousand Oaks: Sage.

Division of Health Psychology (2020). *Annual General Meeting booklet and slides.* Leicester: British Psychological Society.
Division of Health Psychology (2021). *Annual General Meeting booklet and slides.* Leicester: British Psychological Society.
Engel, G. L. (1977). The need for a new medical model: A challenge for biomedicine. *Science, 196*, 129–135.
Engel, G. L. (1980). The clinical application of the biopsychosocial model. *American Journal of Psychiatry, 137*, 535–544.
Epton, T., Ghio, D., Keyworth, C., Whittaker, E., Armitage, C. J., Hart, J., O'Connor, D., Shorter, G., Perriard-Abdoh, S., Lewis, L., Drury, J., Kamal, A., Arden, M., Byrne-Davis, L., McBride, E., Chadwick, P., Swanson, V. & Chater, A. (2020). *Delivering effective public health campaigns during Covid-19.* Leicester: British Psychological Society.
Epton, T., Lawes-Wickwar, S., Ghio, D., Shorter, G., Whittaker, E., Arden, M., Armitage, C. J., Byrne-Davis, L., Chadwick, P., Drury, J., Hart, J., Lewis, L., McBride, E., O'Connor, D., Swanson, V., Kamal, A., & Chater, A. (2020). *Optimising vaccination uptake for Covid-19.* Leicester: British Psychological Society.
European Health Psychology Society. (2023). Ari Haukkala mentoring programme. https://ehps.net/mentoring/#:~:text=The%20EHPS%20Ari%20Haukkala%20mentoring,this%20space%20for%20more%20information! [Accessed 13th February 2023].
Family, H., Chater, A. M., Linton, M.-J., Howlett, N., Gittins, R., Hines, L., Scott, J., Jenkinson, E., Swanson, V., Epton, T., Knowles, N., Abdin, S., Hart, J., Kamal, A., Byrne-Davis, Armitage, C. J., Arden, M. A., Whittaker, E., Chadwick, P., Lewis, L., O'Connor, D. B. L., Drury, J., McBride, E. & Shorter, G. W. (2022). *Covid-19 public health road map: Opioid substitution treatment (OST) adherence.* Leicester: British Psychological Society.
Hart, J., Byrne-Davis, L., Epton, T., Ghio, D., Drury, J., Armitage, C. J., Shorter, G., Arden, M. A., Chadwick, P., Kamal, A., Lewis, L., McBride, E., O'Connor, D., Swanson, V., Whittaker, E. & Chater, A. (2021). *Optimising physical distancing to reduce the spread of Covid-19: Behavioural science and disease prevention guidance for public health.* Leicester: British Psychological Society.
Jenkinson, E. (2022). *Applying a health psychology approach to workforce redesign.* https://blogs.uwe.ac.uk/research-business-innovation/communication-toolkit-health-psychology-for-workforce-transformation-programme/ [Accessed on 14th June 2023].
Jenkinson, E., Ellis, J., Chater, A., Whittaker, E., Hart, J., Byrne-Davis, L., Armitage, C., Kamal, A., Epton, T., Arden, M. A., Drury, J., McBride, E., O'Connor, D., Swanson, V., Thompson, S., Chadwick, P., Lewis, L., Shorter, G. (2020). *COVID-19 Public Health Road Map: Sleep Hygiene.* Leicester: British Psychological Society.
Johnston, M., Weinman, J. & Chater, A. (2011). A quarter century of health psychology. *The Psychologist, 24*(12), 890–902.
Karekla, M., Höfer, S., Plantade-Gipch, A., Neto, D. D., Schjødt, B., David, D., Schütz, C., Eleftheriou, A., Pappová, P. K., Lowet, K., McCracken, L., Sargautytė, R., Scharnhorst, J., & Hart, J. (2021). The role of psychologists in healthcare during the COVID-19 pandemic. *European Journal of Psychology Open, 80*(1–2), 5–17. https://doi.org/10.1024/2673-8627/a000003 [Accessed on 10th October 2023].
Kazak, A. E. (2020). Psychology is an essential science: American Psychologist highlights the role of psychology in understanding and addressing COVID-19. *American Psychologist, 75*(5), 605–606. https://doi.org/10.1037/amp0000682
Knowles, N., Chater, A., Lewis, L., Jenkinson, E., Byrne-Davis, L., Hart, J., Armitage, C., Epton, T., Arden, M. A., Kamal, A., O'Connor, D., Whittaker, E., Chadwick, P., Swanson, V., McBride, E., Thompson, S., Drury, J., Shorter, G. (2020). *COVID-19 Public Health Road Map: Stopping smoking.* Leicester: British Psychological Society.

Lewis, L., Adbin, S., Shorter, G. W., Jenkinson, E., Howlett, N., McBride, E., Hart, J., O'Connor, D. B., Arden, M. A., Armitage, C. J., Epton, T., Byrne-Davis, L., Chadwick, P., Drury, J., Kamal, A., Swanson, V., Whittaker, E. & Chater, A. M. (2022). *Covid-19 public health road map: Accessing appropriate healthcare*. Leicester: British Psychological Society.

McBride, E., Hart, J., O'Connor, D., Shorter, G., Arden, M. A., Armitage, C. J., Epton, T., Byrne-Davis, L., Chadwick, P., Drury, J., Kamal, A., Lewis, L., Swanson, V., Whittaker, E. & Chater, A. (2021). *Behavioural science investment needed to mitigate long-term health impacts of COVID-19*. Leicester: British Psychological Society.

McSharry, J., Chater, A., Lucanin, J. D., Hofer, S., Paschali, A. & Warner, L. M. (2017). Health Psychology education and training in countries represented by the EHPS. *The European Health Psychologist, 19*(6), 375–380.

Michie, S., Atkins, L., & West, R. (2014). *The behaviour change wheel. A guide to designing interventions*. 1st ed. Great Britain: Silverback Publishing.

Michie, S., van Stralen, M. M. & West, R. (2011). The Behaviour Change Wheel: A new method for characterizing and designing behaviour change interventions. *Implementation Science, 6*(42). https://doi.org/10.1186/1748-5908-6-42

Moffat, A., Cook, E. J., & Chater, A. M. (2022). Examining the influences on the use of behavioural science within UK local authority public health: Qualitative thematic analysis and deductive mapping to the COM-B model and Theoretical Domains Framework. *Frontiers in Public Health, 3742*.

Public Health England. (2018). *Improving People's Health: Applying Behavioural and Social Sciences to Improve Population Health and Wellbeing in England*. London: Public Health England.

Quinn, F., Chater, A & Morrison, V. (2020). An oral history of UK Health Psychology. *British Journal of Health Psychology. 25*(3), 502–518. https://doi.org/10.1111/bjhp.12418

Shorter, G., Knowles, N., Abdin, S., Jenkinson, E., Armitage, C., Epton, T., Hart, J., Kamal, A., Byrne-Davis, L., Arden, M. A., Whittaker, E., Chadwick, P., Lewis, L., O'Connor, D., Swanson, V., Drury, J., Thompson, S., McBride, E., Chater, A. (2020). *COVID-19 Public Health Road Map: Alcohol Consumption*. Leicester: British Psychological Society.

Smith, J. A. (2004) Reflecting on the development of interpretative phenomenological analysis and its contribution to qualitative research in psychology. *Qualitative Research in Psychology, 1*(1), 39–54.

Stone, G. C., Adler, N. E. & Cohen, F. (1979). *Health psychology: A handbook: Theories, applications, and challenges of a psychological approach to the health care system*. San Francisco: Jossey-Bass.

Swanson, V. (2017). Adding value to health in Scotland: Big contributions from a small training programme for health psychologists. *Health Psychology in Public Health, 1*(2), 3–4.

Tashakkori, A. & Teddlie, C. (2003). *Handbook of mixed methods in social and behavioural research*. London: Cassell.

Whittaker, E., Howlett, N., Abdin, S., Chadwick, P., Shorter, G., Hart, J., Armitage, C., Epton, T., Byrne-Davis, L., Arden, M. A., Kamal, A., Lewis, L., Drury, J., McBride, E., O'Connor, D., Swanson, V., Thompson, S. & Chater, A. (2020). *COVID-19 Public Health Road Map: Eating Behaviour*. Leicester: British Psychological Society.

SECTION 2

Theories and Methodology

6

HOW TO WORK WITH THEORIES OF HEALTH BEHAVIOUR CHANGE

Lisa Marie Warner and Ines Pfeffer

Introduction

Unhealthy lifestyles are a serious public health problem globally. Even after decades of research, explaining and changing health behaviours are still a challenge. This chapter explains how theories of behaviour change evolve, and some of the most prominent theories of behaviour change are briefly described. The term *health behaviours* includes all behaviours that impact health in a good way – so-called *health-promoting behaviours* (e.g., exercise, healthy nutrition, vaccination, attendance at health screenings) – or a bad way – so-called *health-risk behaviours* (e.g., smoking, unprotected sex or sun exposure). Health behaviours are a function of a person and their environment. When we think about our health behaviours, we often use our own concepts, such as "My *willpower* diminished", or "I just lost *faith in myself* to maintain jogging". To build and test a theory about determinants that actually play a part in most peoples' health behaviours, these determinants need to be defined, and "how" and "why" they affect health behaviours needs to be described. Any health psychological theory hence (1) includes defined and measurable determinants and (2) allows deducting testable causal associations between these determinants and health behaviours.

In the last decades, theories to explain health behaviours were developed and empirically tested abundantly. In this chapter, we explain the evolution of such theories; describe a few of the numerous available theories of health behaviour change; provide guidance on *why* to use them, *how* to *choose*, *use*, and *test* them; and end with some critical perspectives on past and current psychological theorising forward.

 DOI: 10.4324/9781003318026-8

How Theories Emerge and Evolve

One of the aims of health psychology is to *explain* and *promote* health-enhancing behaviours and reduce health-risk behaviours. Most of these behaviours require sustained effort to yield health effects – e.g., involve several steps to prepare, initiate and maintain them – so long-term behaviour change is difficult for most people. Therefore, laypeople and researchers alike wonder what it takes to initiate and maintain health behaviours. Often, personal observations or scientific experiments of a phenomenon spark ideas of what could contribute to acting healthily or unhealthily (e.g., "When I see my friends smoking, my urge to smoke becomes maddening"). In the *observation phase* of the so-called *empirical cycle* (Figure 6.1) to test these ideas, the generation and formulation of new and specific phenomena, patterns or relationships is the primary objective (hypothetico-deductive method; de Groot, 1956/2014).

In the *induction* phase, these observations are formulated more generally – an induction is made about associations assumed to hold for everyone in principle (e.g., "smoking likelihood increases if smokers perceive social cues to smoke") – now a theory has emerged. To test this new theory, predictions need to be made about the phenomena, patterns, or relationships induced in the *deduction* phase. Such testable sentences are called *hypotheses* (e.g., "self-reported urges and videotaped smoking behaviour increase, if smokers see others smoking"). As it is not sufficient for scientific research to formulate intuitively plausible hypotheses from one-time observations, hypotheses must be checked against *empirical data* (e.g., systematic observations or self-reports under naturally occurring or manipulated conditions, see Chapter 8, "Research Design: Overview and Recommendations"). In the deduction phase, plans are made for *how* to test the hypotheses. In this phase, potentially involved psychological concepts – the

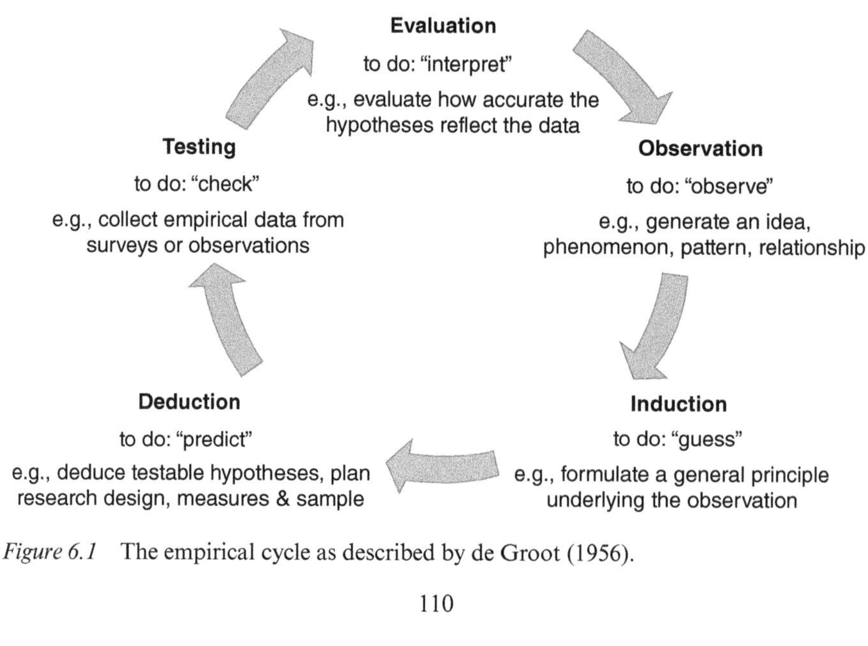

Figure 6.1 The empirical cycle as described by de Groot (1956).

so-called *social-cognitive constructs* or *determinants* of behaviour – are named and defined (e.g., the concept "*urges*" is measurable through self-report questionnaires; see Chapter 9, "Measurement in Health Psychology"). Thus, in the deduction phase, a research design to test the hypotheses is specified.

In the *testing phase*, empirical data is collected, and statistical tests are performed to check the hypotheses' accuracy in predicting the patterns found in the collected data (e.g., smoking likelihood should be higher when smokers observe others smoke). In the final *evaluation phase*, the patterns found in the empirical data are compared to the predictions derived from the theory. It is hence interpreted how accurate the hypotheses were in predicting the observed patterns and whether the hypotheses need to be adjusted or tested under different conditions (e.g., different contexts, samples). If the hypotheses derived from the theory hold up to empirical testing, the scientific belief in the theory is strengthened. However, a whole theory cannot be *proven*, as the statistical tests are usually based on the interpretation of probabilities. Furthermore, the independent manipulation of several constructs of a theory and testing the effects on behaviour is challenging and complex. One empirical cycle can only offer provisional support for a theory before more knowledge is accumulated in further cycles. Behaviour change theories have therefore been described to

> summarise what is known about *constructs* in the process of change, attempt to explain and predict *when*, *why* and *how* behaviour (change) occurs or does not occur, in addition to proposing both *mechanisms of action* and *moderators of change* along various *causal pathways*.
>
> *(Michie et al., 2018, p. 502)*

Why Use Theories?

Using theories for health psychological research and intervention programmes and explicitly stating them brings several benefits to advance knowledge in behavioural science (Bartholomew & Mullen, 2011; Dalgetty et al., 2019):

Theories...

- span a framework, which helps identifying specific determinants of behaviour change but also supports the consideration of other important factors for a behaviour;
- provide a common language and therefore enable the accumulation of empirical evidence;
- describe logical and causal links between constructs and changes in behaviour;
- help selecting methods and modes of delivery for interventions;
- support evaluation and reporting of the results in terms of predefined change objectives and theoretical mediating constructs (active ingredients of the intervention); and
- allow the deduction of hypotheses if novel health threats occur or new or uncertain contexts are to be investigated.

Given these advantages of theoretically based projects, it is logical to think that the use of theories increases the effectiveness of health behaviour change interventions. However, empirical evidence does not (yet) show a strong link between the naming of a theoretical foundation and the strength of the evidence derived from a study. For example, systematic meta-reviews on intervention studies across multiple health behaviours (Dalgetty et al., 2019) and physical activity (Rhodes et al., 2017) did not find support for the hypothesis that programmes are more effective if they mention a theory guiding intervention development. This can either mean that theoretical foundations are still weak or that intervention developers (e.g., researchers, practitioners, policymakers) overlook mentioning the theoretical basis they used explicitly or even *implicitly* (e.g., by remembering formal theories, Dalgetty et al., 2019).

In an effort to accelerate behaviour science (instead of inventing the wheel over and over again, e.g., new names for similar determinants), the use of common labels and transparent reporting of theoretical foundations is well justified. However, as some authors criticise, theories provide a 'menu' of potentially relevant constructs, but they do not specify which ones are the most effective if targeted in interventions (Rothman & Sheeran, 2020). After giving an overview of some prominent theories of behaviour change, we will therefore come back to how to choose the theory that best fits the research question or health problem to tackle.

Prominent Theories in Health Psychology

One broad distinction among health behaviour change theories is whether they focus on processes *outside the individual* (e.g., ecological models) or influences from *within the individual* (e.g., suggesting social-cognitive constructs). For recent overviews of the following theories, how to use them and how effective they have proven in empirical research, see the *Handbook of Behaviour Change* by Hagger et al., 2020.

Theories Focusing on Context

Ecological models define individual health behaviours as being embedded in and shaped by social, community, organisational, and policy layers surrounding the individual. Several such models have been defined, some for explaining behaviour in general (e.g., miso,- meso-, exo-, macrosystem influences; Bronfenbrenner, 1977) and others for health behaviours (e.g., intrapersonal, interpersonal, institutional, community, public policy level; McLeroy et al., 1988). The central notion of ecological models is that influencing individual factors alone will not change behaviour without changing external factors, such as accessibility, availability, attractiveness, or pricing in individuals' environments. One such model was proposed by Dahlgren and Whitehead (2021), specifying the association between the individual, the environment, and health. The authors distinguish between four layers of determinants influencing each other and, finally, health: (1) biology (e.g., age, sex, constitution), (2) individual lifestyles (e.g., physical activity, diet, sleep), (3) social and community networks (e.g., social support, marital status), and (4) general socio-economic, cultural, and environmental conditions (e.g., education, work environment, health care services). This model posits that lifestyles are substantially structurally determined and that links between the social, economic, and cultural determinants and those of lifestyle (i.e., health behaviour) should be examined more intensively.

Another perspective of social influences on health behaviours is *social practice theories* (Blue et al., 2016). Social practices are behavioural patterns differing at specific *times* and *places* (e.g., “morning cigarette”, “work-break-cigarette”). According to this approach, targeting social determinants in specific settings would lead to reflective but also automatic individual change (e.g., if drinking alcohol at work events becomes forbidden, social practices of drinking at work become less normalised; just as smoking in public buildings became unthinkable after smoking bans).

Ecological models suggest changing peoples’ environments as well as how they interact with them to prompt health behaviour change. One such behaviour change strategy in public policymaking has become popular under the name of *nudging*, which aims at changing choice architectures, e.g., by making healthier food choices more easily available or presenting them more prominently. Many ecological models provide very good frameworks to help detect enabling or hindering factors in individuals’ environments and to embed and implement health behaviour interventions into contexts. As they less often name specific variables to change and mechanisms of action toward behaviour change, they are often used in addition to theories that focus on processes within the individual.

Theories Focusing on Processes within the Individual

Continuum Models

The most prominent theories in health psychology are those that aim to explain and change health behaviours by means of defining social-cognitive determinants (e.g., self-efficacy) that are thought to predict health behaviour. The more pronounced the determinant is, the more likely the behaviour will be performed. Models assuming such a linear relationship between determinants and behaviour are called *continuum models*. If environmental determinants are named in these approaches, they are usually conceptualised as being filtered through the lens of the individual (e.g., degree of individual *knowledge* of healthy food choices). Theories focusing on the individual can be classified along numerous axes – e.g., whether they focus on *building* or *executing* intentions (i.e., motivational vs. volitional models), on *reflective* or *habitual* determinants of behaviour (or both in dual-process theories), define behaviour change as a *process* with distinct mindsets (e.g., stage/process models), or *integrate* several of the aforementioned approaches (*integrated models*).

The most frequently used individual theories are *motivational theories* (Michie et al., 2014b; Pfeffer et al., 2023). They primarily focus on explaining how conscious decisions towards changing behaviour develop, hence how *intentions* are built. These models assume intentions to be the most important determinant of behaviour, define social-cognitive constructs to predict intentions, and posit that behaviour change happens, if any or all determinants increase. Prominent representatives of this category are the *reasoned action approach* (RAA; Fishbein & Ajzen, 2009), *social-cognitive theory* (SCT; Bandura, 2004), and *self-determination theory* (SDT; Deci & Ryan, 1985).

In the current conceptualisation of the *RAA*, intentions are built upon favourable *attitudes* (i.e., beliefs about behavioural consequences) and *subjective norms* (i.e., beliefs about what important others appreciate) if the individual has also established *perceived behavioural control* (i.e., their beliefs in capability to perform the behaviour). Intentions are the most proximal determinant of behaviour, which can only be implemented if *actual* behavioural control is present (external barriers/facilitators). Other (e.g., biological, social, environmental, economic, cultural) influences are hypothesised to affect behaviour via one of the theory's variables.

SCT differs from other continuum models in its emphasis on *self-efficacy* – belief in one's capabilities to perform an action required to attain a desired outcome. Together with *outcome expectancies* – beliefs about the consequences of behaviours – they determine *goals* (i.e., intentions) that precede behaviour. Self-efficacy can also have a direct impact on behaviour and is assumed to derive from the four main sources: mastery experiences, vicarious experiences, verbal persuasion, physiological and affective states, which can each be targeted in interventions. A special feature is the explicit mentioning of socio-structural influences, which may either be filtered through individual cognitions or function as direct facilitators and impediments (e.g., health systems, Bandura, 2004).

A much broader theoretical scope is taken by *SDT*, which posits that the three basic human motives of *autonomy*, *competence*, and *relatedness* guide motivation and behaviour. This theory focuses on the *quality* of motivation and suggests that individuals can be *autonomously motivated* – when they freely choose a goal – or *controlled motivated*, e.g., due to social pressures. *Autonomously motivated* behaviour change is expected to be more effective, along with goals that make people feel *competent* and *related* to others.

Stage and Process Models

One major disadvantage of continuum models is that they are good at explaining intentions but much less so at helping individuals overcome the *intention-behaviour gap* – the phenomenon that often intentions are not translated into behaviours (Sheeran, 2002). Stage models, in contrast, propose that it is not enough to build intentions but that people move between qualitatively different psychological mindsets – the so-called *stages of behaviour change* (Figure 6.2): different cognitions are prevalent, and different intervention strategies are needed in different phases of the behaviour change process. A common postulation of stage models is that building an intention is an important first step but that this *motivational phase* needs to be followed by a *volitional phase* in which behaviour

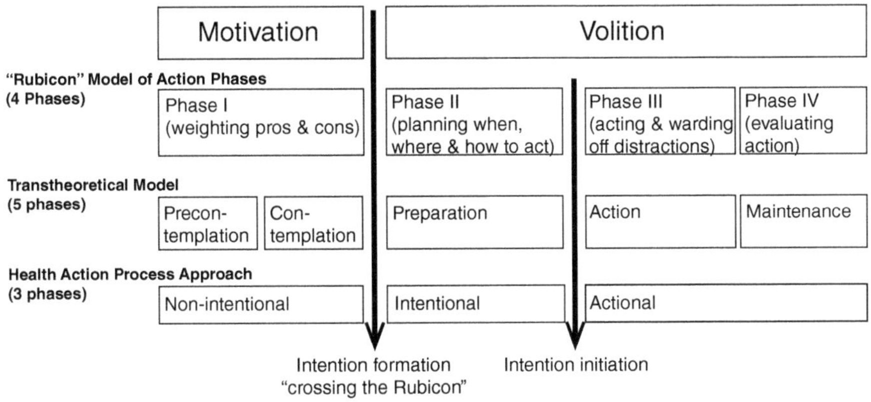

Figure 6.2 Example stage models of behaviour change positing that once an intention is built, individuals enter the volitional mindset (like crossing the river Rubicon revealed Caesar's intentions).

initiation is prepared and planned. One of the first models to propose these two overarching phases was the *"Rubicon" model of action phases* (Heckhausen & Gollwitzer, 1987). According to this and other stage models, building intentions concerns the "why" question (i.e., reasons to make a decision), whereas pursuing intentions needs a "how" oriented approach. Initiating and maintaining behaviour change is assumed to work best if *implementation intentions* are formulated ("if-then"-plans, e.g., "if situation X comes up, then I will perform behaviour Y") to plan *when*, *where*, and *how* the behaviour will be shown. This behaviour change strategy helps recognising *situational cues* (e.g., good opportunities to act, risky situations to avoid) upon which the previously planned behavioural response is enacted more easily than without planning (Hagger et al., 2020).

A prominent stage model developed in the clinical context is the *transtheoretical model* (TTM; Prochaska & DiClemente, 1982). In the TTM, individuals move along the five stages of pre-contemplation, contemplation, preparation, action, and maintenance. Several *experiential* and *behavioural processes of change* (e.g., consciousness raising, stimulus control) are defined that are assumed to prompt progress through the stages.

A hybrid model combining ideas from continuum models and stage models is the *health action process approach* (HAPA, Schwarzer, 1992). It posits that *risk perception* (e.g., awareness of risks of a sedentary lifestyle), *outcome expectancies*, and *self-efficacy* determine intentions, which translate into behaviour via *action planning* (when/where/how to act), *coping planning* (how to overcome difficulties), and *action control* (e.g., self-monitoring of progress). Individuals without intention are in the *pre-intender phase*; those who develop an intention in the *intender phase*, and those who initiate the behaviour are called *actors*. Self-efficacy plays a central role in the HAPA by differentiating between *action*, *coping* and *recovery* self-efficacy along the stages. Also, barriers and resources (e.g., social support) are included as moderators in the HAPA.

One assumed advantage of stage models over continuum models is that stage-matched interventions are more parsimonious as they are better tailored to individuals' needs by only targeting constructs relevant to the current phase. For example, there is no need to provide information about the negative consequences of smoking for people in the preparation stage, as they already decided to quit. Empirical evidence on whether stage-matched approaches are superior is, however, limited (Romain et al., 2018). Another critique is that stages might not represent qualitatively different mindsets but describe continuous processes, e.g., steadily increasing intentions (Warner & Lippke, 2008).

Integrative and Dual-Process Models and Models for Specific Domains

Most individual health behaviour change theories assume rationally built intentions that are enacted if conscious preparatory efforts are successful. Such a well-thought-through process can be the case for one-time health behaviours, where individuals act upon very strong intentions, e.g., buying a new toothbrush. However, for long-term behaviour change, where new behaviours need to be kept up under strong contextual influences, people do not always act rationally upon their intentions. For example, snack binges despite plans to diet or unprotected sex on a one-night stand seldom represent rational decisions.

Dual-process or dual systems theories offer a framework to understand such *impulses* in addition to *reflective* choices. The most prominent is the *reflective-impulsive model* (RIM; Strack & Deutsch, 2004). As the *reflective system* comprises deliberate cognitive processes – e.g., decisions based on attitudes and capability beliefs – it relies on the availability of cognitive resources to control behaviour. It is therefore comparatively slower, effortful, and less efficient than the *impulsive system*, which operates with little cognitive capacities and enables fast, automatic behavioural responses (e.g., snacking crisps as "default" while watching TV). The impulsive system can activate behavioural schemata, even in circumstances in which individuals possess low mental capacities, e.g., tiredness, distractedness, drunkenness, time pressure. These habit-like processes are assumed to be activated upon *internal* (e.g., hunger, mood) or *external cues* (e.g., situations, odours, social norms) learned by positive evaluation and repetition in the past (e.g., pleasant memories of deliciously tasting crisps in front of TV activating snacking). The development of implicit cue-behaviour links hence routes in learning theory of classical and evaluative conditioning (e.g., foremost unconditioned stimulus of the TV becomes conditioned stimulus to activate conditioned behaviour of snacking). According to dual-process models, health behaviours with automatic cue-response associations can be less effectively changed by RAAs but need *stimulus control strategies* (e.g., avoiding bars, work breaks, or stress-triggering smoking), *reward reductions* for behaviours (e.g., nicotine patches to reduce immediate pleasantness of smoking), or *counterconditioning* (e.g., chewing a nicotine gum, approach/avoidance trainings) until new behaviours are established. Whether the impulsive or reflective system is activated depends on boundary conditions such as working memory capacity or habitualness of the behaviour (see Hofmann, Friese & Wiers, 2008); however, at least considering impulsive in addition to reflective processes should make behaviour change efforts more effective.

Integrative theories combine constructs and mechanisms from multiple theories to more effectively predict health behaviour, be more parsimonious, reduce redundancies, or address weaknesses in existing theories. Some integrative theories have summarised core constructs of individual motivational theories (e.g., COM-B model, see the following section); others extended previous theories with pathways of less deliberative cognitive processes. The *prototype willingness model* (Gibbons & Gerrard, 1997), for example, assumes a *social-reactive pathway* with influences on *willingness* to perform a health behaviour formed upon the desire to resemble *prototypes* (influential role models are viewed as similar and favourable) in addition to a *reasoned route* (with social-cognitive constructs). The *integrated behaviour change model* (Hagger & Chatzisarantis, 2014) extended the TPB with *autonomous* and *implicit* forms of *attitudes* and *motivation* that represent a *nonconscious route* besides a *reasoned route* while also adopting the motivational and volitional phase from stage models.

Most of the previously named theories have been used to explain different health behaviours but there are also theories that focus on specific health problems, such as theories of specific health behaviours (e.g., the *physical activity adoption and maintenance (PAAM) model*, Strobach et al., 2020), multiple health behaviour change (e.g., see Chapter 13), illness perception and self-regulation (see Chapter 7), self- or group-identity processes (*identity-value model*; *social identity approach*), effects of *social support* on health, or various models on the development and outcomes of *loneliness*.

However, with more than 100 theories focusing on behavioural *maintenance* alone (Kwasnicka et al., 2016) – how to choose a theory?

How to Choose Theories

It has been argued that some of the most common determinants of intentions and behaviour are very similar – attitudes and outcome expectations, for example, go back to evaluations of behavioural outcomes, also perceived behavioural control and self-efficacy both describe subjective capabilities (Lippke & Ziegelmann, 2008; Rothman & Sheeran, 2020). The *theoretical domains framework* (TDF; Michie, Atkins, & West, 2014a) summarises typical components of behaviour change theories in an integrated meta-theory and defines and categorises them into the overarching *COM-B model*. COM-B postulates that ***behaviour*** is based on ***capability***, ***opportunity***, and ***motivation*** (Figure 6.3).

Considering that no theory includes all constructs, routes, or phases that might be needed to explain behaviour change, assessing the (subjective) realities of (new) target groups is an important step. To determine which of the

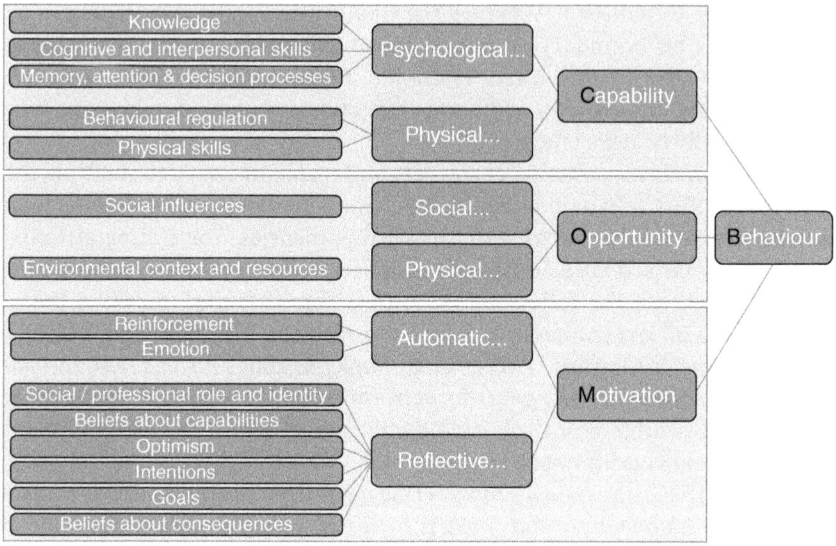

Figure 6.3 COM-B model linked to the TDF (own graphical re-design of the behaviour change wheel, Figure 1.7, page 92 in Michie, Atkins, & West, 2014a).

constructs would need to be targeted to change the health behaviour in a specific context and population, the TDF offers questions, e.g., "What do you think will happen if you do the behaviour?" to elicit beliefs about consequences, or "Do you know how to behave?" to elicit whether cognitive, social, and physical skills are available to the specific population (Michie, Atkins, & West, 2014a). Integrated into the *behaviour change wheel*, the *COM-B model* summarises knowledge on health behaviour change and links it to implementation science and policymaking (e.g., to public regulations, policies, social and environmental planning). This method might result in choosing multi-theory approaches to plan complex health behaviour change interventions (see Chapter 29, "Health Behaviour Change Interventions").

Endeavours to change health behaviour can broadly be categorised into being theory-driven or problem-driven. *Theory-driven* research focuses on explaining the psychological processes involved in changing or maintaining health behaviours and usually follow the *empirical cycle* (focus on testing hypotheses). A pragmatic approach for *problem-driven* projects can be to choose particularly effective *behaviour change techniques* (BCTs) for the target behaviour and population from the scientific literature (e.g., self-monitoring, planning, Michie et al., 2009) and refer back to theories that contain these BCTs in order to review further determinants these theories suggest (not focusing on testing *one* theory, as no theory explains all variance in a certain behaviour anyway; see Ruiter & Crutzen, 2020, as well as Rahaman, Ramos, Harter, & Mosler, 2022, for examples).

How to Use Theories

Practitioners often use a rather *problem-driven approach* that starts by analysing the problem at hand (e.g., low hand hygiene in hospitals, a health-compromising youth trend), followed by applying theory to build interventions that lessen this problem. This approach does not focus on confirming theoretical assumptions or improving theories but evaluates its effectiveness in terms of the reduction of the health problem. It still provides useful insights into health psychological theory building as it tests the *ecological validity* of theories, hence whether they generalise to different behaviours, contexts (e.g., schools, hospitals, online programmes) and populations (e.g., cultures, life phases, minorities). As a starting point, systematic approaches to intervention planning and evaluation are very useful (e.g., *intervention mapping*, *behaviour change wheel*, *PRECEDE-PROCEED*). Based on needs assessments, these approaches incorporate at least one step in which associations between relevant and changeable determinants and behaviours are identified on a theoretical basis, and specific BCTs targeting these determinants are selected.

Once an explicit theoretical foundation has been selected and the study or programme conducted, empirical data on whether and how this theory 'performed' can be analysed. In order to undertake confirmatory (hypothesis-testing) research, well-derived hypotheses from the chosen theory should be pre-registered (Kwasnicka et al., 2021). Pre-registering hypotheses together with study methods and plans for statistical analyses has many advantages and ensures that the predictions are informed by the theory only without knowledge of what the data reveal (see Osborne & Norris, 2022 for open science in health psychology, and Chapter 8, "Research Design: Overview and Recommendations" in this volume).

If the theory does not predict or change the behaviour, one possible conclusion would be that the theory is wrong. However, many other reasons can lead to lacking effects, for example, that a specific theory does not generalise to the tested behaviours, context, delivery methods, or population, that it does not specify concrete BCTs to change its theoretical constructs, also suboptimal measurement, or strong comparison groups can lead to small effects (for further possibilities, see Dalgetty et al., 2019). Based on empirical findings, some of the aforementioned theories were reworked over the years; for example, the TPB derived from the *theory of reasoned action* that lacked the construct of perceived behavioural control. Also, TPB explicitly mentions *interactions*, not just additive effects between its constructs in its latest version. To systematically test theoretical foundations for effective interventions, the aforementioned frameworks help define the boundary conditions under which theories should be able to produce meaningful effects with measurable outcomes (see Chapter 9 in this volume).

Critical Perspectives on Behaviour Change Theories and Ways Forward

Critical perspectives on health behaviour change theories are not new (Lippke & Ziegelmann, 2008). Motivational theories assuming rational choices were criticised for overlooking affective, habitual, and externally triggered behaviours, as well as their lack of consideration of *time* as an explicit variable (Scholz, 2019). One theory to integrate time is the *temporal self-regulation theory* (Hall & Fong, 2007), which specifies a *motivational sphere* (including classic social-cognitive variables), but models a *momentary sphere* as well. In this momentary sphere, the ecological context, such as acute urges or cues from the environment that trigger behaviours, is considered.

As individuals have limited time and energy at their disposal, goal priorities might need to be considered in future theories (health-related intentions often compete with other intentions, e.g., exercising and studying both require time; Hagger et al., 2020). In order to understand dynamically changing determinants and varying self-regulatory capacities, more and more momentary ecological assessment studies, as well as just-in-time interventions, have been conducted to help overcome momentary challenges (see Chapter 9, "Research Design: Overview and Recommendations" and Nahum-Shani et al., 2015). Stage theories, on the other hand, have been criticised for supposedly arbitrary stage categorisation on time criteria (TTM suggested that the maintenance stage would be reached after six months of action), possibly also masking continuous progress (Warner & Lippke, 2008). A lot of this critique has been taken up by theory modifications and integrations, as well as by the development of dual-process and temporal theories.

Other critiques concern the *measurability* of determinants of behaviour change because only a few theories explicitly publish accompanying guidelines for questionnaire constructions, such as the RAA (see https://a-bc.gitlab.io/dct-raa/ and Chapter 9). Debates on overlap between outcome expectancies, self-efficacy, and intention measures, for example, lead to more refined questionnaire items.

More precise *reporting* of BCTs was enabled by BCT taxonomies (Michie et al., 2009); however, the categorisation, homogenisation and focusing on processes *within* individuals was critiqued for bearing the risk of losing theoretical variability and professional flexibility to produce practically relevant behaviour change (Ogden, 2016).

Chalabaev et al. (2023) advocate focusing more on *diverse populations* and *contexts* in which theories of behaviour change effectively explain and predict health behaviour. Or as Chamberlain and Lyons state, "[I]n attempting to develop universal theories, much behaviour change research has been the subject of ongoing critique for side-lining the social contexts in which people live their lives" (p. 432; Chamberlain & Lyons, 2020). Using theories that put individuals into context, explicitly investigating health inequalities due to environmental, structural, or socio-economic barriers, as well as being open to participatory approaches might stimulate new perspectives.

Psychological theorising in general has been criticised for focusing heavily on *testing* instead of *formally developing* theories in a mathematical, computational, or systems theories manner (Borsboom et al., 2021). An approach to overcome this shortfall is to aim for collective theory-building units, such as establishing a sub-discipline of *theoretical health psychology* instead of rebranding old constructs and processes over again. This might help overcome the *toothbrush problem*, meaning that "[p]sychologists treat other peoples' theories like toothbrushes – no self-respecting person wants to use anyone else's" (Mischel, 2008; p.1, para. 3). New theories should either be formulated more formally (more precisely), be broader in scope, and/or more parsimonious, close knowledge gaps, or offer new perspectives, such as concrete information about mediators (e.g., active ingredients) or moderators (e.g., time, context, populations), and take health inequalities and contextual boundary conditions into account. Building new or modified theories will advance scientific progress best if guidelines for psychological theory building in general (Borsboom et al., 2021) and theory description in health psychology are used (Michie et al., 2014b), open science principles implemented (Kwasnicka et al., 2021), and criteria for assessing theory quality applied (Davis et al., 2015), while keeping an open mind to the development of new health BCTs that might feedback into theorising – so not an easy task.

Further Reading

Hagger, M. S., Cameron, L. D., Hamilton, K., Hankonen, N., & Lintunen, T. (2020a). *The handbook of behavior change*. Cambridge University Press.

Michie, S., Campbell, R., Brown, J., & West, R. (2014). *ABC of behaviour change theories*. Silverback Publishing.

Sallis, J. F., Owen, N., & Fisher, E. (2015). Ecological models of health behavior. In K. Glanz, B. K. Rimer, & K. Viswanath (Eds.), *Health behavior: Theory, research, and practice* (5th ed., pp. 43–64). John Wiley & Sons.

References

Bandura, A. (2004). Health promotion by social cognitive means. *Health Education & Behavior*, *31*(2), 143–164. https://doi.org/10.1177/1090198104263660

Bartholomew, L. K., & Mullen, P. D. (2011). Five roles for using theory and evidence in the design and testing of behavior change interventions. *Journal of Public Health Dentistry*, *71*(1), 20–33. https://doi.org/10.1111/j.1752-7325.2011.00223.x

Blue, S., Shove, E., Carmona, C., & Kelly, M. P. (2016). Theories of practice and public health: Understanding (un)healthy practices. *Critical Public Health*, *26*(1), 36–50. https://doi.org/10.1080/09581596.2014.980396

Borsboom, D., van der Maas, H. L., Dalege, J., Kievit, R. A., & Haig, B. D. (2021). Theory construction methodology: A practical framework for building theories in psychology. *Perspectives on Psychological Science*, *16*(4), 756–766. https://doi.org/10.1177/1745691620969647

Bronfenbrenner, U. (1977). Toward an experimental ecology of human development. *American Psychologist*, *32*(7), 513–531. https://doi.org/10.1037/0003-066X.32.7.513

Chamberlain, K., & Lyons, A. (2020). Critical and Qualitative Approaches to Behavior Change. In M. S. Hagger, L. D. Cameron, K. Hamilton, N. Hankonen, & T. Lintunen (Eds.), *The Handbook of Behavior Change* (pp. 430–442). Cambridge University Press. https://doi.org/10.1017/9781108677318.030

Chalabaev, A., Cheval, B., Maltagliati, S., Saoudi, I., & Sniehotta, F. (2023). Beyond individual cognitions: Time for intervention science to focus on health context and audience. *Journal of Physical Activity and Health*, *20*(6), 465–470. https://doi.org/10.31234/osf.io/khw6a

Dahlgren, G., & Whitehead, M. (2021). The Dahlgren-Whitehead model of health determinants: 30 years on and still chasing rainbows. *Public Health*, *199*, 20–24. https://doi.org/10.1016/j.puhe.2021.08.009
Dalgetty, R., Miller, C. B., & Dombrowski, S. U. (2019). Examining the theory-effectiveness hypothesis: A systematic review of systematic reviews. *British Journal of Health Psychology*, *24*(2), 334–356. https://doi.org/10.1111/bjhp.12356
Davis, R., Campbell, R., Hildon, Z., Hobbs, L., & Michie, S. (2015). Theories of behaviour and behaviour change across the social and behavioural sciences: A scoping review. *Health Psychology Review*, *9*(3), 323–344. https://doi.org/10.1080/17437199.2014.941722
Deci, E. L., & Ryan, R. M. (1985). *Intrinsic motivation and self-determination in human behavior*. New York: Plenum Press.
De Groot, A. D. (1956/2014). The meaning of "significance" for different types of research [translated and annotated by eric-jan wagenmakers, denny borsboom, josine verhagen, rogier kievit, marjan bakker, angelique cramer, dora matzke, don mellenbergh, and han lj van der maas]. *Acta Psychologica*, *148*, 188–194. https://doi.org/10.1016/j.actpsy.2014.02.001
Fishbein, M., & Ajzen, I. (2009). *Predicting and changing behavior: The reasoned action approach* (1st ed.). Psychology Press. https://doi.org/10.4324/9780203838020
Gibbons, F. X., & Gerrard, M. (1997). Health images and their effects on health behavior. In B. Buunk & F. X. Gibbons (Eds.), *Health, coping and well-being: Perspectives from social comparison theory* (pp. 63–94). Lawrence Erlbaum Associates. https://doi.org/10.4324/9780203774106
Hagger, M. S., & Chatzisarantis, N. L. (2014). An integrated behavior change model for physical activity. *Exercise and Sport Sciences Reviews*, *42*(2), 62–69. https://doi.org/10.1249/JES.0000000000000008
Hagger, M. S., Cameron, L. D., Hamilton, K., Hankonen, N., & Lintunen, T. (2020). *The handbook of behavior change*. Cambridge University Press.
Hall, P. A., & Fong, G. T. (2007). Temporal self-regulation theory: A model for individual health behavior. *Health Psychology Review*, *1*, 6–52. https://doi.org/10.1080/17437190701492437
Heckhausen, H., & Gollwitzer, P. M. (1987). Thought contents and cognitive functioning in motivational versus volitional states of mind. *Motivation and Emotion*, *11*(2), 101–120. https://doi.org/10.1007/BF00992338
Hofmann, W., Friese, M., & Wiers, R. W. (2008). Impulsive versus reflective influences on health behavior: A theoretical framework and empirical review. *Health Psychology Review*, *2*(2), 111–137. https://doi.org/10.1080/17437190802617668
Kwasnicka, D., Dombrowski, S. U., White, M., & Sniehotta, F. (2016). Theoretical explanations for maintenance of behaviour change: a systematic review of behaviour theories. *Health Psychology Review*, *10*(3), 277–296. https://doi.org/10.1080/17437199.2016.1151372
Kwasnicka, D., Ten Hoor, G. A., van Dongen, A., Gruszczyńska, E., Hagger, M. S., Hamilton, K., … Luszczynska, A. (2021) Promoting scientific integrity through open science in health psychology: Results of the synergy expert meeting of the European Health Psychology Society. *Health Psychology Review*, *15*(3), 333–349. https://doi.org/10.1080/17437199.2020.1844037
Lippke, S., & Ziegelmann, J. P. (2008). Theory-based health behavior change: Developing, testing, and applying theories for evidence-based interventions. *Applied Psychology*, *57*(4), 698–716. https://doi.org/10.1111/j.1464-0597.2008.00339.x
McLeroy, K. R., Bibeau, D., Steckler, A., & Glanz, K. (1988). An ecological perspective on health promotion programs. *Health Education Quarterly*, *15*(4), 351–377.
Michie, S., Abraham, C., Whittington, C., McAteer, J., & Gupta, S. (2009). Effective techniques in healthy eating and physical activity interventions: A meta-regression. *Health Psychology*, *28*(6), 690–701. https://doi.org/10.1037/a0016136

Michie, S., Carey, R. N., Johnston, M., Rothman, A. J., De Bruin, M., Kelly, M. P., & Connell, L. E. (2018). From theory-inspired to theory-based interventions: A protocol for developing and testing a methodology for linking behaviour change techniques to theoretical mechanisms of action. *Annals of Behavioral Medicine*, *52*(6), 501–512. https://doi.org/10.1007/s12160-016-9816-6
Michie, S. F., West, R., Campbell, R., Brown, J., & Gainforth, H. (2014b). *ABC of behaviour change theories*. Silverback publishing.
Michie, S., Atkins, L., & West, R. (2014a). *The behaviour change wheel. A guide to designing interventions* (1st ed.). Silverback Publishing.
Mischel, W. (2008, December 1). *The toothbrush problem*. APS Observer, 21(11). https://www.psychologicalscience.org/observer/the-toothbrush-problem
Nahum-Shani, I., Hekler, E. B., & Spruijt-Metz, D. (2015). Building health behavior models to guide the development of just-in-time adaptive interventions: A pragmatic framework. *Health Psychology*, *34*(Suppl), 1209–1219. https://doi.org/10.1037/hea0000306
Ogden, J. (2016). Celebrating variability and a call to limit systematisation: The example of the behaviour change technique taxonomy and the behaviour change wheel. *Health Psychology Review*, *10*(3), 245–250. https://doi.org/10.1080/17437199.2016.1190291
Osborne, C., & Norris, E. (2022). Pre-registration as behaviour: Developing an evidence-based intervention specification to increase pre-registration uptake by researchers using the behaviour change wheel. *Cogent Psychology*, *9*(1), 2066304. https://doi.org/10.1080/23311908.2022.2066304
Pfeffer, I., Hamilton, K., Hannan, T. & Wegner, M. (2023). Models to explain and change health behavior and physical activity. In J. Schüler et al. (Eds.), *Sport and Exercise Psychology: Theory and Application* (pp. 617–647). Springer. https://doi.org/10.1007/978-3-031-03921-8_25
Prochaska, J. O., & DiClemente, C. C. (1982). Transtheoretical therapy: Toward a more integrative model of change. *Psychotherapy: Theory, Research & Practice*, *19*(3), 276–288. https://doi.org/10.1037/h0088437
Rahaman, K. S., Ramos, S., Harter, M., & Mosler, H. J. (2022). Determination of psychosocial factors of drinking chlorinated water to design behavior change interventions in Rohingya Camps in Bangladesh. *The American Journal of Tropical Medicine and Hygiene*, *106*(4), 1126–1134. https://doi.org/10.4269/ajtmh.21-0313
Rhodes, R. E., Janssen, I., Bredin, S. S., Warburton, D. E., & Bauman, A. (2017). Physical activity: Health impact, prevalence, correlates and interventions. *Psychology & Health*, *32*(8), 942–975. https://doi.org/10.1080/08870446.2017.1325486
Romain, A. J., Bortolon, C., Gourlan, M., Carayol, M., Decker, E., … Bernard, P. (2018). Matched or nonmatched interventions based on the transtheoretical model to promote physical activity: A meta-analysis of randomized controlled trials. *Journal of Sport and Health Science*, *7*(1), 50–57. https://doi.org/10.1016/j.jshs.2016.10.007
Rothman, A. J., & Sheeran, P. (2020). What is slowing us down? Six challenges to accelerating advances in health behavior change. *Annals of Behavioral Medicine*, *54*(12), 948–959. https://doi.org/10.1093/abm/kaaa090
Ruiter, R. A. C., & Crutzen, R. (2020). Core Processes: How to Use Evidence, Theories, and Research in Planning Behavior Change Interventions. *Frontiers in Public Health*, *8*, 247. https://doi.org/10.3389/fpubh.2020.00247
Scholz, U. (2019). It's time to think about time in health psychology. *Applied Psychology: Health and Well-Being*, *11*(2), 173–186. https://doi.org/10.1111/aphw.12156
Schwarzer, R. (1992). Self-efficacy in the adoption and maintenance of health behaviors: Theoretical approaches and a new model. In R. Schwarzer (Ed.), *Self-efficacy: Thought control of action* (pp. 217–243). Hemisphere.
Sheeran, P. (2002). Intention—Behavior relations: A conceptual and empirical review. *European Review of Social Psychology*, *12*(1), 1–36. https://doi.org/10.1080/14792772143000003

Strack, F., & Deutsch, R. (2004). Reflective and impulsive determinants of social behavior. *Personality and Social Psychology Review*, *8*(3), 220–247. https://doi.org/10.1207/s15327957pspr0803_1
Strobach, T., Englert, C., Jekauc, D., & Pfeffer, I. (2020). Predicting adoption and maintenance of physical activity in the context of dual process theories. *Performance Enhancement and Health*, *8*(1), 100162. https://doi.org/10.1016/j.peh.2020.100162
Warner, L. M., & Lippke, S. (2008). Psychological stage models of physical exercise – Research advances. In M. P. Simmons & L. A. Foster (Eds.), *Sport and exercise psychology – research advances* (pp. 19–51). Nova Science Publishers.

7

ILLNESS PERCEPTIONS AND CULTURE

A Common Sense Model Approach

Smita C. Banerjee, Shweta Chawak, Matsungshila Pongener, and Mahati Chittem

Introduction

Understanding illness representations, an integral part of Leventhal's Common Sense Model (CSM), is crucial in explaining health outcomes and health promotion behaviours. The current chapter focuses on cultural understandings of illness perceptions and is divided into four sections. First, we introduce illness representations in the context of health and illness, followed by a brief description of the CSM. Further, it explains the uniqueness of the CSM compared to other health behaviour models by emphasising its multi-level concepts and including socio-cultural and individual contexts to understand illness perceptions. Second, we present a scoping review of research in CSM from across the world, published in the last five years (2018–2022), to highlight the possible impact of the various CSM domains on psychosocial factors and the need to integrate these constructs to develop interventions for the patients. Third, we describe two interventions that have used the CSM: to foster self-monitoring of blood glucose and glycaemic control and lymphoma survivorship care planning, respectively. These interventions show the CSM's advantage in adapting flexibly to contextual and cultural factors to understand different illness perceptions. Finally, we conclude with a review of research in the context of the CSM in India to underscore culturally derived perspectives of illness representations and present limitations and future directions.

Illness perceptions are cognitions about illnesses that include subjective beliefs of a health threat, its potential outcomes, and control over the threat. These individual beliefs, such as the susceptibility of a disease (high or low risk of cancer diagnosis), its causal factors (smoking, alcohol, and pollution), its duration (short or long term), and seriousness (low or heightened) shape health behaviours which are crucial in the management of an illness. Illness perceptions were conceptualised as a result of Leventhal's CSM of illness representations

 DOI: 10.4324/9781003318026-9

(Leventhal et al., 1984). Illness perceptions or illness representations, interchangeably used throughout this chapter, are crucial to understand, as they can affect the maintenance of adherence to treatment regimens (Safo et al., 2015) and the willingness to engage in health promotion behaviours (Vollmann & Salewski, 2021). For example, only when an individual has the belief that their health behaviours have an influence in the prevention or management of chronic illness will they act on it accordingly. The CSM of illness representations is a theoretical framework that examines the perceptual, behavioural, and cognitive processes to understand how individuals make sense of a health threat (Leventhal et al., 1984; Leventhal et al., 2016). It is posited that individuals form mental representations (cognitive and emotional aspects) and personal ideas about a health threat, which then determines the initiation and maintenance of subsequent health behaviours (Leventhal et al., 2016).

The CSM is conceptualised as a parallel processing model, such that one arm is dedicated to processing the *cognitive* aspects of the health threat, whereas the other is focused on processing the *emotional* aspects. Under the *cognitive aspects* of the model, illness representations may be elicited through internal cues (e.g., bodily experience), such as prior experiences with health and illness, or of an imagined disease (e.g., migraine) and external cues (e.g., family, health-care providers, media) (Diefenbach & Leventhal, 1996; Leventhal et al., 1980). The model proposes five cognitive dimensions of illness representations. First, the *identity* dimension refers to the symptoms, labels, and other indicators that represent the illness (e.g., cough). Second, the *causes* dimension refers to an individual's perceptions about the aetiology of the illness (e.g., is the cough caused due to poor immune system (internal factor) or after being exposed to the flu from a crowded public space (external factor) or through hereditary (family history of cancer)?). Third, the *timeline* or a person's perception of the likely duration of the illness and expectations about the course of the health problem (e.g., if the cough is acute, it might be labelled as a flu; if the cough is chronic, it might be interpreted as cancer; or if the cough is cyclical, it might be labelled as a seasonal allergy). Fourth, the *consequences* dimension is conceptualised as an individual's beliefs about the severity of the illness and its impact on the person's physical, emotional, psychological, and socioeconomic functioning (e.g., depending on the timeline of the cough, an individual will label its severity). For acute and cyclical timelines, an individual might resort to over-the-counter medication for the flu or use antihistamines for the seasonal allergy. However, for the chronic timeline, an individual may identify the cough as a symptom of cancer and label it as life-threatening. Lastly, the fifth dimension is *cure/control*, which taps into the individual's beliefs about the curability of their illness and the amount of control they have over their illness (e.g., the timeline and consequence help the individual identify whether the cough can be cured (flu) or controlled (seasonal allergy and cancer) through treatments).

Similarly, the *emotional aspects* of the CSM run parallel and correspond to its cognitive dimensions (Diefenbach & Leventhal, 1996). An individual with a sore throat may identify it as a cough, which might be initially represented in the form of irritability due to discomfort, loss of sleep, or having to call in sick. Next, depending on the symptoms of the cough, the causal factors (internal or external factors or hereditary) may give rise to worry. If the timeline of the cough persists for a longer period, an individual might start to have anxiety, and their representations of cancer may be activated at the same time. This is further fuelled by fear if the consequences of the cough are severe or life-threatening. Once the anxiety and fear are activated due to representations of cancer, depending on the control/curability of the illness, an individual may attempt to reduce these emotional reactions or may be driven to take action to diagnose and start treatment to improve their quality of life. Coping strategies are thus employed and appraisal of the illness is performed through the emotional reactions of the threat and the cognitive aspects that activate the representations of the illness threat. Coping refers to the cognitive and behavioural efforts made by an individual in the face of a stressor. Two types of coping strategies have been defined: emotion focused or problem-focused coping.

Given the dynamic nature of the CSM, the framework allows for bi-directional, multi-level, bottom-up, and top-down approaches across the stages in the presence of a health threat (Diefenbach & Leventhal, 1996; see Figure 7.1). For instance, the appraisal of an illness symptom is influenced by the prototypes (memory structures) and mental representations (perceptual stage), which transforms the representation of an illness (response stage), leading to a change in the coping strategies employed; this process is a feedback loop which is revisited at each stage of the model (Diefenbach & Leventhal, 1996). Distinct from other health behaviour models such as Health Belief Model (HBM) and the Theory of Planned Behaviour (TPB; see Chapter 6, "How to Work with Theories of Health

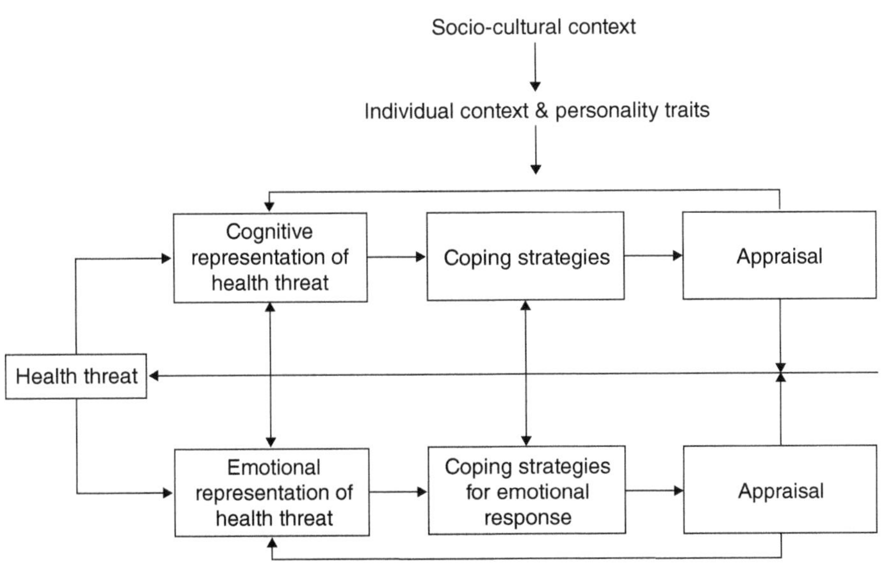

Figure 7.1 A flowchart of the CSM of illness representations.

Behaviour Change" in this volume), the dynamics of the CSM bridge the mechanisms (e.g., "*What factors allow self-efficacious individuals to undergo mammogram?*") and processes (e.g., "*How do self-efficacious older individuals adhere to yearly mammogram?*") of health behaviours and health outcomes in multi-level concepts rather than focusing on a specific abstract concept (e.g., self-efficacy in HBM or behavioural intention in TPB) (Leventhal et al., 2016).

Illness Representation across the World

Studies on understanding illness perception that use the CSM have been carried out across many countries, various research sites, and illness conditions. They explored the relationship between illness perception, quality of life (QoL), psychological distress, cognition, coping, social support, and attitude towards illness. We searched for published articles in the last five years (i.e., from 2018 to 2022) using Google Scholar databases and keywords such as "common sense model" and "Leventhal's CSM". The initial screening yielded 6,155 articles, of which 11 were selected on the basis of relevance to and fulfilment of selection criteria: (i) original and empirical research, (ii) recent research (2018–2022), and (iii) research carried out globally. Table 7.1 provides a detailed description of the articles retained for this chapter.

Illness Perception, Study Design, and Research Site

Of the 11 chosen studies, eight were quantitative studies, whilst three studies used qualitative research designs (see Chapter 8, "Research Design: Overview and Recommendations"). Two studies were multisite and carried out among individuals from different countries. For example, the study by Koert et al. (2018) assessed participants from 79 countries, with a sample size greater than 100 in 18 countries. Similarly, Willemse et al. (2019) included 25 countries, with the majority of participants from the UK, USA, Netherlands, Canada, and Australia. The studies were conducted in 16 languages: Danish, French, German, Italian, Spanish, Portuguese (European and Brazilian), Turkish, Japanese (Nihongo), Hindi, Russian, Chinese (Mandarin and Cantonese), Bahasa (Indonesia), Malay, Tamil, Dutch, and English. We deliberately chose studies carried out across various continents (i.e., Europe, North America, Asia, Australasia, and Africa). Also, the context in which the studies were conducted varies significantly, from recruitment via social media/library/news, approaching children at school, as well as patients from mental health services, hospitals, primary care, a pulmonary rehabilitation centre, or a multiple sclerosis unit, to conducting household surveys.

Participants' Details and Medical Condition

The sample size for the qualitative studies ranged from 14 to 43, and for the quantitative studies, from 113 to 10,045. Participants were patients, children and young adults, the general adult population, older adults, and married couples

Table 7.1 Overview of studies (N = 11) using the CSM model

Study	*Study Design*	*Country*	*Recruitment*	*N*	*Participants*	*Illness*	*Instruments*	*Language*	*Outcome*
Achstetter et al., 2019	Quantitative	Germany	Pulmonary rehabilitation centre	113	Adults	Asthma	IPQ-R Short version ACT		Personal control and conseq predict asthma control
Bassi et al., 2020	Quantitative	Italy	MS Unit	680	Adults	MS	IPQ-R Brief COPE Multidimensional scale of perceived social support Satisfaction with life scale MSQoL Beck Depression Inventory-II		Personal and treatment control associated with better adjustment Emotional rep and timeline associated with worse adjustment
Brooks et al., 2022	Qualitative	Indonesia	MH services	43	Children	MH	Semi-structured interviews Photo elicitation	Bahasa Indonesian	Personal control related to development and treatment of MH

(*Continued*)

Table 7.1 (Continued)

Study	*Study Design*	*Country*	*Recruitment*	*N*	*Participants*	*Illness*	*Instruments*	*Language*	*Outcome*
Haines et al., 2019	Quantitative	UK (129) USA (8) Canada (2) Egypt (1) South Africa (1) Australia (1)	Hospital Online	143	Adolescents	CFS T1DM JIA	BIPQ Children's Anxiety & Depression scale RAND-36 Chalder Fatigue Questionnaire		CFS (vs T1DM & JIA) greater identity, lowered perceived control, chronic timeline, and understanding of illness
Koert et al., 2018	Quantitative	International (79 countries)	Online research panels Fertility clinic	10,045	Married couples trying to be pregnant	Fertility	Descriptive	English Translated into 12 languages	72% provided inaccurate causal explanations Women: causal explanation associated with feeling responsible and self-blame
Moosa et al., 2021	Qualitative	Singapore	Public primary care clinic	17	Older adults (+65 years)	Chronic pruritus	In-depth interviews	Chinese Malay Tamil English	Identity, cause, and chronicity determined behaviour of controlling the problem Controllability led to problem-focused coping

Ringer, 2021	Qualitative	Sweden	School	14	Children	ADHD	In-depth interviews		Children construct beliefs about identity, conseq, timeline, and personal control Additional dimension to CSM for ADHD illness
Shiloh et al., 2021	Quantitative	Israel	Population based	511	Adults	COVID-19	COVID-19 threat appraisal COVID-19 worries BIPQ STAI Health Anxiety Questionnaire		Threat appraisal and worries explained variance in IP Emotional rep was explained by threat appraisal
Vollmann & Salewski, 2021	Quantitative	Netherlands	Social media	584	Young adults	COVID-19	BIPQ Willingness to receive the COVID-19 vaccine Perceptions about COVID-19 vaccination	Dutch	Personal control and concern related to willingness to receive vaccine

(*Continued*)

Table 7.1 (Continued)

Study	*Study Design*	*Country*	*Recruitment*	*N*	*Participants*	*Illness*	*Instruments*	*Language*	*Outcome*
Willemse et al., 2019	Quantitative	25 countries USA (60) UK (60) Netherlands (38) Canada (28) Australia (15)	Online survey	243	Adults	Alopecia Areata	Dermatology Life Quality Index BIPQ Brief COPE	English Dutch	IP (except timeline/ treat control) associated with QoL Avoidant coping partially mediated between IP and QoL
Woodhouse et al., 2018	Quantitative	Australia USA	Social Media	179	Adults	Gastroparesis	BIPQ Brief COPE DASS-21 Gastroparesis Cardinal Symptom Index Patient Assessment of Upper Gastrointestinal Disorders: QoL	English	Symptom severity directly influenced IPs and QoL IPs directly influenced maladaptive, coping, psychological distress, and QoL

Notes: ACT asthma control test, ADHD attention-deficit hyperactivity disorder, BIPQ Brief Illness Perception Questionnaire, CFS chronic fatigue syndrome, Conseq consequences, COVID-19 coronavirus disease, CSM Common Sense Model, DASS-21 Depression, Anxiety, and Stress Scale-21, IP illness perception, IPQ-R Revised Illness Perception Questionnaire, JIA juvenile idiopathic arthritis, MS multiple sclerosis, MSQoL multiple sclerosis quality of life, MH mental health, QoL quality of life, Rep representation, STAI State-Trait Anxiety Inventory, T1DM type I diabetes mellitus.

wishing to have children. Various conditions were investigated: asthma, mental health, COVID-19, type 1 diabetes, multiple sclerosis, fertility issues, chronic pruritus, alopecia areata, gastroparesis, chronic fatigue syndrome, juvenile idiopathic arthritis, and ADHD.

Instruments and Language Translations

The most often used instrument implemented to measure illness perceptions in quantitative studies was the *Brief Illness Perception Questionnaire* (used by five studies, see Table 7.1); others used the *Illness Perception Questionnaire-Revised* (IPQ-R) and *IPQ-R Short Version*. The correlates included general and disease-specific assessments of the *QoL* (e.g., *SF-36*, *MS Quality of Life-54 Inventory*); psychological symptoms (e.g., *Beck Depression Inventory-II*, *Depression Anxiety Stress Scale*); satisfaction with life, coping, social support, and symptoms severity (e.g., *Asthma Control Questionnaire*); physical and mental fatigue (*Gastroparesis Cardinal Symptom Index*); and attitudes towards treatment (e.g., willingness to receive COVID-19 vaccine).

Illness Perception and Outcomes of the Review

From this literature review on illness perception, several associations suggested by the CSM can be extracted: For example, individuals with higher personal control beliefs and more positive identity perceptions of their illnesses reported having higher symptom control (such as asthma control; Achstetter et al., 2019). On the other hand, patients who perceived severe consequences of their illness tended to report higher distress and showed lesser improvement in efforts to control their illness (Achstetter et al., 2019). Interestingly, a study conducted in Singapore by Moosa et al. (2021) reported that uncertainty in knowing the cause of the illness due to a lack of information shared by their physician was associated with patients' perception of treatment control. This experience of lack of information regarding their illness may be deep-rooted in the physician-centred communication style practised in Asian cultures (Chawak et al., 2022). This study emphasises the need to consider socio-cultural influence in understanding illness perception.

Another study also suggested that the *perceived severity* of one's symptoms is associated with poorer illness perceptions, greater engagement in maladaptive coping, increased psychological distress, and poorer QoL (Woodhouse et al., 2018). A study by Willemse et al. (2019) reported that engaging in avoidant coping (such as self-distractions, denial, behavioural engagement, self-blame, and substance use) mediated between individuals' experiences of their illness (identity) and poor QoL. This could, for example, mean that if someone perceives their illness to be overwhelming, their ability to manage the disease actively may be reduced, which could lead to further deterioration in QoL. Further, individuals with higher perceptions of *personal* and *treatment control* were more likely to engage in *problem-focused* coping (e.g., taking their medication instead of trying to distract themselves; Moosa et al., 2021). *Personal control* and *treatment control* were associated with better psychological adjustment, whilst more negatively perceived *emotional representation* and longer *perceived duration of the illness* were associated with worse psychological adjustment (Bassi et al., 2020).

Koert et al. (2018) suggest that higher perceptions of *illness threat* were a predictor for illness perceptions, especially negative *emotional representations*, which may evoke negative emotions, creating a vicious cycle. For example, abortions, miscarriages, and birth control use may be associated with a lack of fertility/pregnancy despite a lack of conclusive evidence to create causation. This may evoke a feeling of self-blame and responsibility for the lack of pregnancy. Illness perceptions were also associated with patients' health behaviours, such as adherence to medication, compliance with treatments to control or cure symptoms, and willingness to receive the COVID-19 vaccine (Moosa et al., 2021; Vollmann & Salewski, 2021). Further, patients who recognised the *benefits* of the treatment more often adhered to the medical plan (Moosa et al., 2021).

A review of these studies highlights the possible impact of the various CSM domains on psychosocial factors, such as QoL, psychological distress, attitude towards an illness, and treatment adherence. Although there are limited studies focusing on socio-cultural factors in illness perception, these studies have emphasised the need to incorporate cultural aspects in understanding illness perception using the CSM. This emphasises the need to integrate constructs from the CSM into research aiming to understand individuals' perceptions of the illness but also their active or passive behaviour towards coping with it, on the one hand, and, on the other, into the development of culturally appropriate interventions to improve cognition, health behaviours and ultimately psychosocial and somatic outcomes for patients themselves.

Interventions Using CSM

One of the key aims of any health psychology theory is to provide avenues or targets of intervention for either the prevention or the treatment or control of chronic illnesses. The CSM includes a dynamic, self-regulative (feedback) control feature and its system structure, which is posited to serve as the foundation for developing interventions for improving management of chronic illnesses (McAndrew et al., 2008). Illness representations, i.e., patients' beliefs and expectations about an illness or somatic symptom, are key concepts of the theory (Leventhal et al., 1980) and provide avenues for intervention development. According to McAndrew et al. (2008),

> [T]he active processing or assignment of meaning and the creation of emotional reactions to somatic stimuli affects the selection of coping mechanisms, and the creation of plans for specific actions and expectations respecting the consequences (feedback from) these actions; (e.g. symptom decline within an expected time frame). Coping decisions will differ as a function of the meaning individuals assign to their symptoms (i.e. their

> illness representation) and this interpretive process will reflect their past illness experience, societal expectations, information from friends, media, and medical practitioners.
>
> *(p. 196)*

Focusing on illness representations, prior research has shown that causal cognitive attributions affect an individual's sense of control of a disease. For example, if a patient attributes their disease to a specific modifiable cause(s) with a target for action, their sense of control may instigate coping towards that cause, as has been observed in cancer survivorship research. Cancer survivors who identify modifiable causal attributions are more likely to make behavioural changes to target the believed cause of cancer (Rabin & Pinto, 2006).

Although past research has been prolific in describing how people utilise different mental tools to form illness representations and how this affects care-seeking and self-management (e.g., Brand et al., 2021; Richardson et al., 2017), very few intervention studies have been designed to influence the process of self-regulatory illness management. One study focused on an intervention encouraging self-monitoring of blood glucose and glycaemic control (McAndrew et al., 2008). The intervention was designed to allow patients to teach themselves to become expert self-managers of self-monitoring of blood glucose by focusing on somatic cues. In particular, the intervention aimed at teaching patients to see how specific behaviours, such as types and amounts of food intake, raise blood glucose levels and how specific activities (e.g., walking) and the combination of food intake and activities can lower the elevations of glucose from eating by using self-monitoring of blood glucose. Specific intervention components included patient education for self-monitoring of blood glucose, selecting actions and timeframes for self-monitoring of blood glucose, and developing an action plan to conduct self-monitoring of blood glucose in one's daily environment. This study provides an appropriate example of how interventions can be culturally adapted to the participants in the study. Doing a qualitative investigation of culturally appropriate foods and activities and tying that into patient education can help make the connections relevant for the participants.

Moving away from patient population to provider population, one intervention study developed a clinician-targeted communication skills intervention titled "Transitioning a Lymphoma Patient to Survivorship." The goal of the training intervention was

> [t]o facilitate the patient's adaptation to their new role as a cancer survivor after they have completed their primary anti-cancer treatment through i) review of their diagnosis, treatment and prognosis to promote integration of knowledge; ii) creation of a continuing care plan covering anti-cancer monitoring, cancer screening and health promotion, potential late or long-term effects from treatment and any lifestyle implications for their future; and iii) promotion of their sense of efficacy and confidence in their future.
>
> *(p. 394; Banerjee et al., 2015)*

This intervention was developed based on prior research from both empirical data and clinical observations that mental models of cancer and treatment change as patients go through different steps of the cancer treatment plan, i.e., from initial discovery through different forms of treatment and to survivorship. Survivors often shift their illness representation with a new focus on prevention and long-term health promotion and adopt an active problem-solving approach to prevent potential relapses. The results described that patients whose providers participated in the intervention reported higher knowledge about their lymphoma and showed greater adherence to physician recommendations for influenza vaccinations and colonoscopy as compared to the patients whose physicians were in the control group (Parker et al., 2018). This study also highlights the intersection of medical knowledge combined with the cultural nuances of the patient population and using that in provider education.

As illustrated in this chapter, research on illness representations can be conducted in any culture and on any health condition. The flexibility of the CSM is an advantage in adapting its constructs to each context and population, and the contextual and cultural factors are very important to understand different illness perceptions depending on the context (also see Chapter 9, "Measurement in Health Psychology"). Therefore, interventions have to be adapted to specific cultural beliefs and cannot be easily transferred to a different patient population or country. India was chosen as the exemplar culture as it brings to the fore the highly relevant discussion on culture and the CSM, as well as delimiting the focus on a mainly Western approach to understanding and applying psychological/behavioural theories.

Cultural Contexts of the CSM: India

Research emerging from India which used the CSM to understand illness representations, behaviours, and self-regulatory efforts is relatively recent, with the earliest studies being published in 2012 (Chittem et al., 2012) and focused on the chronic illnesses of cancer (five empirical studies and one review; Ali et al., 2017; Birudu & Reddy, 2020; Chittem et al., 2012; Chittem et al., 2015; Epton et al., 2020; Kumari & Dubey, 2020), diabetes (two studies; Abraham et al., 2015; Murugesan & Sundaramoorthy, 2018), asthma (one study; Gowda & Damodar; 2015), paediatric neurological conditions (one study; Kelada et al., 2021), and non-alcoholic fatty liver disease (one study; Dhaliwal et al., 2021).

The cancer studies examined the role of nondisclosure of cancer diagnosis on the psychological outcomes of anxiety, depression, coping, and perceived social support, with each of the studies reporting differing links between the individual dimensions of the CSM and these outcomes. Nondisclosure of cancer diagnosis and prognosis is a common, accepted practice in India wherein family relatives intercept the physician before the medical consultation with requests to not reveal the truth to the patient mainly to protect them from the psychological/emotional harm this information may cause (see Chittem et al., 2020). Interestingly, although nondisclosure is almost exclusively initiated by family members, there are no studies using the CSM to better understand families' perceptions of cancer. As determined by Ali et al. (2017), a central dimension of the CSM – illness identity – rests on an individual being aware of their illness and correctly labelling it (e.g., being aware of one's cancer diagnosis and being able to label it as glioblastoma). They argued that without awareness of the cancer diagnosis, it may be difficult to draw meaningful conclusions as it becomes difficult to ascertain whether the individual's appraisal is regarding their "actual" illness or what they assume the illness to be. Yet, all the authors of the five empirical studies confirmed the usefulness of applying the CSM to better understand and explain psychological responses and coping behaviours, and emphasised the need to adapt existing CSM interventions to Indian cancer populations so as to challenge and correct negative illness perceptions whilst strengthening positive illness perceptions.

Reflecting this, the empirical studies examining the other illness types (i.e., diabetes, dental/oral health, brain injury, asthma, paediatric neurological conditions, mental disorders, non-alcoholic fatty liver disease, and COVID-19) underscored the cultural adaptability of the CSM in explaining psychological well-being, self-care practices, help-seeking, and coping among Indians. Both the diabetes studies, for instance, showed that the CSM dimensions of personal control, treatment control, and illness coherence were directly associated with patients' self-care behaviours, suggesting that barriers to self-care need to be addressed through exploring and intervening in these areas of illness appraisal (Abraham et al., 2015; Murugesan & Sundaramoorthy, 2018). Causal attribution of illness was, as the authors argued, the most culturally unique aspect of the CSM which revealed key information on how their participants were self-regulating or seeking care services. For example, in their study evaluating the CSM of periodontal disease, Ali et al. (2022) found that less than half the participants reported poor medical care to be a major cause for their illness (the other causes being stress and increased work pressure), thus suggesting the need to improve awareness about oral health through educational health messages.

All the CSM studies conducted in India were quantitative, and of the 16 empirical studies, nine studies used the Brief Illness Perceptions Questionnaire (BIPQ), 6 studies used the Illness Perceptions Questionnaire – Revised (IPQ-R), and only 1 study used the IPQ-R specifically for oral health (OH) (i.e., IPQ-R-OH; Shulamithi et al., 2022). Most of the studies emerging from India either engaged in individual translation and back-translation of the questionnaires that they used to conduct the CSM studies or made no explicit mention of the language used to administer the questionnaire. There are 22 officially recognised languages in India (Department of Official Language, Ministry of Home Affairs, 2022); therefore, it is critical that the CSM questionnaires should be translated and back-translated following the international guidelines of the World Health Organisation so homogeneity in the administration of the questionnaires is maintained, ease in conducting the studies can be ensured, and the time taken to develop and conduct the study is reduced (also see Chapter 9, "Measurement in Health Psychology").

Further, there are no qualitative studies which use the CSM framework to understand illness perceptions in India. This is problematic, as qualitative research is particularly helpful in making sense of cultural contexts of health and illness (Nicholls, 2009) and, when complemented with quantitative research – i.e., mixed methods (see Chapter 8, "Research Design: Overview and Recommendations"), lends itself to a more comprehensive approach to the ensuing interventions. Given that the existing quantitative research in India overwhelmingly points to the cultural adaptability of the CSM, it is important to ascertain this through qualitative research as well and to unpack the nuances of the findings. For example, Gowda and Damodar (2015) reported that whilst a large proportion of their participants who had asthma reported symptoms of wheezing and breathlessness, only a marginal number of them connected these symptoms to asthma, thus showing poor illness identity (particularly towards symptom identification). However, it would have been helpful to expand on this finding by exploring how the participants make sense of their symptoms through their personal, family, and community narratives regarding illness experiences, their thoughts at the time of experiencing these symptoms, and so on.

Conclusion

This chapter on cultural understandings of illness perceptions highlights three important conclusions: (1) CSM is a dynamic theory that bridges the mechanisms and processes of health behaviours and health outcomes in multi-level concepts; (2) CSM has been studied in a number of health behaviours and with a focus on the impact of the various CSM domains on psychosocial factors such as QoL, psychological distress, attitude towards an illness, and treatment adherence; and (3) CSM provides a rich foundation for designing interventions; however, interventions have to be adapted to the specific cultural beliefs and cannot be easily transferred to a different patient population or country. With a focus on CSM-focused research emerging from India, there is a paucity of qualitative studies that utilise CSM framework to understand illness perceptions in India. Future work should focus on a greater effort to understand illness perceptions and the cultural context in order to not only describe the illness representation but also identify avenues for behaviour change, taking into account the cultural values.

Further Reading

Benyamini, Y., & Leventhal, H. (2019). Beliefs and perceptions of health and illness. In C. D. Llewellyn, S. Ayers, C. McManus, S. Newman, K. J. Petrie, T. A. Revenson, & J. Weinman (Eds.), *Cambridge handbook of psychology, health and medicine* (3rd ed., pp. 106–109). Cambridge: Cambridge University Press.

Cameron, L., & Leventhal, H. (Eds.). (2002). *The self-regulation of health and illness behaviour* (1st ed.). London, UK: Routledge.

Martin, R., Rothrock, N., Leventhal, H., & Leventhal, E. (2003). Common sense models of illness: Implications for symptom perception and health-related behaviors. In J. Suls & K. A. Wallston (Eds.), *Social psychological foundations of health and illness* (pp. 199–225). Malden, MA: Blackwell Publishing.

References

Abraham, A. M., Sudhir, P. M., Philip, M., & Bantwal, G. (2015). Illness perceptions and perceived barriers to self-care in patients with type 2 diabetes mellitus: An exploratory study from India. *International Journal of Diabetes in Developing Countries*, *35*, 137–144.

Achstetter, L. I., Schultz, K., Faller, H., & Schuler, M. (2019). Leventhal's common-sense model and asthma control: Do illness representations predict success of an asthma rehabilitation? *Journal of Health Psychology*, *24*(3), 327–336.

Ali, A. A., Kohli, N., & Yadav, S. (2017). A systematic review of illness perceptions and coping among cancer patients in India. *Indian Journal of Health & Wellbeing*, *8*(11), 1309–1319.

Ali, A. R., Kapoor, A., Chatterjee, D., Gautam, K., Choudhary, A., & Jain, R. L. (2022). Psychometric approach to evaluate periodontal disease using Revised Illness Perception Questionnaire. *Journal of Indian Society of Periodontology*, *26*(1), 69–74.

Banerjee, S. C., Matasar, M. J., Bylund, C. L., Horwitz, S., McLarney, K., Levin, T., Jacobsen, P. B., Parker, P., Astrow, A., & Kissane, D. W. (2015). Survivorship care planning after participation in communication skills training intervention for a consultation about lymphoma survivorship. *Translational Behavioral Medicine*, *5*(4), 393–400. https://doi.org/10.1007/s13142-015-0326-z

Bassi, M., Cilia, S., Falautano, M., Grobberio, M., Niccolai, C., Pattini, M., Pietrolongo, E., Quartuccio, M. E., Viterbo, R. G., Allegri, B., Amato, M. P., Benin, M., De Luca, G., Gasperini, C., Minacapelli, E., Patti, F., Trojano, M., & Delle Fave, A. (2020). Illness perceptions and psychological adjustment among persons with multiple sclerosis: The mediating role of coping strategies and social support. *Disability and Rehabilitation*, *42*(26), 3780–3792.

Birudu, R., & Reddy, K. (2020). Illness perceptions and perceived social support among glioblastoma survivors during hospitalization. *Journal of Cancer Research and Therapeutics*, *16*(6), 1449–1453.

Brand, H., Speiser, D., Besch, L., Roseman, J., & Kendel, F. (2021). Making sense of a health threat: Illness representations, coping, and psychological distress among BRCA1/2 mutation carriers. *Genes*, *12*(5), 741. https://doi.org/10.3390/genes12050741

Brooks, H., Windfuhr, K., Prawira, B., Desyadi Putriningtyas, D. A., Lovell, K., Bangun, S. R., Syarif, A. K., Manik, C. G., Tanjun, I. S., Salim, S., Renwick, L., Pedley, R., & Bee, P. (2022). Children and young people's beliefs about mental health and illness in Indonesia: A qualitative study informed by the common sense model of self-regulation. *PloS One*, *17*(2), e0263232.

Chawak, S., Chittem, M., Dhillon, H., Huilgol, N., & Butow, P. (2022). Treatment-related communication experiences and expectations among Indian cancer patients receiving radiation therapy and their family members: A qualitative study. *Patient Education and Counseling*, *105*(9), 2913–2922.

Chittem, M., Norman, P., & Harris, P. R. (2012). Relationships between perceived diagnostic disclosure, patient characteristics, psychological distress and illness perceptions in Indian cancer patients. *Psycho-oncology*, *22*(6), 1375–1380. https://doi.org/10.1002/pon.3149

Chittem, M., Norman, P., & Harris, P. R. (2015). Illness representations and psychological distress in Indian patients with cancer: Does being aware of one's cancer diagnosis make a difference? *Psycho-Oncology*, *24*(12), 1694–1700.

Chittem, M., Norman, P., & Harris, P. (2020). Primary family caregivers' reasons for disclosing versus not disclosing a cancer diagnosis in India. *Cancer Nursing*, *43*(2), 126–133. https://doi.org/10.1097/NCC.0000000000000669

Dhaliwal, H. S., Singh, R., Abraham, A. M., Sharma, R., Goyal, N. K., Soloman, R., Bansal, P., & Goyal, A. (2021). Perception of illness and its association with treatment willingness in patients with newly diagnosed nonalcoholic fatty liver disease. *Digestive Diseases and Sciences*, *66*(12), 4197–4207. https://doi.org/10.1007/s10620-020-06794-2

Diefenbach, M. A., & Leventhal, H. (1996). The common-sense model of illness representation: Theoretical and practical considerations. *Journal of Social Distress and the Homeless*, *5*(1), 11–38.

Epton, T., Chittem, M., Tanikella, R., Rajappa, S., Sinha, S., & Harris, P. R. (2020). Indian patient use of cancer euphemisms: Association with psychological outcomes and health behaviours. *Psycho-oncology*, *29*(7), 1193–1200. https://doi.org/10.1002/pon.5408

Gowda, G., & Damodar, A. S. (2015). Illness perception among bronchial asthma patients attending a tertiary care hospital in Bengaluru, South India. *Scholars Journal of Applied Medical Sciences*, *3*(3H), 1605–1607.

Haines, C., Loades, M., & Davis, C. (2019). Illness perceptions in adolescents with chronic fatigue syndrome and other physical health conditions: Application of the common sense model. *Clinical Child Psychology and Psychiatry*, *24*(3), 546–563.

Kelada, L., Wakefield, C. E., Muppavaram, N., Lingappa, L., & Chittem, M. (2021). Psychological outcomes, coping and illness perceptions among parents of children with neurological disorders. *Psychology & Health*, *36*(12), 1480–1496. https://doi.org/10.1080/08870446.2020.1859113

Koert, E., Harrison, C., Bunting, L., Gladwyn-Khan, M., & Boivin, J. (2018). Causal explanations for lack of pregnancy applying the common sense model of illness representation to the fertility context. *Psychology & Health*, *33*(10), 1284–1301.

Kumari, N., & Dubey, A. (2020). Coping with cancer: What illness perceptions do? *Cross Current International Journal of Medical and Biosciences*, *2*(10), 165–171. https://doi.org/10.36344/ccijmb.2020.v02i10.003

Leventhal, H., Meyer, D., & Nerenz, D. (1980). The common sense representation of illness danger. In S. Rachman (Ed), *Medical psychology* (pp. 7–30). Pergamon Press.

Leventhal, H., Nerenz, D. R., & Steele, D.J. (1984). Illness representations and coping with health threats. In A. Baum, S.E. Taylor, & J. E. Singer (Eds.), *Handbook of psychology and health* (pp. 219–52). Erlbaum.

Leventhal, H., Phillips, L. A., & Burns, E. (2016). The Common-Sense Model of Self-Regulation (CSM): a dynamic framework for understanding illness self-management. *Journal of Behavioral Medicine*, *39*(6), 935–946.

Department of Official Language, Ministry of Home Affairs. (2022, May 17). *Languages included in the Eight Schedule of the Indian Constitution*. National Informatics Centre. https://rajbhasha.gov.in/en/languages-included-eighth-schedule-indian-constitution

McAndrew, L. M., Musumeci-Szabó, T. J., Mora, P. A., Vileikyte, L., Burns, E., Halm, E. A., Leventhal, E. A., & Leventhal, H. (2008). Using the common sense model to design interventions for the prevention and management of chronic illness threats: From description to process. *British Journal of Health Psychology*, *13*(Pt 2), 195–204. https://doi.org/10.1348/135910708X295604

Moosa, A. S., Leng, N. S. Y., Kum, C. L., & Tan, N. C. (2021). A qualitative research study on the illness perception of chronic pruritus in older Asian adults based on the Common-Sense Model of self-regulation. *Health Expectations*, *24*(5), 1801–1811.

Murugesan, M., & Sundaramoorthy, J. (2018). Type II diabetic patients' illness perception and self-care behaviour: Does comorbidity make any difference? *International Journal of Behavioral Sciences*, *12*(3), 114–124.

Nicholls, D. (2009). Qualitative research: Part two-methodologies. *International Journal of Therapy and Rehabilitation*, *16*(11), 586–592.
Parker, P. A., Banerjee, S. C., Matasar, M. J., Bylund, C. L., Rogers, M., Franco, K., Schofield, E., Li, Y., Levin, T. T., Jacobsen, P. B., Astrow, A. B., Leventhal, H., Horwitz, S., & Kissane, D. (2018). Efficacy of a survivorship-focused consultation versus a time-controlled rehabilitation consultation in patients with lymphoma: A cluster randomized controlled trial. *Cancer*, *124*(23), 4567–4576.
Rabin, C., & Pinto, B. (2006). Cancer-related beliefs and health behaviour change among breast cancer survivors and their first-degree relatives. *Psychooncology*, *15*(8), 701–712. https://doi.org/10.1002/pon.1000
Richardson, E. M., Scott, J. L., Schüz, N., Sanderson, K., & Schüz, B. (2017). 'It was all intertwined': Illness representations and self-management in patients with cancer and anxiety/depression. *Psychology & Health*, *32*(9), 1082–1108. https://doi.org/10.1080/08870446.2017.1324970
Ringer, N. (2021). Utilizing the Common-Sense model of illness representations to explore children's perceptions of, and coping with ADHD. *Journal of Mental Health*, *30*(2), 216–223.
Safo, S. A., Batchelder, A., Peyser, D., & Litwin, A. H. (2015). The common sense model applied to hepatitis C: A qualitative analysis of the impact of disease comparison and witnessed death on hepatitis C illness perception. *Harm Reduction Journal*, *12*(1), 1–8.
Shiloh, S., Peleg, S., & Nudelman, G. (2021). Making sense of COVID-19: a longitudinal investigation of the initial stages of developing illness representations. *Psychology & Health*, *37*(12), 1–17.
Shulamithi, P. S., Kulkarni, S., Doshi, D., Reddy, M. P., Srilatha, A., & Satyanarayana, D. (2022). Oral health illness perception and dental caries: A cross-sectional study among adult dental patients, Hyderabad, Telangana, India. World *Journal of Dentistry*, *13*(6), 545–550.
Vollmann, M., & Salewski, C. (2021). To get vaccinated, or not to get vaccinated, that is the question: illness representations about COVID-19 and perceptions about COVID-19 vaccination as predictors of COVID-19 vaccination willingness among young adults in The Netherlands. *Vaccines*, *9*(9), 941.
Willemse, H., van der Doef, M., & van Middendorp, H. (2019). Applying the Common Sense Model to predicting quality of life in alopecia areata: The role of illness perceptions and coping strategies. *Journal of Health Psychology*, *24*(11), 1461–1472.
Woodhouse, S., Hebbard, G., & Knowles, S. R. (2018). Exploring symptom severity, illness perceptions, coping styles, and well-being in gastroparesis patients using the common sense model. *Digestive Diseases and Sciences*, *63*(4), 958–965.

8
RESEARCH DESIGN
Overview and Recommendations

Nicola O'Brien

Introduction

The blueprint of a new house provides a detailed plan of all the construction specifications, including the size, materials, and methods needed for the build. An accurate blueprint also serves to plan the resources (e.g., time, materials, skills) needed at each stage of construction. Research design is the blueprint of the research. It therefore serves the purpose of defining the activities, methods, and resources needed to conduct the planned research effectively and efficiently. In the same way as a poor blueprint for a house can jeopardise the success of a building project (e.g., inaccurate resource planning), a poor research design can jeopardise the success of a research project. Success in this context does not concern the outcome of the research as such but whether it is possible to answer the research question of interest. A research project that has been poorly designed may fail to collect reliable and valid data (see Chapter 9, "Measurement in Health Psychology") and even fail to answer the intended research question. In contrast, good research design facilitates the likelihood that the research objectives are achieved in a timely and effective manner and provides robust data to answer the research question. Thorough consideration of one's research design is therefore critical regardless of the project type or size (i.e., dissertations, theses, service evaluations, audits, or large multicomponent studies).

This chapter covers why good research design is critical to ensuring that data collected can answer the research question effectively and with research integrity. The different research designs and associated methods commonly used in health psychology are described and discussed in relation to important methodological decisions. Examples of mixed methods studies in health psychology are given, illustrating how quantitative and qualitative research can be combined to provide a richer and more nuanced answer to research questions. Recommendations for good practice in research design are provided.

DOI: 10.4324/9781003318026-10

Choosing a Research Design

There is great diversity of research designs and methods available for application in health sciences research in general and health psychology specifically, which promotes innovation and flexibility over how research questions are answered. Accompanying the overall research design are multiple interrelated decisions including, but not limited to, the research paradigm and methodologies, study population, sampling methods, data collection, and analysis. It may be the case that the optimal and most efficient way to conduct research is by using multiple designs and methods within one project. For example, in a randomised controlled trial (RCT) of a peer-led intervention for individuals at high risk of sexually transmitted infections, the baseline data could comprise a cross-sectional survey of determinants of sexual risk behaviours, an embedded N-of-1 (single-case) study exploring within-individual determinants over time, an embedded mixed methods process evaluation assessing how and why the intervention is successful or not, and the RCT comparator group comprising a cohort study exploring behaviours over time.

Each research design has its own strengths and limitations that need to be considered. Research can be problem or theory-driven, meaning that it starts from an identified problem or theory, respectively. Regardless of the starting point, other factors can contribute to the research, such as a problem-driven study using theory and/or existing data to inform design decisions. Theory-driven research typically involves hypothesis testing, such as a study testing whether social cognitive theory variables mediate the effects of an intervention to retain blood donors. Research can also generate hypotheses, such as a population-based cohort study collecting data on potential risk factors or 'exposure variables' for type 2 diabetes (e.g., age, ethnicity, lifestyle) to identify potential avenues for future hypothesis-testing research (see Chapter 6, "How to Work with Theories of Health Behaviour Change," and Chapter 9, "Measurement in Health Psychology," in this volume).

Choice of research design may also be driven or influenced by the availability of study resources such as funding, time and experience. As a result, some designs may be ruled out due to resource constraints. In contrast, significant experience using a particular design may result in it being favoured over other designs due to its familiarity, even though it may not be optimal to answer the research question. Efforts should be made to ensure that methodological rigour, ethical research practice, and research governance are at the forefront of design decisions so that funding (largely public sector money) is maximised to conduct research with a high level of integrity (i.e., rigour, transparency and without undue participant burden). The value of researcher experience using a particular design should not be dismissed, however, as that experience is likely to include important insights into the design's strengths and limitations, which can inform the decision about whether and how to use that design.

Adding to the complexities of choosing a research design is that, like the earlier example of an RCT of a sexual health intervention, research can have multiple components that occur in parallel or in succession, or where one component is embedded within a larger one. This added complexity means that the strengths and limitations of a given design need to be concurrently considered with the strengths and limitations of the other proposed design components.

Types of Research Designs

As previously stated, the choice of research design should primarily be driven by the suitability and ability of the design to answer the research question. It can be helpful to first define whether a descriptive or analytical approach, and a quantitative, qualitative or a mixed methods research paradigm are more fit for purpose.

Descriptive versus Analytical

Descriptive studies are used to describe the distribution of variables (concerning behaviours, phenomena, or psychological constructs) occurring in a given population without manipulation, such as a cross-sectional survey of the prevalence of asthma in children aged 6–7 years. In contrast, analytical (inferential) studies go beyond description. They are typically hypothesis testing, quantifying the relationship between two or more variables and possibly establishing causation, such as an RCT of an alcohol reduction intervention or a qualitative interview study of cognitions and smoking behaviour in pregnant women.

Quantitative versus Qualitative

In a simplistic manner, it can be said that quantitative research collects numerical data that is statistically analysed, whilst qualitative research collects data in the form of words, images, and behaviours that are analysed to generate themes and categories. Mixed methods research collects both quantitative and qualitative data, which are interpreted together to answer the research question (see mixed methods below).

Types of Research Methods

Research methods are a key part of research design. In health psychology, there is a wealth of methods that are commonly used for data collection that have different strengths and limitations (see Chapter 9, "Measurement in Health Psychology"). The majority of methods are primarily employed within analytical studies but can also be employed within descriptive studies. Depending on the research aims and priorities, methods either fall within a quantitative, a qualitative, or a quantitative *and* qualitative paradigm. Table 8.1 details common methods of data collection in health psychology and how they align with quantitative and qualitative paradigms, descriptive and analytical approaches, and designs.

Table 8.1 Common data collection research methods in health psychology

Research Methods	*Paradigm*	*Approach*	*Designs*
Interview	Qualitative	Descriptive or analytical	• Qualitative study • Cross-sectional • Longitudinal • Single case
Focus group	Qualitative	Descriptive or analytical	• Qualitative study • Cross-sectional • Longitudinal
Observation	Qualitative or quantitative	Descriptive or analytical	• Cross-sectional • Longitudinal • Single case
Questionnaire or survey	Quantitative or qualitative	Descriptive or analytical	• Qualitative study • Cross-sectional • Longitudinal • Single case
Experiment or intervention	Quantitative	Analytical	• Experimental • Natural (quasi-) experimental • Single case
N-of-1	Quantitative	Analytical	• Single case
Participatory research	Quantitative or qualitative	Action research	• All
Secondary research	Quantitative or qualitative	Descriptive or analytical	• Evidence synthesis • Meta-analysis • Analysis of existing dataset

Interviews and focus groups are common methods of data collection in qualitative research to study the nature of phenomena. They can be used flexibly with participants, collecting data in-person, via telephone or video call, to generate rich information that could not have been achieved within a purely quantitative paradigm. Limitations of interviews and focus groups are that they are often resource intensive (requiring substantial researcher time for data collection and analysis) and subject to concerns of generalisability.

Interviews can be unstructured (i.e., questions and order are flexibly determined as the interview progresses), structured (i.e., questionnaires), or, most used in health psychology, semi-structured (i.e., blend of structured and unstructured with an interview plan but flexibility in questions and order). Semi-structured interviews involve a series of open-ended questions asked in accordance with predefined topics set out in an interview schedule or topic guide. Interviews can be used within cross-sectional research to gain insight into participants' thoughts, feelings, motivations, and experiences at a moment in time, such as exploring treatment needs of people recently diagnosed with bowel cancer (Browne et al., 2011). Interviews can also be part of longitudinal research where follow-up interviews are conducted with the same, or subset of, participants to explore changes in experiences over time or to further interrogate data collected previously (Murray et al., 2009). Interviews can also be used in single-case research comprising all or part of a case report or case series of individuals' experience of a phenomenon (Brookes et al., 2007).

Focus groups are small group interviews where views and experiences of a given topic are collected through guided group discussion. Views and experiences can be shared, compared, and contrasted, and interactions between participants can be analysed. Focus groups require careful facilitation to ensure all participants are heard and share their views. Participants are often purposively sampled to share similar demographic characteristics (e.g., age, where they live) or experiences (e.g., eligible to participate in a cardiac rehabilitation programme (Okwose et al., 2020)) in order to create a more homogenous group to understand the phenomenon of interest. Focus group methods, like interviews, can be used within cross-sectional and longitudinal research. A special issue in the journal *Health Psychology* demonstrates the breadth and impact of qualitative health psychology research (Gough & Deatrick, 2015).

Observation, survey, and questionnaire methods of data collection are used in qualitative and quantitative research. Data can be collected in-person or remotely via telephone, video call, or online platforms. Surveys and questionnaires can be a cost- and time-efficient way to collect large amounts of data (particularly with online platforms), compared to observations, which can involve data collection over many months.

Observations allow behaviour to be studied. They can be conducted in a controlled laboratory setting where all conditions and procedures are determined. Observations can take a descriptive approach, such as watching and reporting naturally occurring variability in EEG data of a healthy brain, or an analytical approach, such as manipulating a healthy brain by inducing fear of health consequences and recording subsequent changes in EEG data. Data can be recorded and coded on a predefined structured observation schedule (form). In contrast, naturalistic observations are conducted in natural surroundings and behaviour studied can be more spontaneous. Naturalistic observations are non-participatory, where the observer records behaviour without interacting or interfering with participants. A remote data collection example is observing when, how, and between whom interactions occur in an online health chat room without the observer contributing to any discussions. An in-person example is unobtrusively recording the number of people picking up health information leaflets in a clinic waiting room. When the observer takes a participatory role, it is known as 'participant observation'. Using an example of exploring shared decision-making practices in a multidisciplinary clinical team, a 'passive participant observer' observes the interactions and asks follow-up questions afterwards (e.g., Hahlweg et al., 2017), whereas an 'active participant observer' would conduct the observations as part of their interactions with the team during clinical practice. Ethnographic research exploits 'participant observation' as a key method and enables the study of the theory-practice gap in health care (Cubellis et al., 2021).

Surveys or questionnaires are common methods of quantitative data collection in correlational study designs, where a naturally occurring relationship between two or more variables is studied. Correlational studies can broadly be grouped into cross-sectional and longitudinal designs. Longitudinal designs include cohort and time-series designs, which can use questionnaires to measure the variables of interest at multiple time points in a group (cohort) or individual (single case, see N-of-1), respectively. In correlational studies, the variables measured in the questionnaire or survey are not manipulated. They can be defined as independent (e.g., degree of nicotine dependence) and dependent (e.g., number of cigarettes per day), thereby specifying a potential causal relationship. Surveys can also be employed in experimental and quasi-experimental designs where causation rather than correlation is explored or inferred, such as a questionnaire administered before and after a smoking intervention measuring the effect on self-reported smoking behaviour and behavioural cognitions ((quasi-)experimental designs are described on p. 149). Surveys can be an easy and cost-efficient method, flexibly administered via paper (mail), telephone or through online survey providers, websites, or apps (see Safdar et al., 2016 for an overview of the advantages and disadvantages of surveys). Surveys can also be part of qualitative studies, typically structured interviews, where the researcher asks questions and records the numerical responses (e.g., "How many cigarettes do you smoke per day?").

Experimental or interventional methods typically fall within a quantitative research paradigm and include laboratory-based studies with manipulation, RCTs, and natural experimental studies (for mixed methods research in experiments on p. 150). Experimental designs allow testing of cause-and-effect relationships by manipulating the independent variable(s), potentially controlling all other variables, and studying the effect of manipulation on the dependent variable(s), typically referred to as outcomes in health intervention studies.

Laboratory-based (lab) experiments are the classic experiment, which boast a highly controlled environment to conduct the study. Lab-based experiments have been positioned as providing a bridge between correlational and large-scale population interventional health psychology research (Mullan et al., 2014). Lab-based experiments have high internal validity; apart from the independent variable(s) that is manipulated, all other variables are controlled for (e.g., no distraction by noise), meaning that any changes in the dependent variable(s) were caused by the independent variable(s). In terms of developing behaviour change science, a lab-based experiment can unpick and test potential mechanisms of behaviour change. For example, a 2 × 2 factorial lab-based experiment of the main and interaction effects of behavioural demonstration and feedback intervention techniques on handwashing efficacy to remove potentially infectious pathogens by randomly assigning participants to one of four conditions: (1) control condition (neither intervention technique), (2) demonstration of handwashing only, (3) feedback on handwashing efficacy only, and (4) demonstration and feedback together. The results could indicate possible additive or synergistic effects of techniques, which in turn could inform the design of more effective handwashing interventions. They could also help inform de-implementation of interventions that have no or minimal impact, thus avoiding resource waste. The highly controlled environment of lab-based experiments is often tainted with concerns about the generalisability of findings in a 'real-world' setting (i.e., lower ecological validity). For example, the lab environment and researcher involvement might impact results through sampling bias and participant demand characteristics (Holleman et al., 2020).

RCTs are often referred to as the gold standard for testing medical and health interventions (Schulz et al., 2010). RCTs that are said to be more pragmatic aim to inform healthcare decisions by producing data applicable to situations beyond the precise trial setting (Treweek & Zwarenstein, 2009), which is generally the case in health psychology intervention research. Jones and Podolsky (2015) provide an overview of the history behind the term 'gold standard' for RCTs and discuss its defensibility alongside the burgeoning field of personalised medicine, where interventions are based on individual, rather than population, needs and characteristics (see N-of-1 RCTs on p. 149). Population-based RCTs often have strict inclusion criteria to form a homogenous group of individuals and setting, and thus do not align well with systems thinking, another increasingly popular field, where differing and interconnected characteristics of individuals and environments are explored.

Methodological rigour is intrinsic to RCTs through the random allocation of participants to two or more groups, with at least one group serving as a control or comparator group. Trial outcomes are compared between the intervention group(s), and the comparator group(s). Sometimes, clusters of participants (e.g., school classes, communities, hospital wards) are randomised to the intervention or comparator group (i.e., cluster RCTs) because randomisation of individual participants is unfeasible. In addition to random allocation and the presence of a comparator group, other features of methodological rigour of RCTs include blinding of researchers, participants, and outcome assessors; assessing deviations from the trial protocol in the intervention or analyses; and intention-to-treat analyses (i.e., analyses according to original treatment allocation even if participants did not adhere, e.g., skipped sessions, failing to take the medicine). An appraisal of the risk of bias associated with these and other RCT methodological features is often part of a systematic review of RCTs (e.g., Sterne et al., 2019).

Pilot RCTs are a subset of RCTs used as a precursor to test trial procedures, detect trial problems, and, in cases where the sample size allows accurate estimation, assess preliminary effects before determining intervention efficacy (Eldridge et al., 2016; Viechtbauer et al., 2015). Feasibility studies are similar to pilot studies, generally conducted in advance of an RCT; however, feasibility studies often have the primary aim of determining the feasibility and acceptability of the intervention and RCT. Many feasibility studies test the intervention without randomisation to a comparator group and often utilise mixed methods (Aschbrenner et al., 2022) to collect qualitative (e.g., experiences of treatment) and quantitative (e.g., pain rating) data (discussed on p. 145).

Natural and quasi-experiments are often favoured over randomised experiments and RCTs in applied health psychology and public health research where experimental manipulation is not completely possible. Natural experiments involve exposure to an intervention determined naturally, meaning that intervention allocation is not controlled by the research, such as a study of smoking behaviour and lung function covering the time after introducing nationwide indoor smoking bans (Strassmann et al., 2022). The ability to make causal claims from natural experiments depends on the strength of the 'as-if randomisation' assumption where it can be argued that even though experimental manipulation was not used for intervention allocation, the allocation process was as if by random and thus has not affected the intervention outcomes. Natural experiments are often called quasi-experiments. de Vocht et al. (2021) provide a discussion of different natural and quasi-experimental designs in public health research and a framework to appraise the strength of causal claims.

N-of-1 methods (single-case designs) involve the study of within-individual processes, relationships, and intervention effects by repeatedly quantitatively measuring the variables of interest in one individual (or an individual unit) over time. N-of-1 methods align with the personalised medicine agenda, resulting in conclusions about an individual. In health psychology, they play an important and unique role in developing behaviour change science, producing knowledge and understanding about within-individual behaviour change processes to complement what is already known about between-individual processes derived from more common between-subjects (group-based) designs. In addition to studying the natural history of behaviour and behavioural determinants over time and testing theory within individuals (e.g., Hobbs et al., 2013), N-of-1 methods can evaluate intervention effects for an intervention, including using an N-of-1 RCT design (e.g., Nyman et al., 2016; Sniehotta et al., 2012). Systematic reviews of N-of-1 methods in health behaviour research (McDonald et al., 2017) and randomised N-of-1 trials in health psychology (Shaffer et al., 2018) provide overviews of the N-of-1 literature and discussions of the associated challenging methodological and analytical issues.

Participatory research is described as an umbrella term for partnered research approaches, including community-based participatory research, participatory action research, and participatory evaluation (Cargo & Mercer, 2008). Participatory methods are part of action research rather than a descriptive or analytical study approach. They are predominantly qualitative in nature, eliciting views, ideas and experiences, but can also collect quantitative data (e.g., surveys). Participatory methods can be employed at one or more research stages (e.g., study prioritisation, design, conduct, data analysis, interpretation, dissemination, implementation) and during any activities designed to actively involve key stakeholders. Arnstein's Ladder of Citizen Participation (1969) considers the degrees of involvement of people in decision-making processes and how redistribution of power is essential for meaningful and influential participation of all parties involved. The active and meaningful involvement of patients, public, and other stakeholders in health research is advocated internationally (e.g., United States Patient Centred Outcomes Research Institute, United Kingdom Public Involvement Standards Development Partnership).

In health psychology research, participation of key stakeholders often refers to that of patients, public, service users, carers, health professionals, commissioners, etc., with the aim of incorporating their voices, knowledge, and experiences to better understand and address the needs and challenges of their respective 'communities'. In the United Kingdom, this active participation is referred to as patient and public involvement and engagement (PPI or PPIE). Within the context of intervention research (see Section 6 chapters), co-design participatory approaches can be used to engage stakeholders in intervention development.

Secondary research includes a set of methods in health psychology involving secondary analysis of data, i.e., primary data that have been collected but not for the purpose of answering the research question(s) of the current study. They can be descriptive or analytical and employed in qualitative or quantitative research. Evidence synthesis methods (e.g., systematic, narrative, realist reviews) and meta-analyses provide valuable summaries of evidence on a particular topic to inform future healthcare decisions, interventions, and services. For example, a systematic review of RCTs of habit interventions for lifestyle behaviour change in ethnic minority communities could provide a detailed summary of previous studies in accordance with prespecified PICO characteristics (Population, Intervention, Comparison, Outcome). If data are available and suitable for statistical aggregation, then a meta-analysis of studies can provide a quantitative summary of the magnitude of (intervention) effects. Another type of secondary research that can be low cost and reduce research waste is the analysis of existing datasets, such as those routinely collected in healthcare settings and services.

Even though in health psychology and health sciences more generally, secondary research is more likely to analyse quantitative data, qualitative data can also be re-analysed with new questions. For example, qualitative systematic reviews can synthesise qualitative data on a particular topic, and existing textual, visual, or multimedia datasets can be qualitatively analysed.

Mixed Methods Research Design

Mixed methods designs are popular in health sciences research. Multiple definitions and varying terms exist (e.g., multi-methods); however, general agreement is that mixed methods involve quantitative and qualitative research and multiple methods, which are integrated or combined to answer questions that require detailed contextual understandings and multiple perspectives (NIH Office of Behavioral and Social Sciences, 2018). The temporal order of the quantitative and qualitative research varies, with some research using a sequential approach where a quantitative component precedes a qualitative one or vice versa. The first component may inform the design of the second component, such as quantitative survey findings informing the focus or sampling strategies of subsequent qualitative interviews or qualitative findings informing an RCT or survey. The data from each component are integrated or combined and may serve as standalone findings. Where there is dependency between components, a successful earlier component may provide valuable data to maximise the likelihood of the success of later components. However, if that earlier component fails to deliver the data required, then subsequent components may also fail, and the overarching research question may go unanswered.

In contrast to the sequential approach in mixed methods, is the convergent (contemporaneous) approach where quantitative and qualitative components occur at the same time, such as a quantitative population-based survey and qualitative interviews targeting population subgroups known to disengage with surveys. Data are either merged for analysis or analysed separately and then integrated. The convergent approach removes the risk of research failure associated with dependency between components and is more efficient in terms of less time and research costs.

Overviews of the theoretical and practical benefits and challenges of conducting mixed methods research in health sciences, and health psychology specifically, exist (Dures et al., 2011; NIH Office of Behavioral and Social Sciences, 2018). Mixed methods are increasingly viewed as an important approach to the evaluation of health interventions. Together, qualitative and quantitative research can generate unique insight about the feasibility, effectiveness and implementation of health interventions that would not have been evident with one approach only. Mixed methods process evaluations are recognised as crucial to understanding an intervention's potential mechanisms of change and reasons for its success or failure (Moore et al., 2015). The results of quantitative and qualitative research components of an intervention evaluation do not always align, but mixed methods allow discrepancies to be examined (Moffatt et al., 2006; Tonkin-Crine et al., 2016), which may involve a triangulation protocol or other techniques (see O'Cathain et al., 2010 for a discussion of integrating mixed methods data).

Examples of Mixed Methods Research

To illustrate how mixed methods can be used to integrate and combine different sources and types of evidence to provide a richer and more contextualised answer to the research question, four examples of mixed methods research, relevant to health psychology, are presented in Box 8.1.

Research Design Good Practice

Having provided an overview of the critical decisions in relation to research design and methods that health psychology researchers face when designing and planning research, some recommendations for good practice can be given.

Box 8.1 Example Mixed Methods Studies in Health Psychology

Example A: A mixed methods participatory intervention design process to support healthy eating and physical activity of children and adolescents at school and home (Erzse et al., 2022)

Aim: To develop healthy eating and physical activity interventions, and inform food and built environment priorities at schools and home.

Design: Sequential mixed methods: (1) secondary analysis of qualitative data to identify contextual behavioural determinants, (2) theoretical mapping of evidence-based interventions to determinants, (3) Delphi survey with stakeholders to prioritise the interventions.

Data integration: Data from each component is used to inform the design of the subsequent.

Benefit of mixed methods: Application of quantitative and qualitative theoretical methods, with participatory methods to identify and prioritise context-specific interventions targeting behavioural determinants.

Example B: Co-design of a web-based lifestyle intervention in retirement informed by mixed methods research (O'Brien et al., 2016)

Aim: To integrate scientific evidence, expert experience and stakeholder involvement in the development of a lifestyle intervention in retirement.

Design: Convergent and sequential mixed methods: (1) three systematic reviews (two with meta-analyses), (2) qualitative interviews and focus groups, (3) review of wider behaviour change evidence base and expert consultation, (4) intervention co-design workshops.

Data integration: Data from components 1–3 analysed separately, combined and integrated to derive evidence statements to inform components.

Benefit of mixed methods: Integration of descriptive, context-rich narratives and discrete evidence for a more nuanced understanding of the intervention context to develop an evidence-based and co-designed intervention.

Example C: Mixed methods process evaluation of a digital intervention for asthma embedded within a feasibility RCT (Greenwell et al., 2021)

Aim: To explore user engagement and experiences of the intervention to support and refine the intervention programme theory.

Design: Convergent mixed methods: (1) intervention usage data, (2) intervention satisfaction questionnaire (quantitative and qualitative data), (3) qualitative interviews.

Data integration: Data analysed separately then triangulated.

Benefit of mixed methods: Ability to explore different aspects of intervention engagement using different quantitative and qualitative methods.

Reporting Guidelines

Reporting guidelines intend, as the name suggests, to improve the reporting of research studies. The EQUATOR Network is an international initiative for more accurate and transparent reporting of health research. EQUATOR is a repository of reporting guidelines for the main research designs discussed in this chapter, including CONSORT (RCTs, pilot, feasibility, and N-of-1 trials), PRISMA (systematic reviews), COREQ (qualitative research), and STROBE (observational studies). Even though these guidelines exist to improve research reporting, they can also be useful tools to consult when designing research. The guidelines detail key methodological features that need to be reported, and therefore, they can be used in research team discussions to determine whether all methodological features have been adequately considered in the research design.

Research Protocols and Study Registration

Once a study has been designed, a detailed research protocol that documents the background, rationale, aims, objectives, design, methods, procedures, analysis, and management of the research process should be developed. The protocol serves as a reference document that can be consulted at different stages of the study to confirm the methodological features (e.g., sampling strategies, analysis plans) and monitor study progress. Research protocols are often required by research ethics committees when applying for approval to conduct a study. In health sciences, it is good practice to make trial and systematic review protocols publicly available through peer-reviewed publication, trial registration (e.g., ISRCTN, ClinicalTrials.gov, EU Clinical Trials Register), review registries (e.g., PROSPERO) or the Open Science Framework. Registering a trial prospectively can prevent study duplication and, in turn, reduce research waste. It can also reduce potential bias in research conduct and reporting as pre-specification of the design, aims, and analyses, etc., means that unplanned analyses and selective reporting of findings cannot go unnoticed. Such open science ethical research practices support transparency and replicability of research findings (Kwasnicka et al., 2021) and confidence in the evidence generated.

Conclusions

Like the blueprint of a new house which specifies what is needed for the build, research design is the blueprint of the research specifying the plan, resources, and methods needed to answer the research question effectively and efficiently. Following good practice recommendations, together with careful and thorough consideration of research design and the associated strengths and limitations of designs and methods, will maximise the likelihood that robust data are generated, research objectives are achieved, and research integrity is upheld.

Further Reading

Creswell, J.W. & Plano Clark, V.L. (2017) *Designing and Conducting Mixed Methods Research*, 3rd Edition. SAGE Publications.

Vaughn, L.M., & Jacquez, F. (2020). Participatory research methods – Choice points in the research process. *Journal of Participatory Research Methods*, *1*(1). https://doi.org/10.35844/001c.13244

References

Arnstein, S.R. (1969). A ladder of citizen participation. *Journal of the American Institute of Planners*, *35*(4), 216–224. https://doi.org/10.1080/01944366908977225

Aschbrenner, K.A., Kruse, G., Gallo, J.J., & Plano Clark, V.L. (2022). Applying mixed methods to pilot feasibility studies to inform intervention trials. *Pilot and Feasibility Studies*, *8*(1), 217. https://doi.org/10.1186/s40814-022-01178-x

Brookes, S.T., Biddle, L., Paterson, C., Woolhead, G., & Dieppe, P. (2007). "Me's me and you're you": Exploring patients' perspectives of single patient (n-of-1) trials in the UK. *Trials*, *8*(1), 10. https://doi.org/10.1186/1745-6215-8-10

Browne, S., Dowie, A., Mitchell, E., Wyke, S., Ziebland, S., Campbell, N., & Macleod, U. (2011). Patients' needs following colorectal cancer diagnosis: where does primary care fit in? *British Journal of General Practice*, *61*(592), e692–699. https://doi.org/10.3399/bjgp11X606582

Cargo, M., & Mercer, S.L. (2008). The value and challenges of participatory research: Strengthening its practice. *Annual Review of Public Health*, *29*(1), 325–350. https://doi.org/10.1146/annurev.publhealth.29.091307.083824

Cubellis, L., Schmid, C., & von Peter, S. (2021). Ethnography in health services research: Oscillation between theory and practice. *Qualitative Health Research*, *31*(11), 2029–2040. https://doi.org/10.1177/10497323211022312

de Vocht, F., Katikireddi, S.V., McQuire, C., Tilling, K., Hickman, M., & Craig, P. (2021). Conceptualising natural and quasi experiments in public health. *BMC Medical Research Methodology*, *21*(1), 32. https://doi.org/10.1186/s12874-021-01224-x

Dures, E., Rumsey, N., Morris, M., & Gleeson, K. (2011). Mixed methods in health psychology: Theoretical and practical considerations of the third paradigm. *Journal of Health Psychology*, *16*(2), 332–341. https://doi.org/10.1177/1359105310377537

Eldridge, S.M., Lancaster, G.A., Campbell, M.J., Thabane, L., Hopewell, S., Coleman, C.L., & Bond, C.M. (2016). Defining feasibility and pilot studies in preparation for randomised controlled trials: development of a conceptual framework. *PLOS ONE*, *11*(3), e0150205. https://doi.org/10.1371/journal.pone.0150205

Erzse, A., Rwafa-Ponela, T., Kruger, P., Wayas, F.A., Lambert, E.V., Mapa-Tassou, C., Ngwa, E., Goldstein, S., Foley, L., Hofman, K.J., Teguia, S., Oni, T., Assah, F., Shung-King, M., & Abdool Karim, S. (2022). A mixed-methods participatory intervention design process to develop intervention options in immediate food and built environments to support healthy eating and active living among children and adolescents in Cameroon and South Africa. *International Journal of Environmental Research and Public Health*, *19*(16), 10263. https://www.mdpi.com/1660-4601/19/16/10263

Gough, B., & Deatrick, J.A. (2015). Qualitative health psychology research: Diversity, power, and impact. *Health Psychology*, *34*(4), 289–292. https://doi.org/10.1037/hea0000206

Greenwell, K., Ainsworth, B., Bruton, A., Murray, E., Russell, D., Thomas, M., & Yardley, L. (2021). Mixed methods process evaluation of my breathing matters, a digital intervention to support self-management of asthma. *npj Primary Care Respiratory Medicine*, *31*(1), 35. https://doi.org/10.1038/s41533-021-00248-6

Hahlweg, P., Härter, M., Nestoriuc, Y., & Scholl, I. (2017). How are decisions made in cancer care? A qualitative study using participant observation of current practice. *BMJ Open*, *7*(9), e016360. https://doi.org/10.1136/bmjopen-2017-016360

Hobbs, N., Dixon, D., Johnston, M., & Howie, K. (2013). Can the theory of planned behaviour predict the physical activity behaviour of individuals? *Psychology & Health*, *28*(3), 234–249. https://doi.org/10.1080/08870446.2012.716838

Holleman, G.A., Hooge, I.T.C., Kemner, C., & Hessels, R.S. (2020). The 'real-world approach' and its problems: A critique of the term ecological validity. *Frontiers in Psychology*, *11*, 721. https://doi.org/10.3389/fpsyg.2020.00721

Jones, D.S., & Podolsky, S.H. (2015). The history and fate of the gold standard. *Lancet*, *385*(9977), 1502–1503. https://doi.org/10.1016/s0140-6736(15)60742-5

Kwasnicka, D., ten Hoor, G.A., van Dongen, A., Gruszczyńska, E., Hagger, M.S., Hamilton, K., Hankonen, N., Heino, M.T.J., Kotzur, M., Noone, C., Rothman, A.J., Toomey, E., Warner, L.M., Kok, G., Peters, G.-J., & Luszczynska, A. (2021). Promoting scientific integrity through open science in health psychology: Results of the Synergy Expert Meeting of the European health psychology society. *Health Psychology Review*, *15*(3), 333–349. https://doi.org/10.1080/17437199.2020.1844037

McDonald, S., Quinn, F., Vieira, R., O'Brien, N., White, M., Johnston, D.W., & Sniehotta, F.F. (2017). The state of the art and future opportunities for using longitudinal n-of-1 methods in health behaviour research: A systematic literature overview. *Health Psychology Review*, *11*(4), 307–323. https://doi.org/10.1080/17437199.2017.1316672

Moffatt, S., White, M., Mackintosh, J., & Howel, D. (2006). Using quantitative and qualitative data in health services research – What happens when mixed method findings conflict? [ISRCTN61522618]. *BMC Health Services Research*, *6*, 28. https://doi.org/10.1186/1472-6963-6-28

Moore, G.F., Audrey, S., Barker, M., Bond, L., Bonell, C., Hardeman, W., Moore, L., O'Cathain, A., Tinati, T., Wight, D., & Baird, J. (2015). Process evaluation of complex interventions: Medical Research Council guidance. *BMJ*, *350*, h1258. https://doi.org/10.1136/bmj.h1258

Mullan, B., Todd, J., Chatzisarantis, N.L., & Hagger, M.S. (2014). Experimental methods in health psychology in Australia: Implications for applied research. *Australian Psychologist*, *49*(2), 104–109. https://doi.org/10.1111/ap.12046

Murray, S.A., Kendall, M., Carduff, E., Worth, A., Harris, F.M., Lloyd, A., Cavers, D., Grant, L., & Sheikh, A. (2009). Use of serial qualitative interviews to understand patients' evolving experiences and needs. *BMJ*, *339*, b3702. https://doi.org/10.1136/bmj.b3702

NIH Office of Behavioral and Social Sciences. (2018). *Best practices for mixed methods research in the health sciences*. 2nd Ed. National Institutes of Health.

Nyman, S.R., Goodwin, K., Kwasnicka, D., & Callaway, A. (2016). Increasing walking among older people: A test of behaviour change techniques using factorial randomised N-of-1 trials. *Psychology & Health*, *31*(3), 313–330. https://doi.org/10.1080/08870446.2015.1088014

O'Brien, N., Heaven, B., Teal, G., Evans, E.H., Cleland, C., Moffatt, S., Sniehotta, F.F., White, M., Mathers, J.C., & Moynihan, P. (2016). Integrating evidence from systematic reviews, qualitative research, and expert knowledge using co-design techniques to develop a web-based intervention for people in the retirement transition. *Journal of Medical Internet Research*, *18*(8), e210. https://doi.org/10.2196/jmir.5790

O'Cathain, A., Murphy, E., & Nicholl, J. (2010). Three techniques for integrating data in mixed methods studies. *BMJ*, *341*, c4587. https://doi.org/10.1136/bmj.c4587

Okwose, N.C., O'Brien, N., Charman, S., Cassidy, S., Brodie, D., Bailey, K., MacGowan, G.A., Jakovljevic, D.G., & Avery, L. (2020). Overcoming barriers to engagement and adherence to a home-based physical activity intervention for patients with heart failure: A qualitative focus group study. *BMJ Open*, *10*(9), e036382. https://doi.org/10.1136/bmjopen-2019-036382

Safdar, N., Abbo, L.M., Knobloch, M.J., & Seo, S.K. (2016). Research methods in healthcare epidemiology: Survey and qualitative research. *Infection Control & Hospital Epidemiology*, *37*(11), 1272–1277. https://doi.org/10.1017/ice.2016.171

Schulz, K.F., Altman, D.G., & Moher, D. (2010). CONSORT 2010 Statement: Updated guidelines for reporting parallel group randomised trials. *BMJ*, *340*, c332. https://doi.org/10.1136/bmj.c332

Shaffer, J.A., Kronish, I.M., Falzon, L., Cheung, Y.K., & Davidson, K.W. (2018). N-of-1 randomized intervention trials in health psychology: A systematic review and methodology critique. *Annals of Behavioral Medicine*, *52*(9), 731–742. https://doi.org/10.1093/abm/kax026

Sniehotta, F.F., Presseau, J., Hobbs, N., & Araújo-Soares, V. (2012). Testing self-regulation interventions to increase walking using factorial randomized N-of-1 trials. *Health Psychology*, *31*(6), 733–737. https://doi.org/10.1037/a0027337

Sterne, J.A.C., Savović, J., Page, M.J., Elbers, R.G., Blencowe, N.S., Boutron, I., Cates, C.J., Cheng, H.Y., Corbett, M.S., Eldridge, S.M., Emberson, J.R., Hernán, M.A., Hopewell, S., Hróbjartsson, A., Junqueira, D.R., Jüni, P., Kirkham, J.J., Lasserson, T., Li, T., McAleenan, A., Reeves, B.C., Shepperd, S., Shrier, I., Stewart, L.A., Tilling, K., White, I.R., Whiting, P.F., & Higgins, J.P.T. (2019). RoB 2: A revised tool for assessing risk of bias in randomised trials. *BMJ*, *366*, l4898. https://doi.org/10.1136/bmj.l4898

Strassmann, A., Çolak, Y., Serra-Burriel, M., Nordestgaard, B.G., Turk, A., Afzal, S., & Puhan, M.A. (2022). Nationwide indoor smoking ban and impact on smoking behaviour and lung function: a two-population natural experiment. *Thorax*, *78*,144–150. https://doi.org/10.1136/thoraxjnl-2021-218436

Tonkin-Crine, S., Anthierens, S., Hood, K., Yardley, L., Cals, J.W., Francis, N.A., Coenen, S., van der Velden, A.W., Godycki-Cwirko, M., Llor, C., Butler, C.C., Verheij, T.J., Goossens, H., & Little, P. (2016). Discrepancies between qualitative and quantitative evaluation of randomised controlled trial results: Achieving clarity through mixed methods triangulation. *Implementation Science*, *11*, 66. https://doi.org/10.1186/s13012-016-0436-0

Treweek, S., & Zwarenstein, M. (2009). Making trials matter: Pragmatic and explanatory trials and the problem of applicability. *Trials*, *10*(1), 37. https://doi.org/10.1186/1745-6215-10-37

Viechtbauer, W., Smits, L., Kotz, D., Budé, L., Spigt, M., Serroyen, J., & Crutzen, R. (2015). A simple formula for the calculation of sample size in pilot studies. *Journal of Clinical Epidemiology*, *68*(11), 1375–1379. https://doi.org/10.1016/j.jclinepi.2015.04.014

9

MEASUREMENT IN HEALTH PSYCHOLOGY

Alexandra Lelia Dima

"How are you? Have you been sleeping well lately? Have you been doing your daily walks since we last spoke? How are you getting on with your medication?" These questions and others like them are common in everyday conversations. You have asked them yourself in your personal life, for example, during a visit to an elderly relative, or to a friend who has been unwell lately, or even to yourself to reflect on how you have been managing your health and what you could improve. Health-care professionals, including health psychologists, ask similar questions to individuals they treat or support in managing their health. Researchers in health sciences, including health psychology, collect data on health behaviours and health status indicators of individuals from their study population. The type of information sought is similar when these questions are asked in personal life, clinical practice, and research. Yet, their aims are different in many respects in these three contexts and, consequently, so is the level of accuracy needed in the responses received. This chapter gives an overview of the process of measuring phenomena of interest in health psychology practice and research, such as *health behaviours*, *behaviour determinants*, and *health-related outcomes*, as well as *behaviour change interventions*. It attempts to give practical answers and guidance on *how we can measure better in health psychology* and *how we can know if we did a good job or not*. Different types of measures are discussed, including self-report, biomarkers, sensors, behaviour observation, quantitative content analysis, and routinely collected health-care data, as well as methods for testing and improving their measurement properties and recommendations for good measurement practices. To measure well, we need to understand what measurement is, what constraints apply, and what options we have to make it work under certain constraints.

 DOI: 10.4324/9781003318026-11

What Is Measurement in Health Psychology?

In research and clinical practice, there are several purposes for which we might need answers to questions about health: making clinical decisions (regarding individuals, intervention programmes), describing patient/user populations, predicting outcomes, testing theories (Karademas et al., 2015). Several terms have been used to refer to this process of questioning, depending on its goals and criteria for judging responses: *assessment* denotes a process-oriented inquiry guided by internally defined goals and flexible criteria (e.g., to assess progress towards an individual goal), *evaluation* is aimed at decision-making based on fixed and externally set criteria (e.g., to evaluate effectiveness of an intervention), while *measurement* refers to describing the attributes of an entity (individual, organisation, event, etc.) via quantitative methods (Luszczynska et al., 2018b). This chapter focuses on the latter since generating meaningful and precise quantitative data on the realities of health and illness is central to health psychology, irrespective of the purposes for which data are used.

Measurement is often highlighted as an issue in need of improvement in health and social sciences, to the extent that it has been deemed a key reason for the currently debated 'replication crisis' (Lilienfeld & Strother, 2020), i.e., the failure to reproduce results of empirical studies following the specifications of the original research. While this crisis has numerous interrelated causes, it has also stimulated reflection on how we can address limitations in common measurement practices. For example, a recurring concern in methodological literature is the pervasiveness of the *jingle-jangle fallacy*, or *construct identity fallacy*, i.e., using the same label for two different constructs or different labels for identical or very similar constructs (Larsen & Bong, 2016). Other recurring concerns refer to the insufficient consideration and reporting on measure selection and validation (Crutzen & Peters, 2015; Eronen & Bringmann, 2021; Lilienfeld & Strother, 2020). These practices are closely related to how we develop and test theories and how we build evidence for action in real-life practice. Thus, suboptimal measurement has been considered a major barrier in building a good-quality evidence base in many research areas, such as medication adherence (Dima et al., 2021), mental health (Fried et al., 2022), and self-regulation (Enkavi et al., 2019), to name but a few.

Improving measurement practices has been the focus of many efforts in recent years. General frameworks have been proposed to guide the choice of measurement purpose (Karademas et al., 2015) or to locate the phenomena of study within specific health psychology domains, each with their specific measurement challenges, e.g., health behaviour and prevention, stress and disease, or medical illness and care (Smith, 2011b). Practical advice has been put forward to guide the process of measurement. For example, (Luszczynska et al., 2018b) proposed five steps to guide the planning, selection, and implementation of a measurement instrument in research: (1) choice of general framework, (2) considering the target population, (3) deciding on the type of measurement, (4) considering psychometric properties, and (5) considering implementation of the instrument, and provide pointers to resources and examples to guide researchers through the process. Flake & Fried (2020) proposed six questions to guide researchers, as well as users of research, to identify questionable measurement practices and avoid them by focusing on (1) understanding the construct, (2) the reasons and process of measure selection, (3) operationalisation, (4) administration, (5) quantification, and (6) reporting on measure modification or new developments. Core Outcome Sets, i.e., "agreed standardised sets of outcomes that should be measured and reported in all trials for a specific clinical area", have been developed via consensus methodologies in many different health conditions and patient populations to coordinate the selection and measurement of constructs and thus facilitate evidence accumulation (Williamson et al., 2017). Repositories of health-related measures are now available to facilitate the use of measures that have followed established development and validation procedures, and the assessment and comparison of the quality of these procedures (see examples at the end of the chapter).

These improvement efforts have been directed essentially towards changing the still prevalent belief that measurement is a single decision with limited consequences on theory and practice which consists mainly of taking an already developed tool 'off-the-shelf' or writing some questions *ad hoc* to add to a survey. Instead, they aim to promote a more helpful approach to measurement as continuously evolving in sync with theory and practice to generate and improve knowledge in a particular field. Particular attention has been given to improving the psychometric properties of self-report questionnaires, mostly those including multiple items. However, researchers and practitioners have a broader range of sources of information on health-related phenomena: biomarkers, sensors, quantitative content analysis, and routinely collected health-care data. This diversity is important to consider when deciding on the most appropriate measurement strategy, as the optimal strategy for one's purpose might not be the first that comes to mind. While each strategy might be subject to unique constraints and sources of error or bias, they have in common the general process of measurement, which we will outline next.

To measure a construct, one needs to follow three steps: (1) identify and define the construct – *definition*, (2) determine the set of operations by which this construct is isolated and observable – *operationalisation*, and (3) determine a set of procedures by which observations are transformed into quantitative statements of degree or amount – *quantification* (Thorndike & Thorndike-Christ, 2009). Table 9.1 includes examples of constructs discussed in other chapters in this book, with their definition, operationalisation, and quantification. The next sections discuss each step and how one can make the most of it to improve measurement.

Defining a Construct – What's in a Name?

Constructs are born in the observation and induction phases of the empirical cycle (see Chapter 6, "How to Work with Theories of Health Behaviour Change," in this volume). They are components of psychological theories, together with

Table 9.1 Examples of definition, operationalisation, and quantification of health psychology constructs

Construct	*Definition*	*Operationalisation*	*Quantification*
1. Illness timeline representation	"[A] person's perception of the likely duration of the illness and expectations about the course of the health problem".	Self-reported timeline beliefs by persons living with the illness as measured by the single item from the IPQ questionnaire: "How long do you think your illness will continue?" (Broadbent et al., 2006).	Ordinal variable as per scoring of the response scale provided: 0 (a very short time) to 10 (forever)
2. Medication initiation	Medication adherence behaviour that refers to the first actual dosing event of a prescribed treatment.	Patients with at least one medication pharmacy refill recorded within ten weeks after the first dispensing event, according to data extracted from patient records (Dima et al., 2021).	Binary variable: yes/no
3. Obesity (Chapter 14)	"[T]he accumulation of excess adipose tissue (fat) which presents a risk to health".	Persons with a body mass index (BMI) of 30 or higher as measured by data collected in routine care and accessed from patient records (see Ch 3.4. for uses and limitations of this proxy measure of obesity).	Binary variable: yes/no

(*Continued*)

Table 9.1 (Continued)

Construct	*Definition*	*Operationalisation*	*Quantification*
4. Action planning behaviour change technique (BCT)	"A goal directed BCT that involves making a detailed plan for the performance of the behaviour, which must include at least one of context, frequency, duration or intensity" (Marques et al., 2023).	An app for physical activity support includes a function that opens a window with an action plan, where the user is invited to specify when, where, and how they plan to perform a given activity (Wang et al., 2021).	Binary variable: yes/no
5. Intervention adoption (Chapter 30)	Implementation outcome referring to "how many providers (clinicians or organisations) deliver an intervention".	Proportion of primary care centres participating in a specific new screening programme of the total number of centres eligible in the target area.	Continuous variable: percentage of participation

statements about their relationships with other constructs. Their labels and definitions evolve together with theories through repeated empirical cycles and application to different practice settings. Beyond specific theories, construct labels and definitions also represent anchoring points in a shared representation of a domain of research and practice. Therefore, elaborating explicit and precise definitions of the concepts investigated is essential for organising existing knowledge and integrating new findings into an increasing body of knowledge (Kaplan & Beatty, 2022). In this regard, advances in psychology have been hampered by the limited reporting of construct definitions in published studies (Lilienfeld & Strother, 2020).

There have been several notable initiatives to improve psychological and health sciences by creating ontologies, i.e., explicit, formal specifications of shared conceptualisations in the form of systematic sets of terms and explications of their interrelations (Kaplan & Beatty, 2022). These ontologies range from simple lists of terms and definitions to formally specified sets of entities and relationships. For example, the Metathesaurus of the Unified Medical Language System (UMLS) includes terms and definitions of constructs used in health psychology, among other domains in health sciences, with unique identifiers for constructs and terms in different languages designed for use by developers of information technology systems for health-care practice and research and curated by the United States National Library of Medicine ("Metathesaurus," 2021). The Behaviour Change Intervention Ontology (BCIO) is a formally specified ontological system with a narrower scope, aiming to facilitate efficient accumulation and use of behavioural knowledge by creating a common language to describe interventions and constructs, interoperable with other ontologies and computer-readable in order to ultimately automatise the synthesis and interpretation of research evidence in this field (Michie et al., 2021). These ontologies are intended as evolving resources to be used in conjunction with specific methods to produce and use evidence.

In health psychology, the BCIO is currently articulated with two notable methodologies for representing and testing theories and constructs. A formal system for representing theories has been proposed to improve the clarity and consistency of their statements and thus their development and use; preliminary tests on five theories commonly used in health psychology show promise, and a wider application is encouraged (West et al., 2019). The Science of Behaviour Change (SOBC) programme has adopted a methodology for generating evidence on mechanisms of action (MoAs) in behaviour change that involves MoA identification, measure development and/or validation, experimental manipulation, and testing its effect on behaviour (Sumner et al., 2018). Thus, the first step to measuring well is taking informed decisions on the concepts to measure regarding their labels and definitions and the evidence-generation methodologies to follow throughout.

Operationalisation – How the Construct Can Be Observed?

Once a construct is identified and defined, operationalisation – the process of finding or inventing the operations that will isolate and display the construct of interest – takes place. The description of how the construct is measured represents its 'operational definition' (Thorndike & Thorndike-Christ, 2009). While commonly consisting of developing or selecting a questionnaire, formulating an operational definition is not always straightforward. It requires a deeper incursion into the construct to understand how it manifests in the real-life measurement setting and explore the range of possible operations that can be applied to elicit it in this setting. Constructs may present different variability in time (e.g., state versus trait attributes), may manifest differently in different groups of people (e.g., younger versus older people, questionnaires in different languages or cultures), may be accessible in or observable by different people to different extents (e.g., patient versus carer, child versus parent), by different cognitive processes (e.g., self-report versus implicit association test) or technologies (e.g., self-report versus device monitoring). Reflecting on these properties of a construct leads to selecting, adapting, or designing measures more appropriate in specific measurement contexts (see (Dima et al., 2021, for an example of construct operationalisation).

Quantification – From Observations to Numbers

Operationalisation is decided in conjunction with quantification, which specifies how observations are transformed into numbers (e.g., intensity of agreement, frequency of occurrence). For example, if a construct is operationalised via a multi-item self-report measure, quantification may be the total score calculated following the recommendations of the measure developers (e.g., sum score, weighted mean score). However, quantification benefits from exploring a broader range of options depending on the construct properties and the different sources of variation unrelated to the construct that each type of measure is subject to. The researcher's or practitioner's task is to identify and reduce them to an acceptable level for their measurement purpose. An overview of different types of measures follows, with brief pointers on applicable measurement properties and validation methods.

Types of Measures

Good operational definitions and quantifications are the result of weighing measurement precision and feasibility in relation to the measurement aims. In health psychology, we can differentiate between two broad categories of measures: self-report and capturing behavioural performance. All types of measures reviewed next would have their strengths and limitations; there is no 'best' type of measure for a particular construct but rather multiple options to consider in the context of the research study or clinical practice.

Self-Report Measures

Self-report (example 1 in Table 9.1) is the most common type of measurement in psychology due to its feasibility in many settings, adaptability to verbal (face-to-face or telephone), paper or digital formats, and applicability to various research designs. Self-report is used in most cross-sectional surveys, longitudinal cohort studies, as well as ecological momentary assessment (EMA) approaches. It can collect both factual information, such as socio-demographic characteristics, and the respondents' subjective experience, opinions, and beliefs towards health-related phenomena, which are less accessible via performance measures.

Data quality of self-reports relies fundamentally on how respondents can access the information relevant to the construct in the moment of reporting. The theory of survey response (Tourangeau, 2018) is a valuable guide to questionnaire development and validation and stipulates that, for an individual to answer a survey question, they need to (1) understand the question, (2) retrieve the relevant information from memory or other sources, (3) judge this information in relation to the question to estimate an answer, and, finally, (4) produce a response by mapping the answer on the response format proposed by the survey. Facilitating each response phase goes a long way towards improving data quality – for example, by ensuring clear question wording, supporting recall, reducing social desirability, and matching response options with the question wording. In this process, qualitative research (see Chapter 8 in this volume) plays an important role, from concept elicitation in interviews and focus groups to cognitive interviews to test and improve response processes and measurement properties (Ricci et al., 2019). Good self-report starts with clear, relevant, balanced questions and response options.

Multi-item Measures

Many constructs may have different observable manifestations, each subject to various other sources of variation beyond the construct itself. Selecting several such manifestations when elaborating on self-report items increases measurement precision. Therefore, multi-item measures are strongly recommended if feasible in the measurement context. The repositories mentioned at the end of this chapter include such instruments for constructs in behavioural and health sciences. How do we judge their quality to select the best? The COSMIN guidelines (Consensus-Based Standards for the Selection of Health Status Measurement Instruments) proposed a taxonomy of measurement properties and detailed recommendations for assessing them in health-related, patient-reported outcomes (Mokkink et al., 2010). The COSMIN taxonomy groups four main properties under the label of 'quality': reliability (including internal consistency, reliability, and measurement error), validity (including content, criterion, and construct validity, the latter including structural validity, hypothesis testing, and cross-cultural validity), responsiveness, and interpretability.

The COSMIN platform (https://www.cosmin.nl/) currently provides resources for developing COS (Core Outcome Sets; in collaboration with COMET (Core Outcome Measures in Effectiveness Trials)), searching available measures, and studying measurement properties. Among these properties, structural validity has attracted the most attention and debate, and it is most closely related to quantification. Most multi-item measures are developed and validated under the assumption that items are either interchangeable attempts to measure a 'true score' reflecting the construct (classical test theory) or are causally influenced to different extents by the same non-observable construct (latent variable theory) (Dima, 2018). However, these assumptions are not always applicable, and thus multi-item measures are not the answer for every construct. For example, behaviour measures may aim to capture the frequency of event occurrence within a time window (Dima et al., 2017), and behaviour determinants of BCTs may be better visualised via network models (Heino et al., 2019) or profiles identified via clustering methods (Smit et al., 2018).

Single-Item Measures

Multi-item measures are not feasible or appropriate in all circumstances but are suitable, for example, in intensive longitudinal design requiring repeated experience sampling (such as EMA), in population surveys measuring many constructs, in populations with limited time availability or cognitive functioning, or simply when the construct has a narrow scope that cannot be expressed in sufficiently distinct items. In these situations, single-item measures (Example 1 in Table 9.1) obtain better quality data by reducing burden and thus increasing participation and accuracy of reports. Several measurement properties common to multi-item measures can be evaluated, such as face validity, criterion validity (convergent, predictive, concurrent), and test-retest reliability for constructs theorised as stable over time; moreover, single-item measures are more likely to be used in practice and therefore their use in research would facilitate knowledge transfer (Allen et al., 2022).

Performance Measures

One major limitation of self-reported measures is that they draw respondents' attention to the phenomenon under study and thus risk interfering with how they experience what the measure aims to capture. Measurement reactivity (measurement resulting in changes in the people being measured) has been shown to impact self-reported behaviours, emotions, and cognitions, which may negatively affect the validity of health psychology research (French & Sutton, 2010). Fortunately, there is an ever-increasing diversity of instruments that go beyond what people remember, think, or feel about themselves and their behaviour to measure more directly what people do.

Performance Tasks

Developed in the field of experimental psychology in controlled laboratory settings, performance tasks (also called cognitive-behavioural tasks) such as the dot-probe task or the Stroop task have become established in many applied areas, including health psychology and also used in the study of individual differences (Parsons et al., 2019). In experimental designs, the experimental manipulation may consist of adaptations of these tasks and thus integrate the operationalisation of the construct whose causal effect is in focus. The SOBC repository includes numerous examples of performance measures. These (primarily laboratory) measures have gained an aura of being inherently scientific and precise, which paradoxically reduced efforts to validate, improve, and report their measurement properties (Lilienfeld & Strother, 2020). Guidelines for assessing and reporting measurement properties of performance tasks are a promising development in this area (e.g., Parsons et al., (2019) on reliability). Moreover, transferring tasks from laboratory to real-world settings involves important practical and psychometric challenges. A review of the real-world use of automatic processing computerised tasks showed their increased use as behaviour change interventions, such as alcohol and tobacco use and mental health, although low engagement and the likely presence of distractors remain unaddressed (Jayasinghe et al., 2020). Game-based assessment may provide future solutions for valid and reliable measurement of performance, yet these claims are still in need of investigation (Kato & de Klerk, 2017).

Biomarkers

Biomarkers are objectively measured indicators of physiological or biological processes or responses. In health psychology, they are increasingly used to measure health status, e.g., cytokine concentrations as markers of inflammatory processes related to various health problems, or health behaviours, e.g., level of expired carbon dioxide to measure short-term exposure to tobacco, plasma levels of vitamin C or carotenoids to measure food intake, or levels of drug metabolites in blood or urine to measure medication adherence (Luszczynska et al., 2018b). A construct that benefited from a considerable development of biomarker measures is stress: cortisol has become an established measure of the stress response via the activation of the hypothalamus-pituitary-adrenal axis, either a current systemic concentration in saliva or blood, or as cumulative secretion over time as detected in urine or hair. More recently, salivary alpha-amylase has been used as a marker for the activation of the autonomic nervous system in response to stress stimuli as well (Nater et al., 2013). While they are valued for circumventing reporting biases inherent to self-reports, they are usually limited to measuring the effects of behaviour on single short time windows and represent less proximal measures of behaviour since they are also influenced by variations in subsequent processes, e.g., how substances ingested are metabolised in the case of food intake measurement. The measurement properties of biomarkers are the focus of rapid development as technologies evolve and research designs adjust to constant innovation.

Sensors/Digital Biomarkers

Similar to biomarkers, recent years have witnessed a rapid diversification of digital technologies to capture physiological function and health behaviours in real time in laboratory or ambulatory settings. We now have accelerometers to capture physical activity and sleep patterns, heart/pulse rate sensors monitoring heart rate or blood pressure, smart medication dispensers recording the exact times of opening for medication intake, and many other types of devices for diverse purposes in diverse populations and clinical areas (Motahari-Nezhad et al., 2022). An important strength of these measures is collecting fine-grained data automatically without the participant's active effort to obtain and process it, which opens new possibilities for studying behaviour longitudinally in diverse naturalistic settings. They can also be integrated with other types of measures and with intervention components in complex eHealth behaviour change interventions adaptable to the needs of specific populations. However, this flexibility brings many challenges to data quality that need to be addressed through careful research design (see Chapter 8, "Research Design: Overview and Recommendations"). Unlike the types of measures discussed earlier, completeness of sensor data is influenced by battery life, technical failure, and usage patterns. Reliability, validity, and feasibility of measurement vary depending on the research design and the specific properties of the behaviour in the study population. For example, for good data quality on physical activity, it is recommended to wear accelerometers continuously for at least seven days for ten hours daily, which represents a considerable participation burden for children or persons with disability (Luszczynska et al., 2018b).

Quantitative Content Analysis

A time-tested measurement method in health psychology is quantitative content analysis, a process of systematic coding and quantification of written, visual, or oral content by assigning content to categories according to predefined rules. This method is characterised by the operationalisation of the constructs of interest via a coding scheme that represents the central element of the research design guiding the selection of units of analysis and sample of materials, and the process of coding, data quality monitoring, and improvement, and data analysis and hypothesis testing (Huxley, 2020). One example is the use of methods related to the BCIO to describe behaviour change content of health apps (e.g., Simões et al., 2018) and examine intervention delivery fidelity (e.g., Cross et al., 2022). See example 4 in Table 9.1 for a practical application.

An established content analysis method in behavioural sciences is systematic behavioural observation: capturing behaviours occurring in real life by a systematic process of recording and quantifying occurrences by external observers. It can be performed while witnessing behaviours in real time but also in video or audio recordings of real-life or research-generated situations. While of minimal burden to participants, behavioural observation requires good-quality recordings representative of the behaviours studied and involves a complex process of selecting or designing a coding system taking into account contextual, behavioural, and temporal considerations, implementing it with the input from selected, trained, and carefully monitored coders, and evaluating and improving its reliability in an iterative manner (Furr & Funder, 2007). A coding system widely used in health psychology is the Roter Interaction Analysis System (RIAS) for the study of patient-provider interactions and measuring various constructs related to task-focused and socio-emotional dialogue; its measurement properties have been subject to sustained examination along the years (Roter & Larson, 2002). Currently, the SOBC measures repository includes several observation measures for interpersonal interaction constructs.

Routinely Collected Data

Another recent opportunity in the health psychology measures toolkit is the secondary use of real-world data. We have an unprecedented amount of data produced daily as people search to understand and manage their health and illness via social media, using mobile apps or internet platforms, or interacting with the health-care system. Accessing and using these data to measure health-related constructs represents an active area of methodological research, with much potential and many unknowns (see examples 2 and 3 in Table 9.1). Digital Trace Data (DTD) collection via Application Programming Interfaces (APIs), data donations, or tracking can now provide information on the health-related content users generate or are exposed to. However, they bring important theoretical, methodological, and ethical challenges for which solutions have just started being proposed (Ohme et al., 2023). App use and internet browsing have become essential behaviours for self-managing health and illness, and accessing app logs and browsing histories is an area of rapid methodological development in health psychology measurement (Bach & Wenz, 2020). Health-care service delivery is now recorded systematically for administrative, financial, and clinical monitoring purposes. The use of these data in research requires thorough investigation of data quality dimensions of completeness, correctness, concordance, plausibility, and currency; methods of checking and improving data quality continue to be developed (Weiskopf & Weng, 2013).

Conclusion – Measuring Well

This chapter, instead of providing a failproof cookbook of measures, has aimed to present measurement as an area of active methodological development in close collection to health psychology theories and evidence base. Measurement innovation in health psychology is a necessary endeavour, given the societal transformations we are experiencing and the changes in how we construct health in our society. If innovation continues, most of the information in this chapter will soon become of historical interest. I would therefore propose as guiding principles six summary points more likely to stand the test of time (Figure 9.1). First, think of measurement as a process and of constructs as evolving entities: keep an eye on how your decisions may impact what your measures can tell you about the phenomenon of interest. Second, understand your setting and its

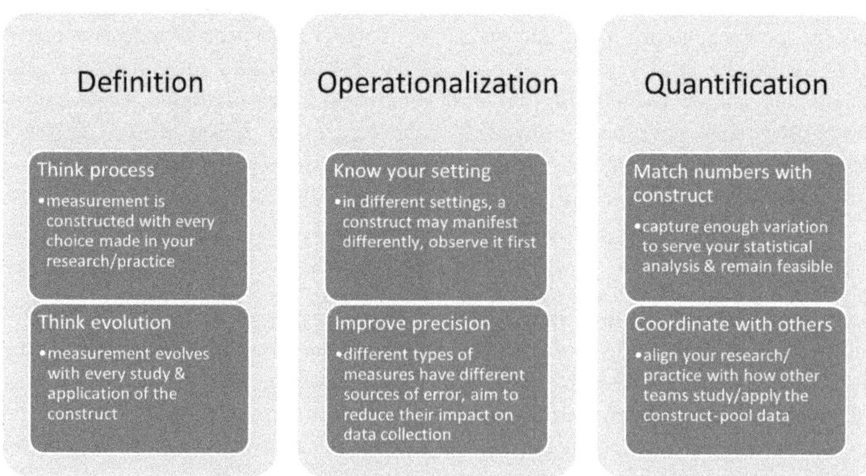

Figure 9.1 Six guiding principles for good measurement in (health) psychology.

constraints and affordances on how the phenomenon may be observed: these will tell you which type of data is more appropriate and how you could limit interference from other factors. Third, decide on how to count your observations with two aims in mind, the data structure necessary for your analysis and the feasibility of data collection, and one meta-aim: collaborative science. By giving careful thought to each phase in the measurement process, you are increasing your chances of obtaining good-quality data that would inform better decisions and contribute to the advancement of the field.

Resources

HealthMeasures – the reference repository for patient-reported measures globally, hosted by Northwestern University and funded by the National Institutes of Health (NIH), United States (https://www.healthmeasures.net/search-view-measures). Includes questionnaires on physical, mental, and social health, and sensory, motor, and cognitive performance tests in different languages. It includes the PROMIS (Patient-Reported Outcomes Measurement Information System), Neuro-QoL (focusing on neurological conditions), ASCQ-Me (sickle cell disease), and NIH Toolbox (general population and chronic conditions).

BiblioPRO – the largest repository of Patient Reported Outcomes and Health-Related Quality of Life Questionnaires in the Spanish language, with over 2,400 records to date (https://www.bibliopro.org/buscador/). Developed and hosted by the Health Services Research Group at the Medical Research Institute of the Hospital del Mar (IMIM) and funded by the Epidemiology and Public Health Research Network (CIBERESP), Spain.

The SOBC Measures – repository of the Science of Behaviour Change Research Network focusing on the measurement of potential targets for behaviour change, with over 180 records to date (https://measures.scienceofbehaviorchange.org/). It is hosted by the Columbia University Medical Center and funded by the NIH. While the BiblioPRO and PROMIS focus on self-reported questionnaires and tests in health research and practice, the SOBC repository includes experimental tasks and observational measures. It includes only measures validated or currently following validation research in line with the SOBC approach.

COMET – the Core Outcome Measures in Effectiveness Trials (COMET) initiative (https://www.cometinitiative.org/) offers a database of Core Outcome Sets developed following a standardised methodology for different disease categories, target populations, and interventions (including psychological, behavioural, or communication interventions) for a range of use scenarios, such as clinical research, practice, or registries. It is currently hosted by the University of Liverpool and funded by the UK National Institute for Health Research (NIHR), Medical Research Council (MRC), and the European Commission.

Further Reading

Benyamini, Y., Karademas, E., & Johnston, M. (2016). *Assessment in Health Psychology*. Hogrefe.
Johnston, M., Weinman, J., & Ozakinci, G. (2021). Measurement in health psychology research and practice. *Oxford Bibliographies in Psychology*. https://doi.org/10.1093/OBO/9780199828340-0270
Luszczynska, A., Kruk, M., & Boberska, M. (2018a). *Measurement in Health Psychology Research*. Routledge Handbooks Online. https://doi.org/10.4324/9781315167534-3
Smith, T. W. (2011a). Measurement in health psychology research. In *The Oxford handbook of health psychology* (pp. 42–72). Oxford University Press.

References

Allen, M. S., Iliescu, D., & Greiff, S. (2022). Single item measures in psychological science. *European Journal of Psychological Assessment*, *38*(1), 1–5. https://doi.org/10.1027/1015-5759/a000699
Bach, R. L., & Wenz, A. (2020). Studying health-related internet and mobile device use using web logs and smartphone records. *PLOS ONE*, *15*(6), e0234663. https://doi.org/10.1371/journal.pone.0234663
Broadbent, E., Petrie, K. J., Main, J., & Weinman, J. (2006). The brief illness perception questionnaire. *Journal of Psychosomatic Research*, *60*(6), 631–637. https://doi.org/10.1016/j.jpsychores.2005.10.020
Cross, R., Greaves, C. J., Withall, J., Rejeski, W. J., & Stathi, A. (2022). Delivery fidelity of the REACT (REtirement in ACTion) physical activity and behaviour maintenance intervention for community dwelling older people with mobility limitations. *BMC Public Health*, *22*(1), Article 1. https://doi.org/10.1186/s12889-022-13496-z
Crutzen, R., & Peters, G.-J. Y. (2015). Scale quality: Alpha is an inadequate estimate and factor-analytic evidence is needed first of all. *Health Psychology Review*, *0*(0), 1–6. https://doi.org/10.1080/17437199.2015.1124240
Dima, A. L. (2018). Scale validation in applied health research: Tutorial for a 6-step R-based psychometrics protocol. *Health Psychology and Behavioral Medicine*, *6*(1), 136–161. https://doi.org/10.1080/21642850.2018.1472602
Dima, A. L., Allemann, S. S., Dunbar-Jacob, J., Hughes, D. A., Vrijens, B., & Wilson, I. B. (2021). TEOS: A framework for constructing operational definitions of medication adherence based on Timelines–Events–Objectives–Sources. *British Journal of Clinical Pharmacology*, *n/a*(n/a). https://doi.org/10.1111/bcp.14659
Dima, A. L., van Ganse, E., Laforest, L., Texier, N., de Bruin, M., & The Astro-Lab Group, null. (2017). Measuring medication adherence in asthma: Development of a novel self-report tool. *Psychology & Health*, 1–20. https://doi.org/10.1080/08870446.2017.1290248
Enkavi, A. Z., Eisenberg, I. W., Bissett, P. G., Mazza, G. L., MacKinnon, D. P., Marsch, L. A., & Poldrack, R. A. (2019). Large-scale analysis of test–retest reliabilities of self-regulation measures. *Proceedings of the National Academy of Sciences*, *116*(12), 5472–5477. https://doi.org/10.1073/pnas.1818430116
Eronen, M. I., & Bringmann, L. F. (2021). The theory crisis in psychology: How to move forward. *Perspectives on Psychological Science*, *16*(4), 779–788. https://doi.org/10.1177/1745691620970586
Flake, J. K., & Fried, E. I. (2020). Measurement Schmeasurement: Questionable Measurement Practices and How to Avoid Them. *Advances in Methods and Practices in Psychological Science*, *3*(4), 456–465. https://doi.org/10.1177/2515245920952393
French, D. P., & Sutton, S. (2010). Reactivity of measurement in health psychology: How much of a problem is it? What can be done about it? *British Journal of Health Psychology*, *15*(3), 453–468. https://doi.org/10.1348/135910710X492341

Fried, E. I., Flake, J. K., & Robinaugh, D. J. (2022). Revisiting the theoretical and methodological foundations of depression measurement. *Nature Reviews Psychology*, *1*(6), Article 6. https://doi.org/10.1038/s44159-022-00050-2

Furr, R. M., & Funder, D. C. (2007). Behavioral observation. In *Handbook of research methods in personality psychology* (pp. 273–291). The Guilford Press.

Heino, M. T. J., Knittle, K., Fried, E., Sund, R., Haukkala, A., Borodulin, K., Uutela, A., Araujo-Soares, V., Vasankari, T., & Hankonen, N. (2019). Visualisation and network analysis of physical activity and its determinants: Demonstrating opportunities in analysing baseline associations in the Let's Move It trial. *Health Psychology and Behavioral Medicine*, *7*(1), 269–289. https://doi.org/10.1080/21642850.2019.1646136

Huxley, K. (2020). Content analysis, quantitative. In *SAGE research methods foundations*. SAGE Publications Ltd. https://doi.org/10.4135/9781526421036880564

Jayasinghe, H., Short, C. E., Braunack-Mayer, A., Merkin, A., & Hume, C. (2020). Evidence regarding automatic processing computerized tasks designed for health interventions in real-world settings among adults: Systematic scoping review. *Journal of Medical Internet Research*, *22*(7), e17915. https://doi.org/10.2196/17915

Kaplan, R. M., & Beatty, A. S. (Eds.). (2022). *Ontologies in the behavioral sciences: Accelerating research and the spread of knowledge*. National Academies Press. https://doi.org/10.17226/26464

Karademas, E., Benyamini, Y., & Johnston, M. (2015). Introduction: Assessment in health psychology. In *Assessment in health psychology* (pp. 3–16). Hogrefe.

Kato, P. M., & de Klerk, S. (2017). *Serious Games for Assessment: Welcome to the Jungle. 18*.

Larsen, K. R., & Bong, C. H. (2016). A Tool for Addressing Construct Identity in Literature Reviews and Meta-Analyses. *MIS Quarterly*, *40*(3), 529–552.

Lilienfeld, S. O., & Strother, A. N. (2020). Psychological Measurement and the Replication Crisis: Four Sacred Cows. *Canadian Psychology*, *61*(4), 281–288. https://doi.org/10.1037/cap0000236

Luszczynska, A., Kruk, M., & Boberska, M. (2018b). Measurement in health psychology research. In T. A. Revenson & R. A. R. Gurung (Eds.), *Handbook of Health Psychology* (1st ed., pp. 27–40). Routledge. https://doi.org/10.4324/9781315167534-3

Marques, M. M., Wright, A. J., Corker, E., Johnston, M., West, R., Hastings, J., Zhang, L., & Michie, S. (2023). The Behaviour Change Technique Ontology: Transforming the Behaviour Change Technique Taxonomy v1. *Wellcome Open Research*, *8*, 308. https://doi.org/10.12688/wellcomeopenres.19363.1

Metathesaurus. (2021). In *UMLS® Reference Manual [Internet]*. Bethesda, MD: National Library of Medicine (US). https://www.ncbi.nlm.nih.gov/books/NBK9684/

Michie, S., West, R., Finnerty, A. N., Norris, E., Wright, A. J., Marques, M. M., Johnston, M., Kelly, M. P., Thomas, J., & Hastings, J. (2021). Representation of behaviour change interventions and their evaluation: Development of the upper level of the behaviour change intervention ontology. *Wellcome Open Research*, *5*, 123. https://doi.org/10.12688/wellcomeopenres.15902.2

Mokkink, L. B., Terwee, C. B., Patrick, D. L., Alonso, J., Stratford, P. W., Knol, D. L., Bouter, L. M., & de Vet, H. C. W. (2010). The COSMIN study reached international consensus on taxonomy, terminology, and definitions of measurement properties for health-related patient-reported outcomes. *Journal of Clinical Epidemiology*, *63*(7), 737–745. https://doi.org/10.1016/j.jclinepi.2010.02.006

Motahari-Nezhad, H., Fgaier, M., Abid, M. M., Péntek, M., Gulácsi, L., & Zrubka, Z. (2022). Digital biomarker–based studies: Scoping review of systematic reviews. *JMIR mHealth and uHealth*, *10*(10), e35722. https://doi.org10.2196/35722

Nater, U. M., Skoluda, N., & Strahler, J. (2013). Biomarkers of stress in behavioural medicine. *Current Opinion in Psychiatry*, *26*(5), 440. https://doi.org/10.1097/YCO.0b013e328363b4ed

Ohme, J., Araujo, T., Boeschoten, L., Freelon, D., Ram, N., Reeves, B. B., & Robinson, T. N. (2023). Digital trace data collection for social media effects research: APIs, data donation, and (screen) tracking. *Communication Methods and Measures*, *0*(0), 1–18. https://doi.org/10.1080/19312458.2023.2181319

Parsons, S., Kruijt, A.-W., & Fox, E. (2019). Psychological science needs a standard practice of reporting the reliability of cognitive-behavioral measurements. *Advances in Methods and Practices in Psychological Science*, *2*(4), 378–395. https://doi.org/10.1177/2515245919879695

Ricci, L., Lanfranchi, J.-B., Lemetayer, F., Rotonda, C., Guillemin, F., Coste, J., & Spitz, E. (2019). Qualitative methods used to generate questionnaire items: A systematic review. *Qualitative Health Research*, *29*(1), 149–156. https://doi.org/10.1177/1049732318783186

Roter, D., & Larson, S. (2002). The Roter interaction analysis system (RIAS): Utility and flexibility for analysis of medical interactions. *Patient Education and Counseling*, *46*(4), 243–251. https://doi.org/10.1016/S0738-3991(02)00012-5

Simões, P., Silva, A. G., Amaral, J., Queirós, A., Rocha, N. P., & Rodrigues, M. (2018). Features, behavioral change techniques, and quality of the most popular mobile apps to measure physical activity: Systematic search in app stores. *JMIR mHealth and uHealth*, *6*(10), e11281. https://doi.org10.2196/11281

Smit, E. S., Brinkhues, S., de Vries, H., & Hoving, C. (2018). Subgroups among smokers in preparation: A cluster analysis using the I-change model. *Substance Use & Misuse*, *53*(3), 400–411. https://doi.org/10.1080/10826084.2017.1334062

Smith, T. W. (2011b). Measurement in health psychology research. In *The Oxford handbook of health psychology* (pp. 42–72). Oxford University Press.

Sumner, J. A., Carey, R. N., Michie, S., Johnston, M., Edmondson, D., & Davidson, K. W. (2018). Using rigorous methods to advance behaviour change science. *Nature Human Behaviour*, *2*(11), Article 11. https://doi.org/10.1038/s41562-018-0471-8

Thorndike, R. M., & Thorndike-Christ, T. M. (2009). *Measurement and Evaluation in Psychology and Education* (8th edition). Pearson.

Tourangeau, R. (2018). The survey response process from a cognitive viewpoint. *Quality Assurance in Education*, *26*(2), 169–181. https://doi.org/10.1108/QAE-06-2017-0034

Wang, Y., König, L. M., & Reiterer, H. (2021). A smartphone app to support sedentary behavior change by visualizing personal mobility patterns and action planning (SedVis): Development and pilot study. *JMIR Formative Research*, *5*(1), e15369. https://doi.org/10.2196/15369

Weiskopf, N. G., & Weng, C. (2013). Methods and dimensions of electronic health record data quality assessment: Enabling reuse for clinical research. *Journal of the American Medical Informatics Association*, *20*(1), 144–151. https://doi.org/10.1136/amiajnl-2011-000681

West, R., Godinho, C. A., Bohlen, L. C., Carey, R. N., Hastings, J., Lefevre, C. E., & Michie, S. (2019). Development of a formal system for representing behaviour-change theories. *Nature Human Behaviour*, *3*(5), 526. https://doi.org/10.1038/s41562-019-0561-2

Williamson, P. R., Altman, D. G., Bagley, H., Barnes, K. L., Blazeby, J. M., Brookes, S. T., Clarke, M., Gargon, E., Gorst, S., Harman, N., Kirkham, J. J., McNair, A., Prinsen, C. A. C., Schmitt, J., Terwee, C. B., & Young, B. (2017). The COMET Handbook: Version 1.0. *Trials*, *18*(3), Article 3. https://doi.org/10.1186/s13063-017-1978-4

10

PERSONALITY AND HEALTH

The Role of Individual Differences in Theory, Methods, and Intervention

Christina M. Juchem and Eva Asselmann

Introduction

'To good health and happiness' is universally valued. However, individuals differ widely in their physical and mental well-being. Explaining these differences has long been pondered, dating back to the Hippocratic tradition, positioning the concept of four 'bodily humours'. While the notion that diseases can be attributed to black and yellow bile has now long been discredited, contemporary research recognises the interplay of three broad domains: individual dispositions (e.g., a family history of breast cancer), lifestyle (e.g., smoking), and environmental factors (e.g., air pollution), including social relationships (e.g., social support). In brief, health is determined by a variety of biological, psychological, and social factors that can vary substantially between individuals.

How can between-person differences be captured? Common categories used to describe interindividual variation are demographic characteristics such as age, gender, socioeconomic status, or ethnicity. However, demographic categories have little explanatory value when it comes to psychological differences. The goal of personality psychology is to study individuals' enduring and relatively consistent patterns of thoughts, feelings, and behaviours across situations that make individuals unique and different, including those relevant to health and health behaviour.

The emerging field of 'personalised medicine' recognises not only the need but also the potential of considering individual differences in health care. This approach aims to tailor medical treatments to the unique genetic, molecular, and clinical characteristics of individual patients with the goal of optimising treatment outcomes and increasing patient satisfaction. The concept has expanded beyond biological markers to include patient-specific environmental and lifestyle factors (Holden et al., 2019). Personality traits have also been proposed to

DOI: 10.4324/9781003318026-12

personalise treatment to increase adherence and efficacy (e.g., for treating obesity and metabolic diseases, Boersma et al., 2011). As the efficacy of health (behaviour) interventions varies widely between individuals (Strömmer et al., 2020), the consideration of personality characteristics may indeed prove valuable throughout the entire health-care process, spanning from targeted prevention to personalised treatment (Cohen et al., 2021).

In this chapter, we aim to further encourage the consideration of personality characteristics in both health research and practice. We will (1) explain the concept of personality and (2) provide a brief overview of the current state of research on the relationship between personality and health. We then delve into the main content of this chapter by discussing (3) theories and mechanisms (how does personality relate to health?), (4) current and future avenues for research (how to examine the link between personality and health?), and (5) practical implications (how can personality research improve health interventions?).

What Is Personality?

Personality *traits* refer to individual differences in thoughts, feelings, and behaviours that are relatively stable across situations and over time. Personality traits show moderate to high rank-order consistency,[1] with correlations ranging between .40 and .60 (Roberts & Yoon, 2022). Despite this remarkable consistency, personality can – and does – change across the lifespan, although these changes are small on average (Bleidorn et al., 2022). Personality is shaped by gene-environment interactions (Roberts & Jackson, 2008) and manifests in (or emerges from) cognitive and affective processes. Environmental factors (e.g., stressful events) can influence personality. At the same time, personality influences which environments people select and how they react to these environments.

The most common taxonomies of personality traits are the Big Five or Five-Factor Model (John et al., 2008; McCrae & Costa, 2008) and the HEXACO Model (Ashton et al., 2014). Both describe a large proportion of between-person differences and are characterised by a hierarchical structure. The top level consists of the Big Five domains openness to experience, conscientiousness, extraversion, agreeableness, and emotional stability (reverse neuroticism). The HEXACO Model includes a sixth factor honesty-humility (for a comparison, see Ashton & Lee, 2018). Each domain can be divided into several facets (e.g., conscientiousness includes competence, dutifulness, striving for achievement, self-discipline, orderliness, and deliberation), which in turn can be measured by several items (e.g., "I am a productive person who always gets the job done"). The Big Five and the HEXACO factors have received extensive empirical support and have been replicated across different methods, samples, and cultures. Other personality traits of particular relevance to health include, for example, self-efficacy, which refers to people's beliefs in their ability to perform tasks and achieve goals (Bandura, 1986), and locus of control, which describes the extent to which individuals attribute events and outcomes to their own actions (internal locus of control) or to external factors (external locus of control; Rotter, 1966).

Personality is multifaceted and dynamic – features that are often neglected. First, research on personality is not limited to the Big Five or HEXACO traits but includes other domains such as motives (i.e., goals, values, and interests), abilities (i.e., cognitive and socioemotional skills), and narratives (i.e., subjective experiences and their integration into one's identity) (Roberts & Wood, 2006). Second, personality traits are not static (e.g., Bruinsma & Crutzen, 2018) but can change over longer (e.g., years) and intermediate (e.g., months) time periods, and personality states can change even in the short term (e.g., within one day). This latter aspect is emphasised in so-called trait-state models of personality (e.g., Rauthmann, 2021; Steyer et al., 2015), which distinguish between enduring personality characteristics (traits) and situation-dependent expressions of these traits (states). In other words, individuals may deviate from their characteristic behavioural pattern depending on the context and situation (e.g., under time pressure, even a highly conscientious person may slip a task). In sum, personality captures not only differences between individuals but also variations within individuals, making it a compelling variable in the context of health research and health promotion.

Personality Traits and Health Outcomes

The relationship between personality and health is well established. At this point, we provide a brief overview of the vast body of research that has contributed to this area. Because the Big Five have received by far the most attention, this chapter will focus particularly on these traits. Specifically, the current state of research has yielded several meta-analyses, including a comprehensive meta-synthesis (Strickhouser et al., 2017). This synthesis included 150 meta-analytic effects of the Big Five personality traits on a broad range of health outcomes grouped into physical health, mental health, and health behaviour. Across all outcomes, associations were strongest for emotional stability ($\bar{r}$ = .20), conscientiousness ($\bar{r}$ = .19), and agreeableness ($\bar{r}$ = .17), while correlations were much weaker for extraversion ($\bar{r}$ = .08) and openness to experience ($\bar{r}$ = .05). Notably, the relationship between personality and health varied by health outcome, with mental health outcomes showing the strongest relationships with personality traits ($\bar{r}$ = .35),[2] followed by health behaviour ($\bar{r}$ = .18) and physical health ($\bar{r}$ = .06).

Mental Health

Associations with mental health indicators were strongest for emotional stability ($\bar{r}$ = .27), followed by conscientiousness ($\bar{r}$ = .22), and agreeableness ($\bar{r}$ = .21). Weakest links were found for extraversion ($\bar{r}$ = .11) and openness ($\bar{r}$ = .06) (Strickhouser et al., 2017). These associations varied by mental health outcome. For example, subjective well-being (Anglim et al., 2020) was most strongly associated with higher emotional stability and extraversion, whereas psychopathy (Miller & Lynam, 2012) was most strongly associated with lower conscientiousness and lower agreeableness. It has even been argued that the Big Five lie on the same spectra as mental disorders. The Hierarchical Taxonomy of Psychopathology posits five dimensions of psychopathology that are considered maladaptive variants of the Big Five (i.e., negative affectivity-emotional stability, detachment-extraversion, psychoticism-openness, antagonism-agreeableness, and disinhibition-conscientiousness) (Widiger et al., 2019). Overall, this underscores the close connection, or even conceptual overlap, between personality and mental health.

Health Behaviours

Health behaviours were most strongly associated with higher conscientiousness ($\bar{r} = .12$), agreeableness ($\bar{r} = .10$), and emotional stability ($\bar{r} = .07$), while associations with extraversion ($\bar{r} = -.02$) and openness ($\bar{r} < .01$) were negligible (Strickhouser et al., 2017). Consistently, higher conscientiousness relates to positive treatment outcomes such as medication adherence (Bucher et al., 2019) and lower conscientiousness relates to virtually all types of health risk behaviours, such as physical inactivity, alcohol use, and risky driving (Bogg & Roberts, 2004). In particular, low agreeableness appears to be associated with sexual risk-taking (Hoyle et al., 2000) and lower emotional stability with higher substance use (e.g., Malouff et al., 2007).

Physical Health

Personality traits showed the weakest associations with physical health indicators, with small associations for conscientiousness ($\bar{r} = .03$), extraversion ($\bar{r} = -.02$), agreeableness ($\bar{r} = -.01$), openness ($\bar{r} = .01$), and emotional stability ($\bar{r} = .00$) (Strickhouser et al., 2017). In a multiple cohort study, all-cause mortality was robustly associated with lower conscientiousness but not with any of the other Big Five traits (Jokela et al., 2013). These findings are echoed in studies on intermediate health markers such as inflammatory cytokines, which were also associated with lower conscientiousness (Luchetti et al., 2014). Notably, in Asian populations, higher levels of extraversion and higher agreeableness – but not conscientiousness – were associated with physical health (i.e., higher BMI in men), highlighting the importance of considering cultural and socialisation aspects when examining the relationship between personality and health (Sutin et al., 2015).

Beyond the Big Five, self-efficacy predicts a variety of positive health outcomes, whereas findings on health locus of control are mixed. Specifically, higher self-efficacy has been associated with various health behaviours, such as smoking cessation or dieting (Holden, 1991), and with better physical health, particularly among the elderly (Stretton et al., 2006). Internal locus of control was primarily associated with higher physical activity and healthier dietary choices but showed little association with substance use (Cheng et al., 2016).

Having summarised this, three additional aspects are worth noting: first, personality traits interact with each other. For example, individuals with higher conscientiousness and lower emotional stability experience better health outcomes than those with higher conscientiousness alone – a pattern labelled 'healthy neuroticism' (Turiano et al., 2013). Second, health domains (e.g., mental vs. physical health) are not clear-cut but related. For example, heavy substance use may be both a health risk behaviour and a mental health problem. Third, given that both personality and health are dynamic processes, correlated changes between personality and health have been reported (e.g., Kornadt et al., 2018). This has raised questions about the direction of causality. Do changes in personality (e.g., decreased emotional stability) lead to changes in health, or do changes in health (e.g., chronic pain) lead to changes in personality? In fact, research suggests that personality and health exert a mutual influence on each other (for an overview, see Jackson et al., 2017).

In summary, self-efficacy and conscientiousness emerge as key personality traits associated with health behaviour and physical health, and emotional stability in particular is associated with mental health. However, much unexplained variability remains. Researchers have therefore shifted their focus from investigating *whether* to examining *why* personality is related to health.

Theories and Mechanisms: How Personality Relates to Health

Multiple mechanisms underlying the relationship between personality and health have been proposed, but only some have been incorporated into theoretical models. The most prominent are (a) health behaviour, (b) stress response, (c) social relationships, and (d) environmental factors.

Health Behaviour

As proposed by several theories on health behaviour and health behaviour change (e.g., the Health Behavior Model in Smith, 2006), personality relates to specific behaviours that are favourable or unfavourable for health. For instance, people who frequently experience anxiety and negative affect (i.e., low levels of emotional stability) may turn to substances like alcohol or cannabis to alleviate these feelings temporarily (Suh et al., 2008). People who are well organised and disciplined (i.e., high levels of conscientiousness) are more likely to engage in regular physical activity, eat a healthy diet, and seek preventive health care (Bogg & Roberts, 2004). These behaviours, in turn, are beneficial to health and can explain a lower average risk of disease and mortality.

Stress Response

The detrimental effects of stress on mental and physical health have long been recognised. The Stress Moderation Model (Smith, 2006) posits that personality affects how individuals cope with stress, which in turn affects their physical health. Consistent with this idea, there is strong empirical evidence that personality influences whether individuals experience stress and how they cope with it. For example, lower emotional stability relates to higher negative affect, which promotes stress (Moyle, 1995), whereas higher extraversion relates to higher positive affect, which attenuates stress (van Steenbergen et al., 2021). Conscientiousness remains linked to beneficial health behaviours even in high-stress conditions (Korotkov, 2008). Meta-analytic work has shown that higher conscientiousness, extraversion, and openness were associated with favourable coping strategies (e.g., problem-solving and seeking social support), whereas lower emotional stability was associated with unfavourable coping strategies (e.g., withdrawal and substance use; Connor-Smith & Flachsbart, 2007). Taken together, these individual differences in stress experience and stress coping may explain the relationship between personality and health.

Social Relationships

Better social relationships promote well-being, prevent stress, and provide individuals with important resources to cope with stress (e.g., through emotional, informational, and practical social support), which promotes health (Berkman et al., 2000). Conversely, loneliness and social isolation are central risk factors for mortality across all ages and are associated with poor health outcomes such as poor sleep habits, depressive symptoms, increased risk of suicide, and cardiovascular disease (Bhatti & ul Haq, 2017; Holt-Lunstad et al., 2015). Previous research has shown that personality is related to the type, quality, and duration of social relationships. For example, more extraverted individuals tend to have larger social networks and are more likely to seek social support when needed (Swickert et al., 2002). In intimate relationships, higher levels of extraversion, emotional stability, conscientiousness, and agreeableness have been associated with greater relationship satisfaction (Malouff et al., 2010). Dyadic data suggests that an individual's personality also predicts the health of their partner, suggesting, for example, that high levels of conscientiousness in one partner may benefit the health of the other beyond their own conscientiousness levels (Roberts et al., 2009).

Environment

Environmental factors play a major role in health (Sallis et al., 2015), and personality traits can determine which environment an individual selects into, how they interact with it, and are affected by their environment in return. The concept of person-environment fit suggests that the alignment between one's personality and their surroundings can foster well-being, for instance, when a person's personality matches the prevalent traits of their city's inhabitants (Bleidorn et al., 2016) or aligns with their organisation's culture at work (Iyer et al., 2020). In models linking personality and health, environmental features are typically considered through the pathway of stress, but they can also have direct effects. For example, research consistently shows that people's geographical preferences correspond to their personality traits: Introverted individuals prefer mountain areas (Oishi et al., 2015), while those high in extraversion and openness tend to live in metropolitan areas (Militaru et al., 2023; Walmsley, 1982), increasing their susceptibility to health risks like traffic noise and air pollution. Furthermore, there is robust evidence that people low in conscientiousness, low in agreeableness, and high in extraversion (particularly sensation seeking, Zhang et al., 2019) are more frequently involved in accidents (Clarke & Robertson, 2005) because they are more likely to select into high-risk environments and less likely to adhere to safety regulations in such situations. This example also emphasises that the mechanisms between personality and health are multifaceted and often act in concert.[3]

Personality in Theories on Health Behaviour and Health Behaviour Change

Many theories of health behaviour and health behaviour change include components in which personality can be placed or which account for specific aspects of individual differences. Some models (e.g., Theory of Planned Behaviour, Health Belief Model) include personality as a very broad and undefined *distal* factor that, in combination with other external factors, may influence more *proximal* factors such as beliefs, attitudes, or motivation. Other models explicitly refer to specific personality traits such as self-efficacy (e.g., Health Action Process Approach, Social Cognitive Theory) or self-regulation (e.g., COM-B framework). These specific traits are considered to be determinants of either motivational (i.e., self-efficacy) or volitional (i.e., self-regulation) aspects. However, although it is widely recognised that there are considerable individual differences in health behaviour (change), theories rarely consider personality traits in their multifaceted nature (Bogg, 2008).

In applied behavioural science, it is not uncommon to create novel personality profiles, sometimes called 'personae'. For example, in health-care decision-making, individual differences are often considered in the form of preferences. Patients are then grouped based on these preferences, such as the extent to which they want to be involved in treatment selection (e.g., 'autonomists' vs. 'delegators') (Flynn et al., 2006). While such personae can inform treatment decisions and even improve outcomes, their utility is often limited to the specific problem. Regarding theory development, this also holds the risk of overfitting (i.e., models become overly tailored to a specific context or population), limiting broader application and understanding of general processes (i.e., lack of generalisability).

Taken together, there is a broad consensus that relatively stable individual differences (whether termed traits, preferences, or tendencies) play a critical role in health and health behaviour. Health theories typically refer either to personality as a broad and unspecific category, very specific personality traits (e.g., self-efficacy), or problem-specific personality types. Thus, what is known about multiple personality traits is not always explicitly considered. To better integrate personality into health theories and inform interventions, a deeper understanding of the precise mechanisms is needed.

Methods: How to Examine the Relationship between Personality and Health

Research Designs

Appropriate research designs are needed to examine the underlying mechanisms and causal relationship between personality and health. Although the number of longitudinal studies has increased, most studies have been limited to two measurement occasions, which makes it difficult to examine nuanced (e.g., discontinuous) changes over time or underlying mechanisms.[4] Large-scale panel studies with multiple assessments offer a more nuanced understanding by allowing modelling of short- and long-term continuous and discontinuous changes in personality and health, including their reciprocal interrelationships. For causal inference, experimental designs, including randomised control trials, are considered the gold standard (see Chapter 8 in this volume). For example, intervention studies can test whether increasing self-efficacy causes changes in health. Finally, given the crucial role of social relationships in the relationship between personality and health, dyadic and social network analyses are essential. They can be used, for example, to examine how one's relationship with one's partner, family members, friends, or even one's health-care providers influence individual health outcomes.

Measurement

The choice of assessment tools affects the aspect of personality that is captured. Most research to date has focused on domain-level assessments, and longitudinal studies have typically used brief scales because more comprehensive personality inventories are longer and more time-consuming (consider that the NEO PI-R, one of the earliest comprehensive measures of the Five-Factor Model, consists of 240 items). However, research has shown that specific personality facets often serve as more accurate predictors of distinct aspects of mental well-being (Anglim et al., 2020) and physical health (Arumäe et al., 2022) when compared to domain-level assessments. Furthermore, to measure facets and nuances, much shorter scales with narrow content are sufficient (McCrae & Mõttus, 2019), rendering them a promising avenue for future research and interventions.

While self-reports are cost-effective and useful for capturing subjective experiences, they can be subject to retrospective recall, memory, and reporting biases and should therefore be ideally complemented with other reports (e.g., by a friend, partner, or parent). Data can be collected directly in daily life using ambulatory assessments, which reduce bias and allow for temporal (e.g., short-term fluctuations over the course of the day) and contextual (e.g., a person's current environment) factors to be taken into account. Specifically, ambulatory assessments provide high-frequency measures of momentary thoughts, feelings, and behaviours in everyday contexts, enabling the distinction between personality traits, states, and situational influences and their association with diverse health outcomes.

Practical Implications: How Personality Research Can Improve Health Interventions

Personality research considers (a) stable between-person differences in personality traits and (b) context- and situation-dependent within-person fluctuations in personality traits and states. Both approaches can improve the efficacy of existing health interventions and provide guidance for the development of new ones.

Personality *traits* are important in health interventions for several reasons. First, health-related personality traits (e.g., self-efficacy) can be enhanced to facilitate health behaviour change. For example, there is evidence that self-efficacy interventions are effective in supporting smoking cessation and physical activity (Sheeran et al., 2016). Second, personality traits can serve as indicators of risk or resilience and are therefore useful for identifying high-risk groups who might benefit from closer monitoring and targeted prevention. For example, individuals with low emotional stability could be screened more frequently for mental health problems or offered targeted stress management training. Third, information on personality traits can be used not only to identify target groups for interventions but also to tailor the intervention itself. Tailored interventions flexibly adjust the content, dose, or sequence of intervention elements to meet the individual's unique needs. For example, in a health promotion programme, individuals with low conscientiousness might receive more frequent reminders to complete their training sessions or homework assignments. Such an individualised approach could increase overall effectiveness, especially in heterogeneous target groups. Meta-analyses suggest that tailored health behaviour interventions are successful overall (Krebs et al., 2010; Noar et al., 2007; Tong et al., 2021), although much of the research is still in its infancy and their superiority to standardised care requires further investigation. In particular, personality-based tailored health interventions have been scarce to date, but initial findings are promising (e.g., De Vries et al., 2017; Debenham et al., 2021).

In addition, research on personality *states* (or persons-in-situations) can provide insights for health interventions. For example, individuals who report high levels of self-regulation (at the trait level) rarely find themselves in situations where they actually self-regulate (at the state level) (Inzlicht et al., 2021). Consequently, an effective intervention approach may be to help individuals avoid situations that require challenging self-regulation in the first place rather than train momentary self-regulatory strategies. Studies have examined the separation of trait and state components in relation to other health behaviours, such as dietary choices (Wahl et al., 2020) and alcohol use (Nealis et al., 2016). The latter study showed that situational factors have a greater influence on heavy drinking among younger individuals, while trait-like factors become more prominent with age, findings that may also inform tailored intervention strategies. In summary, integrating findings from personality research, particularly through a trait-state lens, may prove valuable in gaining a deeper understanding of target groups and designing more effective health promotion interventions.

Conclusion

In this chapter, we have shown that personality and health are intertwined and that the strength of this association varies depending on the traits and health outcomes under examination. Advances in technology and methods, including large-scale, long-term panel studies and ambulatory assessments, will continue to deepen our understanding of the underlying mechanisms. Approaching health behaviour through the lens of personality research can enhance both theory and intervention development by considering both between-person differences in personality traits and within-person fluctuations in personality states. In particular, the consideration of personality characteristics allows for the tailoring of interventions, which, in most cases, may be superior to simple one-size-fits-all approaches to health promotion.

Notes

1 Rank-order consistency refers to an individual's *relative* position or rank (e.g., on a specific personality scale) compared to others.
2 Since both personality and mental health outcomes are typically measured via self-report, common-method-variance may contribute largely to this finding. We discuss further methodological issues later in this chapter.
3 The pathways of social relationships, stress, and health behaviour have recently been integrated into the Personality and Health Processes Model (Turiano et al., 2021). Their model also accommodates the bidirectional association between health and personality.
4 For an in-depth discussion on testing personality-health mechanisms, see Turiano et al. (2021).

Further Reading

Anglim, J., Horwood, S., Smillie, L. D., Marrero, R. J., & Wood, J. K. (2020a). Predicting psychological and subjective well-being from personality: A meta-analysis. *Psychological Bulletin, 146*(4), 279–323. https://doi.org/10.1037/bul0000226
Bleidorn, W., Hopwood, C. J., Ackerman, R. A., Witt, E. A., Kandler, C., Riemann, R., … Donnellan, M. B. (2020). The healthy personality from a basic trait perspective. *Journal of Personality and Social Psychology, 118*(6), 1207–1225. https://doi.org/10.1037/pspp0000231
Luchetti, M., Barkley, J. M., Stephan, Y., Terracciano, A., & Sutin, A. R. (2014a). Five-factor model personality traits and inflammatory markers: New data and a meta-analysis. *Psychoneuroendocrinology, 50*, 181–193. https://doi.org/10.1016/j.psyneuen.2014.08.014

References

Anglim, J., Horwood, S., Smillie, L. D., Marrero, R. J., & Wood, J. K. (2020). Predicting psychological and subjective well-being from personality: A meta-analysis. *Psychological Bulletin, 146*(4), 279–323. https://doi.org/10.1037/bul0000226
Arumäe, K., Vainik, U., & Mõttus, R. (2022). Body mass is linked with a broad range of personality nuances, but especially those with behavioral content: A multi-sample exploration. *Personality Science, 3*, 1–26. https://doi.org/10.5964/ps.7583

Ashton, M. C., & Lee, K. (2018). How well do Big Five measures capture HEXACO scale variance? *Journal of Personality Assessment*, 567–573. https://doi.org/10.1080/00223891.2018.1448986
Ashton, M. C., Lee, K., & De Vries, R. E. (2014). The HEXACO honesty-humility, agreeableness, and emotionality factors: A review of research and theory. *Personality and Social Psychology Review*, *18*(2), 139–152.
Bandura, A. (1986). Social foundations of thought and action: A social cognitive theory. Prentice-Hall, (23–28).
Berkman, L. F., Glass, T., Brissette, I., & Seeman, T. E. (2000). From social integration to health: Durkheim in the new millennium. *Social Science & Medicine*, *51*(6), 843–857. https://doi.org/10.1016/S0277-9536(00)00065-4
Bhatti, A. B., & ul Haq, A. (2017). The pathophysiology of perceived social isolation: Effects on health and mortality. *Cureus*, *9*(1). https://doi.org/10.7759/cureus.994
Bleidorn, W., Schönbrodt, F., Gebauer, J. E., Rentfrow, P. J., Potter, J., & Gosling, S. D. (2016). To live among like-minded others: Exploring the links between person-city personality fit and self-esteem. *Psychological Science*, *27*(3), 419–427. https://doi.org/10.1177/0956797615627133
Bleidorn, W., Schwaba, T., Zheng, A., Hopwood, C. J., Sosa, S. S., Roberts, B. W., & Briley, D. (2022). Personality stability and change: A meta-analysis of longitudinal studies. *Psychological Bulletin*, *148*(7–8), 588. https://doi.org/10.1037/bul0000365
Boersma, G. J., Benthem, L., Van Beek, A. P., Van Dijk, G., & Scheurink, A. J. W. (2011). Personality, a key factor in personalized medicine? *European Journal of Pharmacology*, *667*(1–3), 23–25. https://doi.org/10.1016/j.ejphar.2011.05.079
Bogg, T. (2008). Conscientiousness, the transtheoretical model of change, and exercise: A neo-socioanalytic integration of trait and social-cognitive frameworks in the prediction of behavior. *Journal of Personality*, *76*(4), 775–802. https://doi.org/10.1111/j.1467-6494.2008.00504.x
Bogg, T., & Roberts, B. W. (2004). Conscientiousness and health-related behaviors: A meta-analysis of the leading behavioral contributors to mortality. *Psychological Bulletin*, *130*(6), 887–919. https://doi.org/10.1037/0033-2909.130.6.887
Bruinsma, J., & Crutzen, R. (2018). A longitudinal study on the stability of the need for cognition. *Personality and Individual Differences*, *127*, 151–161.
Bucher, M. A., Suzuki, T., & Samuel, D. B. (2019). A meta-analytic review of personality traits and their associations with mental health treatment outcomes. *Clinical Psychology Review*, *70*, 51–63. https://doi.org/10.1016/j.cpr.2019.04.002
Cheng, C., Cheung, M. W. L., & Lo, B. C. Y. (2016). Relationship of health locus of control with specific health behaviours and global health appraisal: A meta-analysis and effects of moderators. *Health Psychology Review*, *10*(4), 460–477. https://doi.org/10.1080/17437199.2016.1219672
Clarke, S., & Robertson, I. T. (2005). A meta-analytic review of the Big Five personality factors and accident involvement in occupational and non-occupational settings. *Journal of Occupational and Organizational psychology*, *78*(3), 355–376. https://doi.org/10.1348/096317905X26183
Cohen, Z. D., Delgadillo, J., & DeRubeis, R. J. (2021). Personalized treatment approaches. In *Bergin and Garfield's handbook of psychotherapy and behavior change: 50th anniversary edition*, 7th ed. (pp. 673–703). John Wiley & Sons, Inc.
Connor-Smith, J. K., & Flachsbart, C. (2007). Relations between personality and coping: A meta-analysis. *Journal of Personality and Social Psychology*, *93*(6), 1080–1107. https://doi.org/10.1037/0022-3514.93.6.1080
De Vries, R. A. J., Truong, K. P., Zaga, C., Li, J., & Evers, V. (2017). A word of advice: How to tailor motivational text messages based on behavior change theory to personality and gender. *Personal and Ubiquitous Computing*, *21*(4), 675–687. https://doi.org/10.1007/s00779-017-1025-1

Debenham, J., Grummitt, L., Newton, N. C., Teesson, M., Slade, T., Conrod, P., & Kelly, E. V. (2021). Personality-targeted prevention for adolescent tobacco use: Three-year outcomes for a randomised trial in Australia. *Preventive Medicine*, *153*, 106794. https://doi.org/10.1016/j.ypmed.2021.106794

Flynn, K. E., Smith, M. A., & Vanness, D. (2006). A typology of preferences for participation in healthcare decision making. *Social Science & Medicine*, *63*(5), 1158–1169. https://doi.org/10.1016/j.socscimed.2006.03.030

Holden, C., Bignell, L., Mukhopadhyay, S., & Jones, C. (2019). The public perception of the facilitators and barriers to implementing personalized medicine: A systematic review. *Personalized Medicine*, *16*(5), 409–420. https://doi.org/10.2217/pme-2018-0151

Holden, G. (1991). The relationship of self-efficacy appraisals to subsequent health related outcomes: A meta-analysis. *Social Work in Health Care*, *16*(1), 53–93. https://doi.org/10.1300/J010v16n01_05

Holt-Lunstad, J., Smith, T. B., Baker, M., Harris, T., & Stephenson, D. (2015). Loneliness and social isolation as risk factors for mortality: A meta-analytic review. *Perspectives on Psychological Science*, *10*(2), 227–237. https://doi.org/10.1177/1745691614568352

Hoyle, R. H., Fejfar, M. C., & Miller, J. D. (2000). Personality and sexual risk taking: A quantitative review. *Journal of Personality*, *68*(6), 1203–1231. https://doi.org/10.1111/1467-6494.00132

Inzlicht, M., Werner, K. M., Briskin, J. L., & Roberts, B. W. (2021). Integrating Models of Self-Regulation. *Annual Review of Psychology*, *72*(1), 319–345. https://doi.org/10.1146/annurev-psych-061020-105721

Iyer, P. V., Oostrom, J. K., Serlie, A. W., van Dam, A., & Born, M. P. (2020). The criterion-related validity of a short commensurate measure of personality-based person-organization fit. *International Journal of Selection and Assessment*, *28*(2), 143–162. https://doi.org/10.1111/ijsa.12276

Jackson, J. J., Weston, S. J., & Schultz, L. H. (2017). Personality development and health. In *Personality development across the lifespan* (pp. 371–384). Elsevier. https://doi.org/10.1016/B978-0-12-804674-6.00023-5

John, O. P., Naumann, L. P., & Soto, C. J. (2008). Paradigm shift to the integrative big five trait taxonomy. *Handbook of Personality: Theory and Research*, *3*(2), 114–158.

Jokela, M., Batty, G. D., Nyberg, S. T., Virtanen, M., Nabi, H., Singh-Manoux, A., & Kivimäki, M. (2013). Personality and all-cause mortality: Individual-participant meta-analysis of 3,947 deaths in 76,150 adults. *American Journal of Epidemiology*, *178*(5), 667–675. https://doi.org/10.1093/aje/kwt170

Kornadt, A. E., Hagemeyer, B., Neyer, F. J., & Kandler, C. (2018). Sound body, sound mind? The interrelation between health change and personality change in old age. *European Journal of Personality*, *32*(1), 30–45. https://doi.org/10.1002/per.2135

Korotkov, D. (2008). Does personality moderate the relationship between stress and health behavior? Expanding the nomological network of the five-factor model. *Journal of Research in Personality*, *42*(6), 1418–1426. https://doi.org/10.1016/j.jrp.2008.06.003

Krebs, P., Prochaska, J. O., & Rossi, J. S. (2010). A meta-analysis of computer-tailored interventions for health behavior change. *Preventive Medicine*, *51*(3), 214–221. https://doi.org/10.1016/j.ypmed.2010.06.004

Luchetti, M., Barkley, J. M., Stephan, Y., Terracciano, A., & Sutin, A. R. (2014). Five-factor model personality traits and inflammatory markers: New data and a meta-analysis. *Psychoneuroendocrinology*, *50*, 181–193. https://doi.org/10.1016/j.psyneuen.2014.08.014

Malouff, J. M., Thorsteinsson, E. B., Rooke, S. E., & Schutte, N. S. (2007). Alcohol involvement and the five-factor model of personality: A meta-analysis. *Journal of Drug Education*, *37*(3), 277–294. https://doi.org/10.2190/DE.37.3.d

Malouff, J. M., Thorsteinsson, E. B., Schutte, N. S., Bhullar, N., & Rooke, S. E. (2010). The five-factor model of personality and relationship satisfaction of intimate partners: A meta-analysis. *Journal of Research in Personality*, *44*(1), 124–127. https://doi.org/10.1016/j.jrp.2009.09.004

McCrae, R. R., & Costa, P. T., Jr. (2008). Empirical and theoretical status of the five-factor model of personality traits. In G. J. Boyle, G. Matthews, & D. H. Saklofske (Eds.), *The SAGE handbook of personality theory and assessment*, Vol. 1. Personality theories and models (pp. 273–294). Sage Publications, Inc. https://doi.org/10.4135/9781849200462.n13

McCrae, R. R., & Mõttus, R. (2019). What personality scales measure: A new psychometrics and its implications for theory and assessment. *Current Directions in Psychological Science*, *28*(4), 415–420. https://doi.org/10.1177/0963721419849559

Militaru, I. E., Serapio-García, G., Ebert, T., Kong, W., Gosling, S. D., Potter, J., Rentfrow, P. J., & Götz, F. M. (2023). The lay of the land: Associations between environmental features and personality. *Journal of Personality*. https://doi.org/10.1111/jopy.12822

Miller, J. D., & Lynam, D. R. (2012). An examination of the Psychopathic Personality Inventory's nomological network: A meta-analytic review. *Personality Disorders: Theory, Research, and Treatment*, *3*(3), 305–326. https://doi.org/10.1037/a0024567

Moyle, P. (1995). The role of negative affectivity in the stress process: Tests of alternative models. *Journal of Organizational Behavior*, *16*(S1), 647–668. https://doi.org/10.1002/job.4030160705

Nealis, L. J., Thompson, K. D., Krank, M. D., & Stewart, S. H. (2016). Shifting patterns of variance in adolescent alcohol use: Testing consumption as a developing trait-state. *Addictive Behaviors*, *55*, 25–31. https://doi.org/10.1016/j.addbeh.2015.12.012

Noar, S. M., Benac, C. N., & Harris, M. S. (2007). Does tailoring matter? Meta-analytic review of tailored print health behavior change interventions. *Psychological Bulletin*, *133*(4), 673–693. https://doi.org/10.1037/0033-2909.133.4.673

Oishi, S., Talhelm, T., & Lee, M. (2015). Personality and geography: Introverts prefer mountains. *Journal of Research in Personality*, *58*, 55–68. https://doi.org/10.1016/j.jrp.2015.07.001

Rauthmann, J. F. (2021). Capturing interactions, correlations, fits, and transactions: A person-environment relations model. In J. F. Rauthmann (Ed.), *The handbook of personality dynamics and processes* (pp. 427–522). Elsevier.

Roberts, B. W., & Jackson, J. J. (2008). Sociogenomic Personality Psychology. *Journal of Personality*, *76*(6), 1523–1544. https://doi.org/10.1111/j.1467-6494.2008.00530.x

Roberts, B. W., Smith, J., Jackson, J. J., & Edmonds, G. (2009). Compensatory conscientiousness and health in older couples. *Psychological Science*, *20*(5), 553–559. https://doi.org/10.1111/j.1467-9280.2009.02339.x

Roberts, B. W., & Wood, D. (2006). Personality Development in the Context of the Neo-Socioanalytic Model of Personality. In D. K. Mroczek & T. D. Little (Eds.), *Handbook of personality development* (pp. 11–39). Lawrence Erlbaum Associates Publishers.

Roberts, B. W., & Yoon, H. J. (2022). Personality psychology. *Annual Review of Psychology*, *73*, 489–516.

Rotter, J. B. (1966). Generalized expectancies for internal versus external control of reinforcement. *Psychological Monographs: General and Applied*, *80*(1), 1–28. https://doi.org/10.1037/h0092976

Sallis, J. F., Owen, N., & Fisher, E. (2015). Ecological models of health behavior. *Health Behavior: Theory, Research, and Practice*, *5*(43–64).

Sheeran, P., Maki, A., Montanaro, E., Avishai-Yitshak, A., Bryan, A., Klein, W. M., Miles, E., & Rothman, A. J. (2016). The impact of changing attitudes, norms, and self-efficacy on health-related intentions and behavior: A meta-analysis. *Health Psychology*, *35*(11), 1178–1188.

Smith, T. W. (2006). Personality as risk and resilience in physical health. *Current Directions in Psychological Science*, *15*(5), 227–231. https://doi.org/10.1111/j.1467-8721.2006.00441.x

Steyer, R., Mayer, A., Geiser, C., & Cole, D. A. (2015). A theory of states and traits—Revised. *Annual Review of Clinical Psychology*, *11*(1), 71–98. https://doi.org/10.1146/annurev-clinpsy-032813-153719

Stretton, C. M., Latham, N. K., Carter, K. N., Lee, A. C., & Anderson, C. S. (2006). Determinants of physical health in frail older people: The importance of self-efficacy. *Clinical rehabilitation*, *20*(4), 357–366. https://doi.org/10.1191/0269215506cr946oa

Strickhouser, J. E., Zell, E., & Krizan, Z. (2017). Does personality predict health and well-being? A metasynthesis. *Health Psychology*, *36*(8), 797–810. https://doi.org/10.1037/hea0000475

Strömmer, S., Lawrence, W., Shaw, S., Correia Simao, S., Jenner, S., Barrett, M., Vogel, C., Hardy-Johnson, P., Farrell, D., Woods-Townsend, K., Baird, J., Morrison, L., Sloboda, D. M., Inskip, H., & Barker, M. (2020). Behaviour change interventions: Getting in touch with individual differences, values and emotions. *Journal of Developmental Origins of Health and Disease*, *11*(6), 589–598. https://doi.org/10.1017/s2040174420000604

Suh, J. J., Ruffins, S., Robins, C. E., Albanese, M. J., & Khantzian, E. J. (2008). Self-medication hypothesis: Connecting affective experience and drug choice. *Psychoanalytic Psychology*, *25*(3), 518–532. https://doi.org/10.1037/0736-9735.25.3.518

Sutin, A. R., Stephan, Y., Wang, L., Gao, S., Wang, P., & Terracciano, A. (2015). Personality traits and body mass index in Asian populations. *Journal of Research in Personality*, *58*, 137–142. https://doi.org/j.jrp.2015.07.006

Swickert, R. J., Rosentreter, C. J., Hittner, J. B., & Mushrush, J. E. (2002). Extraversion, social support processes, and stress. *Personality and Individual Differences*, *32*(5), 877–891. https://doi.org/10.1016/S0191-8869(01)00093-9

Tong, H. L., Quiroz, J. C., Kocaballi, A. B., Fat, S. C. M., Dao, K. P., Gehringer, H., Chow, C. K., & Laranjo, L. (2021). Personalized mobile technologies for lifestyle behavior change: A systematic review, meta-analysis, and meta-regression. *Preventive Medicine*, *148*, 106532. https://doi.org/10.1016/j.ypmed.2021.106532

Turiano, N. A., Mroczek, D. K., Moynihan, J., & Chapman, B. P. (2013). Big 5 personality traits and interleukin-6: Evidence for "healthy Neuroticism" in a US population sample. *Brain, Behavior, and Immunity*, *28*, 83–89. https://doi.org/10.1016/j.bbi.2012.10.020

Turiano, N. A., Silva Belanger, N. M., Damitz, R. L., Hill, P. L., & Mroczek, D. K. (2021). Chapter 49 - Health processes in personality. In J. F. Rauthmann (Ed.), *The Handbook of Personality Dynamics and Processes* (pp. 1251–1271). Academic Press. https://doi.org/10.1016/B978-0-12-813995-0.00049-2

van Steenbergen, H., de Bruijn, E. R. A., van Duijvenvoorde, A. C. K., & van Harmelen, A.-L. (2021). How positive affect buffers stress responses. *Current Opinion in Behavioral Sciences*, *39*, 153–160. https://doi.org/10.1016/j.cobeha.2021.03.014

Wahl, D. R., Villinger, K., Blumenschein, M., König, L. M., Ziesemer, K., Sproesser, G., Schupp, H. T., & Renner, B. (2020). Why we eat what we eat: Assessing dispositional and in-the-moment eating motives by using ecological momentary assessment. *JMIR mHealth and uHealth*, *8*(1), e13191. https://doi.org/10.2196/13191

Walmsley, D. (1982). Personality and regional preference structures: A study of introversion-extraversion. *The Professional Geographer*, *34*(3), 279–288. https://doi.org/10.1111/j.0033-0124.1982.00279.x

Widiger, T. A., Sellbom, M., Chmielewski, M., Clark, L. A., DeYoung, C. G., Kotov, R., Krueger, R. F., Lynam, D. R., Miller, J. D., & Mullins-Sweatt, S. (2019). Personality in a hierarchical model of psychopathology. *Clinical Psychological Science*, *7*(1), 77–92. https://doi.org/10.1177/2167702618797105

Zhang, X., Qu, X., Tao, D., & Xue, H. (2019). The association between sensation seeking and driving outcomes: A systematic review and meta-analysis. *Accident Analysis & Prevention*, *123*, 222–234. https://doi.org/10.1016/j.aap.2018.11.023

SECTION 3

Health Behavior

11

DEFINING AND SPECIFYING HEALTH BEHAVIOUR – CONCEPTUAL OVERVIEW

Stephan U. Dombrowski and Gerard J. Molloy

Behaviour for Health and Beyond

The behaviours we engage in matter on an individual, interpersonal, societal, and environmental level. Most sources of modern health and disease can be traced to behaviour. Behaviours such as eating, moving, drinking alcohol, or taking medication are critical in determining health outcomes. Consequently, guidelines have been developed to suggest the types and magnitude of behaviours to be performed to increase the chances of desired health outcomes and minimise disease and premature mortality.

The importance of behaviour in influencing health and disease is undisputed, and has been established across different behaviours, populations, and contexts. A prospective population study, for example, examined the combined impact of four behavioural variables (physical activity, not smoking, moderate alcohol intake, and fruit and vegetable consumption) on mortality in 20,244 men and women aged 45–79 years without cardiovascular disease or cancer (Khaw et al., 2008). Participants who did not perform any of the health behaviours were four times more likely to die over an average follow-up period of 11 years compared to those who performed all four. The risk of mortality decreased with an increase in the number of health behaviours performed, indicating that changes in any of the four health behaviours would reduce mortality risk. Another prospective cohort study examined the relationship between five behaviour and behaviour-related variables (never smoking, 'normal' body mass index, being physically active, moderate alcohol intake, and higher diet quality) and life expectancy free of diabetes, cardiovascular disease, and cancer (Li et al., 2020). Higher behavioural adherence scores were associated with a longer life expectancy free of major chronic diseases, suggesting protective effects of behaviours from disease onset.

DOI: 10.4324/9781003318026-14

Experimental evidence supports the link between behaviour and health. The Diabetes Prevention Programme, for example, demonstrated that an intervention targeting behaviour change can prevent or delay the onset of type 2 diabetes in people at high risk for the disease (Knowler et al., 2002). Participants were randomly assigned to (i) a 'lifestyle modification programme' focused on changing physical activity and eating-related behaviours and weight, (ii) a drug intervention (metformin), or (iii) a placebo control group. After an average follow-up time of 2.8 years, the 'lifestyle' and drug intervention groups had a 58% and 31% lower chance, respectively, of developing type 2 diabetes compared to the placebo control group. This underlines the potential for behaviour change to influence the disease process in higher-risk individuals. Longer-term follow-up studies confirmed that 'lifestyle' group participants continued to show delayed onset of diabetes after 10 and 15 years (Diabetes Prevention Program Research Group, 2015; Knowler et al., 2009).

Despite evidence outlining the importance of behaviours and guidelines outlining key behaviours for health, this knowledge has not readily translated into widespread adoption at the population level. For example, the World Health Organization (WHO) estimates that more than one in four adults and more than 80% of adolescents do not meet the recommended levels of physical activity for optimum health, a figure that has remained relatively stable and unchanged over time (World Health Organization, 2022). Similarly, evidence on the prevalence of fruit and vegetable intake has shown room for improvement (Micha et al., 2015), whilst consumption of ultraprocessed foods is high and increasing (Monteiro et al., 2013).

Beyond the well-established link between behaviour and individual health outcomes, behaviour can lead to social and environmental consequences which indirectly impact health (Chevance et al., 2023b; Page & Page, 2014). For example, an increasing focus on the climate emergency and its potential to increase adverse ecological, economic, and societal consequences has shifted perspective on established individual health behaviours (e.g., eating or physical activity) and given rise to a new set of behaviours previously not considered as related to health (e.g., food waste or travelling). Researchers have started to highlight the bi-directional association between climate change and behaviours, whereby changes in climate-related aspects (e.g., rising temperatures) impact health behaviours (e.g., reduced physical activity), and health behaviours (e.g., active transport) impact climate change (e.g., reduced air pollution; Chevance et al., 2023b). It may be beneficial to widen the scope of what one considers to be health behaviours to include those with evidence of direct as well as indirect impact on health outcomes.

New health behaviours are continuously being established and refined in response to changes in infectious disease threats, sociocultural change, and emerging research findings. For example, the COVID-19 pandemic refocused global attention on a variety of different health behaviours related to the emerging global health threat, such as handwashing, obtaining vaccinations, and social distancing, with evidence for the link between behavioural performance and health outcomes evolving over time (West et al., 2020). Moreover, societal and technological changes enable new behaviours with potential links to health outcomes. For example, the possibility of streaming television content on an increasing number of available screens has given rise to 'binge-watching' behaviour, where individuals can consume large volumes of television content in a single sitting whilst being largely sedentary (Walton-Pattison et al., 2018). Research in this area has focused on establishing labels, measures, and definitions for this new behaviour to systematically study the link between behavioural performance and health outcomes.

What Are 'Behaviour' and 'Behaviour Change'?

Psychology is the scientific study of the mind and behaviour (American Psychological Association, 2023b), and several definitions of behaviour exist. However, behaviour as a phenomenon and theoretical construct often remains undefined. To date, no widely agreed definition of behaviour exists, and defining behaviour remains a topic of academic debate (Bergner, 2016; Henriques & Michalski, 2020).

Behaviour has been defined by the American Psychological Association (APA) as "*an organism's activities in response to external or internal stimuli, including objectively observable activities, introspectively observable activities, and nonconscious processes*" (American Psychological Association, 2023a). In a recent exercise to define human behaviour, an expert group suggested that behaviour was "*anything a person does in response to internal or external events. Actions may be overt (motor or verbal) and directly measurable or, covert (activities not viewable but involving voluntary muscles) and indirectly measurable; behaviours are physical events that occur in the body and are controlled by the brain*" (p. 327, Davis et al., 2015).

These two definitions stress that behaviour has a starting point, such as an internal or external stimuli or event, and is observable or measurable. The starting point and measurability criteria of the behavioural definitions are critical and allow for behaviour to be a subject of scientific investigation. Without the ability to identify the beginning or 'initiation' and means of assessment, behaviour would be a continuous flow of activity (Heckhausen & Heckhausen, 2008). Figure 11.1 contextualises behaviour as distinct from the external or internal determinants that precede it and the consequences that follow.

The previous definitions mostly cover approach behaviours (doing something). However, often evidence suggests that avoidance behaviours (not doing something) are important for health outcomes. Although not drinking alcohol is observable, at any one moment in time, people are not performing every possible behaviour, except for a small set of behaviours they engage in. Thus, the category of avoidance behaviours requires consideration of context and/or past behaviour. For example, not smoking cigarettes is considered a health behaviour, but observing it requires contexts in which smoking could be enacted (e.g., being offered a cigarette). Not smoking cigarettes is a meaningful behavioural target

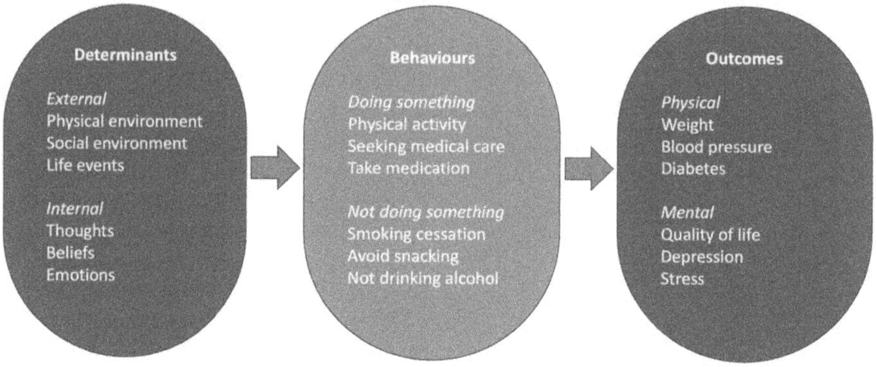

Figure 11.1 Behaviour in context, including an initiation point (determinants) and possible end points or outcomes (consequences).

for individuals who smoked cigarettes in the past but may lack meaning for those who have never smoked. Avoidance behaviours are often considered in the context of behaviour change, where alteration of past behavioural performance is included in the concept of the behaviour. The definition of behaviour could be amended as "*any action that a person does in response to internal or external events, or refrains from doing when the action is possible or when they have done it in the past*".

When considering behaviour change, where past behaviour is included as a reference point, the distinction between approach and avoidance behaviours becomes less critical. Behaviour change can be viewed as the alteration of past actions or action tendencies in response to internal or external events. This typically includes changes in duration, frequency, quality, or intensity of behaviours. Behaviour change can include any of the following elements: increasing (e.g., going for walks more often), decreasing (e.g., reducing consumption of the number of discretionary snacks), cessation (e.g., stopping alcohol intake), initiation (e.g., starting to run regularly), or replacing (e.g., ordering a salad instead of fish and chips).

What are 'Health Behaviour' and 'Health Behaviour Change'?

Health behaviours are a sub-type of behaviour. Similar to defining 'behaviour', variation exists when defining 'health behaviour'. One typical definition suggests that health behaviour is "*any activity undertaken for the purpose of preventing or detecting disease or for improving health and well-being*" (p. 2, Conner & Norman, 2015). This definition highlights the connection between behaviour and health-related outcomes for preventing disease onset or detecting existing disease, implying that disease detection leads to treatments that improve health. An assumption of this definition is that health behaviour requires an intentional and conscious engagement in behaviours for health-based motives. However, motives for behavioural performance are varied and are often not based on health considerations nor accessible to awareness. Another definition suggests, "*Health behaviors refer to any behaviors that impact on people's physical and mental health and quality of life*" (p. 2, Tombor & Michie, 2017). This definition is inclusive of behaviours performed for non-health motives and highlights a variety of different health outcomes, including physical, mental, and quality of life in a non-directional manner, i.e., including desirable or undesirable outcomes. This definition defines health behaviour using the term 'behaviour', leaving open the need to define behaviour.

Combining the aforementioned considerations, health behaviour can be defined as

> *anything a person does in response to internal or external events, or refrains from doing when the action is possible or when they have done it in the past, that directly or indirectly impacts on the person's health including physical, mental, and quality of life outcomes, including actions undertaken for the purpose of improving health.*

This definition provides descriptive accounts of health (physical, mental, and quality of life outcomes), behaviour (anything a person does in response to internal or external events or refrains from doing), and their relationship (direct or indirect impact or performed to bring about an impact). It is inclusive of non-traditional health behaviours which can indirectly affect health and includes behaviours performed with the intention to improve health, which might not have evidence of an impact on health outcomes, e.g., vitamin supplements are taken for health motives, even though there is sometimes limited measurable impact on health outcomes (O'Connor et al., 2022).

Given the link between health behaviour and desired outcomes, a key task is to support behaviour change. Based on the previous definitions, health behaviour change can be defined as

> *the alteration of past actions or action tendencies in response to internal or external events which directly or indirectly impacts on the person's health including physical and mental and quality of life outcomes, including actions undertaken for the purpose of improving health.*

Figure 11.2 outlines the relationship between the behavioural concepts outlined in this section. Central to the figure is 'behaviour', which can be considered a 'health behaviour' when focusing on the impact that a behaviour has on health. 'Behaviour change' requires the consideration of 'past behaviour' as a reference point for detecting change, and the concept of 'health behaviour change' includes the consideration of behaviour in the context of past behaviour and its impact on health.

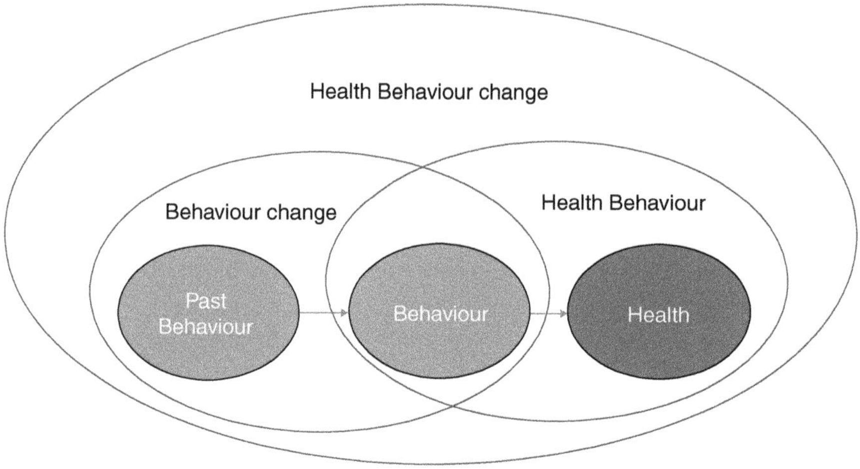

Figure 11.2 Relationship between behavioural concepts, including behaviour, health behaviour, behaviour change, and health behaviour change.

Language around (Health) Behaviour

Language is critical when communicating about scientific constructs such as behaviour. Behaviour-related communication has been hampered by at least three issues: (i) failing to label behaviour as behaviour, (ii) using synonyms for behaviour, and (iii) the use of behavioural descriptors. These issues are outlined in the following sections and visually represented in Figure 11.3a–c.

The Call Behaviour 'Behaviour' Issue

A common occurrence in communications about behaviour is the use of different terms. Johnston and Dixon (2008) noted that health psychologists frequently use various labels specific to forms and context, such as 'walking', 'adherence', or 'physical activity' (Johnston & Dixon, 2008). They suggest to label behaviour 'behaviour' to ensure that health psychological evidence and theory are considered and consulted. This can often be achieved by combining existing labels with the term behaviour, e.g., walking behaviour, adherence behaviour, or physical activity behaviour.

The Behavioural Synonym Issue

Behavioural synonyms that go beyond the definition of behaviour as a construct can interfere with understanding. A prominent example is the term 'lifestyle', which in the context of health is frequently used to refer to someone's way of living and the activities that a person or group of people do, i.e., behaviour. The use of the term lifestyle in a health-related context has been the subject of debate (see Box 11.1).

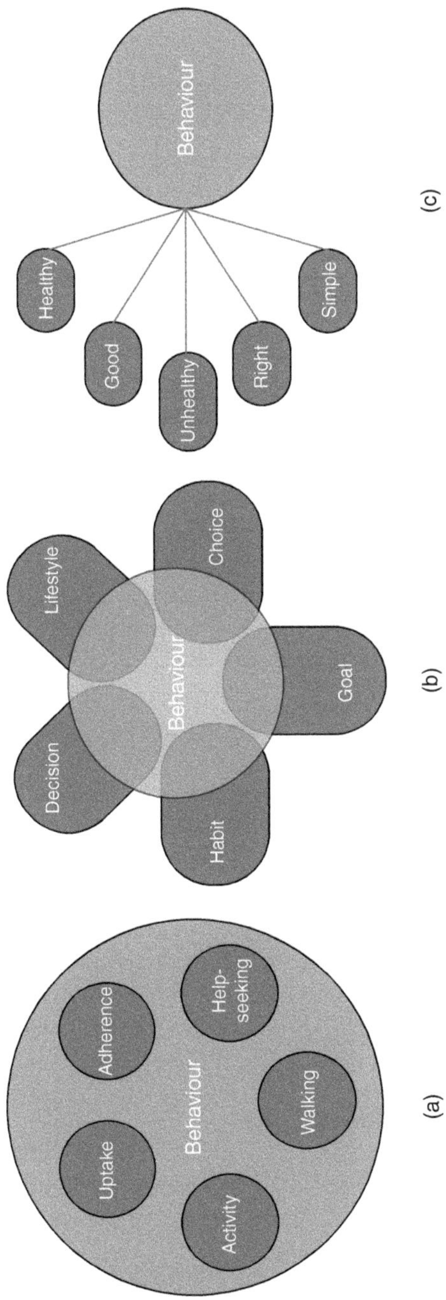

Figure 11.3 (a) The call behaviour behaviour issue, (b) the behavioural synonym issue, (c) the behavioural descriptor issue.

Box 11.1 Should We Use the Term 'Lifestyle' in the Context of Health Behaviour?

'Lifestyle' is a common term used in everyday conversations, as well as academic literature and scientific research, including health psychology (for an in-depth narrative review of the use of 'lifestyle' in health psychology, see Brivio et al., 2023).

Critical reflections on the term 'lifestyle' have been consistently voiced across academic disciplines and include statements that the term 'lifestyle' is "lazy language" (Robinson & Smith, 2023), "one of the most abused words in the English language" (Sobel, 2013), which is fundamentally a political concept with symbolic power that legitimises certain ways of thinking, feeling and acting at the expense of others (Korp, 2008). Some have called for an abandonment of the concept altogether within health-related contexts (de Gruchy, 2019; Lincoln, 2015). The following is an examination of the advantages and disadvantages of using the term 'lifestyle' in the context of behaviour-related research and practice.

Advantages of Using the Term 'Lifestyle'

- **Multi-behavioural**: 'Lifestyle' can be used to refer to multiple behaviours using one term. Multiple health-related behaviours often cluster together within an individual to affect health and well-being (Spring et al., 2012). The term 'lifestyle' can be used as a shorthand to refer to clusters or bundles of behaviours.
- **Multidimensionality**: 'Lifestyle' is a multidimensional concept which has attracted attention from a variety of disciplines such as sociology, marketing, psychology, epidemiology, and anthropology. As a result, a rich body of literature, concepts, frameworks, and theories can be drawn on when examining 'lifestyle'. These concepts go beyond the focus on individual health behaviours and include the economic, cultural, and social environment.
- **Inequity potential**: A 'lifestyle' perspective can provide insights into individual and social conditions in relation to health inequalities, with the potential to provide solutions or targets to tackle inequity (Blaxter, 1990; Cockerham, 2017). For example, socially disadvantaged neighbourhoods may simultaneously make it more likely that residents engage in multiple health-harming behaviours (Pampel et al., 2010).

Disadvantages of Using the Term 'Lifestyle'

- **Definitional fuzziness**: 'Lifestyle' is often poorly defined, which is of particular concern for an expansive and generic concept which has been described as a "hotchpotch category for almost everything that somehow has to do with social behaviour and health" (p. 54, Abel et al., 2002) and a "buzzword for all kinds of perspectives" (p. 807, Korp, 2010).

- **Lack of specificity**: 'Lifestyle' is often conceptualised using a combination of behavioural, cognitive, and social factors, confounding and conflating behaviour with other relevant explanatory factors, such as determinants, behaviour, outcomes (see Figure 11.1). This lack of specificity can hamper advancement and clarity in understanding health-related phenomena.
- **(Mis)interpretation**: 'Lifestyle' is often used as a synonym for health behaviours, whereas conceptualisations and definitions typically include additional elements such as cognitive, environmental, cultural, economic, and social factors as part of the concept (Blaxter, 1990; Cockerham, 2017). The concept of 'lifestyle' is frequently (mis)interpreted as an agency-advocating construct whereby individuals freely choose their particular 'lifestyle' from a menu of options (Nunan et al., 2021). Such narrow (mis)interpretations of the term 'lifestyle' are often at the heart of false dichotomies (Sniehotta et al., 2017b), such as 'individual vs population approaches', 'agency vs social structure', or 'behaviour vs environmental change', which are largely fruitless and unresolvable debates.

When communicating about behaviour, the term 'behaviour' should be used rather than 'lifestyle', which carries additional meaning. 'Behaviour' typically refers to a narrower and more focused construct and carries less risk of being used as a 'hotchpotch category' and 'buzzword' for a plethora of factors influencing health. Where communication uses the term 'lifestyle' to refer to factors including but beyond behaviour, it is advisable to accompany the use of the term with an explicit definition given the number of different (mis)interpretations. Given the 'conceptual baggage' of the term 'lifestyle', the variety of (mis)interpretations need to be kept in mind to avoid confusion.

Using synonyms for behaviour which carry additional meaning or interpretation potential can impede progress in understanding and changing behaviour and may lead to unhelpful interpretations and unintended consequences. For instance, using the term 'habit' instead of behaviour might narrow the scope of behavioural explanations and underestimates the volitional control individuals can exert over the behaviour. From a theoretical perspective, referring to behaviour as habits is not in line with definitions of habits as a psychological process (Gardner, 2015) and is unlikely to advance scientific or lay understanding of behavioural phenomena. For additional examples of behavioural synonyms and their inherent confusion potential, see Table 11.1.

The Behavioural Descriptor Issue

The term 'behaviour' is often accompanied by descriptors which can uncover implicit underlying assumptions, some of which may require reflection and consideration. For example, the Canadian government lists the term 'healthy

Table 11.1 Behavioural synonyms alongside explanations and reflections on inherent confusion potential

Behavioural Synonym	*Explanation*	*Confusion Potential*
Habit	Frequently used term typically referring to repeatedly performed behaviours.	Habits are a psychological process and not a behaviour *per se* (Gardner & Lally, 2022). Using the term 'habits' might narrow the scope of explanations considered for behaviour.
Goal	A versatile term usually referring to the attainment of a desired outcome.	Goals are a behaviourally unspecific term which may or may not refer to behaviour, and covers a range of factors, including cognitions, behaviours, outcomes, or events.
Action	A common term used to refer to a specific behaviour or subset of a behaviour.	Actions are usually references to observable acts and thus in line with the definition of behaviour. The use of the term 'action' instead of behaviour has little confusion potential, but it should be noted that action is part of behaviour as a concept.
Lifestyle	A summary term for a variety of behaviours or clusters of behaviours alongside other factors.	Lifestyle is an indiscriminate term for a range of phenomena and processes. Many of these are not behavioural in nature and are not within an individual's control. Lifestyle is frequently interpreted as implying a degree of autonomy to constructing one's life. For a full list of advantages and disadvantage of the term 'lifestyle', see Box 11.1.
Choice	A term describing the selection of a behaviour in the presence of several alternative modes of action.	Choice implies a deliberate selection of a behaviour for performance. This can overestimate the degree to which individuals engage in deliberate decision-making and overstate the degree of awareness individuals have over their performed behaviours. Moreover, having made a choice is itself not the enactment of that choice but is a cognitive process with behavioural enactment implied.

(*Continued*)

Table 11.1 (Continued)

Behavioural Synonym	*Explanation*	*Confusion Potential*
Decision	The product of a deliberation process that weighs the pros and cons of a behaviour, as well as possible alternatives used frequently when the intention is to emphasise personal responsibility of the actor.	Decisions are often seen as the results of a deliberation process, often based on the gathering of relevant information, overstating the degree to which individuals engage in conscious deliberations. A decision is a psychological process which may not be related to behavioural performance.

behaviours' as one of 12 determinants of health. The term 'healthy' suggests that other behaviours can be readily categorised as 'not healthy' or 'unhealthy'. 'Healthy behaviours' is an ambiguous term. Describing a behaviour as 'healthy' suggests that it is desirable to perform and implies a universal direction of impact (healthy = always beneficial). However, not all 'healthy behaviours' are necessarily 'healthy' across all contexts and individuals. For instance, eating an apple is usually considered to be a 'healthy behaviour'. Those individuals diagnosed with an apple allergy might not consider apple consumption to be a 'healthy behaviour'. Moreover, using the term 'healthy' can lead to moralising, bias, and judgement of individuals who, for a variety of reasons, are not engaging in these 'healthy behaviours'. Other behavioural descriptors can have a similar impact, including 'good behaviour' (where performance implies being a good person), 'right behaviour' (where performance implies doing the right thing), or 'simple behaviour' (which minimises the degree of difficulty some experience in behavioural performance).

Language around behaviour can be complex, which is further amplified by combinations of the aforementioned terms. For example, one might come across phrases such as 'healthy lifestyle habits', which combine a variety of terms and concepts that may or may not refer to behaviour. Being aware of the natural diversity of language around the construct of behaviour is useful for health psychologists to obtain clarity in their own communication, the interpretation of evidence and theory, and to question existing accounts of behaviour, including implicit underlying assumptions.

Having examined instances of communication around the concept of behaviour, the next section covers different aspects of communication and language when individuals use the term behaviour, focusing on behavioural components and dimensions.

Behavioural Components, Dimensions, and Categories

Behaviour as a concept is often used to refer to different but related phenomena which reflect distinct aspects of the construct. Figure 11.4 outlines four different behavioural components underlying the use of the term behaviour, which are outlined in turn.

The first component is '*behaviour proper*', which is most closely aligned with the previous definition of behaviour as "*anything a person does in response to internal or external events or refrains from doing when the action is possible or when they have done it in the past*". Behaviour proper is observable in the moment and refers to what an individual does. For instance, it is possible to observe someone going for a walk. Behaviour proper can be further sub-divided into smaller units of behaviour (such as putting on shoes or opening the door) which form an observable action unit performed at a specific moment in time. This level of conceptualisation allows behaviour to be explored within context and examined in detail and is a useful level of conceptualisation when developing interventions for change.

The second component is the '*behavioural category*', which consists of higher-level descriptors of behaviours, groups, or patterns of behaviours performed over time. For example, physical activity is not an 'in the moment' behaviour (i.e., behaviour proper). However, physical activity comprises a variety of different behaviours which fall under the definition of physical activity as "*bodily movement produced by skeletal muscles that results in energy expenditure, and increases heart rate and breathing*" (Canadian Society for Exercise Physiology, 2023). Given the plethora of physical activity behaviours that one could engage in, the

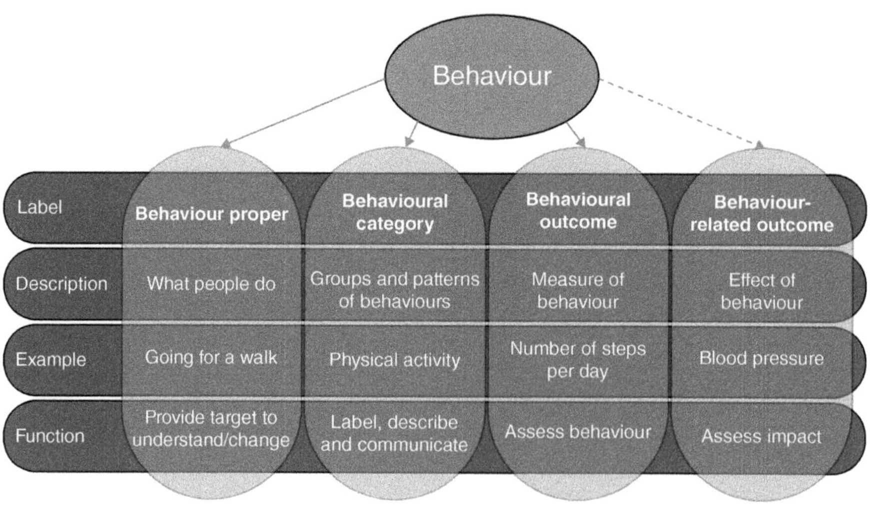

Figure 11.4 Different behavioural components underlying the use of the term behaviour. Note that behaviour-related outcomes are not behaviour (indicated by the dashed line).

behavioural category label is typically employed. Behavioural categories are useful for labelling groups or patterns of behaviours.

The third component is the '*behavioural outcome*'. Behavioural outcomes aim to provide an assessment of behaviour to quantify or measure performance. The number of steps walked in a day, for instance, is an assessment of physical activity (behavioural category) and is achieved through the performance of various movements throughout the day, such as going for a walk (behaviour proper). Behavioural outcomes require assessment of the behaviour (e.g., by using a pedometer) and are often compared to behavioural outcome goals (10,000 steps a day). Behavioural recommendations in guidelines are typically formulated at the behavioural outcome level (e.g., eat five portions of fruit and vegetables) to provide individuals with targets to aspire to, which can be achieved through a plethora of behaviours, e.g., eating an apple at lunch, eating broccoli at dinner.

The fourth component are '*behaviour-related outcomes*'. Behaviour-related outcomes are not behaviours. They are outcomes linked to behavioural performance, although often, these outcomes are influenced by factors other than behaviour. Outcomes, such as blood pressure or weight, can be influenced through eating and physical activity behaviours, but these are not the sole determinants of these outcomes. Behaviour-related outcomes are frequently assessed as a proxy measure of an underlying disease process (e.g., hypertension or obesity) but should not be confused with the other behavioural concepts outlined earlier.

Various attempts have been made to describe and classify health behaviours to facilitate theorising and communication. A common distinction is between health-promoting behaviours, such as physical activity (also referred to as 'approach behaviours', 'health protective behaviours', 'health enhancing behaviours', and 'positive health behaviours'), and health risk behaviour, such as smoking tobacco (also referred to as 'avoidance behaviours', 'behavioural pathogens', 'health impairing behaviours', or 'negative health behaviours'). Several ways to classify different health behaviours have been identified.

McEachan et al. (2010) attempted to classify 20 health behaviours promoted in government guidelines (e.g., eating five fruits and vegetables per day). They identified 11 distinct key characteristics which can be used to describe health behaviour, such as 'approach – avoid', effort, or emotionality. To examine possible clusters of characteristics, principal components analysis indicated behaviours were perceived along three key dimensions: 'easy immediate pay-offs' versus 'effortful long-term pay-offs', 'private unproblematic' versus 'public and problematic', and 'important routines' versus 'unimportant one-offs' (McEachan et al., 2010).

Nudelman and Shiloh (2015) developed a taxonomy that represents how members of the public conceptualise 45 health behaviours. The study found two meta-clusters of health behaviours which were physical and psychosocial (Nudelman & Shiloh, 2015). The physical cluster was divided into risk avoidance (including substance abuse, danger avoidance, and environmental risk factors), health maintenance (including sleep, medical practices, and bodily routines), and nutrition. The psychosocial cluster covered general well-being (including enjoyment and meaning, relationships, and work) and included various items which could be considered behaviour-related outcomes (e.g., reducing stress) or general life goals (e.g., learning and expanding one's horizons) rather than behaviours *per se* as defined earlier. This common-sense taxonomy replicated the common distinction between health-promoting behaviours (represented by the clusters of health maintenance and nutrition) and health risk behaviours (represented by the category risk avoidance).

Health behaviours can be described and classified in a variety of ways. The most common distinction which repeatedly emerges is between approach behaviours (doing an action) and avoidance behaviours (not doing an action). This might be the result of approach/avoidance behaviour conceptualisations implicitly including the dimension of health impact (approach = obtain positive impact on health; avoidance = prevent negative impact on health), as well as the frequency (approach = start or increase; avoid = decrease or stop). However, the way behaviour is described and classified is dependent on the practical or research context, and different aspects are relevant for different purposes.

Lifespan Perspective on Behaviour

A lifespan perspective is necessary for understanding health behaviour, as behaviour is influenced by both internal and external factors that change throughout people's lives. For example, the extent to which health-relevant behaviour can be changed through internal self-regulatory mechanisms varies across the human lifespan (J. Heckhausen et al., 2010). Self-regulatory capacity develops throughout childhood, adolescence, and early adulthood. The related neuroscientific understanding of the developing brain has elucidated changes to both the structure and function of the neural circuitry underlying key executive functions, such as planning, working memory, and impulse control, that are ongoing during the first three decades of life (Blakemore & Robbins, 2012). Therefore, there are good theoretical and empirical reasons for having developmentally informed health behaviour change approaches (Miller et al., 2020).

The limited capacity for self-regulation of behaviour in early life has been recognised long before the neuroscientific details of the developing brain have been established. This can be seen in the long-standing legally enforced age limits in access to some health-harming products in most jurisdictions, e.g., tobacco and alcohol. Similarly, early life contexts such as school settings often implement nutritious eating policies that prohibit access to some health-harming foods (Story et al., 2009). Such autonomy reducing, i.e., low agency, dietary interventions (Adams et al., 2016) are usually seen as an acceptable and equitable means of shaping health behaviours at a stage in life where reliance on self-regulation could be considered neglectful to younger people from a public health perspective.

One of the key lifespan considerations for health behaviour change concerns an analysis of whether interventions might support or inhibit the developmental needs or goals of any potential target group (J. Heckhausen et al., 2010, 2019).

For example, in the context of an infectious disease pandemic where interventions that aim to increase physical distancing are implemented, the benefits and harms of such interventions might vary across the lifespan. During adolescence and early adulthood social connections and contact outside the family home context are critical for psychological development. Therefore any prolonged disruption to ongoing social relationships during this part of the lifespan has the potential to negatively impact key developmental processes such as identity development, establishing independence, establishing career goals, and the formation of intimate relationships outside of the family.

In those living with life-long chronic illnesses such as type 1 diabetes (Berg et al., 2017) or asthma (Murphy et al., 2021), there is a particular ongoing developmental transition throughout adolescence and early adulthood characterised by gradual development of the capacity to engage in medical self-care with reduced support from both caregivers and health-care providers. Health behaviour change interventions for such groups need to be attuned to the developmental needs of those in emerging adulthood and, in particular, the often abrupt reduction in health-care support that can accompany the transition from paediatric to adulthood medical care. There are recent examples of co-design of behavioural interventions with young people living with type 1 diabetes that demonstrate how these can be developmentally informed to meet the needs and goals of those living with this illness at this life stage (Morrissey et al., 2021).

A lifespan perspective on health behaviour later in life is also critical, as health behaviour change interventions can impact factors that become more salient during midlife and older adulthood. The time spent engaging in group-based physical activity with relative strangers, for example, might displace time previously used for investing in close relationships with one's partner, children, or close friends. The nature of these social opportunity costs varies throughout life. For example, the evidence supporting the socioemotional selectivity theory of lifespan motivation (Carstensen et al., 1999) indicates that as humans age, they prioritise a smaller number of social relationships with close social partners that satisfy their emotional needs. Therefore a lifespan perspective on the social contexts and costs that accompany physical activity behaviour change may be required. This can help ensure that health behaviour change does not disrupt developmental needs in midlife and older adulthood.

In addition, these variable impacts might interact with contextual risk factors such as socio-economic status. Indeed, there is evidence beginning to accumulate showing that school closures that were enforced during the COVID-19 pandemic to enhance physical distancing had outsized negative impacts on younger people from socially deprived backgrounds (Luijten et al., 2021; O'Connor et al., 2021). Primary prevention public health interventions that aim to change the behaviour of whole populations need to consider the benefits and harms of any interventions from a lifespan perspective. This is critical as an intervention that might immediately and clearly reduce morbidity metrics for people at higher health risk later in life could potentially simultaneously increase the risk for psychological morbidity among younger people at developmentally sensitive periods of the lifespan. The health consequences of such harms may take considerably more time to transpire. Any analysis of population health behaviour change needs to avoid the present bias that may fixate on immediate health outcomes, e.g., hospital bed occupancy this week, over those that may be similarly consequential but take more time to produce a public health signal, e.g., adolescent and young adult mental health service use in five years' time.

In summary, describing, predicting, explaining, and intervening in health-relevant behaviour requires a developmental perspective. This needs to be more nuanced than the paediatric and adult dichotomy that pervades much of healthcare organisation. Lumping together the 7-month-old and the 17-year-old and the 18- and 80-year-old into developmentally meaningful categories is at odds with the psychological science of human development. Health behaviour change approaches need to foster agency and motivation to promote health across the lifespan. Achieving this will require parallel analysis of developmental needs and goals in the design of behaviour change interventions.

Summary and Link to Chapters in the Section

Having examined in detail health behaviour as a construct and contextualised it within a lifespan perspective, the following chapters will build on and illustrate the conceptual points made in the current chapter. Chapter 12 will introduce in detail what it means to adopt a behavioural perspective when examining a variety of behaviour-related issues in practice and contrast what a behavioural perspective adds to other existing approaches. Chapter 13 will build on and extend the notion that health behaviours cluster at the individual and population level, and showcase the psychological processes that have been explored to understand and change several behaviours. Chapter 14 uses the pressing public health issue of obesity to provide an example of health behaviour as a critical aspect when attempting to understand a complex disease process within a multidisciplinary approach. Lastly, Chapter 15 provides an in-depth example of developments in relation to the understanding of the traditional health behaviour of medication taking, illustrating how a seemingly 'simple' and straightforward health behaviour is complex, dynamic, but ultimately changeable. Overall, this section demonstrates that focusing on health behaviour as a concept in health psychology affords a unique perspective, which has led to advancements in the understanding of the contribution of behavioural factors in complex issues that affect human health and well-being.

Further Reading

Brivio, F., Viganò, A., Paterna, A., Palena, N., & Greco, A. (2023). Narrative Review and Analysis of the Use of "Lifestyle" in Health Psychology. *Int J Environ Res Public Health*, *20*(5). doi:10.3390/ijerph20054427

Chevance, G., Fresán, U., Hekler, E., Edmondson, D., Lloyd, S. J., Ballester, J., … Bernard, P. (2023). Thinking Health-Related Behaviors in a Climate Change Context: A Narrative Review. *Ann Behav Med*, *57*(3), 193–204. doi:10.1093/abm/kaac039

Sniehotta, F. F., Araújo-Soares, V., Brown, J., Kelly, M. P., Michie, S., & West, R. (2017). Complex Systems and Individual-Level Approaches to Population Health: A False Dichotomy? *Lancet Public Health*, *2*(9), e396–e397. doi:10.1016/s2468-2667(17)30167-6

References

Abel, T., Cockerham, W. C., & Niemann, S. (2002). A Critical Approach to Lifestyle and Health. In S. Platt & J. Watson (Eds.), *Researching Health Promotion* (pp. 70–98): Routledge.

Adams, J., Mytton, O., White, M., & Monsivais, P. (2016). Correction: Why Are Some Population Interventions for Diet and Obesity More Equitable and Effective Than Others? The Role of Individual Agency. *PLOS Medicine*, *13*(5), e1002045. https://doi.org/10.1371/journal.pmed.1002045

American Psychological Association. (2023a). Behaviour. Retrieved from https://dictionary.apa.org/behavior

American Psychological Association. (2023b). Psychology. Retrieved from https://dictionary.apa.org/psychology

Berg, C. A., Butner, J., Wiebe, D. J., Lansing, A. H., Osborn, P., King, P. S., … Butler, J. M. (2017). Developmental Model of Parent-Child Coordination for Self-Regulation across Childhood and into Emerging Adulthood: Type 1 Diabetes Management as an Example. *Dev Rev*, *46*, 1–26. https://doi.org/10.1016/j.dr.2017.09.001

Bergner, R. M. (2016). What Is Behavior? And Why Is It Not Reducible to Biological States of Affairs? *J Theor Philos Psychol*, *36*(1), 41.

Blakemore, S. J., & Robbins, T. W. (2012). Decision-Making in the Adolescent Brain. *Nat Neurosci*, *15*(9), 1184–1191. https://doi.org/10.1038/nn.3177

Blaxter, M. (1990). *Health and Lifestyles* (Vol. 1). Routledge.

Brivio, F., Viganò, A., Paterna, A., Palena, N., & Greco, A. (2023). Narrative Review and Analysis of the Use of "Lifestyle" in Health Psychology. *Int J Environ Res Public Health*, *20*(5). https://doi.org/10.3390/ijerph20054427

Canadian Society for Exercise Physiology. (2023). Https://Csepguidelines.Ca/Resources/Glossary/. Retrieved from https://csepguidelines.ca/resources/glossary/

Carstensen, L. L., Isaacowitz, D. M., & Charles, S. T. (1999). Taking Time Seriously. A Theory of Socioemotional Selectivity. *Am Psychol*, *54*(3), 165–181. https://doi.org/10.1037//0003-066x.54.3.165

Chevance, G., Fresán, U., Hekler, E., Edmondson, D., Lloyd, S. J., Ballester, J., … Bernard, P. (2023b). Thinking Health-Related Behaviors in a Climate Change Context: A Narrative Review. *Ann Behav Med*, *57*(3), 193–204. https://doi.org/10.1093/abm/kaac039

Cockerham, W. C. (2017). Health Lifestyle Theory. In B. S. Turner (Ed.), *The Wiley-Blackwell Encyclopedia of Social Theory* (pp. 1–3).

Conner, M., & Norman, P. (2015). *Research and Practice with Social Cognition Models*: Open University Press.

Davis, R., Campbell, R., Hildon, Z., Hobbs, L., & Michie, S. (2015). Theories of Behaviour and Behaviour Change across the Social and Behavioural Sciences: A Scoping Review. *Health Psychol Rev*, *9*(3), 323–344. https://doi.org/10.1080/17437199.2014.941722

de Gruchy, J. (2019). The Lazy Language of 'Lifestyles' – Let's Rid This from Our Talk About Prevention. Retrieved from https://www.adph.org.uk/2019/04/the-lazy-language-of-lifestyles-lets-rid-this-from-our-talk-about-prevention/

Diabetes Prevention Program Research Group. (2015). Long-Term Effects of Lifestyle Intervention or Metformin on Diabetes Development and Microvascular Complications over 15-Year Follow-Up: The Diabetes Prevention Program Outcomes Study. *Lancet Diabetes Endocrinol*, *3*(11), 866–875. https://doi.org/10.1016/S2213-8587(15)00291-0

Gardner, B. (2015). A Review and Analysis of the Use of 'Habit' in Understanding, Predicting and Influencing Health-Related Behaviour. *Health Psychol Rev*, *9*(3), 277–295. https://doi.org/10.1080/17437199.2013.876238

Gardner, B., & Lally, P. (2022). Habit and Habitual Behaviour. *Health Psychol Rev*, 1–7. https://doi.org/10.1080/17437199.2022.2105249

Heckhausen, J., Wrosch, C., & Schulz, R. (2010). A Motivational Theory of Life-Span Development. *Psychol Rev*, *117*(1), 32–60. https://doi.org/10.1037/a0017668

Heckhausen, J., Wrosch, C., & Schulz, R. (2019). Agency and Motivation in Adulthood and Old Age. *Annu Rev Psychol*, *70*, 191–217. https://doi.org/10.1146/annurev-psych-010418-103043

Heckhausen, J. E., & Heckhausen, H. E. (2008). *Motivation and Action*: Cambridge University Press.

Henriques, G., & Michalski, J. (2020). Defining Behavior and Its Relationship to the Science of Psychology. *Integr Psychol Behav Sci*, *54*, 328–353.

Johnston, M., & Dixon, D. (2008). Current Issues and New Directions in Psychology and Health: What Happened to Behaviour in the Decade of Behaviour? *Health Psychol*, *23*(5), 509–513.

Khaw, K. T., Wareham, N., Bingham, S., Welch, A., Luben, R., & Day, N. (2008). Combined Impact of Health Behaviours and Mortality in Men and Women: The Epic-Norfolk Prospective Population Study. *PLoS Med*, *5*(1), e12. https://doi.org/10.1371/journal.pmed.0050012

Knowler, W. C., Barrett-Connor, E., Fowler, S. E., Hamman, R. F., Lachin, J. M., Walker, E. A., & Nathan, D. M. (2002). Reduction in the Incidence of Type 2 Diabetes with Lifestyle Intervention or Metformin. *N Engl J Med*, *346*(6), 393–403. https://doi.org/10.1056/NEJMoa012512

Knowler, W. C., Fowler, S. E., Hamman, R. F., Christophi, C. A., Hoffman, H. J., Brenneman, A. T., … Nathan, D. M. (2009). 10-Year Follow-up of Diabetes Incidence and Weight Loss in the Diabetes Prevention Program Outcomes Study. *Lancet*, *374*(9702), 1677–1686. https://doi.org/10.1016/s0140-6736(09)61457-4

Korp, P. (2008). The Symbolic Power of 'Healthy Lifestyles'. *Health Social Rev*, *17*(1), 18–26. https://doi.org/10.5172/hesr.451.17.1.18

Korp, P. (2010). Problems of the Healthy Lifestyle Discourse. *Social Compass*, *4*(9), 800–810. https://doi.org/10.1111/j.1751-9020.2010.00313.x

Li, Y., Schoufour, J., Wang, D. D., Dhana, K., Pan, A., Liu, X., … Hu, F. B. (2020). Healthy Lifestyle and Life Expectancy Free of Cancer, Cardiovascular Disease, and Type 2 Diabetes: Prospective Cohort Study. *BMJ*, *368*, l6669. https://doi.org/10.1136/bmj.l6669

Lincoln, P. (2015). Lifestyle: A Plea to Abandon the Use of This Word in Public Health. Retrieved from https://ukpublichealthnetwork.org.uk/lifestyle-a-plea-to-abandon-the-use-of-this-word-in-public-health/

Luijten, M. A. J., van Muilekom, M. M., Teela, L., Polderman, T. J. C., Terwee, C. B., Zijlmans, J., … Haverman, L. (2021). The Impact of Lockdown During the Covid-19 Pandemic on Mental and Social Health of Children and Adolescents. *Qual Life Res*, *30*(10), 2795–2804. https://doi.org/10.1007/s11136-021-02861-x

McEachan, R. R., Lawton, R. J., & Conner, M. (2010). Classifying Health-Related Behaviours: Exploring Similarities and Differences Amongst Behaviours. *Br J Health Psychol*, *15*(Pt 2), 347–366. https://doi.org/10.1348/135910709x466487

Micha, R., Khatibzadeh, S., Shi, P., Andrews, K. G., Engell, R. E., & Mozaffarian, D. (2015). Global, Regional and National Consumption of Major Food Groups in 1990 and 2010: A Systematic Analysis Including 266 Country-Specific Nutrition Surveys Worldwide. *BMJ Open*, *5*(9), e008705.

Miller, A. L., Lo, S. L., Bauer, K. W., & Fredericks, E. M. (2020). Developmentally Informed Behaviour Change Techniques to Enhance Self-Regulation in a Health Promotion Context: A Conceptual Review. *Health Psychol Rev*, *14*(1), 116–131. https://doi.org/10.1080/17437199.2020.1718530

Monteiro, C. A., Moubarac, J. C., Cannon, G., Ng, S. W., & Popkin, B. (2013). Ultra-Processed Products Are Becoming Dominant in the Global Food System. *Obes Rev*, *14*(Suppl 2), 21–28. https://doi.org/10.1111/obr.12107

Morrissey, E. C., Casey, B., Hynes, L., Dinneen, S. F., & Byrne, M. (2021). Supporting Self-Management and Clinic Attendance in Young Adults with Type 1 Diabetes: Development of the D1 Now Intervention. *Pilot Feasibility Stud*, *7*(1), 186. https://doi.org/10.1186/s40814-021-00922-z

Murphy, J., McSharry, J., Hynes, L., Matthews, S., Van Rhoon, L., & Molloy, G. J. (2021). Prevalence and Predictors of Adherence to Inhaled Corticosteroids in Young Adults (15–30 Years) with Asthma: A Systematic Review and Meta-Analysis. *J Asthma*, *58*(5), 683–705. https://doi.org/10.1080/02770903.2020.1711916

Nudelman, G., & Shiloh, S. (2015). Mapping Health Behaviors: Constructing and Validating a Common-Sense Taxonomy of Health Behaviors. *Soc Sci Med*, *146*, 1–10. https://doi.org/10.1016/j.socscimed.2015.10.004

Nunan, D., Blane, D. N., & McCartney, M. (2021). Exemplary Medical Care or Trojan Horse? An Analysis of the 'Lifestyle Medicine'movement. *Br J Gen Pract*, *71*(706), 229–232.

O'Connor, R. C., Wetherall, K., Cleare, S., McClelland, H., Melson, A. J., Niedzwiedz, C. L., … Robb, K. A. (2021). Mental Health and Well-Being During the Covid-19 Pandemic: Longitudinal Analyses of Adults in the Uk Covid-19 Mental Health & Wellbeing Study. *Br J Psychiatry*, *218*(6), 326–333. https://doi.org/10.1192/bjp.2020.212

O'Connor, E. A., Evans, C. V., Ivlev, I., Rushkin, M. C., Thomas, R. G., Martin, A., & Lin, J. S. (2022). Vitamin and Mineral Supplements for the Primary Prevention of Cardiovascular Disease and Cancer: Updated Evidence Report and Systematic Review for the Us Preventive Services Task Force. *JAMA*, *327*(23), 2334–2347. https://doi.org/10.1001/jama.2021.15650

Page, N., & Page, M. (2014). Climate Change: Time to Do Something Different. *Front Psychol*, *5*, 1294. https://doi.org/10.3389/fpsyg.2014.01294

Pampel, F. C., Krueger, P. M., & Denney, J. T. (2010). Socioeconomic Disparities in Health Behaviors. *Annu Rev Sociol*, *36*, 349–370. https://doi.org/10.1146/annurev.soc.012809.102529

Robinson, M., & Smith, J. A. (2023). The Lazy Language of 'Lifestyles'. *Health Promot J Austr*, *34*(1), 3–5. https://doi.org/10.1002/hpja.677

Sniehotta, F. F., Araújo-Soares, V., Brown, J., Kelly, M. P., Michie, S., & West, R. (2017b). Complex Systems and Individual-Level Approaches to Population Health: A False Dichotomy? *Lancet Public Health*, *2*(9), e396-e397. https://doi.org/10.1016/s2468-2667(17)30167-6

Sobel, M. E. (2013). *Lifestyle and Social Structure: Concepts, Definitions, Analyses*. Elsevier.

Spring, B., Moller, A. C., & Coons, M. J. (2012). Multiple Health Behaviours: Overview and Implications. *Journal of Public Health*, *34*(suppl_1), i3–i10. https://doi.org/10.1093/pubmed/fdr111

Story, M., Nanney, M. S., & Schwartz, M. B. (2009). Schools and Obesity Prevention: Creating School Environments and Policies to Promote Healthy Eating and Physical Activity. *Milbank Q*, *87*(1), 71–100. https://doi.org/10.1111/j.1468-0009.2009.00548.x

Tombor, I., & Michie, S. (2017). *Methods of Health Behavior Change*. Oxford University Press.

Walton-Pattison, E., Dombrowski, S. U., & Presseau, J. (2018). 'Just One More Episode': Frequency and Theoretical Correlates of Television Binge Watching. *J Health Psychol*, *23*(1), 17–24. https://doi.org/10.1177/1359105316643379

West, R., Michie, S., Rubin, G. J., & Amlôt, R. (2020). Applying Principles of Behaviour Change to Reduce Sars-Cov-2 Transmission. *Nat Hum Behav*, *4*(5), 451–459. https://doi.org/10.1038/s41562-020-0887-9

World Health Organization. (2022). *Global Status Report on Physical Activity 2022*. Geneva: World Health Organization.

12

A BEHAVIOURAL PERSPECTIVE ON HEALTH

Julia Allan

Introduction

Every day, people engage in behaviours that impact their health: what they eat, how much they move, what they do at work, how they spend their free time, whether they take recreational drugs, smoke tobacco, spend time with friends, engage in unprotected sex, drink alcohol, wear sunscreen, use dental floss, wear a seatbelt, get vaccinated, attend screening; the list goes on. These behaviours extend beyond the individual, impacting the behaviours and health of other people – parents give their children food to eat, teenagers encourage each other to take risks, people pick up behaviours from their friends. When illness strikes, behaviours are again key: whether people seek help for symptoms, take medication as prescribed, attend appointments, rest, stay active, change what they eat, and whether health professionals wash their hands, adhere to clinical guidelines, attend training, or go on strike. Behaviours across the health system have an impact: whether healthcare managers implement (or not) policies that protect patient safety and staff well-being, whether the grounds crew clear hospital paths on icy mornings, whether the cleaning staff disinfect surfaces regularly. Ultimately, in every moment of every day, people at every level of society engage in behaviours that impact their own health and the health of others. Put simply, behaviour matters (Fisher et al., 2011).

Behaviour plays a "*broad and central role in health*" (Fisher et al., 2011) as a determinant of health outcomes, in the prevention and management of health conditions (Matarazzo, 1982), and in the delivery and evaluation of healthcare (Mokdad et al., 2004; Belloc & Breslow, 1972; Matarazzo, 1982; Kaplan, 1990; Fisher et al., 2011). Consequently, efforts to understand and improve health can be advanced by taking a behavioural perspective. This chapter considers what it

DOI: 10.4324/9781003318026-15

means to take a behavioural perspective and outlines the advantages and limitations of this approach. It also contrasts the behavioural perspective commonly used in health psychology and behavioural medicine with complementary perspectives from other health-relevant disciplines such as medicine, epidemiology, sociology, cognitive science, and economics. Examples for illustrating the behavioural perspective in action can be found in the box at the end of this chapter.

Taking a Behavioural Perspective

Taking a behavioural perspective on health means focusing on what people do, why they do it, and how these behaviours impact processes and outcomes in the context of health, illness, and health care. In his seminal 1990 paper, Kaplan argued that "*the only important indicators of health and wellness are behavioural*", and so efforts to improve health and healthcare should focus on behavioural rather than biomedical outcomes. He contended that behavioural outcomes are more important than disease categories because people only care about having a disease if it leads their behaviour to stop (death) or changes their behaviour in ways that compromise their quality of life (Kaplan, 1990). This focus on the importance of behavioural consequences reflected a broader behavioural focus that had emerged in the 1970s and 80s from the development of health psychology and behavioural medicine as distinct academic disciplines.

Drawing on research and practice from psychological, health, and social science disciplines, health psychology and behavioural medicine advocated the application of behavioural theory and methods to the promotion and maintenance of health; to the prevention, diagnosis, and treatment of illness; and to the improvement of healthcare policies, systems, and practices (Matarazzo, 1980; Johnston, 1994; Schwartz & Weiss, 1978). This behavioural focus evolved largely in response to changes in the health challenges facing society – for example, an ageing population, a shift from infectious to chronic diseases, and a growing recognition that population-level behaviour change would be key in managing these challenges. As behaviour change is within the psychological rather than medical expertise domain (Schwarzer & Gutierrez-Dona, 2000), health psychology, and the behavioural perspective it brought, became increasingly valued and recognised (Johnson & Acabchuk, 2018). The value of a behavioural perspective is now recognised in many health-relevant policies and guidelines which explicitly prioritise behaviour change (e.g., the World Health Organisation's Behavioural Sciences for Better Health Initiative; Ghebreyesus, 2021; House of Lords Science & Technology Select Committee, 2011). Governments and healthcare providers have invested in the development and application of training and competency frameworks to upskill health professionals in the delivery of strategies to promote health behaviour change (e.g., Dixon & Johnston, 2010; Haighton et al., 2021). This shift towards wider acceptance of the behavioural perspective reflects recognition of the many advantages of this approach.

Advantages of the Behavioural Perspective

Describing, Predicting, Explaining, and Changing

As argued by Johnston (1997), a key strength of health psychology's behavioural perspective is that it enables better description, prediction, explanation, and changing of health-relevant phenomena. Describing health-relevant phenomena in behavioural terms opens new opportunities for understanding. For example, while disability was traditionally conceptualised biomedically as the outcome of physical impairment from disease or injury (WHO, 1980), reconceptualising it as a behaviour helped researchers to understand why people with equivalent levels of physical impairment might show different levels of disability and/or recover at different rates (Johnston & Dixon, 2014). By focusing on what people do differently when impaired and why, rather than on the impairment itself, researchers and practitioners can separate out difficulties related to psychological factors, such as fear of movement, and those related to physical factors, such as inability to move in a particular way. They can also use behavioural theories to differentiate between factors that predict outcomes of interest but do not explain them (e.g., demographics) and those which predict and explain them and are potentially modifiable (e.g., illness beliefs), which can then be targeted for change in an intervention.

Understanding based on a behavioural perspective allows the development of transparent and coherent interventions. In recent years, there have been huge advances in the classification of techniques that can be used to change behaviour once clear targets are identified. For example, the behaviour change techniques taxonomy defines the different techniques that can be used to change behaviour (Michie et al., 2013; Marques et al., 2023), leading to an increased ability to recognise and synthesise evidence about the 'active ingredients' of behavioural interventions. Similarly, the MAP (Motivation, Action, Prompt) mnemonic (Dixon & Johnston, 2020) describes the three primary routes to behaviour change and helps non-specialists to select appropriate behaviour change techniques for behaviours they are trying to address with interventions.

Objectivity and Quantification

Behaviour has been defined as "*those activities of an organism that can be observed by another organism or by an experimenter's instruments*" (Atkinson et al., 1987). This definition highlights two key scientific advantages of the behavioural perspective – behaviours are observable and therefore relatively objective, and they are measurable and therefore quantifiable. Consequently, the behavioural perspective moves psychology further towards the objectivity of the natural sciences, where variables can be accurately measured and findings can be reliably tested and replicated. Indeed, Watson wrote in 1913, "*[P]sychology as a behaviorist views it [is] a purely objective experimental branch of natural science*" (Watson, 1913).

To be objectively measured, behaviours must be clearly specified, as they are multi-faceted and typically more complex in nature than variables in the natural sciences. It is a common oversight, for example, to think about behaviour purely in terms of an action. As highlighted by Presseau et al. (2019), behaviours should be thought of in terms of someone (actor), somewhere (context) doing something (action). This level of additional specificity is essential when trying to identify behaviours that are problematic, that are targets for change, or that would be suitable measures for evaluation purposes. For example, if we want to accurately measure, understand, or change the behaviour 'prescribing antibiotics', it would not be sufficient to focus only on the action. Rather, we need to expand this specification to include other relevant aspects.

Fishbein and Ajzen (2010) originally proposed that behaviours be specified in terms of their target, action, context, and timing (TACT). This TACT principle has been expanded in recent years with the suggestion that behaviours be specified in terms of what, who, when, where, and how (Michie & Johnston, 2004) or action, actor, context, target, time (AACTT; Presseau et al., 2019). If we consider again the example 'prescribing antibiotics', this behaviour could be further specified as a primary care physician [actor] prescribing antibiotics [action], in the doctor's office [context], during a consultation [timing], to a patient with a sore throat [target]. Outlining a behaviour with such increased specificity enables accurate measurement and identification of a clear target for change.

Similarly, specification of behaviours may give a more objective way of assessing subjective phenomena that are otherwise difficult to quantify and compare across individuals. If we view pain through a behavioural lens, for example – rather than asking people to subjectively describe the nature and intensity of pain, we can observe and record pain behaviours, such as grimacing, and pain-related changes to functioning, such as altered gait. This focus on concrete, observable behaviours enables us to standardise the information that we are gathering across individuals in a way that is difficult or impossible with subjective reports of experiences.

Recognition of a Complicated Reality

Despite its focus on specific behaviours, the behavioural perspective does not imply a simplistic view of health. Rather, it enables the development of theories and methods which move us towards being able to describe, predict, and change behaviours that arise as the result of a complex interplay of cognitions, emotions, and external conditions and stimuli. For example, Marmot (2006) famously described the well-established gradient between socioeconomic status and health as 'status syndrome'. Viewing this through a behavioural lens makes clear that it is not social position that is problematic per se; rather, it is what social position means for what people do and can do in society. Relative to those living in affluent circumstances, people in lower socioeconomic groups are more likely, on average, to have jobs with low levels of autonomy, to work long hours, to eat cheaper foods, and to have fewer opportunities to participate in social and physical activities that are beneficial to health. This shift of perspective moves us towards a deeper understanding of why a socioeconomic health gradient might exist and to the identification of actionable targets for change.

Similarly, a behavioural focus helps to move thinking about health away from what people 'should do' (i.e., what common sense, knowledge-based, or rational models suggest should happen) and towards a more nuanced and ecologically valid mapping of what people actually do and why. As this approach focuses on behaviours rather than people, it helps to move discourse away from the unhelpful position that health is an individual responsibility. One example of this position is evidenced in the discussion around obesity. Weight, particularly in the mainstream press, is often reduced to a problem of individual responsibility, and negative characteristics are ascribed to those who struggle to achieve and maintain a 'normal' weight. By focusing on the behaviours involved in weight gain instead of the qualities or attributes of the person performing these behaviours, behaviour itself is identified as the clear target for intervention. This helps to make clear that change can occur via individual-, group-, community-, or population-level routes. Consequently, the behavioural perspective can help to promote the understanding that people are products of the environments and social structures that they live in, and that behaviours and outcomes have many determinants (Heino et al., 2021).

A Focus on Outcomes That Matter

Clinical trials and epidemiological studies typically focus on so-called hard endpoints, such as disease diagnoses or mortality rates, as the outcomes of interest. Although these outcomes are clearly important in the study of health and illness, a behavioural perspective helps us to identify outcomes that may matter more to people and to society more broadly: what will people be able to *do* as a result of a diagnosis? Will they be able to take care of their children? Walk again? Live independently? Return to work? Drive?

Viewing outcomes through a behavioural lens encourages us to think more broadly about the kinds of outcomes that matter to those affected and to identify clusters of behaviours that contribute to broader constructs that people value, such as functional independence and quality of life. Similarly, behavioural variables are often more impactful in the overall hierarchy of importance than other (e.g., knowledge-based or emotional) variables. Does it matter more if someone knows what a balanced diet is or that they eat nutritious food? Does it matter more if patients feel anxious before a procedure or if they do not attend their procedure because they are anxious? Does it matter more if doctors score 20/20 during their infection control training or that they consistently engage in appropriate hand hygiene behaviours? A behavioural perspective helps us to focus in on the outcomes with the greatest potential for benefit. In the context of healthcare, this focus on what matters aligns with the long-standing ethical imperative to deliver person and patient-centred care (Eklund et al., 2019).

Complementary and Contrasting Perspectives to the Behavioural Perspective on Health

The behavioural perspective can be viewed as complementary to, and overlapping with, many alternative perspectives but also distinct in its focus (see Figure 12.1). Some common overlapping perspectives are reviewed briefly here.

Biomedical Perspective

The most common contrast to the behavioural perspective is the traditional biomedical model. Health defined purely biomedically, is the absence of disease or impairment, although most medical models today embrace the broader biopsychosocial perspective which emphasises the interactions between biomedical, environmental, psychological, and social determinants of health (Engel, 1977). A pure biomedical perspective on health is often insufficient to maximise health and well-being (Wade & Halligan, 2004). For example, a colorectal cancer patient who has been surgically treated and is cancer-free has, according to the biomedical model, been returned to a state of health. However, if the same patient has not resumed their normal sex life (behaviour) due to self-consciousness about a stoma, avoids the foods they love (behaviour), and has stopped engaging in social activities (behaviour) due to fears about stoma leakage and toilet access, the behavioural perspective would identify that they are not yet in a state of 'health'

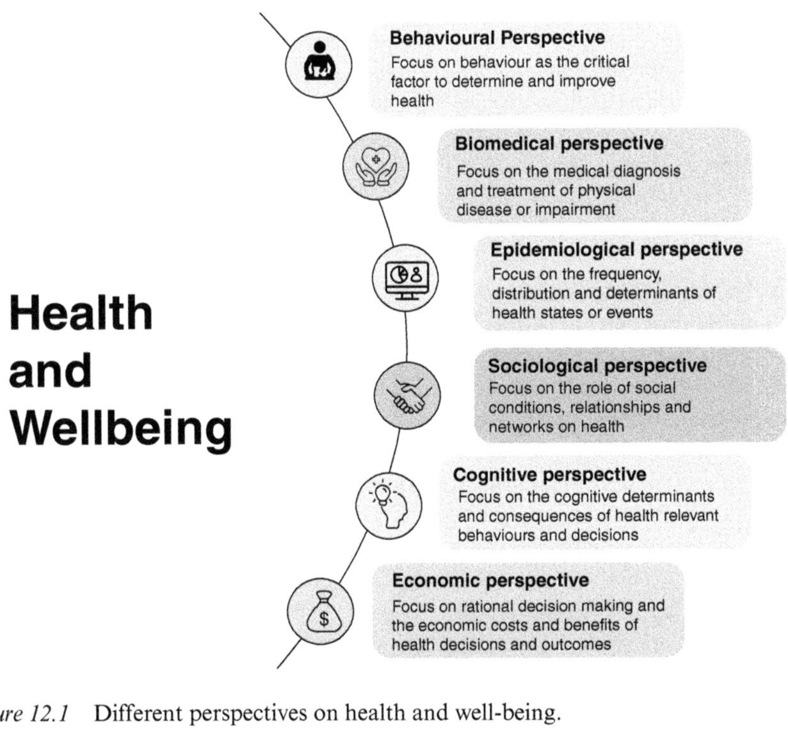

Figure 12.1 Different perspectives on health and well-being.

and would highlight behaviours that could be modified to improve outcomes. The biomedical and behavioural perspectives are typically complementary rather than contradictory: many health problems require medical treatment to resolve – for example, a badly broken ankle may need surgery – but a focus on the behavioural aspects (e.g., walking with a limp after recovery, avoiding important activities) can highlight where the medical resolution has not been enough for a full return to health.

Epidemiological Perspective

Epidemiology is the study of the distribution and determinants of health-related states or events (including disease) and the application of this study to the control of diseases and other health problems (WHO, 2017). While the epidemiological perspective is primarily focused on describing the prevalence, incidence, and distribution of disease, it is also concerned with identifying the determinants of health states and events, many of which are behavioural. Consequently, there is substantial overlap between epidemiological and behavioural perspectives. One of the classic epidemiology cases, for example, is John Snow tracing the cause of a devastating cholera outbreak in London in 1854 by meticulously mapping patterns of behaviour in people within areas with different rates of disease prevalence. This mapping exercise revealed that those who were dying of cholera had two consistently shared behaviours – they were washing in and collecting drinking water from the same Broad Street water pump. It also revealed that large groups of people living in high-prevalence areas who had not contracted cholera used private water supplies (e.g., workers in factories with their own wells). This led not only to the effective management of the outbreak in question but also to a more accurate understanding of cholera transmission as waterborne rather than airborne (Ruths, 2009).

Sociological Perspective

Medical sociology focuses on social factors in the context of health and illness, for example, studying the association between health and social relationships in areas of life such as the workplace and the family, and investigating social inequalities in health outcomes and care (Peter, 2013). Sociology more broadly is focused on social connections, conditions, and influences. Sociological approaches frequently involve an explicit focus on behaviour and can therefore often be usefully integrated into work from a predominantly behavioural perspective. For example, using interventions that capitalise on existing or newly created social networks to create or enhance change in health behaviours (Hunter et al., 2019). One example of this was the use of social identity in combination with behavioural science to leverage engagement and behaviour change in the successful Football Fans in Training intervention (Hunt et al., 2014a), an intervention which capitalised on men's social identification with football teams to support change in dietary and activity behaviours. This integration of behavioural and sociological perspectives created a holistic intervention that successfully reduced weight in participants, and critically, which attracted, retained, and was enjoyed by participants from a hard-to-reach group who were at elevated risk of future ill health (Hunt et al., 2014b). This combination of sociological and psychological perspectives is often neglected but has considerable potential for developing sustainable community-led health behaviour change (Haslam et al., 2018; Steffens et al., 2021).

Cognitive Perspective

Cognitive science is the study of how people think and process information and of specific mental processes such as attention, memory, and decision-making. When applied to the health context, the cognitive perspective is often complementary to the behavioural perspective, as it helps researchers to understand key cognitive determinants of health-relevant decisions and behaviours. For example, a cognitive perspective helps to explain the presence of bias in medical decision-making (Allan et al., 2019), the attentional processes involved in the rapid visual assessment of scan images (Evans et al., 2016), the cognitive processes needed to initiate and maintain effortful health behaviours over time (e.g., Allan et al., 2016, Caes et al., 2021), and the effects of cognitively framing health information to make different aspects more salient (Tversky & Kahneman, 1981). Understanding the cognitive processes underlying health-relevant decisions and behaviours enables the development of interventions that manipulate or capitalise on these factors to make target health behaviours cognitively easier and therefore more likely to be performed (e.g., Murchie et al., 2015; Allan & Powell, 2020).

Economic Perspective

Classical economics emphasises rationality and was originally based on utility theory where actors are seen as rational agents choosing options that maximise their utility. Laterally, this evolved into 'bounded rationality' where rationality is recognised to be limited by conditions such as people's cognitive capacity and the information or time available. Within the broad field of economics is the sub-discipline behavioural economics, which combines theories from economics and psychology to describe, explain, and change behaviour. Behavioural economics consequently overlaps with health psychology and has been popularised in recent decades through books such as *Nudge* (Thaler & Sunstein, 2008) and *Thinking Fast and Slow* (Kahneman, 2011). Economic perspectives on behavioural issues have been influential in highlighting how approaches which change the choice architecture of target environments can change the behaviour of people within those environments (e.g., the TIPPME typology of interventions in microenvironments that can influence the selection, purchase, and consumption of food, alcohol, and tobacco; Hollands et al., 2017). The economic perspective has also highlighted the importance of considering the profile of costs and benefits over time when trying to change behaviour as people typically discount future rewards in favour of more immediate gratification (e.g., Muñoz Torrecillas et al., 2021). Integration of this economic perspective into behavioural science has led to the advancement of theorising about the enactment and maintenance of health behaviours. Many health behaviours have initial costs and only longer-term benefits, but as highlighted by Hall and Fong (2007), traditional behavioural theories have typically failed to take this into account.

There are many alternative perspectives that can be usefully applied to the understanding and changing of health-related processes and outcomes. In most cases these perspectives are complementary to the behavioural perspective and can be integrated with a behavioural approach. The behavioural perspective has some unique strengths over and above other approaches, but this is not to say that it is without limitations. Indeed, a purely behavioural perspective may be viewed as a relatively reductionist approach that underestimates the impacts of sociological, cognitive, and economic factors on behaviours within the complex systems that determine behaviour. There are many examples where insights from related disciplines such as sociology, behavioural economics, and cognitive science supplement the behavioural perspective, helping us to better understand the broader determinants of behaviour and design more effective interventions.

Conclusion

The behavioural perspective offers many advantages to researchers and practitioners aiming to study and improve health. It aligns itself naturally with the health outcomes that matter most to people and to society more generally. It allows us to increase the objectivity and accuracy of our measurement and to enhance our science by facilitating efforts to describe, predict, explain, and change behaviours in the context of health.

The Behavioural Perspective in Action #1: Clinical Guideline Uptake

In 2004, Michie and Johnston applied a behavioural perspective to the problem of clinical guideline implementation. While clinical guidelines include general guidance about practice, Michie and Johnston identified that few clearly state who needs to do what and when in order to implement the guidance. As practitioners are nearly twice as likely to follow specific, precisely worded guidelines than vague, non-specific ones (Grol et al., 1998), and behaviour change is more likely to occur when a clear plan about how and when to act is provided (Gollwitzer, 1999), they advocated changes to guideline phrasing that emphasised the concrete behaviours required for implementation. For example, changing guideline phrasing from "*X should be available as a treatment option for Y in primary care*" to "*all primary care physicians should offer X to patients who present with Y*".

The Behavioural Perspective in Action #2: Infection Control

The behavioural perspective played a key role in the COVID-19 pandemic. As efforts to reduce transmission were largely reliant on the public's adherence to behaviours such as mask-wearing, handwashing, vaccination, and physical distancing, health psychologists used to working from a behavioural perspective were well placed to advise (e.g., Michie et al., 2020; West et al., 2020; Ruiz & Revenson, 2020; Baetsch et al., 2020; Bavel et al., 2020). Building on non-COVID-19 behavioural expertise in adherence, vaccination, hand hygiene, and infection control behaviours, such as condom use, health psychologists were uniquely qualified to predict likely determinants of transmission-related behaviours and to recommend appropriate strategies to support compliance. Studies were quickly established to track and test possible determinants of transmission-related behaviours (e.g., den Daas et al., 2021), with results being fed back in real time to public health teams to inform their messaging and planning. Teams of health psychologists were also instrumental in developing behaviourally informed national guidance throughout the COVID pandemic (e.g., in the UK https://www.bps.org.uk/covid-19-professionals-and-practitioners-resources).

The Behavioural Perspective in Action #3: Healthy, Sustainable Diets

König and Araújo-Soares (2022) have highlighted the need for a behavioural perspective to be taken if national targets around healthy and sustainable diets are to be achieved. While national dietary guidance to date has focused largely on communicating information about the contents of an optimal diet, König and Araújo-Soares highlight that most consumers already have sufficient dietary knowledge (Bucher et al., 2015), and dietary targets still continue to be missed. As the authors highlight, "*[I]t seems to be a doing problem rather than a knowing problem*". Consequently, they advocate for strategies that use behavioural theory to go beyond information provision to prompt and support action – both at the individual and environmental levels through the use of evidence-based behaviour change techniques and changes to the choice architecture and food system. In recent years, the behavioural perspective has started to influence national dietary guidance in this way. For example, Food Standards Scotland has recently worked with health psychologists to integrate evidence-based behaviour change content into national dietary guidance that illustrates *how* to make changes in addition to outlining the changes that should be made (https://www.eatwellyourway.scot/making-a-change/).

The Behavioural Perspective in Action #4: Self-Management of Melanoma

In melanoma (skin cancer), outcomes are heavily dependent on behaviour. The initial risk of developing melanoma is tied to behaviour, most notably to excess sun exposure, inadequate sunscreen use, and regular holidaying in sunny destinations. Treatment of melanoma is also influenced by behaviour, primarily how early a patient has a lesion checked and removed. After treatment, regular high-quality skin checking can reduce mortality from melanoma by as much as 63% (Berwick et al., 1996), but adherence to skin checking is low. Where a behavioural perspective has been applied to this problem, it has enabled adherence to a clearly specified target behaviour (conducting a 'total skin self-examination' or TSSE, once a month) to be monitored over time and determinants of suboptimal adherence identified (Allan et al., 2022). It has also facilitated the development of a behavioural intervention that supports TSSE and improves quality of life by (1) increasing TSSE motivation and self-efficacy, (2) prompting and reminding people to plan and conduct a monthly TSSE, and (3) supporting timely action if and when skin changes are detected (Murchie et al., 2015, 2022).

Further Reading

Fisher, E. B., Fitzgibbon, M. L., Glasgow, R. E., Haire-Joshu, D., Hayman, L. L., Kaplan, R. M., Nanney, M. S., & Ockene, J. K. (2011). Behavior matters. *American Journal of Preventive Medicine*, *40*(5), e15–e30.

Ghebreyesus T. A. (2021). Using behavioural science for better health. *Bulletin of the World Health Organization*, *99*(11), 755.

Johnson, B. T., & Acabchuk, R. L. (2018). What are the keys to a longer, happier life? Answers from five decades of health psychology research. *Social Science & Medicine*, *196*, 218–226.

Johnston, M. (1997). How health psychology makes a difference. *The Irish Journal of Psychology*, *18*, 4–12.

References

Allan, J. L., & Powell, D. J. (2020). Prompting consumers to make healthier food choices in hospitals: a cluster randomised controlled trial. *The International Journal of Behavioral Nutrition and Physical Activity*, *17*(1), 86.

Allan, J. L., McMinn, D., & Daly, M. (2016). A Bidirectional Relationship between Executive Function and Health Behavior: Evidence, Implications, and Future Directions. *Frontiers in Neuroscience*, *10*, 386.

Allan, J. L., Johnston, D. W., Powell, D. J. H., Farquharson, B., Jones, M. C., Leckie, G., & Johnston, M. (2019). Clinical decisions and time since rest break: An analysis of decision fatigue in nurses. *Health Psychology*, *38*(4), 318–324.

Allan, J. L., Johnston, D. W., Johnston, M., & Murchie, P. (2022). Describing, predicting and explaining adherence to total skin self-examination (TSSE) in people with melanoma: a 12-month longitudinal study. *BMJ Open*, *12*(8), e056755.

Atkinson, R. L., Atkinson, R. C., Smith, E. E., & Hilgard, E. R. (1987). *Introduction to psychology* (9th ed.). Harcourt Brace Jovanovich.

Baetsch, C., Wieler, L. H., & Habersaat, K. (2020). Monitoring behavioural insights related to COVID-19. *The Lancet*, *395*(10232), 1255–1256.

Bavel, J. J. V., Baicker, K., Boggio, P. S., Capraro, V., Cichocka, A., Cikara, M., Crockett, M. J., Crum, A. J., Douglas, K. M., Druckman, J. N., Drury, J., Dube, O., Ellemers, N., Finkel, E. J., Fowler, J. H., Gelfand, M., Han, S., Haslam, S. A., Jetten, J., … Willer, R.

(2020). Using social and behavioural science to support COVID-19 pandemic response. *Nature Human Behaviour*, *4*(5), 460–471.
Belloc, N. B., & Breslow, L. (1972). Relationship of physical health status and health practices. *Preventive Medicine*, *1*(3), 409–421.
Berwick, M., Begg, C. B., Fine, J. A., Roush, G. C., & Barnhill, R. L. (1996). Screening for cutaneous melanoma by skin self-examination. *Journal of the National Cancer Institute*, *88*(1), 17–23.
Bucher, T., Müller, B., & Siegrist, M. (2015). What is healthy food? Objective nutrient profile scores and subjective lay evaluations in comparison. *Appetite*, *95*, 408–414.
Caes, L., Dick, B., Duncan, C., & Allan, J. (2021). The cyclical relation between chronic pain, executive functioning, emotional regulation, and self-management. *Journal of Pediatric Psychology*, *46*(3), 286–292.
Den Daas, C., Hubbard, G., Johnston, M., Dixon, D., & CHARIS Consortium (2021). Protocol of the COVID-19 Health and Adherence Research in Scotland (CHARIS) study: understanding changes in adherence to transmission-reducing behaviours, mental and general health, in repeated cross-sectional representative survey of the Scottish population. *BMJ Open*, *11*(2), e044135.
Dixon, D. & Johnston, M. (2010). *The health behaviour change competency framework*. Edinburgh: Scottish Government. Available from: http://www.healthscotland.com/documents/4877.aspx
Dixon, D., & Johnston, M. (2020). MAP: A mnemonic for mapping BCTs to three routes to behaviour change. *British Journal of Health Psychology*, *25*(4), 1086–1101.
Eklund, J. H., Holmström, I. K., Kumlin, T., Kaminsky, E., Skoglund, K., Höglander, J., … & Meranius, M. S. (2019). Same same or different? A review of reviews of person-centered and patient-centered care. *Patient Education and Counseling*, *102*(1), 3–11.
Engel G. L. (1977). The need for a new medical model: a challenge for biomedicine. *Science*, *196*(4286), 129–136.
Evans, K. K., Haygood, T. M., Cooper, J., Culpan, A. M., & Wolfe, J. M. (2016). A half-second glimpse often lets radiologists identify breast cancer cases even when viewing the mammogram of the opposite breast. *Proceedings of the National Academy of Sciences of the United States of America*, *113*(37), 10292–10297.
Fishbein, M., & Ajzen, I. (2010). *Predicting and changing behavior: The reasoned action approach*. Psychology Press.
Fisher, E. B., Fitzgibbon, M. L., Glasgow, R. E., Haire-Joshu, D., Hayman, L. L., Kaplan, R. M., Nanney, M. S., & Ockene, J. K. (2011). Behavior matters. *American Journal of Preventive Medicine*, *40*(5), e15–e30.
Ghebreyesus T. A. (2021). Using behavioural science for better health. *Bulletin of the World Health Organization*, *99*(11), 755.
Gollwitzer, P. M. (1999). Implementation intentions: Strong effects of simple plans. *American Psychologist*, *54*(7), 493–503.
Grol, R., Dalhuijsen, J., Thomas, S., Veld, C., Rutten, G., & Mokkink, H. (1998). Attributes of clinical guidelines that influence use of guidelines in general practice: observational study. *BMJ*, *317*(7162), 858–861.
Haighton, C., Newbury-Birch, D., Durlik, C., Sallis, A., Chadborn, T., Porter, L., Harling, M., & Rodrigues, A. (2021). Optimizing Making Every Contact Count (MECC) interventions: A strategic behavioral analysis. *Health Psychology*, *40*(12), 960–973.
Hall, P. A. & Fong, G.T. (2007). Temporal self-regulation theory: A model for individual health behaviour. *Health Psychology Review*, *1*, 6–52.
Haslam, S. A., McMahon, C., Cruwys, T., Haslam, C., Jetten, J., & Steffens, N. K. (2018). Social cure, what social cure? The propensity to underestimate the importance of social factors for health. *Social Science & Medicine*, *198*, 14–21.
Heino, M. T., Knittle, K., Noone, C., Hasselman, F., & Hankonen, N. (2021). Studying behaviour change mechanisms under complexity. *Behavioral Sciences*, *11*(5), 77.

Hollands, G., Bignardi, G., Johnston, M., Kelly, M.P., Ogilvie, D., Petticrew, M., Prestwich, A., Shemilt, I., Sutton, S., & Marteau, T. (2017). The TIPPME intervention typology for changing environments to change behaviour. *Nature Human Behaviour*, *1*, 0140.

House of Lords Science & Technology Select Committee. (2011). *Report on behaviour change*. London: The Stationery Office.

Hunt, K., Wyke, S., Gray, C. M., Anderson, A. S., Brady, A., Bunn, C., Donnan, P. T., Fenwick, E., Grieve, E., Leishman, J., Miller, E., Mutrie, N., Rauchhaus, P., White, A., & Treweek, S. (2014a). A gender-sensitised weight loss and healthy living programme for overweight and obese men delivered by Scottish Premier League football clubs (FFIT): A pragmatic randomised controlled trial. *The Lancet*, *383*(9924), 1211–1221.

Hunt, K., Gray, C. M., Maclean, A., Smillie, S., Bunn, C., & Wyke, S. (2014b). Do weight management programmes delivered at professional football clubs attract and engage high risk men? A mixed-methods study. *BMC Public Health*, *14*, 50.

Hunter, R. F., de la Haye, K., Murray, J. M., Badham, J., Valente, T. W., Clarke, M., & Kee, F. (2019). Social network interventions for health behaviours and outcomes: A systematic review and meta-analysis. *PLoS Medicine*, *16*(9), e1002890.

Johnson, B. T., & Acabchuk, R. L. (2018). What are the keys to a longer, happier life? Answers from five decades of health psychology research. *Social Science & Medicine*, *196*, 218–226.

Johnston, M., & Dixon, D. (2014). Developing an integrated biomedical and behavioural theory of functioning and disability: adding models of behaviour to the ICF framework. *Health Psychology Review*, *8*(4), 381–403.

Johnston, M. (1997). How health psychology makes a difference. *The Irish Journal of Psychology*, *18*, 4–12.

Johnston, M (1994). Current Trends in Health Psychology. *The Psychologist*, *7*, 114–118.

Kahneman, D. (2011). *Thinking, fast and slow*. Farrar, Straus and Giroux.

Kaplan, R. M. (1990). Behavior as the central outcome in health care. *American Psychologist*, *45*, 1211–1220.

König, L.M. & Araújo-Soares, V. (2022). Will the Farm to Fork strategy be effective in changing food consumption behavior? A health psychology perspective. *Applied Economic Perspectives and Policy*, *45*(2), 785–802.

Marmot, M. (2006). Status syndrome: A challenge to medicine. *Journal of the American Medical Association*, *295*, 1304–1307.

Marques, M.M., Wright, A.J., Corker, E. et al. (2023). The Behaviour Change Technique Ontology: Transforming the Behaviour Change Technique Taxonomy v1. Wellcome Open Res 2023, 8:308. https://doi.org/10.12688/wellcomeopenres.19363.1

Matarazzo, J. D. (1980). Behavioral health and behavioral medicine: Frontiers for a new health psychology. *American Psychologist*, *35*(9), 807–817.

Matarazzo, J. D. (1982). Behavioral health's challenge to academic, scientific, and professional psychology. *American Psychologist*, *37*(1), 1–14.

Michie, S., & Johnston, M. (2004). Changing clinical behaviour by making guidelines specific. *BMJ*, *328*(7435), 343–345.

Michie, S., West, R., Rogers, M. B., Bonell, C., Rubin, G. J., & Amlôt, R. (2020). Reducing SARS-CoV-2 transmission in the UK: A behavioural science approach to identifying options for increasing adherence to social distancing and shielding vulnerable people. *British Journal of Health Psychology*, *25*(4), 945–956.

Michie, S., Richardson, M., Johnston, M., Abraham, C., Francis, J., Hardeman, W., Eccles, M. P., Cane, J., & Wood, C. E. (2013). The behavior change technique taxonomy (v1) of 93 hierarchically clustered techniques: Building an international consensus for the reporting of behavior change interventions. *Annals of Behavioral Medicine*, *46*(1), 81–95.

Muñoz Torrecillas, M. J., Cruz Rambaud, S., & Takahashi, T. (2021). Editorial: Discounting models in behavioral health economics and quantitative health psychology. *Frontiers in Public Health*, *9*, 658808.

Mokdad, A. H., Marks, J. S., Stroup, D. F., & Gerberding, J. L. (2004). Actual causes of death in the United States, 2000. *Journal of the American Medical Association, 291*(10), 1238–1245.

Murchie, P., Allan, J. L., Brant, W., Dennis, M., Hall, S., Masthoff, J., Walter, F. M., & Johnston, M. (2015). Total skin self-examination at home for people treated for cutaneous melanoma: Development and pilot of a digital intervention. *BMJ Open, 5*(8), e007993.

Murchie, P., Constable, L., Hall, S., Brant, W., Allan, J., Johnston, M., Masthoff, J., Lee, A., Treweek, S., Ayansina, D., Proby, C., Rahman, K., Walter, F., Burrows, N., Durrani, A., & Maclennan, G. (2022). The achieving self-directed integrated cancer aftercare intervention for detection of recurrent and second primary melanoma in survivors of melanoma: Pilot randomized controlled trial. *Journal of Medical Internet Research: Cancer, 8*(3), e37539.

Peter, R. (2013). Medical Sociology. In: Gellman, M.D., Turner, J.R. (eds) *Encyclopedia of Behavioral Medicine*. Springer, New York, NY.

Presseau, J., McCleary, N., Lorencatto, F., Patey, A. M., Grimshaw, J. M., & Francis, J. J. (2019). Action, actor, context, target, time (AACTT): A framework for specifying behaviour. *Implementation Science, 14*(1), 102.

Ruiz, J. M., & Revenson, T. A. (2020). Behavioral medicine in the COVID-19 era: Dawn of the golden age. *Annals of Behavioral Medicine, 54*(8), 541–543.

Ruths M. B. (2009). The lesson of john snow and the broad street pump. *The Virtual Mentor, 11*(6), 470–472.

Schwartz, G. E., & Weiss, S. M. (1978). Behavioral medicine revisited: An amended definition. *Journal of Behavioral Medicine, 1*(3), 249–251.

Schwarzer, R. & Gutierrez-Dona, B. (2000). Health psychology. In K. Pawlik & M.R. Rosenweig (Eds.), *The international handbook of psychology*. London: Sage.

Steffens, N. K., LaRue, C. J., Haslam, C., Walter, Z. C., Cruwys, T., Munt, K. A., … Tarrant, M. (2021). Social identification-building interventions to improve health: A systematic review and meta-analysis. *Health Psychology Review, 15*(1), 85–112.

Thaler, R. H., & Sunstein, C. R. (2008). *Nudge: Improving decisions about health, wealth, and happiness*. Yale University Press.

Tversky, A. and Kahneman, D. (1981) The framing of decisions and the psychology of choice. *Science, 211*, 453–458.

Wade, D. T., & Halligan, P. W. (2004). Do biomedical models of illness make for good healthcare systems? *BMJ, 329*(7479), 1398–1401.

Watson, J. B. (1913). Psychology as the behaviorist views it. *Psychological Review, 20*(2), 158–177.

West, R., Michie, S., Rubin, G. J., & Amlôt, R. (2020). Applying principles of behaviour change to reduce SARS-CoV-2 transmission. *Nature Human Behaviour, 4*(5), 451–459

World Health Organisation. (1980). *International classification of impairments, disabilities and handicaps*. WHO: Geneva.

World Health Organization. (2017). *Epidemiology*. Available: http://www.who.int/topics/epidemiology/en/

13

UNDERSTANDING MULTIPLE HEALTH BEHAVIOURS

Lena Fleig, Theda Radtke, and Stephan U. Dombrowski

Introduction

Human life consists of a continuous flow of action. Every day, people engage in multiple behaviours, most of which are performed repeatedly over time. What people do serves a function fulfilling inherent needs and has consequences for the physical and social environment and the individual themselves. Several behaviours individuals routinely perform increase the likelihood of health enhancing or impairing outcomes. Behaviours such as being physically active, eating a balanced diet, refraining from smoking, or digital technology use jointly affect health.

Behaviours are interconnected and co-occur as behavioural clusters, at the individual, group, and social levels. These behavioural clusters can be conceptualised at the behavioural category level (e.g., consuming foods high in fat, sugar, and sodium) or across behavioural categories (e.g., smoking behaviour often co-occurs with physical inactivity). To improve health and well-being, it is critical to understand interconnections between behaviours and the groups and circumstances when these relations apply to support interventions successful at changing more than one behaviour.

Multiple health behaviour change (MHBC) interventions have been defined "*as efforts to promote two or more health behaviours*" (p. 183, Prochaska et al., 2008), with health behaviours defined as "*actions in which individuals engage that influence health … [which] can be negative, as with tobacco […]and risky sexual behaviors, or positive, as with physical activity, fruit and vegetable consumption, and the wearing of helmets[…]*" (p. 183, Prochaska et al., 2008). The 'multiple' aspect of MHBC interventions is – as in this definition typically focused on (interventions that target behaviours from) different behavioural categories (e.g., physical activity (PA) is one behaviour and smoking is another behaviour). The

DOI: 10.4324/9781003318026-16

label 'multiple', however, also applies to interventions that target different actions within a behavioural category which is inherent in every behavioural intervention (e.g., a PA intervention might target going for a walk, using the stairs at work, and engaging in a workout). In addition, the previous definition does not explain behaviour change or avoidance behaviours (not doing something). An amended definition might be: MHBC interventions are "*efforts to change health behaviours from two or more behavioural categories, including performing or increasing future actions or refraining from or decreasing past actions with the aim to maximise behavioural and behaviour-related outcomes*".

Multiple behaviour change typically focuses on behaviours which require repeated performance over time to impact health. The temporal aspect of multiple behaviour change is critical, as individuals usually perform behaviours sequentially (one after the other) and not simultaneously (at the same time). For example, when going for a walk, it is unlikely that one could simultaneously cook a meal. The behaviours that individuals engage in over the course of a day, week, or month compete for resources such as time and self-control. However, engaging in more than one behaviour can create synergies for individual health. Compared to perspectives focusing on changing single behaviours, a multiple behaviour change perspective requires an understanding of change processes for a single behaviour alongside considerations of processes that occur between different behaviours and behavioural categories.

Approaches to Studying Multiple Health Behaviours

Noar et al. (2008) suggest three general approaches to applying behavioural theory to understanding multiple behaviours and multiple behaviour change. Each of the three approaches is outlined briefly alongside a fourth novel approach. Figures 13.1a–d present the approaches visually, and Table 13.1 summarises and contrasts the core features of all approaches, including implications for interventions.

Behaviour Change Principles Approach

The behaviour change principles approach focuses on a common underlying set of key principles to explain behaviour and behaviour change across different categories (see Figure 13.1, panel a). These key principles transcend health behaviours and form the intervention targets for behaviour change.

In line with this approach, Webb and Sheeran (2006) conducted a systematic review examining the common theoretical proposition that intentions lead to behaviour (Webb & Sheeran, 2006), as proposed through social cognition models, such as the theory of planned behaviour. A medium-to-large change in intention ($d = 0.66$) was found to lead to a small-to-medium change in behaviour ($d = 0.36$). In line with the assumption that the influence of intentions on behaviour is a key principle underlying all behaviours, effect size estimates were based on studies targeting a wide range of different behaviours (e.g., sunscreen use, testicular self-examination).

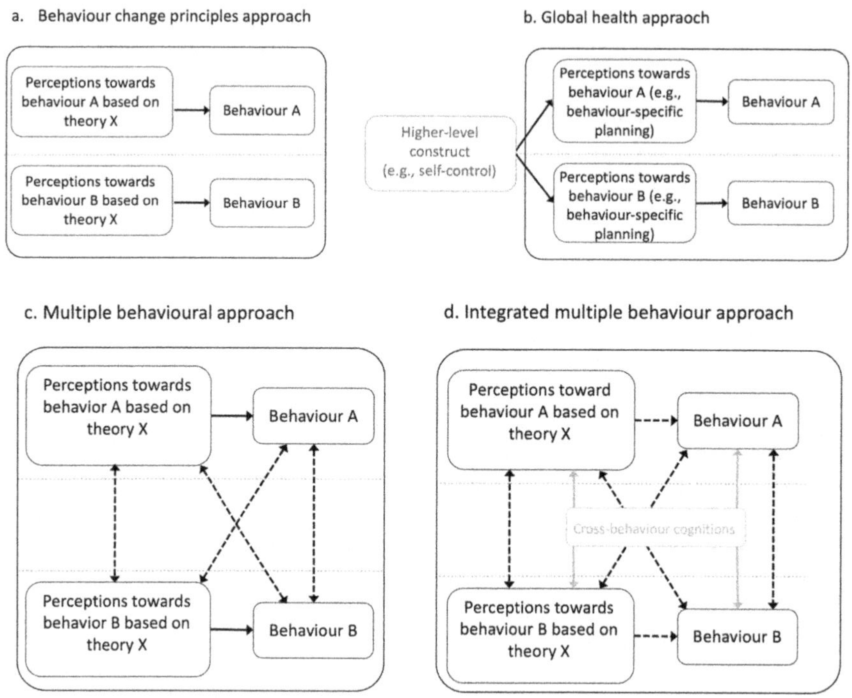

Figure 13.1 Overview of approaches to studying multiple health behaviours, including (a) the behaviour change principles approach, (b) the global health approach, (c) the multiple behavioural approach, and (d) the integrated multiple behaviour approach.

In a meta-analysis, Zhang et al. (2019) examined behavioural categories as moderators of the relationships between variables of the health action process approach (HAPA). The analysis found stronger effects of action self-efficacy on intentions in PA studies, whereas effects of volitional self-efficacy on behaviour were higher for dietary behaviours. These findings suggest that variables based on the same theory may show different predictive patterns for different behaviours. In addition to focusing on the commonalities among behaviours, research in multiple behaviour contexts, should therefore, also consider unique behavioural features.

Global Health Approach

The global health approach focuses on high-level constructs which are assumed to underly performing multiple behaviours (see Figure 13.1, panel b). Broad constructs such as a general health orientation are assumed to be related to several health behaviours and behaviour-specific perceptions.

An example of a general health orientation cognition is health locus of control; the general belief that health is in one's control (internal control) or is not in one's control (external control). Evidence suggests that an internal health locus of control is predictive of the performance of multiple health behaviours (Norman et al., 1998). Similarly, Hankonen et al. (2014) provided an example of how to examine the assumed top-down-processes of this approach. In a mediation model, a link between trait self-control and fruit and vegetable consumption, as well as fast-food consumption, was found to be mediated by behaviour-specific cognitions (e.g., intentions). Besides trait self-control (De Ridder et al., 2012; Hagger et al., 2019), other high-level constructs have been proposed to explain aspects of multiple health behaviours at a general level, including executive function, health goals (e.g., weight reduction; Noar et al., 2008), general self-efficacy (Schutte & Malouff, 2016), self-determination (Mata et al., 2009), and a time perspective (Zimbardo & Boyd, 1999).

Multiple Behavioural Approach

The multiple behavioural approach focuses on the associations between different health behavioural constructs (see Figure 13.1, panel c) and how individuals might change multiple behaviours.

To explore the nature of the association between multiple behaviours one can examine (a) how different health behaviours and relevant predictors are interrelated (e.g., by means of correlational analyses or structural equation modelling), aim to (b) examine whether and how health behaviours group (e.g., by means of factor analyses; Hofstetter et al., 2014), or aim to (c) identify groups of individuals (rather than behaviours) sharing the same behavioural patterns (by means of cluster analyses).

Instead of merely observing within-behaviour correlations (i.e., modelling predictors only for the target behaviour as seen in the common principles approach), the multiple behaviour approach adds a cross-behaviour perspective (see Figure 13.1, panel d). For example, based on the HAPA, Fleig et al. (2015) investigated cross-behaviour associations between fruit and vegetable intake (FVI) and PA, reporting a small and positive association between behaviours (i.e., at the behavioural level) and positive associations of moderate size between PA self-efficacy and FVI self-efficacy (i.e., at the perceptual level). Cross-behaviour associations between PA-related cognitions with FVI were small but higher than the association between FVI-related cognitions and PA. However, results were only of correlational nature. Based on the reasoned action approach, Aulbach et al. (2023) examined within- and cross-behaviour associations between PA and screen time (Aulbach et al., 2023). Structural equation modelling showed assumed within-behaviour predictions, however, no strong associations between the cognitions specific to PA and screen time could be observed. Only intending to engage in PA was weakly related to reduced screen time.

Previous research following the multiple behavioural approach has often examined one health behaviour in relation to another. When three or more health behaviours are under study, one may also examine whether particular behaviours group due to a common underlying factor (Hofstetter et al., 2014). For example, using factor analysis, Lippke et al. (2012) found that nutrition and PA loaded on one factor ('health behaviours'), whereas smoking and alcohol consumption loaded on another ('avoidance behaviours').

To examine the nature of multiple health behaviours, cluster analysis can be used as an exploratory grouping technique to identify homogeneous subgroups of individuals sharing the same behavioural patterns. For example, Nudelman and Yakubovich (2022) found three clusters of engagement in health behaviours which were termed "healthy", "unhealthy", and "mixed". It was observed that young, non and less-educated individuals were more likely to belong to the "unhealthy" cluster.

Each of the three aforementioned analytical approaches has implications for interventions. MHBC interventions can either target particular groups of individuals (i.e., clusters) showing the same behavioural pattern or target possible groups of interrelated behaviours from the same or different behavioural categories. If health behaviours are interrelated and share the same underlying 'source', intervening on one health behaviour may be associated with changes in related health behaviours. For example, if an intervention succeeds, in changing PA, changes in associated behaviours, such as, FVI or smoking, may also occur (e.g., Run to Quit, see Box 13.1).

Box 13.1 Approaches to Studying Multiple Health Behaviours in Practice – The Example of the 'Run to Quit' Intervention

Run to Quit is a multiple behaviour change intervention targeting smoking cessation through group-based running clinics. The 10-week intervention consisted of a smoking cessation component focused on smoking-related topics and strategies, as well as a running component in the form of a progressive learn-to-run programme that incrementally built up to 5 km event over the 10 weeks. The intervention showed promising findings in relation to smoking cessation and PA change (Priebe et al., 2017).

Run to Quit was developed based on the principles of global and multiple behaviour change approaches. For example, the intervention delivery in a group setting was hypothesised as motivating for initiating and maintaining change for both behaviours in line with the principles approach. The intervention also drew on identity theory, attempting to change smoker and runner identities and potentially inducing an identity shift in line with the global approach. Moreover, in line with the multiple behaviour approach, the study noted the incongruency between smoking and PA, drawing on evidence outlining that PA is inversely related to smoking behaviour.

The Run to Quit intervention illustrates that in practice, interventions can draw on several approaches to understanding and changing multiple health behaviours. The integrated multiple behaviour approach outlined in this chapter was not explicitly drawn on in this intervention, demonstrating room for improvement in terms of applying and understanding cross-behaviour cognitions and processes.

Other critical questions refers to how individuals change multiple behaviours and how to best implement interventions targeting more than one health behaviour (e.g., which behaviours should be targeted? How many behaviours should be targeted? In which sequence?). For example, Vandelanotte et al. (2008) evaluated whether there were differences in behaviour change (changes in no, one, or two behaviours) depending on whether individuals were encouraged to change two behaviours (i.e., PA and fat intake) concurrently (i.e., through simultaneous intervention) or through receiving one intervention at a time with several weeks apart (i.e., through sequential intervention). Results indicated that both interventions were equally effective in changing PA and fat intake. A review by Maisano et al. (2020) compared simultaneous and sequential interventions targeting two weight-related behaviours and found no consistent evidence in support of either delivery format. In addition to observational studies (i.e., studying interrelations, common underlying factors, and/or clusters), future experimental studies comparing the efficacy of different sequencing of intervention components (e.g., by examining both stable differences between persons and fluctuations within persons over time) will help advance multiple health behaviour theory and practice.

Summing up, the three approaches to applying theory to multiple behaviour change proposed by Noar et al. (2008) provide cross-cutting (principles approach), overarching (global approach), and immersive (multiple approach) explanations to understand this phenomenon. The *principles approach* is single behaviour focused in nature and examines the application of hypothesised principles to several single behaviours, thereby providing explanations for multiple single behaviours. The *global approach* offers high-level and broad theorising, which are relevant background factors but might be less informative for explaining multiple behaviours and for intervening on behaviour change in specific contexts. The *multiple behavioural approach* is focused on multiple behaviours and their interrelations. However, all approaches lack an explanatory value as to why health behaviours are interrelated and why individuals engage or do not engage in more than one behaviour. Table 13.1 contains an outline of an extended approach – the integrated multiple behaviour approach.

Integrated Multiple Behaviour Approach

The integrated multiple behaviour perspective focuses on perceptions of relationships between different behaviours. These behavioral relationships include perceived associations of variables such as multiple intentions, plans, and behaviours (Fleig et al., 2014; Sniehotta et al., 2016), termed cross-behaviour cognitions (see Figure 13.1, panel d). Rhodes and Blanchard (2008) originally used the term 'cross-behaviour cognitions' to describe potentially competing perceptions relating to a behaviour, which might challenge the implementation of the target behaviour. Intentions to engage in a behaviour other than being physically active (e.g., I intend to watch a television show) would be, according to Rhodes and Blanchard (2008), referred to as cross-behaviour cognitions. However, in this chapter, the term 'cross-behaviour

Table 13.1 Overview of core features of approaches to studying multiple health behaviours

	1. Behaviour Change Principles Approach	*2. Global Health Approach*	*3. Multiple Behavioural Approach*	*4. Integrated Multiple Behaviour Approach*
Key assumption	To explain and change multiple health behaviours, the same single behaviour theory can be used across health behaviours from different behavioural categories (see Figure 13.1, panel a)	To explain and change multiple health behaviours requires identification of higher-level constructs that operate across behaviours from different categories (see Figure 13.1, panel b)	To explain and change multiple health behaviours requires the study of health behaviours and their predictors in the context of one another by considering dynamics regarding the behavioural and perceptual level across behaviours (see Figure 13.1, panel c)	To explain and change multiple health behaviours requires the study of health behaviours and their predictors in the context of one another by considering dynamics at the behavioural and perceptual level across behaviours as well as cross-behaviour cognitions (see Figure 13.1, panel d)

Research questions	Can the same behaviour change principles (e.g., theory-based predictors, behaviour change techniques) be applied to explain or to change health behaviours from different behavioural categories?	Can higher-level, behaviour-unspecific constructs explain changes in different lower-level health behaviours and their predictors?	To what extent are health behaviours and behaviour-specific predictors related to one another? Which health behaviours cluster? How do individuals change multiple health behaviours?	To what extent are health behaviours and behaviour-specific predictors related to one another? Do cross-behaviour cognitions add to the prediction of behaviour beyond behaviour-specific predictors? How do individuals change multiple health behaviours? How can interventions create synergies among change processes? How can cross-behaviour cognitions be targeted in interventions?
Implications for interventions	Foster non-domain specific skills (e.g., how to set goals) and apply these across different behaviours. In addition or as an alternative, to address health behaviours in separate, behaviour-specific intervention components (e.g., planning for PA and planning for FVI)	Target higher-level constructs (e.g., general self-efficacy or higher-level health goals) and not a specific health behaviour. Higher-level construct leads to positive changes in lower-level, behaviour-specific perceptions and specific behaviours	Target health behaviours that hold similarities to one another (those that are positively interrelated on a behavioural and/or perceptual level) Based on interrelations among target behaviours, a rationale for a sequential or simultaneous intervention approach needs to be developed	Target health behaviours that hold similarities to one another and to aim to support synergies among change processes of two or more health behaviours (in addition to supporting behaviour-specific processes) by a supporting transfer (of skills, resources), goal facilitation, and concurrent self-efficacy, and b reducing goal conflict and compensatory health beliefs

(*Continued*)

Table 13.1 (Continued)

<table>
<tr><th></th><th>1. Behaviour Change Principles Approach</th><th>2. Global Health Approach</th><th>3. Multiple Behavioural Approach</th><th>4. Integrated Multiple Behaviour Approach</th></tr>
<tr><td>Advantages</td><td>Efficient intervention design and theory use: one-principle-fits-all-behaviour approach</td><td>Efficient intervention design and theory use: one-global construct-fits-all-behaviour approach</td><td>Addition of a cross-behavioural perspective: consideration of dynamics across behaviours and behaviour-specific perceptions</td><td>Consideration of cross-behaviour cognitions
Efficient intervention design: to build upon positive interrelations between change processes to accelerate MHBC, and to create synergies between behaviour-specific interventions</td></tr>
<tr><td rowspan="2">Limitations</td><td colspan="3">Lacks accounts on why health behaviours are related to one another
Potential psychosocial mechanisms of change are not considered (i.e., perceptions towards how and why health behaviours are related to one another, termed cross-behaviour cognitions)</td><td rowspan="2">This approach overcomes most of the limitations of the other three approaches, but is more complex to implement and has a limited theoretical foundation and is often not the intervention choice due to the novelty of the approach</td></tr>
<tr><td>Neglects potential unique features of health behaviours</td><td>Associations between global higher-level constructs and behavioural outcomes are typically small
Fails to provide an account for lower-level processes of behaviour and behaviour change</td><td></td></tr>
</table>

Source: Adapted from Noar et al. (2008).

cognitions' refers to cognitions that explicitly describe a relational perception between behaviours, in line with Sniehotta et al. (2016) and Fleig et al. (2014). Fleig et al. (2014), for example, found initial evidence to support the hypothesis that transfer cognitions provide a psychological explanation for the positive link between physical exercise and FVI. Other cross-behaviour cognitions are summarised in Table 13.1.

From Single to Multiple Behaviour Theory

The dynamics of behaviour-specific perceptions are outlined in detail by single behaviour theories, such as the theory of planned behaviour and the HAPA. These theories can inform the design of single health behaviour interventions. However, adding a cross-behaviour perspective to the within-behaviour perspective can extend the models' applicability to understanding, predicting, and changing multiple behaviours (Fleig et al., 2015). In health psychology, at least two comprehensive theories aligned with the integrated multiple behaviour approach exist: the Compensatory Health Belief Model (CHBM) and the Compensatory Carry-Over Action Model (CCAM). Both theories include several different cross-behaviour cognitions (see Table 13.2).

Compensatory Health Belief Model

The CHBM seeks to explain how individuals resolve a motivational conflict between the gratification of immediate desires and achieving personal long-term health. For example, an individual may be tempted to eat a calorie-rich, sugary dessert while simultaneously striving to follow a nutritious diet. As a result, the individual finds themselves in a state of cognitive dissonance that requires the use of self-regulatory processes to resolve the conflict.

The CHBM suggests three primary strategies to reduce conflict and cognitive dissonance:

1. ***Resisting the temptation***: Involves resisting the desire to engage in health-compromising behaviour and instead focusing on self-control and willpower to adhere to health goals related to health-enhancing alternative behaviour.
2. ***Adjustment of goal importance***: Adapts perceived risk in relation to the tempting, desirable, and health-compromising behaviour and/or re-evaluates outcome expectancies about that behaviour (e.g., it is not harmful to eat fries today). Adjusting these cognitions can temporarily ease motivational conflict by reducing the significance of the goal for health-enhancing behaviour.
3. ***Justification through cross-behaviour cognitions***: Activates compensatory health beliefs (CHBs), which are defined as cognitive beliefs that the negative effects of a volitional health compromising immediately gratifying behaviour can be compensated for or neutralised by engaging in a volitionally, health-enhancing behaviour. This cognition allows individuals rationalise compromising behaviour by perceiving a balance between health-enhancing and compromising behaviours.

Table 13.2 Overview of important cross-behaviour cognitions in facilitating or compromising MHBC

Cross-Behaviour Cognitions Facilitating MHBC	*Definition*	*Author*	*Assessment*	*Example*	*Theory*
Goal facilitation	*"Intergoal facilitation occurs when the pursuit of one goal simultaneously increases the likelihood of success in reaching another goal" (p. 1511).*	(Riediger & Freund, 2004)	Intergoal Relations Questionnaire (Riediger, 2001)	*How often can it happen that you do something in the pursuit of Goal A that is simultaneously beneficial for Goal B?*	Model of Emotional Goal System
Concurrent self-regulatory efficacy	*"Confidence in one's ability to self-regulate the management of multiple goals" (p. 601).*	(Jung & Brawley, 2013)	Concurrent Self-Regulatory Efficacy Scale (Jung & Brawley, 2013)	*During the next week, how confident are you in your ability to accurately monitor your time so that your progress for both your exercise and your academic activity is effective?*	Social Cognitive Theory

Transfer cognitions	*"Cognitions that the engagement in one behaviour domain supports an increase in behaviour in a different domain by activating self-regulatory strategies (e.g. planning and goal setting)" (p. 1363).*	(Fleig et al., 2014)	Transfer Cognitions Scale (Fleig et al., 2014)	*When I exercise regularly, it is easier for me to make plans for my healthy nutrition.*	Transfer
Carry-over mechanisms (COM)	*"One can measure COM as a mechanism carrying over resources from one domain to another, or in terms of one behaviour serving as a gateway for another" (p. 3).*	(Lippke et al., 2012)	Transfer Cognitions Scale (Fleig et al., 2014)	*If I stick to a balanced diet on a regular basis, it also becomes easier for me to be physically more active.*	CCAM
Higher-level goals/life goals	*"Higher-level goals or so-called life goals are assumed to drive the different single behaviors" (p. 3).*	(Lippke et al., 2012)	Personal Goals (Riediger & Freund, 2004)	*Currently, my main goal in life is changing my weight.*	CCAM, Motivational Theory of Lifespan Development

(Continued)

Table 13.2 (Continued)

Cross-Behaviour Cognitions Facilitating MHBC	*Definition*	*Author*	*Assessment*	*Example*	*Theory*
Compensatory cognitions	*"Compensatory cognitions emerge if individuals perceive a discrepancy between their intentions [...] and their actual behaviour performance [...] CCs can function as intentions, post-hoc explanations or subjective beliefs" (p. 2).*	(Lippke et al., 2012)	General Compensatory Health Beliefs Scale (Knäuper et al., 2004)	*I can eat this piece of cake now because I will exercise this evening.*	CCAM Compensatory Health Belief Model
Compensatory health beliefs	*"Compensatory Health Beliefs (CHBs) are beliefs that the negative effects of an unhealthy behaviour can be compensated for, or 'neutralised,' by engaging in a healthy behaviour" (p. 607).*	(Knäuper et al., 2004)			

Goal conflict/ Goal interference	*"Intergoal interference occurs when the pursuit of one goal impairs the likelihood of success in reaching another goal" (p. 1511).*	(Riediger & Freund, 2004)	Intergoal Relations Questionnaire (Riediger, 2001)	*How often can it happen that you do something in the pursuit of Goal A that is incompatible with Goal B?*	Model of Emotional Goal System
Irrational health beliefs	*"Tendency to appraise health-related situations or experiences in a biased or distorted manner" (p. 170).*	(Christensen et al., 1999)	Irrational Health Belief Scale (Christensen et al., 1999)	*During your last checkup, your cholesterol level was high, and your doctor recommended that you reduce the fat in your diet.* *Today at lunch, you notice that all of your coworkers were eating hamburgers and french fries. You think, "If everybody eats like this, it can't be that bad for you." How similar are these thoughts to how you would think in that situation?*	Health Belief Model; Cognitive Theory of Depression (Beck, 2002)

Source: Adapted from McLellan (2020).

Rabiau et al. (2006) argue that strategies 1 and 2 demand effort and self-control while CHBs are an automatically motivated regulatory process reducing cognitive dissonance by justifying health-compromising behaviour with planned health-enhancing behaviour. CHBs can be activated before or after the health-compromising behaviour has been carried out. Overall, the strategy of CHBs to solve the conflict is hypothesised to be the least resource intensive method, as CHBs permit the performance of the desired behaviour and do not interfere with one's own goals.

The CHB model primarily focuses on explaining CHB formation, with limited exploration of their relationship with intention formation and multiple behavioural change (Radtke et al., 2012). The CCAM expands on this, suggesting that CHBs are crucial in the motivational phase for intention formation. Although this assumption is supported by other research, the role of CHBs in the motivational and volitional phase of behaviour change remains uncertain (Radtke et al., 2012), partly due to the ambiguity regarding whether CHBs are adaptive or maladaptive in health behaviour contexts.

Compensatory Health Beliefs – Beneficial or Detrimental to Health?

CHBs resolve cognitive dissonance, but their impact on health remains uncertain, as CHBs may be correct, partly correct, or incorrect (Rabiau et al., 2006). Categorising them is complex, as compromising behaviours often lead to multiple negative health effects, while compensatory behaviours usually address only one singular consequence, and simultaneously, uncertainties in executing intended compensatory behaviours exist (Knäuper et al., 2004). This phenomenon is due to the potential time gap between CHB activation and executing the intended compensatory behaviour. Consequently, cognitive dissonance experienced and the perceived need to compensate for compromising behaviour may decrease over time. Thus, CHBs can impede intention formation and the successful adherence to various health behaviour changes as illustrated as follows: individuals of different ages holding stronger CHBs seem to drink more alcohol (Matley & Davies, 2018), have a lower intention to stop smoking and consume cigarettes more often (Radtke et al., 2012), have a lower intention to eat a balanced diet and a higher snack consumption (Fleig et al., 2014), engage in internet gratification behaviour more often (Yin & Shen, 2023), or use the mobile phone while driving (Zhou et al., 2016).

Overall, CHBs are a cognitive strategy ('beliefs') to lower cognitive dissonance and have mainly been considered as a trait (Radtke et al., 2014). However, according to the CHBM, CHBs are activated in the moment of temptation and thus function as situational justification in daily life (Amrein et al., 2021). Thus, CHBs as a type of cross-behaviour cognition differ from compensatory behaviour (Radtke & Scholz, 2016), as the implementation of CHBs into behaviour may not occur, particularly when individuals use these in-the-moment rationalisations to justify their behaviour.

Compensatory Carry-Over Action Model

The CCAM outlines the dynamics between different behaviours alongside specifying within-behaviour processes. The CCAM builds upon the basic assumptions of the CHBM and HAPA and combines these with other theoretical approaches. Figure 13.2 illustrates the core features of this model. In line with the global health approach, the CCAM integrates higher-level goals (see Table 13.2), which drive more than one behaviour.

At the within-behaviour level, the CCAM predicts that behaviour change starts with forming an intention (e.g., "I intend to go for a walk more often"). This intention has to be translated into plans (e.g., "I have already planned when and where I will go for a walk"). If individuals link their goal behaviour with specific contextual cues (e.g., time, place), behaviour can be initiated with a higher degree of automaticity. Besides planning, self-efficacy (e.g., "I am confident that I will be able to go for a walk, although I feel tempted to stay at home with my partner") is another important factor that determines behaviour.

At the cross-behaviour level, the CCAM models are compensatory, as well as COM. COM refer to resources and strategies that can be carried from one health behaviour to another, or that one behaviour can initiate another. An example of a carry-over mechanism is transfer (Barnett & Ceci, 2002). Initial efforts to empirically support transfer as a mechanism of regulating more than one health behaviour stem from cross-sectional findings. Lippke et al. (2012), for example, interpreted the clustering of PA and FVI as an indicator of the potential transfer of self-regulatory strategies. Alternatively, individuals' perceptions that the

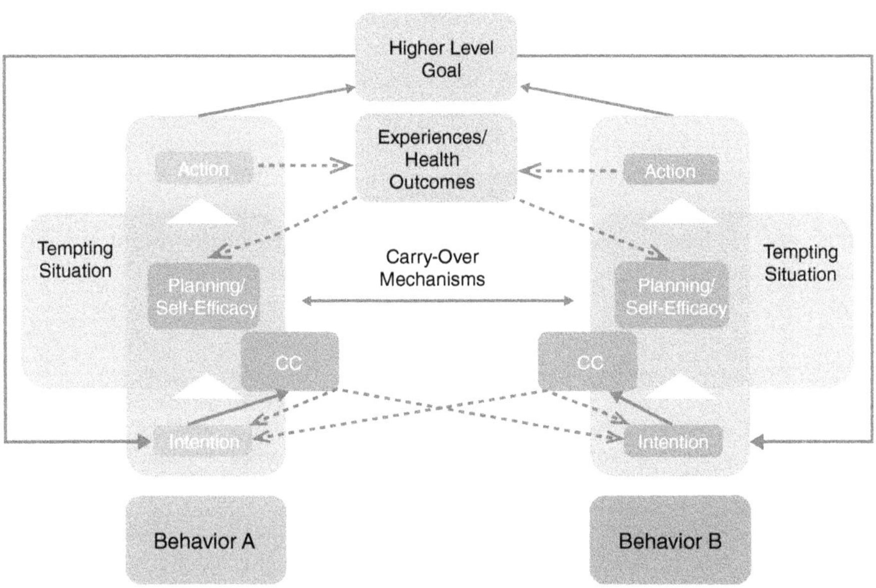

Figure 13.2 The CCAM (adapted from Lippke 2014b). CC = compensatory cognitions.

engagement in one behaviour supports an increase in a different behaviour through activating self-regulatory strategies can be explicitly measured (Fleig et al., 2014). As an extension of the CCAM, Fleig et al. (2014) studied COM in the context of habit formation, as the level of automaticity of one behaviour can have implications for the availability of resources and strategy use. The authors showed that high levels of habit strength in one behaviour facilitate the use of transfer and thereby potential changes in another behaviour. Whereas compensatory mechanisms (i.e., CHBs) are assumed to play a central role in intention formation, COM are assumed to facilitate the use of behaviour-specific resources and strategies of self-regulation in the volitional phase (Fleig et al., 2015).

Although the theoretical advances in understanding multiple behaviour change processes are rich and varied (see Table 13.2), future research is required to test and refine theoretical hypotheses and translate the increase in understanding into effective and scalable interventions that help individuals address the multiple behaviours that impact their health.

Conclusion

Health and well-being are determined by engaging in multiple behaviours. Recent advances in understanding multiple behaviours have evolved from focusing on universal and high-level explanations of single behaviour theories to nuanced, detailed, and reflective accounts of change processes across behaviours alongside accompanying cognitive and emotive dimensions. Future research should examine whether it is more promising to intervene in health behaviours separately (either simultaneously or sequentially), to prioritise supporting the creation of synergies among change processes (e.g., by reducing goal conflict), or to find a combination of both approaches. In addition, future research might uncover when a change in multiple behaviour is most likely to occur, as individuals might be more amenable to restructuring behavioural routines in certain life phases and following specific life events. Further theoretical and empirical perspectives are needed to advance emerging innovative accounts of multiple behaviour change processes such as the CCAM. Lastly, to improve population health, theory and evidence-based interventions are required to ensure recent advances in understanding multiple behaviour benefit society more widely.

Further Reading

Fleig, L., Ngo, J., Roman, B., Ntzami, E., Satta, P., Warner, L. M., Schwarzer, R., & Brandi, M. L. (2015). Beyond single behaviour theory: Adding cross-behaviour cognitions to the health action process approach. *British Journal of Health Psychology*, *20*(4), 824–841. https://doi.org/10.1111/bjhp.12144

Lippke, S. (2014a). Modelling and supporting complex behavior change related to obesity and diabetes prevention and management with the compensatory carry-over action model. *Journal of Diabetes and Obesity*, *1*(2), 39–43. https://doi.org/10.15436/2376-0494.14.009

Noar, S. M., Chabot, M., & Zimmerman, R. S. (2008). Applying health behavior theory to multiple behavior change: Considerations and approaches. *Preventive Medicine*, *46*(3), 275–280. https://doi.org/10.1016/j.ypmed.2007.08.001

Rabiau, M., Knäuper, B. & Miquelon, P. (2006). The eternal quest for optimal balance between maximizing pleasure and minimizing harm: The compensatory health beliefs model. *British Journal of Health Psychology*, *11*, 139–153. https://doi.org/10.1348/135910705X52237

Radtke, T., Scholz, U., Keller, R., & Hornung, R. (2012). Smoking is ok as long as I eat healthily: Compensatory Health Beliefs and their role for intentions and smoking within the Health Action Process Approach. *Psychology & Health*, *27*(sup2), 91–107.

References

Amrein, M. A., Scholz, U., & Inauen, J. (2021). Compensatory health beliefs and unhealthy snack consumption in daily life. *Appetite*, *157*, 104996. https://doi.org/10.1016/j.appet.2020.104996

Aulbach, M. B., Konttinen, H., Gardner, B., Kujala, E., Araujo-Soares, V., Sniehotta, F. F., Lintunen, T., Haukkala, A., & Hankonen, N. (2023). A dual process model to predict adolescents' screen time and physical activity. *Psychology & Health*, 1–20. https://doi.org/10.1080/08870446.2021.1988598

Barnett, S. M., & Ceci, S. J. (2002). When and where do we apply what we learn?: A taxonomy for far transfer. *Psychological Bulletin*, *128*(4), 612.

Beck, A. T. (2002). Cognitive models of depression. In R. L. Leahy & E. T. Dowd (Eds.), *Clinical Advances in Cognitive Psychotherapy: Theory and Application* (pp. 29–61). Springer Publishing Company.

Christensen, A. J., Moran, P. J., & Wiebe, J. S. (1999). Assessment of irrational health beliefs: Relation to health practices and medical regimen adherence. *Health Psychology*, *18*(2), 169–176. https://doi.org/10.1037/0278-6133.18.2.169

De Ridder, D. T., Lensvelt-Mulders, G., Finkenauer, C., Stok, F. M., & Baumeister, R. F. (2012). Taking stock of self-control: A meta-analysis of how trait self-control relates to a wide range of behaviors. *Personality and Social Psychology Review*, *16*(1), 76–99. https://doi.org/10.1177/1088868311418749

Fleig, L., Kerschreiter, R., Schwarzer, R., Pomp, S., & Lippke, S. (2014). 'Sticking to a healthy diet is easier for me when I exercise regularly': cognitive transfer between physical exercise and healthy nutrition. *Psychology & Health*, *29*(12), 1361–1372. https://doi.org/10.1080/08870446.2014.930146

Fleig, L., Küper, C., Lippke, S., Schwarzer, R., & Wiedemann, A. U. (2015a). Cross-behavior associations and multiple health behavior change: A longitudinal study on physical activity and fruit and vegetable intake. *Journal of Health Psychology*, *20*(5), 525–534. https://doi.org/10.1177/1359105315574951

Fleig, L., Ngo, J., Roman, B., Ntzami, E., Satta, P., Warner, L. M., Schwarzer, R., & Brandi, M. L. (2015b). Beyond single behaviour theory: Adding cross-behaviour cognitions to the health action process approach. *British Journal of Health Psychology*, *20*(4), 824–841. https://doi.org/10.1111/bjhp.12144

Gozli, D. G., & Dolcini, N. (2018). Reaching into the unknown: Actions, goal hierarchies, and explorative agency [Perspective]. *Frontiers in Psychology*, *9*. https://doi.org/10.3389/fpsyg.2018.00266

Hagger, M. S., Hankonen, N., Kangro, E. M., Lintunen, T., Pagaduan, J., Polet, J., Ries, F., & Hamilton, K. (2019). Trait self-control, social cognition constructs, and intentions: Correlational evidence for mediation and moderation effects in diverse health behaviours. *Applied Psychology: Health and Well-Being*, *11*(3), 407–437. https://doi.org/10.1111/aphw.12153

Hankonen, N., Kinnunen, M., Absetz, P., & Jallinoja, P. (2014). Why do people high in self-control eat more healthily? Social cognitions as mediators. *Annals of Behavioral Medicine*, *47*(2), 242–248. https://doi.org/10.1007/s12160-013-9535-1

Hofstetter, H., Dusseldorp, E., van Empelen, P., & Paulussen, T. W. G. M. (2014). A primer on the use of cluster analysis or factor analysis to assess co-occurrence of risk behaviors. *Preventive Medicine*, *67*, 141-146. https://doi.org/10.1016/j.ypmed.2014.07.007

Jung, M. E., & Brawley, L. R. (2013). Concurrent self-regulatory efficacy as a mediator of the goal: Exercise behaviour relationship. *Journal of Health Psychology*, *18*(5), 601–611.

Knäuper, B., Rabiau, M., Cohen, O., & Patriciu, N. (2004). Compensatory health beliefs: Scale development and psychometric properties. *Psychology & Health*, *19*(5), 607–624. https://doi.org/10.1080/0887044042000196737

Lippke, S. (2014b). Modelling and supporting complex behavior change related to obesity and diabetes prevention and management with the compefnsatory carry-over action model. *J Diab Obes*. 2014; 1: 1–5. *Journal of Diabetes and Obesity, 1*(2), 39–43.

Lippke, S., Nigg, C. R., & Maddock, J. E. (2012). Health-promoting and health-risk behaviors: Theory-driven analyses of multiple health behavior change in three international samples. *International Journal of Behavioral Medicine*, *19*(1), 1–13. https://doi.org/10.1007/s12529-010-9135-4

Maisano, M. S., Shonkoff, E. T., & Folta, S. C. (2020). Multiple health behavior change for weight loss: a scoping review. *American Journal of Health Behavior*, *44*(5), 559–571.

Mata, J., Silva, M. N., Vieira, P. N., Carraça, E. V., Andrade, A. M., Coutinho, S. R., Sardinha, L. B., & Teixeira, P. J. (2009). Motivational "spill-over" during weight control: Increased self-determination and exercise intrinsic motivation predict eating self-regulation. *Health Psychology*, *28*(6), 709–716. https://doi.org/10.1037/a0016764

Matley, F. A. I., & Davies, E. L. (2018). Resisting temptation: Alcohol specific self-efficacy mediates the impacts of compensatory health beliefs and behaviours on alcohol consumption. *Psychology, Health & Medicine*, *23*(3), 259–269. https://doi.org/10.1080/13548506.2017.1363395

McLellan, J. (2020). *The development of an intervention to support midwives in addressing multiple health behaviours with pregnant women*. University of Stirling.

Noar, S. M., Chabot, M., & Zimmerman, R. S. (2008). Applying health behavior theory to multiple behavior change: Considerations and approaches. *Preventive Medicine*, *46*(3), 275–280. https://doi.org/10.1016/j.ypmed.2007.08.001

Norman, P., Bennett, P., Smith, C., & Murphy, S. (1998). Health locus of control and health behaviour. *Journal of Health Psychology*, *3*(2), 171–180. https://doi.org/10.1177/135910539800300202

Nudelman, G., & Yakubovich, S. (2022). Patterns of health lifestyle behaviours: Findings from a representative sample of Israel. *BMC Public Health*, *22*(1), 2099. https://doi.org/10.1186/s12889-022-14535-5

Priebe, C. S., Atkinson, J., & Faulkner, G. (2017). Run to Quit: An evaluation of a scalable physical activity-based smoking cessation intervention. *Mental Health and Physical Activity*, *13*, 15–21. https://doi.org/10.1016/j.mhpa.2017.08.001

Prochaska, J. J., Spring, B., & Nigg, C. R. (2008). Multiple health behavior change research: an introduction and overview. *Preventive Medicine*, *46*(3), 181–188. https://doi.org/10.1016/j.ypmed.2008.02.001

Rabia, M., Knäuper, B., & Miquelon, P. (2006). The eternal quest for optimal balance between maximizing pleasure and minimizing harm: The compensatory health beliefs model. *British Journal of Health Psychology*, *11*(Pt 1), 139–153. https://doi.org/10.1348/135910705x52237

Radtke, T., Kaklamanou, D., Scholz, U., Hornung, R., & Armitage, C. J. (2014). Are diet-specific compensatory health beliefs predictive of dieting intentions and behaviour? *Appetite*, *76*, 36–43.

Radtke, T., & Scholz, U. (2016). Beliefs are not behavior: The distinction of compensatory health beliefs and compensatory health behavior. *European Journal of Health Psychology*, *24*, 119–129. https://doi.org/10.1026/0943-8149/a000161

Radtke, T., Scholz, U., Keller, R., & Hornung, R. (2012). Smoking is ok as long as I eat healthily: Compensatory Health Beliefs and their role for intentions and smoking within the Health Action Process Approach. *Psychology & Health*, *27*(sup2), 91–107.

Radtke, T., Scholz, U., Keller, R., Knäuper, B., & Hornung, R. (2011). Smoking-specific compensatory health beliefs and the readiness to stop smoking in adolescents. *British Journal of Health Psychology*, *16*(3), 610–625. https://doi.org/10.1348/2044-8287.002001

Rhodes, R. E., & Blanchard, C. M. (2008). Do sedentary motives adversely affect physical activity? Adding cross-behavioural cognitions to the theory of planned behaviour. *Psychology & Health*, *23*(7), 789–805. https://doi.org/10.1080/08870440701421578

Riediger, M. (2001). *On the dynamic relations among multiple goals: Intergoal conflict and intergoal facilitation in younger and older adulthood.*

Riediger, M., & Freund, A. M. (2004). Interference and facilitation among personal goals: Differential associations with subjective well-being and persistent goal pursuit. *Personality and Social Psychology Bulletin*, *30*(12), 1511–1523.

Schutte, N. S., & Malouff, J. M. (2016). General and realm-specific self-efficacy: Connections to life functioning. *Current Psychology*, *35*, 361–369.

Sniehotta, F. F., Presseau, J., Allan, J., & Araújo-Soares, V. (2016). You can't always get what you want: A novel research paradigm to explore the relationship between multiple intentions and behaviours. *Applied Psychology: Health and Well-Being*, *8*(2), 258–275. https://doi.org/10.1111/aphw.12071

Vandelanotte, C., Reeves, M. M., Brug, J., & De Bourdeaudhuij, I. (2008). A randomized trial of sequential and simultaneous multiple behavior change interventions for physical activity and fat intake. *Preventive Medicine*, *46*(3), 232–237.

Webb, T. L., & Sheeran, P. (2006). Does changing behavioral intentions engender behavior change? A meta-analysis of the experimental evidence. *Psychological Bulletin*, *132*(2), 249–268. https://doi.org/10.1037/0033-2909.132.2.249

Yin, B., & Shen, Y. (2023). Compensatory beliefs in the internet gratification behavior: A study of game-based assessment. *Frontiers in Public Health*, *11*. https://doi.org/10.3389/fpubh.2023.997108

Zhang, C. Q., Zhang, R., Schwarzer, R., & Hagger, M. S. (2019). A meta-analysis of the health action process approach. *Health Psychology*, *38*(7), 623–637. https://doi.org/10.1037/hea0000728

Zhou, R., Yu, M., & Wang, X. (2016). Why do drivers use mobile phones while driving? The contribution of compensatory beliefs. *PLoS One*, *11*(8), e0160288. https://doi.org/10.1371/journal.pone.0160288

Zimbardo, P. G., & Boyd, J. N. (1999). Putting time in perspective: A valid, reliable individual-differences metric. *Journal of Personality and Social Psychology*, *77*(6), 1271–1288. https://doi.org/10.1037/0022-3514.77.6.1271

14

THE ROLE OF HEALTH BEHAVIOUR IN OBESITY

Elizabeth H. Evans, Amy L. Ahern, Stephan U. Dombrowski, and Milica Vasiljevic

Introduction

Obesity is an accumulation of excess adipose tissue (fat) which presents a risk to health, including hypertension, cardiovascular disease, type 2 diabetes, and some cancers. Moreover, obesity is bidirectionally associated with poorer mental health. Societal stigmatisation of obesity may account for some negative physical and psychological outcomes (Brown et al., 2022). Both psychosocial and physiological factors make long-term weight loss challenging (Greenway, 2015), yet unrealistically proportioned idealised bodies are socio-culturally promoted as desirable and achievable. This chapter summarises and contextualises the role of health behaviour in obesity and the evidence base for health behaviour interventions, whilst addressing the widespread misconception that obesity results from individual 'choices'. A synergy of interventions at multiple levels is necessary to address an environment in which health-promoting dietary and physical activity behaviours are increasingly difficult.

This chapter uses the term 'persons with obesity' (PWO) to refer to individuals who carry excess adipose tissues. However, preferred terminology around obesity and elevated body weight varies, and practitioners and researchers should adopt terminology most acceptable to the individuals with whom they work (Brown & Flint, 2021).

Prevalence, Measurement, and Conceptualisation of Obesity

Body mass index (BMI) – a ratio of weight to height – is commonly used as a proxy for adiposity at the population level due to its comparative ease of measurement. As a measure, BMI is highly specific, but its current cut-offs have low to moderate sensitivity, i.e., they do not identify approximately 50% of individuals with excess adipose tissue (Okorodudu et al., 2010). BMI does not distinguish

DOI: 10.4324/9781003318026-17

between lean and fat mass or the fat distribution in the body. Other common indices of weight status include waist circumference and body fat percentage measured using bioimpedance; accuracy of adiposity measurement is broadly inversely proportional to the scalability of the measurement method. Globally, obesity affects 11% of men and 15% of women (NCD Risk Factor Collaboration, 2016) and is particularly prevalent in high-income countries. Whilst the mean BMI in high-income countries has begun to stabilise, rates in low- and middle-income countries continue to climb (Chooi et al., 2019).

The World Obesity Federation characterises obesity as a chronic, relapsing, progressive, non-communicable disease (Bray et al., 2017), arguing that elevated adiposity itself constitutes a multisystem pathology; this approach is also adopted by the Centers for Disease Control and Prevention, the Obesity Society, and numerous others. Conversely, it has been argued that obesity is better characterised as a risk factor for diseases rather than a disease itself (Vallgårda et al., 2017). In support of the risk factor perspective, obesity is not synonymous with or deterministic of health status: between 10% and 30% of PWO do not have markers of cardiometabolic disease (Blüher, 2020). Moreover, characterising obesity as a disease may perpetuate the tendency to use weight as a heuristic for health, a weight-normative approach associated with poorer long-term health outcomes for PWO (Hunger et al., 2020). One suggestion for obesity treatment is to focus on health behaviours as the primary endpoint rather than weight.

Causes of Obesity

Obesity is not a health behaviour but a behaviour-related outcome. For decades, obesity was considered the direct product of individual behaviour related to energy intake and expenditure (i.e., eating and physical activity). This perspective, which downplays the role of external factors, remains the dominant view of obesity amongst the general public (Joslyn & Haider-Markel, 2019). However, evidence shows that obesity is multifactorial, resulting from complex interactions amongst biological, psychological, social, behavioural, and environmental variables (see Figure 14.1).

Modern life is increasingly 'obesogenic' (tending to cause obesity), affecting health behaviours and physiological processes related to the development of obesity. Sedentary jobs and leisure pursuits, coupled with readily available transport, predispose low levels of physical activity behaviour. Easily available food and drink, the cheapest and most heavily promoted of which are typically high in fat, sugar, and salt, make it increasingly likely that individuals consume excess energy, leading to excess calories stored as body fat or glycogen (Townshend & Lake, 2017). However, not everyone exposed to the same environment develops obesity. This causal complexity can be illustrated by examining the relationship between biological and behavioural factors.

Weight status is substantially genetically determined. Aside from rare, severe monogenic obesity syndromes, obesity is influenced by hundreds of genetic

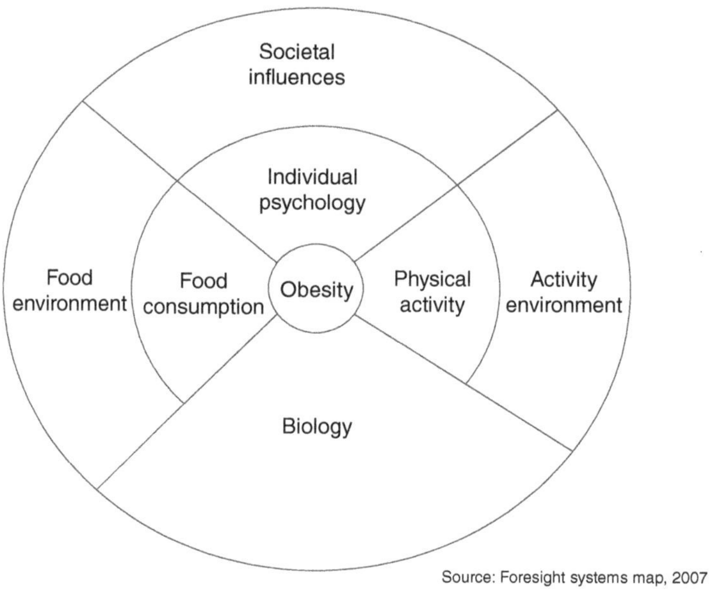

Figure 14.1 Factors causing obesity. (Adapted from Butland et al., 2007).

polymorphisms (typically single-nucleotide polymorphisms) that each have a small effect (Loos & Yeo, 2022). These polymorphisms are found in areas of the genome associated with eating behaviour, weight regulation, and their underlying neuroendocrine processes in both body and brain. Furthermore, many other obesity-linked polymorphisms have yet to be definitively associated with biological functions. These genetic susceptibilities can interact with environmental and behavioural factors to increase or decrease the probability of obesity. For example, humans carry two copies of the FTO allele, which has two variants: one variant confers a higher risk of obesity and the other a lower risk. European white adults who carry one high-risk copy weigh, on average, 1.2 kg more than people with two low-risk copies. Those with two high-risk copies weigh, on average, 3 kg more (Frayling et al., 2007). People with high-risk copies do not differ from people with two low-risk copies in terms of their weight-adjusted resting energy expenditure or levels of physical activity. However, multiple studies show that people with two high-risk copies consume more energy each day, on average, than people without high-risk copies. They also report reduced satiety (fullness) responsiveness and greater preference for high-fat foods (Loos & Yeo, 2014). This indicates a genetic basis for dietary intake behaviours. However, the risks posed by FTO can be at least partially ameliorated behaviourally. Physically active adults with two high-risk copies have a 30% lower obesity risk than sedentary high-risk adults (Kilpeläinen et al., 2011), suggesting that physical activity may attenuate the effects of high genetic risk. Similarly, adults with a lower saturated fat intake show a weaker association between high-risk copies and their risk of obesity (Corella et al., 2011). Several studies also suggest that people with two high-risk copies lose more weight through behaviour change interventions than those with low-risk copies (Xiang et al., 2016), though evidence is mixed.

In summary, obesity results from many factors, amongst which energy-balance behaviours are one part. Behaviours do not 'stand-alone' but are influenced by, and influential in, the expression of genotypes and the surrounding obesogenic environment. This emphasises the importance of health behavioural interventions because energy-balance behaviours can both turn up and turn down the likelihood of obesity developing even when someone is at high genetic risk. Behavioural interventions are an important part of the picture, although they cannot provide a sole solution to high levels of population obesity.

Behavioural Interventions for Obesity

Behavioural interventions that teach skills and strategies to change behaviours can support modest weight loss associated with health benefits (LeBlanc et al., 2018). Changes to physical activity, dietary behaviours, and psychosocial support are also critical to any obesity treatment approach, including bariatric surgery and pharmacotherapy. Moreover, approaches such as bariatric surgery and pharmacotherapy typically influence eating behaviours by changing body structures, which leads to reduced energy intake, or influencing physiological processes, which leads to changes in behaviour. For example, the obesity medication Orlistat prevents absorption of some dietary fat, which can lead to bowel urgency and other side effects when consuming a high-fat diet – thus providing negative reinforcement for the consumption of a low-fat diet.

Behavioural interventions for obesity usually target changes in diet and physical activity–related behaviours, with interventions that tackle both behaviours typically more effective in the long-term than single behaviour interventions. Physical activity–only interventions are ineffective for weight loss but may be critical for weight-loss maintenance. Increasingly, behavioural interventions for obesity tackle additional health behaviours associated with obesity, including sleep hygiene and stress management–related behaviours, acknowledging the wider determinants of obesity and the importance of mental and physical health.

Behavioural treatments for obesity incorporate several behaviour change techniques, such as goal setting, action planning, and self-monitoring, which are congruent with social cognitive theory and self-regulation theory. Some common types of techniques are outlined next.

Goal-Setting Techniques

Goal setting includes the amount of weight change and the short-term behavioural goals that will support weight change, such as daily targets for calorie intake or step counts. Whilst it is generally agreed that short-term goals should be achievable to maintain motivation, there is debate over whether unrealistic weight-loss goals hinder weight loss. Weight loss through behavioural treatment is often substantially less than patients desire (Foster et al., 2001). Whilst unrealistic goals are thought to undermine motivation when expectations are not met, several studies have found larger goals associated with larger weight losses (Calugi et al., 2017). Perhaps what is critical is that goal setting is a dynamic process and that goals are agreed upon collaboratively and are revisited and adjusted throughout treatment.

Self-Regulation Techniques

Once a goal is set, planning how to achieve it becomes relevant. People are more likely to achieve a weight goal if they make a specific and detailed plan of where, when, and how they will achieve it (Dombrowski et al., 2016). It is also important to monitor progress to evaluate whether the action plan is effective. Self-monitoring of weight and behaviours (food intake and physical activity) is a cornerstone of many weight management strategies and is strongly associated with weight loss (Burke et al., 2011). Self-monitoring allows people to notice specific patterns of behaviour and how these are related to changes in body weight. It provides an opportunity for positive reinforcement when goals are reached and allows reflection and change in strategy when goals are not met.

Roadblocks, setbacks, or life events will inevitably happen. Acknowledging the possibility of setbacks during the initial goal-setting stage and developing problem-solving strategies to address these help patients move past these when they happen.

Cognitive Behavioural Techniques

Some behavioural interventions incorporate techniques from cognitive behavioural therapy, which seek to identify and change thinking patterns that undermine weight loss. These include cognitive distortions such as all-or-nothing-thinking, over-generalisations, and must/should statements. For example, cognitive restructuring encourages people to identify when these negative thoughts occur and weigh up the evidence for and against them, leading to a more balanced thought instead.

Some evidence suggests that incorporating strategies from third-wave cognitive behavioural therapies, such as mindfulness and acceptance and commitment therapy (ACT), may improve long-term outcomes of behavioural weight management programmes. The most promising of these is ACT, which focuses on improving psychological flexibility. Whereas cognitive behavioural therapy aims to 'fix' dysfunctional thoughts that underlie behaviours, ACT aims for the non-judgemental acceptance of uncomfortable thoughts and feelings that may accompany health behaviours such as diet and physical activity. The existing evidence base for ACT is promising, but further research is needed (Lawlor et al., 2020).

Behavioural interventions for obesity have accumulated consistent evidence of generating small to medium effects over time. A systematic review and meta-analysis of 67 trials of behavioural weight management programmes found that interventions achieved greater weight loss than control conditions at up to 36-month follow-up, with an average difference in weight loss of 2.4 kg at 12–18 months (LeBlanc et al., 2018). However, there was substantial heterogeneity, with mean weight change in the intervention group ranging from −0.5 kg to −9.3 kg.

Several reviews have examined specific intervention components and individual behaviour change techniques. For example, there is some evidence that interventions that include providing instructions about how to perform a behaviour, self-monitoring, prompting practice, and relapse prevention techniques increase weight loss compared to those that do not use these techniques (Dombrowski et al., 2010). However, this evidence is often limited by vague reporting of intervention content in trials. This challenge is ubiquitous in the field of health behaviour interventions, and standardised reporting templates and taxonomies may enable better evidence synthesis in the future.

Behavioural Weight-Loss Maintenance and Regain

A key challenge for weight loss interventions is weight regain. Most interventions that are successful at supporting the initiation of weight loss report long-term weight regain (Wing & Hill, 2001), which typically starts to occur six months after the intervention (Dombrowski et al., 2010). Despite the widespread prevalence of weight regain, evidence suggests that behavioural interventions reduce cardiometabolic risk factors with effects lasting at least five years (Hartmann-Boyce et al., 2023). Moreover, the provision of maintenance-focused support targeting eating and physical activity behaviours can lead to small changes in the amount of weight individuals regain following clinically significant weight loss (Dombrowski et al., 2014).

A systematic review examining determinants of weight regain identified 67 articles reporting 124 determinants. Behavioural and cognitive determinants that promote a reduction in energy intake, increase in energy expenditure, and monitoring of this balance were predictive determinants, highlighting the central role of health behaviours in long-term weight management (Varkevisser et al., 2019). A narrative review examining over 100 behavioural theories in relation to their explanations of behavioural maintenance reported five themes hypothesised as relevant for long-term maintenance of behaviour change: maintenance motives including satisfaction with behaviour and behavioural outcomes, ongoing support, availability of resources, ongoing self-monitoring, and habit formation (Kwasnicka et al., 2016).

A systematic review examined characteristics of behavioural weight management programmes associated with weight regain and concluded that the best predictor of slower weight regain was continued programme availability (Hartmann-Boyce et al., 2021). This underlines the need for long-term intervention delivery to support behaviour change for weight management in line with the conceptualisation of obesity as a chronic condition.

Mental Health Implications of Behavioural Interventions for Obesity

The association between obesity and mental health is often overlooked. Obesity is stigmatised with a dominant narrative of personal responsibility that ignores complex multifactorial determinants of health behaviours and obesity. This individual responsibility narrative can detrimentally affect the physical and mental well-being of PWO (Tomiyama et al., 2018). Several mental health conditions are more prevalent in PWO, and people with mental health conditions have higher rates of obesity and related illnesses (Avila et al., 2015). Mental health issues and some psychiatric medications promote weight (re)gain and may prevent people from accessing or adhering to potentially beneficial treatments.

A frequent concern raised about obesity treatment is that a focus on weight, and specifically dietary restriction, can worsen mental health and increase risk of eating disorders. Systematic reviews and meta-analyses have found that on average, behavioural interventions have small benefits for mental health and reduce eating disorder symptoms (Jebeile et al., 2023; Jones et al., 2021). However, these are average effects, and people can experience worsening mental health or develop disordered eating during weight management. More research is needed into the individual-level and intervention-level factors that predict those at risk. Qualitative research highlights the desire for more psychological support from people taking part in obesity treatment (Mold & Forbes, 2013). An increased understanding is required of how to best provide behavioural obesity interventions that improve mental and physical health.

Environments and Changing Behaviours Related to Obesity

Environmental interventions target the complex interactions between the individual and the wider environment in relation to obesity-related behaviours (Jackson et al., 2020). Much work historically has focused on the role of the individual in engaging with dietary and physical activity change. However, whilst traditional accounts linked lower engagement with these behaviours amongst those less affluent with individual factors, more recent theorising and empirical work has started to highlight the importance of the wider environment, including fiscal, social, and physical environment (for a discussion, see Adams, 2020). Interventions requiring high levels of individual resources are usually more acceptable to the public but are often less effective and less equitable, with interventions aimed at modifying the environment considered more effective and equitable (see Adams et al., 2016).

Several recent interventions aim at modifying people's environments to increase engagement with dietary and physical activity behaviour change. A framework developed to categorise the different environmental features and cues that may impact people's behaviours is the typology of interventions in proximal physical micro-environments (TIPPME; Hollands et al., 2017). The TIPPME categorises six intervention types, altering either the properties or the placement of objects or stimuli in the environment. For example, the presence (*availability*) and location of objects/stimuli within an environment (*position*) can be manipulated. Other types of interventions examine the properties of objects/cues that can be manipulated within a given environment (e.g., *functionality*, *presentation*, *size*, and *information*). The following discusses the evidence regarding the effectiveness and public acceptability of size, availability and proximity, and nutritional (calorie) labelling interventions to change obesity-related behaviours.

Behaviour Change Interventions Aimed at Modifying the Environment

Size

Reducing the size of food portions, packaging, and tableware has been suggested as a potential intervention to reduce energy intake. A Cochrane Review showed that compared to smaller-sized versions, larger-sized portions, packaging, and/or tableware led to increases in food consumption (Hollands et al., 2015). The review further suggested that if portions, packaging, and tableware were reduced in size, then this would equate to approximately a 12%–16% change in average daily energy intake. These findings were however based on a few randomised studies amongst small samples and rated high in risk of bias. A further meta-analysis disentangling the effects of self-served or pre-served foods found a substantial effect of food size when foods were self-served, with a minimal effect when foods were pre-served (Holden et al., 2016). Since self-serving is an integral part of food intake, the potential of size interventions that could modify self-served foods seems critical. Recent fully powered experiments have provided evidence of effectiveness when manipulating the size of plates/containers when food was self-served in laboratory settings (Clarke et al., 2021).

Availability and Proximity

A Cochrane Review synthesising the evidence regarding altering the availability (the range and/or amount of options) of food products, or their proximity (the distance at which they are positioned) to individuals found evidence of effectiveness (Hollands et al., 2019). The evidence was however deemed of low certainty, with six and 18 studies investigating availability and proximity interventions, respectively. Due to the heterogeneity in this small sample of studies, particularly for availability, the confidence range regarding the potential size of the effect is large, and at present, the change in food consumption arising from these interventions cannot be estimated. Additional studies testing the impact of altering the availability of healthier food options, have found further evidence of effectiveness (see Marteau et al., 2022 for a recent summary). Recent investigations have started elucidating some of the mechanisms of action for these types of intervention, including social norms.

Nutritional (Calorie) Labelling

Nutritional labelling (often in the form of providing energy/calorie information) of food products (either front of pack for pre-packed foods or on menus and displays at point of sale for non-packed foods) has garnered interest amongst the public and policymakers. Findings from a small body of three randomised studies of low-quality evidence synthesised for a Cochrane Review suggest that nutritional labelling comprising energy information on menus may reduce energy purchased in restaurants by about 47 calories (7.8%) per meal on average (Crockett et al., 2018). The evidence regarding consumption was less definite and of low quality. Most of the synthesised studies were conducted in university settings in the USA, with many conducted in laboratory settings relying on hypothetical tasks.

Another systematic review synthesised evidence from 186 mainly US-based studies (including both experimental and non-experimental studies conducted across laboratory or field settings). This synthesis estimated a smaller effect of calorie labelling – approximate reduction of 27 calories (4.6%) per meal – further showing that the effect size of calorie labelling was larger in laboratory (hypothetical-choice) studies and larger amongst women and those who were overweight (Zlatevska et al., 2018). Another systematic review has provided evidence that calorie labelling may be more effective amongst those of higher socioeconomic status (Sarink et al., 2016). These recent systematic reviews suggest that there remains considerable uncertainty about the potential impact of calorie labelling and that calorie labelling may have heterogeneous effectiveness amongst different groups and across intervention settings. More recent studies conducted in UK workplaces found no effect on purchasing and consumption of calorie labelling (Vasiljevic et al., 2018), even for visually enhanced calorie labelling (Vasiljevic et al., 2019).

Acceptability of Environmental Interventions

Intervention effectiveness needs to be considered alongside public acceptability when deciding which interventions to legislate, since public support is consequential for the successful initiation and maintenance of policies. Whilst the evidence for effectiveness of calorie labelling is lowest, public support for legislating calorie labelling on foods is high. Similarly, intervening on availability where robust evidence of effectiveness exists is often hampered by low public support. Even highlighting the role of environments in causing obesity is not sufficient to increase public support for environmental interventions/policies to tackle obesity (Reynolds et al., 2022). These findings support work on the Nuffield ladder, which shows that the public is significantly more in favour of the least intrusive but also least effective policies (Nuffield Council on Bioethics, 2007).

Beyond effectiveness and public acceptability, interventions also affect industry-level outcomes. Thus, for example, even though the evidence of effectiveness of calorie labelling is low, there may be other positive impacts of legislating for calorie labelling on foods. For example, the review by Zlatevska et al. (2018) found upstream evidence of effectiveness whereby calorie labelling impacted industry reformulation of different food products. Similar effects have been found for interventions regarding the sizing of products.

Whilst some environmental interventions have targeted dietary behaviour change, others focused on environmental change to increase physical activity. Some less well-researched interventions altering the extant environment have aimed to modify the physical space that the public inhabits with the intention of increasing physical activity and, more recently, engagement in active travel. For example, various interventions have been designed to discourage lift use and instead encourage greater use of the stairs. The evidence for effectiveness and acceptability of these types of interventions is still at a nascent stage, with some encouraging initial findings.

Weight Stigma

A key barrier to uptake, engagement, retention, and sustainability of behavioural interventions for obesity at the individual and environmental levels is weight stigma. Weight stigma comprises negative attitudes and behaviours towards PWO due to weight or size (Meadows & Calogero, 2018). Weight stigma is typically subdivided into experienced and internalised forms, the latter reflecting stigmatising beliefs that PWO apply to themselves. Stigmatising beliefs about obesity are common among the general population, the media, health-care professionals, and researchers, and in workplaces, schools, and health-care settings (Brown et al., 2022).

Weight stigma is relevant to health behaviour interventions for PWO because it is associated with poorer health outcomes through a number of pathways, independently of BMI. First, weight stigma contributes to poorer quality health-care experiences through providers' attitudes and behaviours and patients' subsequent responses to feeling stigmatised. Second, weight stigma prospectively predicts maladaptive eating behaviours, decreased physical activity, and other obesogenic behaviours (Puhl et al., 2020); it is also associated with physiological changes (such as elevated C-reactive protein), which themselves predict weight gain, morbidity, and mortality (Sutin et al., 2014; Tomiyama et al., 2018). Third, it predicts increased body dissatisfaction (Meadows & Calogero, 2018), which is associated with weight gain and the onset of (sub)clinical mental health conditions, including eating and depressive disorders. Finally, weight stigma both reflects and perpetuates a dominant and counterproductive societal narrative of personal responsibility, blame, and shame around body size/shape and its relationship to health behaviours.

Anti-Stigma Practices in Health Behaviour Interventions for People with Obesity

Health behaviour interventions for PWO should consider adopting an anti-stigma perspective (Rubino et al., 2020). Good practice includes using respectful language (spoken and written) and providing environments that are inclusive of and comfortable to all body sizes (e.g., furniture and research equipment). Images in communication should avoid perpetuating unwarranted stereotypes and be guided by size-positive image banks (e.g., as provided by the World Obesity Federation). Other recommendations suggest avoiding sensationalist or combative language around weight, such as 'the war against obesity' or 'obesity epidemic'. A helpful anti-stigma practice is the inclusion of PWO in designing, implementing, evaluating, and refining health behaviour interventions for PWO (e.g., as advisors, co-investigators, or experts by experience). The weight-inclusive approach to health care for PWO recommends centring the potential for personally meaningful health and well-being gains over weight change and focusing on behavioural and modifiable health indices as primary targets for intervention and support (Tylka et al., 2014).

Conclusions

Individual health behaviour change forms one component of a multilevel approach to obesity. Moreover, individual behaviour is embedded in biogenetic, environmental, socio-economic, and structural drivers. Approaches to obesity on a population level involve a synergy of interventions on multiple levels, the majority of which directly or indirectly influence health behaviours. Interventions at any level benefit from addressing the deleterious effects of weight stigma on the physical and mental health of PWO.

Further Reading

Adams, J., Mytton, O., White, M., & Monsivais, P. (2016). Why Are Some Population Interventions for Diet and Obesity More Equitable and Effective Than Others? The Role of Individual Agency. *PLoS Med*, *13*(4), e1001990. doi:10.1371/journal.pmed.1001990

Lawlor, E. R., Islam, N., Bates, S., Griffin, S. J., Hill, A. J., Hughes, C. A., … Ahern, A. L. (2020). Third-Wave Cognitive Behaviour Therapies for Weight Management: A Systematic Review and Network Meta-Analysis. *Obes Rev*, *21*(7), e13013. doi:10.1111/obr.13013

LeBlanc, E. S., Patnode, C. D., Webber, E. M., Redmond, N., Rushkin, M., & O'Connor, E. A. (2018). Behavioral and Pharmacotherapy Weight Loss Interventions to Prevent Obesity-Related Morbidity and Mortality in Adults: Updated Evidence Report and Systematic Review for the Us Preventive Services Task Force. *Jama*, *320*(11), 1172–1191. doi:10.1001/jama.2018.7777

Loos, R. J., & Yeo, G. S. (2022). The Genetics of Obesity: From Discovery to Biology. *Nat Rev Genet*, *23*(2), 120–133. doi:10.1038/s41576-021-00414-z

Meadows, A., & Calogero, R. M. (2018). Studies on Weight Stigma and Body Image in Higher-Weight Individuals. In M. Cuzzolaro & S. Fassino (Eds.), *Body image, eating, and weight* (pp. 381–400). Cham: Springer. https://doi.org/10.1007/978-3-319-90817-5_28

References

Adams, J. (2020). Addressing Socioeconomic Inequalities in Obesity: Democratising Access to Resources for Achieving and Maintaining a Healthy Weight. *PLoS Med*, *17*(7), e1003243. https://doi.org/10.1371/journal.pmed.1003243

Adams, J., Mytton, O., White, M., & Monsivais, P. (2016). Why Are Some Population Interventions for Diet and Obesity More Equitable and Effective Than Others? The Role of Individual Agency. *PLoS Med*, *13*(4), e1001990. https://doi.org/10.1371/journal.pmed.1001990

Avila, C., Holloway, A. C., Hahn, M. K., Morrison, K. M., Restivo, M., Anglin, R., & Taylor, V. H. (2015). An Overview of Links between Obesity and Mental Health. *Curr Obes Rep*, *4*(3), 303–310. https://doi.org/10.1007/s13679-015-0164-9

Blüher, M. (2020). Metabolically Healthy Obesity. *Endocr Rev*, *41*(3), bnaa004.

Bray, G. A., Kim, K. K., & Wilding, J. P. H. (2017). Obesity: A Chronic Relapsing Progressive Disease Process. A Position Statement of the World Obesity Federation. *Obes Rev*, *18*(7), 715–723. https://doi.org/10.1111/obr.12551

Brown, A., & Flint, S. W. (2021). Preferences and Emotional Response to Weight-Related Terminology Used by Healthcare Professionals to Describe Body Weight in People Living with Overweight and Obesity. *Clin Obes*, *11*(5), e12470. https://doi.org/10.1111/cob.12470

Brown, A., Flint, S. W., & Batterham, R. L. (2022). Pervasiveness, Impact and Implications of Weight Stigma. *EClinicalMedicine*, *47*, 101408. https://doi.org/10.1016/j.eclinm.2022.101408

Burke, L. E., Wang, J., & Sevick, M. A. (2011). Self-Monitoring in Weight Loss: A Systematic Review of the Literature. *J Am Diet Assoc*, *111*(1), 92–102. https://doi.org/10.1016/j.jada.2010.10.008

Butland, B., Jebb, S., Kopelman, P., McPherson, K., Thomas, S., Mardell, J., & Parry, V. (2007). *Tackling obesities: Future choices-project report* (Vol. 10, p. 17). London: Department of Innovation, Universities and Skills.

Calugi, S., Marchesini, G., El Ghoch, M., Gavasso, I., & Dalle Grave, R. (2017). The Influence of Weight-Loss Expectations on Weight Loss and of Weight-Loss Satisfaction on Weight Maintenance in Severe Obesity. *J Acad Nutr Diet*, *117*(1), 32–38. https://doi.org/10.1016/j.jand.2016.09.001

Chooi, Y. C., Ding, C., & Magkos, F. (2019). The Epidemiology of Obesity. *Metabolism*, *92*, 6–10. https://doi.org/10.1016/j.metabol.2018.09.005

Clarke, N., Pechey, E., Pechey, R., Ventsel, M., Mantzari, E., De-Loyde, K., … Hollands, G. J. (2021). Size and Shape of Plates and Size of Wine Glasses and Bottles: Impact on Self-Serving of Food and Alcohol. *BMC Psychol*, *9*(1), 163. https://doi.org/10.1186/s40359-021-00645-z

Corella, D., Arnett, D. K., Tucker, K. L., Kabagambe, E. K., Tsai, M., Parnell, L. D., … Ordovas, J. M. (2011). A High Intake of Saturated Fatty Acids Strengthens the Association between the Fat Mass and Obesity-Associated Gene and Bmi. *J Nutr*, *141*(12), 2219–2225. https://doi.org/10.3945/jn.111.143826

Crockett, R. A., King, S. E., Marteau, T. M., Prevost, A. T., Bignardi, G., Roberts, N. W., … Jebb, S. A. (2018). Nutritional Labelling for Healthier Food or Non-Alcoholic Drink Purchasing and Consumption. *Cochrane Database Syst Rev*, *2*(2), Cd009315. https://doi.org/10.1002/14651858.CD009315.pub2

Dombrowski, S. U., Avenell, A., & Sniehott, F. F. (2010). Behavioural Interventions for Obese Adults with Additional Risk Factors for Morbidity: Systematic Review of Effects on Behaviour, Weight and Disease Risk Factors. *Obes Facts*, *3*(6), 377–396. https://doi.org/10.1159/000323076

Dombrowski, S. U., Endevelt, R., Steinberg, D. M., & Benyamini, Y. (2016). Do More Specific Plans Help You Lose Weight? Examining the Relationship between Plan Specificity, Weight Loss Goals, and Plan Content in the Context of a Weight Management Programme. *Br J Health Psychol*, *21*(4), 989–1005. https://doi.org/10.1111/bjhp.12212

Dombrowski, S. U., Knittle, K., Avenell, A., Araújo-Soares, V., & Sniehotta, F. F. (2014). Long Term Maintenance of Weight Loss with Non-Surgical Interventions in Obese Adults: Systematic Review and Meta-Analyses of Randomised Controlled Trials. *BMJ*, *348*, g2646. https://doi.org/10.1136/bmj.g2646

Foster, G. D., Wadden, T. A., Phelan, S., Sarwer, D. B., & Sanderson, R. S. (2001). Obese Patients' Perceptions of Treatment Outcomes and the Factors That Influence Them. *Arch Intern Med, 161*(17), 2133–2139.

Frayling, T. M., Timpson, N. J., Weedon, M. N., Zeggini, E., Freathy, R. M., Lindgren, C. M., … McCarthy, M. I. (2007). A Common Variant in the Fto Gene Is Associated with Body Mass Index and Predisposes to Childhood and Adult Obesity. *Science, 316*(5826), 889–894. https://doi.org/10.1126/science.1141634

Greenway, F. L. (2015). Physiological Adaptations to Weight Loss and Factors Favouring Weight Regain. *Int J Obes (Lond), 39*(8), 1188–1196. https://doi.org/10.1038/ijo.2015.59

Hartmann-Boyce, J., Theodoulou, A., Oke, J. L., Butler, A. R., Bastounis, A., Dunnigan, A., … Aveyard, P. (2023). Long-Term Effect of Weight Regain Following Behavioral Weight Management Programs on Cardiometabolic Disease Incidence and Risk: Systematic Review and Meta-Analysis. *Circ Cardiovasc Qual Outcomes, 16*(4), e009348. https://doi.org/10.1161/circoutcomes.122.009348

Hartmann-Boyce, J., Theodoulou, A., Oke, J. L., Butler, A. R., Scarborough, P., Bastounis, A., … Aveyard, P. (2021). Association between Characteristics of Behavioural Weight Loss Programmes and Weight Change after Programme End: Systematic Review and Meta-Analysis. *BMJ, 374*, n1840. https://doi.org/10.1136/bmj.n1840

Holden, S. S., Zlatevska, N., & Dubelaar, C. (2016). Whether Smaller Plates Reduce Consumption Depends on Who's Serving and Who's Looking: A Meta-Analysis. *JACR, 1*(1), 134–146. https://doi.org/10.1086/684441

Hollands, G. J., Bignardi, G., Johnston, M., Kelly, M. P., Ogilvie, D., Petticrew, M., … Marteau, T. M. (2017). The Tippme Intervention Typology for Changing Environments to Change Behaviour. *Nat Hum Behav, 1*(8), 0140. https://doi.org/10.1038/s41562-017-0140

Hollands, G. J., Carter, P., Anwer, S., King, S. E., Jebb, S. A., Ogilvie, D., … Marteau, T. M. (2019). Altering the Availability or Proximity of Food, Alcohol, and Tobacco Products to Change Their Selection and Consumption. *Cochrane Database Syst Rev, 9*(9), Cd012573. https://doi.org/10.1002/14651858.CD012573.pub3

Hollands, G. J., Shemilt, I., Marteau, T. M., Jebb, S. A., Lewis, H. B., Wei, Y., … Ogilvie, D. (2015). Portion, Package or Tableware Size for Changing Selection and Consumption of Food, Alcohol and Tobacco. *Cochrane Database Syst Rev, 2015*(9), Cd011045. https://doi.org/10.1002/14651858.CD011045.pub2

Hunger, J. M., Smith, J. P., & Tomiyama, A. J. (2020). An Evidence-Based Rationale for Adopting Weight-Inclusive Health Policy. *Soc Iss Policy Rev, 14*(1), 73–107. https://doi.org/10.1111/sipr.12062

Jackson, S. E., Llewellyn, C. H., & Smith, L. (2020). The Obesity Epidemic - Nature Via Nurture: A Narrative Review of High-Income Countries. *SAGE Open Med, 8*, 2050312120918265. https://doi.org/10.1177/2050312120918265

Jebeile, H., Libesman, S., Melville, H., Low-Wah, T., Dammery, G., Seidler, A. L., … Lister, N. B. (2023). Eating Disorder Risk During Behavioral Weight Management in Adults with Overweight or Obesity: A Systematic Review with Meta-Analysis. *Obes Rev, 24*(6), e13561. https://doi.org/10.1111/obr.13561

Jones, R. A., Lawlor, E. R., Birch, J. M., Patel, M. I., Werneck, A. O., Hoare, E., … Ahern, A. L. (2021). The Impact of Adult Behavioural Weight Management Interventions on Mental Health: A Systematic Review and Meta-Analysis. *Obes Rev, 22*(4), e13150. https://doi.org/10.1111/obr.13150

Joslyn, M. R., & Haider-Markel, D. P. (2019). Perceived Causes of Obesity, Emotions, and Attitudes About Discrimination Policy. *Soc Sci Med, 223*, 97–103. https://doi.org/10.1016/j.socscimed.2019.01.019

Kilpeläinen, T. O., Qi, L., Brage, S., Sharp, S. J., Sonestedt, E., Demerath, E., … Loos, R. J. (2011). Physical Activity Attenuates the Influence of Fto Variants on Obesity Risk: A Meta-Analysis of 218,166 Adults and 19,268 Children. *PLoS Med, 8*(11), e1001116. https://doi.org/10.1371/journal.pmed.1001116

Kwasnicka, D., Dombrowski, S. U., White, M., & Sniehotta, F. (2016). Theoretical Explanations for Maintenance of Behaviour Change: A Systematic Review of Behaviour Theories. *Health Psychol Rev*, *10*(3), 277–296. https://doi.org/10.1080/17437199.2016.1151372

Lawlor, E. R., Islam, N., Bates, S., Griffin, S. J., Hill, A. J., Hughes, C. A., ... Ahern, A. L. (2020). Third-Wave Cognitive Behaviour Therapies for Weight Management: A Systematic Review and Network Meta-Analysis. *Obes Rev*, *21*(7), e13013. https://doi.org/10.1111/obr.13013

LeBlanc, E. S., Patnode, C. D., Webber, E. M., Redmond, N., Rushkin, M., & O'Connor, E. A. (2018). Behavioral and Pharmacotherapy Weight Loss Interventions to Prevent Obesity-Related Morbidity and Mortality in Adults: Updated Evidence Report and Systematic Review for the Us Preventive Services Task Force. *JAMA*, *320*(11), 1172–1191. https://doi.org/10.1001/jama.2018.7777

Loos, R. J., & Yeo, G. S. (2014). The Bigger Picture of Fto: The First Gwas-Identified Obesity Gene. *Nat Rev Endocrinol*, *10*(1), 51–61. https://doi.org/10.1038/nrendo.2013.227

Loos, R. J., & Yeo, G. S. (2022). The Genetics of Obesity: From Discovery to Biology. *Nat Rev Genet*, *23*(2), 120–133. https://doi.org/10.1038/s41576-021-00414-z

Marteau, T. M., Hollands, G. J., Pechey, R., Reynolds, J. P., & Jebb, S. A. (2022). Changing the Assortment of Available Food and Drink for Leaner, Greener Diets. *Bmj*, *377*, e069848. https://doi.org/10.1136/bmj-2021-069848

Meadows, A., & Calogero, R. M. (2018). Studies on Weight Stigma and Body Image in Higher-Weight Individuals. In M. Cuzzolaro & S. Fassino (Eds.), *Body image, eating, and weight* (pp. 381–400). Cham: Springer. https://doi.org/10.1007/978-3-319-90817-5_28

Mold, F., & Forbes, A. (2013). Patients' and Professionals' Experiences and Perspectives of Obesity in Health-Care Settings: A Synthesis of Current Research. *Health Expect*, *16*(2), 119–142. https://doi.org/10.1111/j.1369-7625.2011.00699.x

NCD Risk Factor Collaboration. (2016). Trends in Adult Body-Mass Index in 200 Countries from 1975 to 2014: A Pooled Analysis of 1698 Population-Based Measurement Studies with 19·2 Million Participants. *Lancet*, *387*(10026), 1377–1396. https://doi.org/10.1016/s0140-6736(16)30054-x

Nuffield Council on Bioethics. (2007). Public Health: Ethical Issues. Retrieved from https://www.nuffieldbioethics.org/publications/public-health

Okorodudu, D. O., Jumean, M. F., Montori, V. M., Romero-Corral, A., Somers, V. K., Erwin, P. J., & Lopez-Jimenez, F. (2010). Diagnostic Performance of Body Mass Index to Identify Obesity as Defined by Body Adiposity: A Systematic Review and Meta-Analysis. *Int J Obes (Lond)*, *34*(5), 791–799. https://doi.org/10.1038/ijo.2010.5

Puhl, R. M., Himmelstein, M. S., & Pearl, R. L. (2020). Weight Stigma as a Psychosocial Contributor to Obesity. *Am Psychol*, *75*(2), 274–289. https://doi.org/10.1037/amp0000538

Reynolds, J. P., Vasiljevic, M., Pilling, M., & Marteau, T. M. (2022). Communicating Evidence About the Environment's Role in Obesity and Support for Government Policies to Tackle Obesity: A Systematic Review with Meta-Analysis. *Health Psychol Rev*, *16*(1), 67–80. https://doi.org/10.1080/17437199.2020.1829980

Rubino, F., Puhl, R. M., Cummings, D. E., Eckel, R. H., Ryan, D. H., Mechanick, J. I., ... Dixon, J. B. (2020). Joint International Consensus Statement for Ending Stigma of Obesity. *Nat Med*, *26*(4), 485–497. https://doi.org/10.1038/s41591-020-0803-x

Sarink, D., Peeters, A., Freak-Poli, R., Beauchamp, A., Woods, J., Ball, K., & Backholer, K. (2016). The Impact of Menu Energy Labelling across Socioeconomic Groups: A Systematic Review. *Appetite*, *99*, 59–75. https://doi.org/10.1016/j.appet.2015.12.022

Sutin, A. R., Stephan, Y., Luchetti, M., & Terracciano, A. (2014). Perceived Weight Discrimination and C-Reactive Protein. *Obesity (Silver Spring)*, *22*(9), 1959–1961. https://doi.org/10.1002/oby.20789

Tomiyama, A. J., Carr, D., Granberg, E. M., Major, B., Robinson, E., Sutin, A. R., & Brewis, A. (2018). How and Why Weight Stigma Drives the Obesity 'Epidemic' and Harms Health. *BMC Medicine*, *16*(1), 123. https://doi.org/10.1186/s12916-018-1116-5

Townshend, T., & Lake, A. (2017). Obesogenic Environments: Current Evidence of the Built and Food Environments. *Perspect Public Health*, *137*(1), 38–44. https://doi.org/10.1177/1757913916679860

Tylka, T. L., Annunziato, R. A., Burgard, D., Daníelsdóttir, S., Shuman, E., Davis, C., & Calogero, R. M. (2014). The Weight-Inclusive Versus Weight-Normative Approach to Health: Evaluating the Evidence for Prioritizing Well-Being over Weight Loss. *J Obes*, *2014*, 983495. https://doi.org/10.1155/2014/983495

Vallgårda, S., Nielsen, M. E. J., Hansen, A. K. K., Cathaoir, K., Hartlev, M., Holm, L., … Sandøe, P. (2017). Should Europe Follow the Us and Declare Obesity a Disease?: A Discussion of the So-Called Utilitarian Argument. *Eur J Clin Nutr*, *71*(11), 1263–1267. https://doi.org/10.1038/ejcn.2017.103

Varkevisser, R. D. M., Van Stralen, M. M., Kroeze, W., Ket, J. C. F., & Steenhuis, I. H. M. (2019). Determinants of weight loss maintenance: A systematic review. *Obesity Reviews*, *20*(2), 171–211.

Vasiljevic, M., Cartwright, E., Pilling, M., Lee, M.-M., Bignardi, G., Pechey, R., … Marteau, T. M. (2018). Impact of Calorie Labelling in Worksite Cafeterias: A Stepped Wedge Randomised Controlled Pilot Trial. *Int J Behav Nutr Phys Act*, *15*(1), 41. https://doi.org/10.1186/s12966-018-0671-7

Vasiljevic, M., Fuller, G., Pilling, M., Hollands, G. J., Pechey, R., Jebb, S. A., & Marteau, T. M. (2019). What Is the Impact of Increasing the Prominence of Calorie Labelling? A Stepped Wedge Randomised Controlled Pilot Trial in Worksite Cafeterias. *Appetite*, *141*, 104304. https://doi.org/10.1016/j.appet.2019.05.035

Wing, R. R., & Hill, J. O. (2001). Successful Weight Loss Maintenance. *Annu Rev Nutr*, *21*, 323–341. https://doi.org/10.1146/annurev.nutr.21.1.323

Xiang, L., Wu, H., Pan, A., Patel, B., Xiang, G., Qi, L., … Qi, Q. (2016). Fto Genotype and Weight Loss in Diet and Lifestyle Interventions: A Systematic Review and Meta-Analysis. *Am J Clin Nutr*, *103*(4), 1162–1170. https://doi.org/10.3945/ajcn.115.123448

Zlatevska, N., Neumann, N., & Dubelaar, C. (2018). Mandatory Calorie Disclosure: A Comprehensive Analysis of Its Effect on Consumers and Retailers. *J Retail*, *94*(1), 89–101. https://doi.org/10.1016/j.jretai.2017.09.007

15

MOVING FROM DESCRIPTION TO EXPLANATION

How Well Can We Explain Medication-Taking Behaviour?

Louise Foley and Gerard J. Molloy

Describing Medication Adherence

Treatment adherence has been defined as the extent to which "a person's behaviour – taking medication, following a diet, and/or executing lifestyle changes, corresponds with agreed recommendations from a health care provider" (Sabaté, 2003). This behaviour has been the focus of decades of systematic study in many disciplines (Haynes et al., 1996; DiMatteo, 2004; Stewart et al., 2023b), with many estimates suggesting that up to 50% of people do not use medications as agreed with health-care providers. There are several key reasons why this behaviour has been intensively examined. First, despite the substantial financial investment in developing, testing, and manufacturing medications, variability in medication adherence is one of the key reasons that people do not benefit from the multitude of medicines that have well-established positive impacts on health problems. Second, this behaviour is amenable to behavioural intervention in health care (Brown & Bussell, 2011). Third, due to the ageing population in many contexts, chronic illness and the related long-term medication use often become the norm for many older adults (Barnett et al., 2012; Foley et al., 2021). Therefore, from a lifespan perspective, there is frequently an inevitability and increasing salience of the challenge of medication use for many older people.

Over the last decade, medication adherence has been helpfully disaggregated into a few distinct components. For example, the classification of medication adherence into three major phases has gained increasing currency as an important focus for both research and practice (Vrijens et al., 2012). This disaggregation into (1) initiation of drug treatment, i.e., taking a dose for the first time

 DOI: 10.4324/9781003318026-18

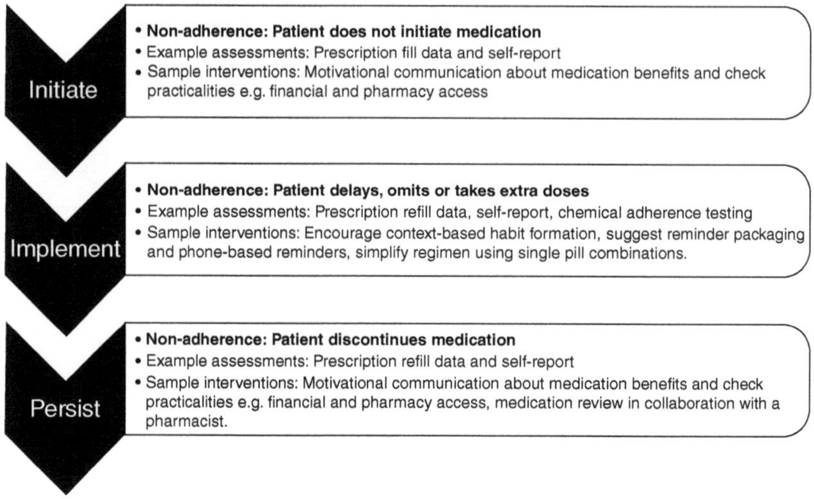

Figure 15.1 A summary of (non-)adherence phases, assessments, and interventions.

(versus not starting a regimen); (2) implementation, i.e., taking doses as prescribed (versus not taking doses as prescribed); and (3) persistence, i.e. continuation with treatment for the prescribed duration (versus discontinuation of treatment), has been helpful, as these represent temporally distinct and unique challenges that are likely to require phase and context-specific assessment and intervention as summarised in Figure 15.1. For example, in the case of chronic illness, initiation of a treatment typically requires a person to firstly present to a prescribing physician with some health need or signs and symptoms of an illness. This is followed by a prescription of a medicine or set of medicines that is then presented by the patient to a pharmacist, often in a different health-care setting, who issues the medicine with specific use recommendations. Finally, the patient usually starts using the medicines in their home, as initially agreed with the prescriber. Therefore, there are several potentially complex behavioural steps involved, and there may be a need for behavioural support at multiple points in this complex sequence.

Measuring Medication Adherence

Our ability to understand and explain adherence to medicines is dependent upon the careful and reliable measurement of medication-related behaviours (Kronish et al., 2021b). A range of measures have been used across the adherence literature, contributing in part to the varied estimates of the prevalence of non-adherence that have been observed among different patient populations (Schoenwald & Garland, 2013). Approaches to measurement have been previously classified as being either objective or subjective (Anghel et al., 2019).

Existing Approaches to Measurement

Objective measures attempt to observe adherence levels without questioning the person directly and involve using resources and methods such as pharmacy records, biochemical assays, pill counts, and electronic monitoring systems (Lam & Fresco, 2015). The data available in pharmacy records can be used to estimate the proportion of medicines available to a person for use within an observation window; biochemical assay can be used to indicate the presence of medications or related markers in samples, such as blood or urine; pill counts can be used to assess the number of remaining pills a person has in their possession relative to how many they would have if fully adherent; and electronic monitoring can be used to record each opening of a pill box. Together, these objective measures may reveal the extent to which a person has engaged with the various phases of adhering to medications, including collecting medicines from the pharmacy, removing medicines from their container, and ingesting medicines (Anghel et al., 2019; Lam & Fresco, 2015).

Subjective measures include the reporting of medication adherence by the person themselves or by relevant others such as caregivers or health-care providers. Several self-report psychometric scales have been developed and validated to measure the constructs related to medication taking, e.g., Medication Adherence Report Scale (Chan et al., 2021; Cohen et al., 2009; Horne & Weinman, 2002). Unlike objective adherence measures, subjective measures often capture some of the reasons for not taking prescribed medicines, such as unintentional forgetting or intentional altering of the medication dose (Stirratt et al., 2015). Choosing the most appropriate measure will depend on the objectives and resources of a programme of research.

Strengths and Limitations of Existing Measures

Existing approaches to measuring medication-taking behaviour have several reported strengths and limitations (Anghel et al., 2019; Jimmy & Jose, 2011; Lam & Fresco, 2015; Lehmann et al., 2014), which will be summarised here. Administrative health data, such as pharmacy claims data, often contain accurate information for many individuals. However, the estimates provided by this type of data can be distorted by both the formulae used to calculate adherence and the potential for individuals to possess medicines without necessarily taking them. At face value, electronic monitoring or pill counts can plausibly provide more insight into how often medicines have been removed from a container; however, estimates of adherence may be impacted by pill sharing or dumping, i.e., disposing of medicines before adherence is measured (Park et al., 2015). Biochemical assay, also known as chemical adherence testing (Lane et al., 2022), is one method which can confirm whether markers of a medicine are present in samples taken directly from an individual. However, this approach is expensive to implement widely and provides only a snapshot of medication-taking behaviour, often at a scheduled point in time. Self-report approaches to assessing medication taking are generally inexpensive to implement at scale. Nonetheless, the limitations inherent to any self-report approach remain relevant to the measurement of adherence in this form. Recall bias, for example, can obscure estimates when individuals are tasked with reporting past behaviour, and social desirability bias can lead to over-reporting of adherence levels. Many existing measures address some but not all phases in the process of adhering to medicines (Gellad et al., 2017). For example, administrative claims data reflects the collection of medications from a pharmacy, electronic monitoring reflects opening the pill container, and pill counts reflect removing pills from the container. Given the complexity of the behaviour, combining multiple measures is offered as a suitable approach to assessing medication adherence to allow for the strengths of one measure to balance the limitations of another (Durand et al., 2017; Sabaté, 2003).

Innovative Methods for Monitoring Adherence

While some of the aforementioned approaches, such as electronic monitoring, reflect the influence of technological advancement in the measurement of adherence, several other technologies exist to monitor medication-taking behaviour (Kim et al., 2020; Mason et al., 2022; McCormick et al., 2018). Digital pills, also referred to as ingestible sensors or digital ingestion monitoring, are medications combined with sensors which are activated by gastric fluid after the medication has been ingested. The time and date of the sensor activation are recorded by a wearable device, providing a record that a medication dose has been taken (Chai et al., 2022). Wearable motion-sensor technologies have also been used to monitor medication-taking behaviours (Lim & Abdullah, 2017). These sensors take the form of wrist-worn devices and use accelerometery to detect the movements which can be attributed to medication taking. While less invasive than digital pills, these wearable devices are limited in their ability to distinguish medication administration motions from other daily motions, such as eating or drinking (Mason et al., 2022). Pairing wearable devices with other monitors capable of detecting proximity to pill boxes is a possible solution (Aldeer et al., 2018). Vision-based systems have also been developed, including camera installations in the home environment which can detect events such as bottle opening, pill picking, pill swallowing, and bottle closing (Aldeer et al., 2018; Valin et al., 2006). Despite these advances, ethical questions remain relating to autonomy, privacy, and confidentiality (Campbell et al., 2016; Rand & Sevick, 2000). Advances in surveillance technologies do present new opportunities for monitoring medication-taking behaviours in naturalistic settings such as the home, with possible strides for understanding adherence from the perspective of increased data accuracy and quantity. However, the potential for the monitoring of behaviour in this way to undermine trust between patients and providers – and prompt a return to more paternalistic constructions of medication-taking behaviour – needs to be carefully considered (McCormick et al., 2018).

Predicting Medication Adherence

A large and disparate body of evidence has attempted to identify factors that reliably predict medication adherence. One review of systematic reviews (Kardas et al., 2013) reported that more than 771 individual factors have been linked to medication taking. This review also identified that few studies have focused on persistence of medication taking, with the majority focusing on the implementation phase of adherence. They also noted a limited number of studies on the determinants of adherence to short-term treatments for acute conditions, e.g., bacterial infection, as opposed to chronic conditions, e.g., hypertension. Therefore, despite a considerable corpus of studies focusing on prediction of medication adherence, there are research gaps on key aspects of medication-taking behaviour.

With such diversity of potential determinants of adherence, it has been somewhat useful to organise these variables into a small number of broad domains. One widely used classification derives from the World Health Organization's (WHO) "five dimensions of adherence" (Sabaté, 2003) – namely, (i) social/economic factors, (ii) therapy-related factors, (iii) patient-related factors, (iv) condition-related factors, and (v) health system/health-care team factors. These dimensions summarise the complexity of the factors operating at multiple levels that can be involved in potentially determining medication-taking behaviour. This WHO five dimensions of adherence framework has been used to distil the multiple barriers and facilitators to medication adherence that have been identified in 102 existing conceptual frameworks in the adherence literature (Peh et al., 2021). The five dimensions are illustrated in Figure 15.2. Such frameworks can help to map out the complexity of the system within which this behaviour occurs.

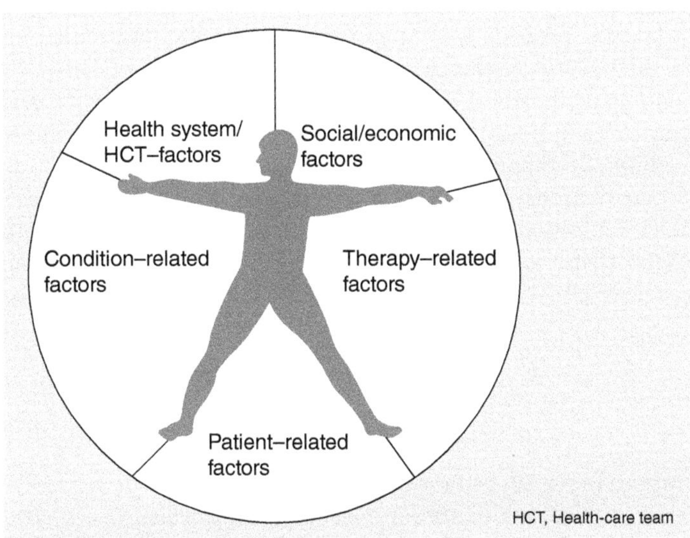

Figure 15.2 WHO's five dimensions of adherence (Sabaté, 2003).

This recognition of multi-level influences can inform the design of interventions at multiple levels, e.g., patient, family, doctor, and pharmacy interactions, to enhance adherence to medication. However, more parsimonious theoretical models of medication adherence are needed to explain why a disparate array of predictors might account for medication adherence in some contexts.

Clarity is needed around more precise mechanisms of action and the related parameters for effectiveness that can explain the process whereby a behavioural intervention works (Carey et al., 2019; Kok et al., 2016). This specification does not preclude the development of complex multi-component behavioural interventions to support adherence; however, it does require researchers to outline the specific pathways whereby an intervention is thought to have a causal effect on medication adherence and the related health outcomes (Band et al., 2017b).

One specific patient-related factor that warrants special attention when considering the predictors of medication adherence concerns key lifespan processes (Molloy and O'Carroll, 2017). These developmental factors are important throughout life but are particularly salient in the first three decades of life (Pharo et al., 2011). While many studies do refer to *age* as a predictor of medication adherence, there is comparatively less consideration of relevant *developmental processes* in the context of medication adherence. For example, the capacity for self-regulation becomes established over the first three decades of life; therefore, developmentally aligned behaviour change approaches should be considered when developing adherence supports earlier in the lifespan (Miller et al., 2020). There is considerable literature on adherence to medications in childhood and adolescence (McGrady and Hommel, 2013; Badawy et al., 2017), while more recently, there has been a growing focus on the period after adolescence that is sometimes referred to as emerging adulthood (Arnett, 2000). Further intensive study of medication adherence among those living with lifelong conditions is needed during this post-adolescent and pre-adulthood point of the lifespan to help ensure that adherence can be supported in ways that align with developmental needs and goals during the transition into adulthood (Murphy et al., 2021; Hynes et al., 2016). Equally, there are developmental needs and goals in midlife and older adulthood that may need to be considered in the design of medication adherence interventions. For example, the socio-emotional needs and goals of those in older adulthood, e.g., the relative focus on emotion-related goals, differ from the earlier phase of adulthood, e.g., the relative focus on knowledge-related goals (Carstensen et al., 1999).

Explaining Medication Adherence

Theory-Based Approaches

In an attempt to move beyond description, several theories have been applied to explain medication-taking behaviours. Among those which have been used are the Common-Sense Model of Self-Regulation (CSM-SR; Leventhal et al., 2016) and the related Necessity-Concerns Framework (NCF; Horne & Weinman,

1999). The CSM is a model describing an individual's perceptions of their illness and their approach to coping (Leventhal et al., 2016). In a review of the relationship between illness perceptions and adherence, beliefs related to the identity, cause, timeline, consequences, control, and emotional representations of an illness were each directly or indirectly related to medication taking (Kucukarslan, 2012). The NCF is a related framework describing the role of beliefs about the necessity of medicines and concerns about medicines in adherence (Horne & Weinman, 1999). While higher necessity beliefs and lower concern beliefs are regularly found to be related to higher levels of adherence (Horne et al., 2013), this relationship is multidimensional, i.e., people can hold positive and negative beliefs simultaneously, and the combination of these beliefs can relate to medication-taking behaviours (Foley et al., 2023; Phillips et al., 2014).

A review of the use of theory in interventions to improve medication adherence reported that social cognitive theory and motivational interviewing were the most commonly applied (Conn et al., 2016). While regularly used, these theories and models have been described as limited due to the predominant focus on perceptual barriers to medication adherence with a relative neglect of key practical barriers, e.g., financial and social support. The Perceptions and Practicalities Approach is a framework which accounts for both patient motivation and patient ability to adhere to medicines, therefore acknowledging the role of such practical barriers (Horne et al., 2019b). The absence of habit theory in adherence interventions has also been noted despite the known role of habit strength in medication taking (Conn et al., 2016; Robinson et al., 2022). The COM-B (Capability, Opportunity, Motivation – Behaviour; Michie et al., 2011) model has been proposed as another encompassing framework which accounts for both the perceptual and practical challenges associated with adherence, as well as the automatic processes that enable or prevent medication taking, such as habit (Easthall & Barnett, 2017).

Exploring Patterns of Non-adherence with Data

When attempting to explain medication taking, some of the common approaches to measurement fail to account for the dynamic and temporal patterns that are inherent to behaviour. Indeed, several of the formulae for calculating adherence levels from pharmacy claims data reduce a complex behaviour observed over a window of time to a single number (Franklin et al., 2013). Yet during this observation window, an individual could encounter a range of experiences that lead them to take or not take their medicines. For example, diuretics are a type of medication that are sometimes used to treat hypertension. The side-effect of urinary frequency may require some people who take this medication to use it in a more variable way, depending on their circumstances (Kronish et al., 2011). It is therefore possible for an array of patterns of medication taking to be observed from one individual to another, or indeed from one medication to another. Some such patterns could include consistent dosing and persistence, discontinuation before a dose is complete, missing several medication doses, or taking most doses but at irregular times (Vrijens et al., 2008). Considering the phases of adherence

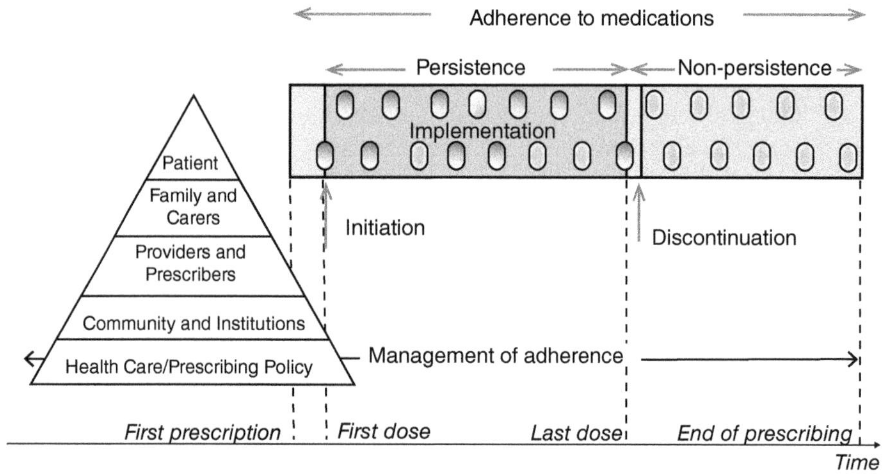

Figure 15.3 Phases of medication adherence (Vrijens et al. 2012).

outlined previously, documenting the variable levels of engagement with medication taking at each phase could contribute to explaining some of this variation. Methods such as trajectory modelling have been used to classify individuals into groups which describe their adherence levels over time (e.g., Walsh et al., 2020). Such statistical methods can identify, for example, groups with high levels of adherence at initiation which (a) remain high throughout implementation and persistence, (b) fall somewhat in the implementation phase, or (c) fall dramatically following initiation. Figure 15.3 provides a visual representation of each of these phases, highlighting the occurrence of non-persistence and discontinuation when medicines are no longer taken as prescribed (Vrijens et al., 2012).

Supporting Medication Adherence

There is now a considerable body of evidence that has developed and evaluated interventions to support medication adherence in randomised controlled trial designs. These kinds of trials that aim to change medication-taking behaviour have been carried out for more than 50 years (Sackett et al., 1975). One of the foremost research syntheses of this evidence is a Cochrane Review that has been updated four times over the last two decades (Nieuwlaat et al., 2014). The current consensus from this review and similar others is that adherence interventions can potentially improve medication-taking behaviour and related health outcomes; however, there remains considerable uncertainty about which specific adherence interventions are most effective for different patient populations and medical conditions. As with many areas of health behaviour change, there is significant heterogeneity in key methodological details such as study designs, measurement approaches, and the complexity and intensity of intervention delivery that contribute to this uncertainty around the efficacy and effectiveness of these interventions.

Cognitive or Behavioural Intervention?

There are however some specific generalisable approaches to support medication adherence that have a reasonably strong evidence base. For example, the use of prompts or reminders in the form mobile phone text messaging has been shown to be effective in several different chronic conditions (Thakkar et al., 2016). Conn and Ruppar (2017) reported that habit-based interventions were associated with larger effect sizes in their meta-analysis of RCTs evaluating medication adherence interventions. Such interventions include linking medication taking with existing habitual behaviours using techniques such as if-then plans, e.g., forming an implementation intention (Robinson et al., 2022; O'Carroll et al., 2013b; Brown et al., 2009). These are usually low-intensity interventions that can be delivered without specialised training in behavioural intervention. However, such approaches are likely to be unsuitable for non-adherence that is intentional, for example, when someone deliberately decides that they will not take a medication because of some concern and/or a perceived lack of necessity to take the medication. For this kind of psychological barrier to medication adherence, a focus on perceptions of medication or the illness may be needed, as opposed to a focus on the practicalities (Horne et al., 2019b). Indeed, it is likely that effective interventions may often need to target both the cognitive and behavioural drivers of medication-taking behaviour, as there may be a combination of intentional and unintentional factors determining adherence (O'Carroll et al., 2013b).

Simplifying Regimens

Simplifying medication regimens has also been shown to have positive impacts on medication adherence for those with more complex medication regimens. For example, there is accumulating evidence showing that combination dosing can improve adherence (Parati et al., 2021; Böhm et al., 2021). Some recent evidence, however, has cast doubt on the efficacy of simplifying complex medication regimens in improving outcomes for those with multiple chronic conditions and using multiple medications (Muth et al., 2018). These intervention approaches of reducing the task complexity of the medication-taking behaviour, e.g., simplifying the medication regimen, can clearly be distilled into well-established behaviour change techniques (Michie et al., 2013), e.g., setting an easier-to-perform task in a graded schedule or conserving mental resources. Such approaches have been successfully applied to behaviour modification in multiple domains for decades. Therefore, following the principle of aiming to reduce the demands on memory, attention, and decision processes seems like an important mechanism of action whereby less complex medication-taking behaviours will in most contexts be desirable for promoting adherence and reducing the overall burden of treatment (Mair & May, 2014).

Digital Interventions

Over the last decade, there has been exponential growth in the development of digital interventions to support medication adherence (Blakey et al., 2018;

Morrissey et al., 2016). One of the challenges for this area of research is the evolving regulatory frameworks that designate some technology supported adherence solutions as medical devices or medical device software (Murphy et al., 2022). Recent changes in the legislative landscape mean that some digital solutions to support medication taking may no longer be seen as ancillary behavioural supports but *de facto* medical devices that could be subject to similar regulatory rigour as surgically implanted medical devices. A key distinguishing feature in this regard is the extent to which these digital interventions are used alone or in combination for "diagnosis, prevention, monitoring, prediction, prognosis, treatment, or alleviation of disease and which does not achieve its main intended purpose by pharmacological, immunological or metabolic means but may be assisted in its function by such means" (European Union, 2017). The interpretation of this and the evolving regulation around the use of artificial intelligence means that future developments in digital health technologies to support medication adherence are in a major phase of transition. However, it seems inevitable that digital technologies incorporating artificial intelligence will offer increasingly sophisticated means of supporting medication adherence (Babel et al., 2021; Fogel and Kvedar, 2018).

Interventions in Real-World Settings

Translating this knowledge on supporting medication adherence into routine health-care practice is challenging for several reasons. First, it can be difficult to definitively establish if someone is not taking their medication in the absence of an objective measurement that captures medication taking over a sufficiently prolonged period. Therefore, assessment of non-adherence to medication usually requires reliable recall from the person prescribed the medication. Framing an adherence conversation in a no-blame way that maintains the relationship with the patient can sometimes seem challenging; therefore, it can be easier to avoid this potentially contentious discussion. Second, health-care providers may not have the knowledge or skills in behavioural intervention to support medication adherence. Some approaches to enhance motivation to take medications, such as motivational interviewing (Palacio et al., 2016), may be seen as outside of the range of competence of some medication prescribers. Finally, the perennial challenge for many prescribers is a shortage of time to carry out the necessary assessment, formulation, and intervention delivery to support medication-taking behaviour. It is often seen as one challenging issue among many competing for time in a time-pressured consultation (Burnier et al., 2021).

Extending How We Think about Medication-Taking Behaviour

Multimorbidity, Polypharmacy, and Treatment Burden

Although adherence to medications is related to and influenced by the specific nuances of individual conditions, many people living with chronic illness are managing two or more concurrent conditions, referred to as multimorbidity

(Barnett et al., 2012). Multimorbidity is closely associated with the use of multiple medicines, i.e., polypharmacy (Sinnott & Bradley, 2015), which adds complexity to our understanding of medication adherence. Specifically, the presence of multimorbidity and polypharmacy impacts both the behaviour of taking medications and our ability to accurately measure that behaviour. When a person is prescribed multiple medicines for multiple health conditions, the workload associated with self-management can increase (Rosbach & Andersen, 2017). This is known as treatment burden, which exists alongside the burden of illness, impacting functioning and well-being (Eton et al., 2015). It has been proposed that some people with multimorbidity engage in a process of prioritisation when faced with increasing treatment burden, leading them to adhere to some medicines more than others (Cheraghi-Sohi et al., 2013; Foley et al., 2021). Reasons for prioritisation may be informed by short-term goals related to symptom relief or daily functioning, or by longer-term goals related to future morbidity and mortality (Cheraghi-Sohi et al., 2013; Morris et al., 2011). Multimorbidity and polypharmacy can also add complexity to medication regimens, requiring medications to be taken at multiple times throughout the day (Mansur et al., 2012). The majority of the existing literature in adherence that has accounted for multimorbidity involves controlling for the presence of multiple conditions within analyses focused on single conditions. Less attention has been attributed to the direct measurement of adherence across all conditions a person is self-managing, with most existing adherence measures designed for single-condition populations (Arnet et al., 2016). While it is feasible to apply these measures in populations with multiple conditions, the estimates of adherence often reflect an average across conditions, leading to a gap in our understanding of whether and why people may be differentially adherent to different medicines (INVOLVE, 2020). To understand medication-taking behaviours as they regularly present in clinical practice, i.e., in the context of multimorbidity and polypharmacy, new measures must be designed which directly account for the associated complexity (Pednekar et al., 2019).

Public and Patient Involvement and Multidisciplinary Collaboration

Our ability to understand and explain complex behaviour like medication taking is limited by the extent to which we have experienced the related challenges ourselves. Often, our appreciation for what determinants, outcomes, measures and interventions are of most relevance is informed by the available literature. Public and Patient Involvement (PPI) reflects an approach to research that goes beyond usual forms of participation by engaging with patients and members of the public actively and regularly throughout the research process (INVOLVE, 2020). This can include, for example, involvement in planning research studies, interpreting analyses, and disseminating findings. In general terms, PPI is reported to increase the relevance and appropriateness of research across these stages of the research cycle (Brett et al., 2014). In the specific context of studies aiming to understand medication adherence or *non*-adherence, PPI can direct researchers towards the most acceptable measures, the most suitable modes of intervention delivery, and the most effective means of communicating about medicines. Indeed, in the creation of digital adherence interventions, the value of engaging with end-users during the development phase is clearly apparent, given the advances made by pervasive technologies which prioritise user experience during the development phases. Likewise, our construction of adherence as a health behaviour is informed by our position as members of the health psychology community. Collaborating with colleagues from disciplines such as pharmacy, general practice, sociology, and health services and policy research will present alternative, and possibly conflicting, ways of making sense of medication adherence. Interrogating and integrating these perspectives across disciplines should lead to more nuanced approaches to explaining and supporting medication-taking behaviour through appropriate intervention.

Conclusions

Following the boundless growth of literature attempting to describe, measure, predict, explain and intervene to improve medication-taking behaviours, it is clear that adherence to prescribed medicines is a complex, dynamic, and changeable health behaviour. Complexity is apparent across the several phases of adherence, requiring individuals to complete numerous related but distinct behaviours in order to achieve optimal use and benefit of their medications. The dynamic nature of medication-taking behaviour is clear in the variability that is observed across individuals, as well as differences within individuals – both day-to-day and across the lifespan. Finally, the changeability of this behaviour has been demonstrated through some successful approaches to intervention, though the translation of this knowledge into practice requires further effort. Each characteristic therefore contributes to the challenge of explaining medication-taking behaviours. Application of theory, acknowledgement of multimorbidity and polypharmacy, involvement of patient and public contributors in our research, and collaboration across disciplines will further strengthen our attempts to explain and ultimately support medication-taking behaviour in the future.

Further Reading

Band, R., Bradbury, K., Morton, K. et al. (2017) Intervention planning for a digital intervention for self-management of hypertension: A theory-, evidence- and person-based approach. *Implementation Science 12*, 25. https://doi.org/10.1186/s13012-017-0553-4

Horne, R., Cooper, V., Wileman, V., & Chan, A. (2019). Supporting adherence to medicines for long-term conditions. *European Psychologist. 24*(1), 82–96. https://doi.org/10.1027/1016-9040/a000353

Kronish, I. M., Thorpe, C. T., & Voils, C. I. (2021). Measuring the multiple domains of medication nonadherence: Findings from a Delphi survey of adherence experts. *Translational Behavioral Medicine, 11*(1), 104–113. https://doi.org/10.1093/tbm/ibz133

O'Carroll, R. E., Chambers, J. A., Dennis, M., Sudlow, C., & Johnston, M. (2013). Improving adherence to medication in stroke survivors: A pilot randomised controlled trial. *Annals of Behavioral Medicine, 46*(3), 358–368. https://doi.org/10.1007/s12160-013-9515-5

Stewart, S. J. F., Moon, Z., & Horne, R. (2023). Medication nonadherence: Health impact, prevalence, correlates and interventions. *Psychology & Health, 38*, 726–765. https://doi.org/10.1080/08870446.2022.2144923

References

Aldeer, M., Javanmard, M., & Martin, R. P. (2018). A review of medication adherence monitoring technologies. *Applied System Innovation, 1*(2), 14. https://doi.org/10.3390/asi1020014

Anghel, L. A., Farcas, A. M., & Oprean, R. N. (2019). An overview of the common methods used to measure treatment adherence. *Medicine and Pharmacy Reports, 92*(2), 117–122. https://doi.org/10.15386/mpr-1201

Arnet, I., Kooij, M. J., Messerli, M., Hersberger, K. E., Heerdink, E. R., & Bouvy, M. (2016). Proposal of standardization to assess adherence with medication records: methodology matters. *The Annals of Pharmacotherapy, 50*(5), 360–368. https://doi.org/10.1177/1060028016634106

Arnett, J. J. (2000). Emerging adulthood: a theory of development from the late teens through the twenties. *American Psychologist, 55*(5), 469–480. https://doi.org/10.1037/0003-066X.55.5.469

Babel, A., Taneja, R., Mondello Malvestiti, F., Monaco, A., & Donde, S. (2021). Artificial intelligence solutions to increase medication adherence in patients with non-communicable diseases. *Frontiers in Digital Health, 69*, 3, https://doi.org/10.3389/fdgth.2021.669869

Badawy, S. M., Barrera, L., Sinno, M. G., Kaviany, S., O'Dwyer, L. C., & Kuhns, L. M. (2017). Text messaging and mobile phone apps as interventions to improve adherence in adolescents with chronic health conditions: a systematic review. *JMIR mHealth and uHealth, 5*(5), e7798. https://doi.org/10.2196/mhealth.7798

Band, R., Bradbury, K., Morton, K. et al. (2017b) Intervention planning for a digital intervention for self-management of hypertension: A theory-, evidence- and person-based approach. *Implementation Science 12*, 25. https://doi.org/10.1186/s13012-017-0553-4

Barnett, K., Mercer, S. W., Norbury, M., Watt, G., Wyke, S., & Guthrie, B. (2012). Epidemiology of multimorbidity and implications for health care, research, and medical education: A cross-sectional study. *The Lancet, 380*(9836), 37–43. https://doi.org/10.1016/S0140-6736(12)60240-2

Blakey, J. D., Bender, B. G., Dima, A. L., Weinman, J., Safioti, G., & Costello, R. W. (2018). Digital technologies and adherence in respiratory diseases: The road ahead. *European Respiratory Journal*, 52(5).

Böhm, A. K., Schneider, U., Aberle, J., & Stargardt, T. (2021). Regimen simplification and medication adherence: Fixed-dose versus loose-dose combination therapy for type 2 diabetes. *PloS one, 16*(5), e0250993. https://doi.org/10.1371/journal.pone.0250993

Brett, J. O., Staniszewska, S., Mockford, C., Herron-Marx, S., Hughes, J., Tysall, C., & Suleman, R. (2014). Mapping the impact of patient and public involvement on health and social care research: A systematic review. *Health Expectations, 17*(5), 637–650. https://doi.org/10.1111/j.1369-7625.2012.00795.x

Brown, M. T., & Bussell, J. K. (2011). Medication adherence: WHO cares? M*ayo Clinic Proceedings, 86, 4*, 304–314. https://doi.org/10.4065/mcp.2010.0575

Brown, I., Sheeran, P., & Reuber, M. (2009). Enhancing antiepileptic drug adherence: A randomized controlled trial. *Epilepsy & Behavior, 16*(4), 634–639.

Burnier, M., Prejbisz, A., Weber, T., Azizi, M., Cunha, V., Versmissen, J., … Working Group on Cardiovascular Therapy and Adherence of the European Society of Hypertension. (2021). Hypertension healthcare professional beliefs and behaviour regarding patient medication adherence: a survey conducted among European Society of Hypertension Centres of Excellence. *Blood Pressure, 30*(5), 282–290. https://doi.org/10.1080/08037051.2021.1963209

Campbell, J. I., Eyal, N., Musiimenta, A., & Haberer, J. E. (2016). Ethical questions in medical electronic adherence monitoring. *Journal of General Internal Medicine, 31*(3), 338–342. https://doi.org/10.1007/s11606-015-3502-4
Carey, R. N., Connell, L. E., Johnston, M., Rothman, A. J., De Bruin, M., Kelly, M. P., & Michie, S. (2019). Behavior change techniques and their mechanisms of action: a synthesis of links described in published intervention literature. *Annals of Behavioral Medicine, 53*(8), 693–707.
Carstensen, L. L., Isaacowitz, D. M., & Charles, S. T. (1999). Taking time seriously: A theory of socioemotional selectivity. *American Psychologist, 54*(3), 165–181
Chai, P. R., Vaz, C., Goodman, G. R., Albrechta, H., Huang, H., Rosen, R. K., ... O'Cleirigh, C. (2022). Ingestible electronic sensors to measure instantaneous medication adherence: A narrative review. *Digital Health*, 8, 20552076221083119. https://doi.org/10.1177/20552076221083119
Chan, A. H. Y., Vervloet, M., Lycett, H., Brabers, A., van Dijk, L., & Horne, R. (2021). Development and validation of a self-report measure of practical barriers to medication adherence: The medication practical barriers to adherence questionnaire (MPRAQ). *British Journal of Clinical Pharmacology, 87*(11), 4197–4211. https://doi.org/10.1111/bcp.14744
Cheraghi-Sohi, S., Morden, A., Bower, P., Kennedy, A., Rogers, A., Richardson, J., Sanders, T., Stevenson, F., & Ong, B. N. (2013). Exploring patient priorities among long-term conditions in multimorbidity: A qualitative secondary analysis. *SAGE Open Medicine, 1*, 2050312113503955. https://doi.org/10.1177/2050312113503955
Cohen, J. L., Mann, D. M., Wisnivesky, J. P., Horne, R., Leventhal, H., Musumeci-Szabó, T. J., & Halm, E. A. (2009). Assessing the validity of self-reported medication adherence among inner-city asthmatic adults: The Medication Adherence Report Scale for Asthma. *Annals of Allergy, Asthma & Immunology, 103*(4), 325–331. https://doi.org/10.1016/S1081-1206(10)60532-7
Conn, V. S., Enriquez, M., Ruppar, T. M., & Chan, K. C. (2016). Meta-analyses of theory use in medication adherence intervention research. *American journal of health behavior, 40*(2), 155–171. https://doi.org/10.5993/AJHB.40.2.1
Conn, V. S., & Ruppar, T. M. (2017). Medication adherence outcomes of 771 intervention trials: systematic review and meta-analysis. *Preventive Medicine*, 99, 269–276. https://doi.org/10.1016/j.ypmed.2017.03.008
DiMatteo, M. R. (2004). Variations in patients' adherence to medical recommendations: a quantitative review of 50 years of research. *Medical Care, 42*, 200–209. https://www.jstor.org/stable/4640729
Durand, H., Hayes, P., Morrissey, E. C., Newell, J., Casey, M., Murphy, A. W., & Molloy, G. J. (2017). Medication adherence among patients with apparent treatment-resistant hypertension: systematic review and meta-analysis. *Journal of Hypertension, 35*(12), 2346–2357. https://doi.org/10.1097/HJH.0000000000001502
European Union (2017). Regulation (EU) 2017/745 of the European Parliament and of the Council of 5 April 2017 on medical devices, amending Directive 2001/83/EC, Regulation (EC) No 178/2002 and Regulation (EC) No 1223/2009 and repealing Council Directives 90/385/EEC and 93/42/EEC. *Official Journal of the European Union, 2017*, 1–175.
Easthall, C., & Barnett, N. (2017). Using theory to explore the determinants of medication adherence; moving away from a one-size-fits-all approach. *Pharmacy, 5*(3), 50. https://doi.org/10.3390/pharmacy5030050
Eton, D. T., Ridgeway, J. L., Egginton, J. S., Tiedje, K., Linzer, M., Boehm, D. H., Poplau, S., Ramalho de Oliveira, D., Odell, L., Montori, V. M., May, C. R., & Anderson, R. T. (2015). Finalizing a measurement framework for the burden of treatment in complex patients with chronic conditions. *Patient Related Outcome Measures, 6*, 117–126. https://doi.org/10.2147/PROM.S78955

Foley, L., Hynes, L., Murphy, A. W., & Molloy, G. J. (2021). 'Just keep taking them, keep hoping they'll work': a qualitative study of adhering to medications for multimorbidity. *British Journal of Health Psychology*, *27*(3), 691–715. https://doi.org/10.1111/bjhp.12568
Fogel, A.L., & Kvedar, J.C. (2018). Artificial intelligence powers digital medicine. *npj Digital Medicine*, *1*, 5. https://doi.org/10.1038/s41746-017-0012-2
Foley, L., Doherty, A. S., Wallace, E., Boland, F., Hynes, L., Murphy, A. W., & Molloy, G. J. (2023). Exploring the multidimensional relationship between medication beliefs and adherence to medications among older adults living with multimorbidity using polynomial regression: an observational cohort study. *Annals of Behavioral Medicine*, kaad004. https://doi.org/10.1093/abm/kaad004
Franklin, J. M., Shrank, W. H., Pakes, J., Sanfélix-Gimeno, G., Matlin, O. S., Brennan, T. A., & Choudhry, N. K. (2013). Group-based trajectory models: a new approach to classifying and predicting long-term medication adherence. *Medical Care*, 789–796. https://www.jstor.org/stable/42568759
Gellad, W. F., Thorpe, C. T., Steiner, J. F., & Voils, C. I. (2017). The myths of medication adherence. *Pharmacoepidemiology and Drug Safety*, *26*(12), 1437–1441. https://doi.org/10.1002/pds.4334
Haynes, R. B., McKibbon, K. A., & Kanani, R. (1996). Systematic review of randomised trials of interventions to assist patients to follow prescriptions for medications. *The Lancet*, *348*(9024), 383–386. https://doi.org/10.1016/S0140-6736(96)01073-2
Horne, R., Cooper, V., Wileman, V., & Chan, A. (2019b). Supporting adherence to medicines for long-term conditions. *European Psychologist*, *24*(1), 82–96. https://doi.org/10.1027/1016-9040/a000353
Horne, R., Chapman, S. C. E., Parham, R., Freemantle, N., Forbes, A., & Cooper, V. (2013). Understanding patients' adherence-related beliefs about medicines prescribed for long-term conditions: a meta-analytic review of the Necessity-Concerns Framework. *PLoS ONE*, *8*(12), e80633. https://doi.org/10.1371/journal.pone.0080633
Horne, R., & Weinman, J. (1999). Patients' beliefs about prescribed medicines and their role in adherence to treatment in chronic physical illness. *Journal of Psychosomatic Research*, *47*(6), 555–567. https://doi.org/10.1016/S0022-3999(99)00057-4
Horne, R., & Weinman, J. (2002). Self-regulation and self-management in asthma: exploring the role of illness perceptions and treatment beliefs in explaining non-adherence to preventer medication. *Psychology and Health*, *17*(1), 17–32. https://doi.org/10.1080/08870440290001502
Hynes, L., Byrne, M., Dinneen, S. F., McGuire, B. E., O'Donnell, M., & Mc Sharry, J. (2016). Barriers and facilitators associated with attendance at hospital diabetes clinics among young adults (15–30 years) with type 1 diabetes mellitus: a systematic review. *Pediatric Diabetes*, *17*(7), 509-518. https://doi.org/10.1111/pedi.12198
INVOLVE. (2020). *INVOLVE*. https://www.invo.org.uk/
Jimmy, B., & Jose, J. (2011). Patient medication adherence: measures in daily practice. *Oman Medical Journal*, *26*(3), 155–159. https://doi.org/10.5001/omj.2011.38
Kardas, P., Lewek, P., & Matyjaszczyk, M. (2013). Determinants of patient adherence: a review of systematic reviews. *Frontiers in Pharmacology*, *4*, 91. https://doi.org/10.3389/fphar.2013.00091
Kim, J., Kassels, A. C., Costin, N. I., & Schmidt, H. (2020). Remote monitoring of medication adherence and patient and industry responsibilities in a learning health system. *Journal of Medical Ethics*, *46*(6), 386–391. https://doi.org/10.1136/medethics-2019-105667
Kok, G., Gottlieb, N. H., Peters, G. J. Y., Mullen, P. D., Parcel, G. S., Ruiter, R. A., … Bartholomew, L. K. (2016). A taxonomy of behaviour change methods: an intervention mapping approach. *Health Psychology Review*, *10*(3), 297–312.
Kronish, I. M., Woodward, M., Sergie, Z., Ogedegbe, G., Falzon, L., & Mann, D. M. (2011). Meta-analysis: impact of drug class on adherence to antihypertensives. *Circulation*, *123*(15), 1611–1621. https://doi.org/10.1161/CIRCULATIONAHA.110.983874

Kronish, I. M., Thorpe, C. T., & Voils, C. I. (2021b). Measuring the multiple domains of medication nonadherence: findings from a Delphi survey of adherence experts. *Translational Behavioral Medicine*, *11*(1), 104–113. https://doi.org/10.1093/tbm/ibz133
Kucukarslan, S. N. (2012). A review of published studies of patients' illness perceptions and medication adherence: lessons learned and future directions. *Research in Social and Administrative Pharmacy*, *8*(5), 371–382. https://doi.org/10.1016/j.sapharm.2011.09.002
Lam, W. Y., & Fresco, P. (2015). Medication adherence measures: an overview. *BioMed Research International*, *2015*, 1–12. https://doi.org/10.1155/2015/217047
Lane, D., Lawson, A., Burns, A., Azizi, M., Burnier, M., Jones, D. J., … Endorsed by the European Society of Hypertension (ESH) Working Group on Cardiovascular Pharmacotherapy and Adherence. (2022). Nonadherence in hypertension: how to develop and implement chemical adherence testing. *Hypertension*, *79*(1), 12–23.
Lehmann, A., Aslani, P., Ahmed, R., Celio, J., Gauchet, A., Bedouch, P., Bugnon, O., Allenet, B., & Schneider, M. P. (2014). Assessing medication adherence: options to consider. *International Journal of Clinical Pharmacy*, *36*(1), 55–69. https://doi.org/10.1007/s11096-013-9865-x
Leventhal, H., Phillips, L. A., & Burns, E. (2016). The Common-Sense Model of Self-Regulation (CSM): A dynamic framework for understanding illness self-management. *Journal of Behavioral Medicine*, *39*(6), 935–946. https://doi.org/10.1007/s10865-016-9782-2
Lim, T. H., & Abdullah, A. H. (2017). Medication adherence using non-intrusive wearable sensors. *EAI Endorsed Transactions on Ambient Systems*, *4*(16). http://dx.doi.org/10.4108/eai.19-12-2017.153484
Mair, F. S., & May, C. R. (2014). Thinking about the burden of treatment. *BMJ*, *349*. https://doi.org/10.1136/bmj.g6680
Mansur, N., Weiss, A., & Beloosesky, Y. (2012). Looking beyond polypharmacy: Quantification of medication regimen complexity in the elderly. *The American Journal of Geriatric Pharmacotherapy*, *10*(4), 223–229. https://doi.org/10.1016/j.amjopharm.2012.06.002
Mason, M., Cho, Y., Rayo, J., Gong, Y., Harris, M., & Jiang, Y. (2022). Technologies for medication adherence monitoring and technology assessment criteria: narrative review. *JMIR MHealth and UHealth*, *10*(3), e35157. https://doi.org/10.2196/35157
McCormick, J. B., Green, M. J., & Shapiro, D. (2018). Medication Nonadherence: There's an App for That! *Mayo Clinic Proceedings*, *93*(10), 1346–1350. https://doi.org/10.1016/j.mayocp.2018.05.029
McGrady, M. E., & Hommel, K. A. (2013). Medication adherence and health care utilization in pediatric chronic illness: a systematic review. *Pediatrics*, *132*(4), 730–740.
Michie, S., Richardson, M., Johnston, M., Abraham, C., Francis, J., Hardeman, W., … Wood, C. E. (2013). The behavior change technique taxonomy (v1) of 93 hierarchically clustered techniques: building an international consensus for the reporting of behavior change interventions. *Annals of Behavioral Medicine*, *46*(1), 81–95. https://doi.org/10.1007/s12160-013-9486-6
Michie, S., van Stralen, M. M., & West, R. (2011). The behaviour change wheel: a new method for characterising and designing behaviour change interventions. *Implementation Science*, *6*(1), 42. https://doi.org/10.1186/1748-5908-6-42
Miller, A. L., Lo, S. L., Bauer, K. W., & Fredericks, E. M. (2020). Developmentally informed behaviour change techniques to enhance self-regulation in a health promotion context: a conceptual review. *Health Psychology Review*, *14*(1), 116–131. https://doi.org/10.1080/17437199.2020.1718530
Molloy, G. J., & O'Carroll, R. E. (2017). Medication adherence across the lifespan: Theory, methods, interventions and six grand challenges. *Psychology & Health*, *32*(10), 1169–1175.
Morris, R. L., Sanders, C., Kennedy, A. P., & Rogers, A. (2011). Shifting priorities in multimorbidity: a longitudinal qualitative study of patient's prioritization of multiple conditions. *Chronic Illness*, *7*(2), 147–161. https://doi.org/10.1177/1742395310393365

Morrissey, E. C., Corbett, T. K., Walsh, J. C., & Molloy, G. J. (2016). Behavior change techniques in apps for medication adherence: a content analysis. *American Journal of Preventive Medicine*, *50*(5), e143–e146. https://doi.org/10.1016/j.amepre.2015.09.034

Murphy, J., McSharry, J., Hynes, L., Matthews, S., Van Rhoon, L., & Molloy, G. J. (2021). Prevalence and predictors of adherence to inhaled corticosteroids in young adults (15–30 years) with asthma: a systematic review and meta-analysis. *Journal of Asthma*, *58*(5), 683–705. https://doi.org/10.1080/02770903.2020.1711916

Murphy, J., McSharry, J., Hynes, L., & Molloy, G. J. (2022). Benefits and Challenges of Evaluating an Existing, Commercially Available Digital Health Intervention: a Self-Management Application for Asthma. ICCHP-AAATE 2022 Open Access Compendium" Assistive Technology, Accessibility and (e) Inclusion" Part II. https://doi.org/10.35011/icchp-aaate22-p2-28

Muth, C., Uhlmann, L., Haefeli, W. E., Rochon, J., van den Akker, M., Perera, R., … Harder, S. (2018). Effectiveness of a complex intervention on Prioritising Multimedication in Multimorbidity (PRIMUM) in primary care: results of a pragmatic cluster randomised controlled trial. *BMJ Open*, *8*(2), e017740.

Nieuwlaat, R., Wilczynski, N., Navarro, T., Hobson, N., Jeffery, R., Keepanasseril, A., … Haynes, R. B. (2014). Interventions for enhancing medication adherence. *Cochrane Database of Systematic Reviews, (11)*. https://doi.org/10.1002/14651858.CD000011.pub4

O'Carroll, R. E., Chambers, J. A., Dennis, M., Sudlow, C., & Johnston, M. (2013b). Improving adherence to medication in stroke survivors: a pilot randomised controlled trial. *Annals of Behavioral Medicine*, *46*(3), 358–368. https://doi.org/10.1007/s12160-013-9515-5

Palacio, A., Garay, D., Langer, B., Taylor, J., Wood, B. A., & Tamariz, L. (2016). Motivational interviewing improves medication adherence: a systematic review and meta-analysis. *Journal of General Internal Medicine*, *31*, 929–940. https://doi.org/10.1007/s11606-016-3685-3

Parati, G., Kjeldsen, S., Coca, A., Cushman, W. C., & Wang, J. (2021). Adherence to single-pill versus free-equivalent combination therapy in hypertension: a systematic review and meta-analysis. *Hypertension*, *77*(2), 692–705.

Park, L. G., Howie-Esquivel, J., & Dracup, K. (2015). Electronic measurement of medication adherence. *Western Journal of Nursing Research*, *37*(1), 28–49. https://doi.org/10.1177/0193945914524492

Pednekar, P., Ágh, T., Malmenäs, M., Raval, A., Bennett, B., Borah, B., Hutchins, D., Manias, E., Williams, A., Hiligsmann, M., Turcu-Stiolica, A., Zeber, J., Abrahamyan, L., Bunz, T., & Peterson, A. (2019). Methods for measuring multiple medication adherence: A systematic review – report of the ISPOR medication adherence and persistence special interest group. *Value Health*, *22*(2), 139–156. https://doi.org/10.1016/j.jval.2018.08.006

Peh, K. Q. E., Kwan, Y. H., Goh, H., Ramchandani, H., Phang, J. K., Lim, Z. Y., … & Thumboo, J. (2021). An adaptable framework for factors contributing to medication adherence: results from a systematic review of 102 conceptual frameworks. *Journal of General Internal Medicine*, *36*, 2784–2795. https://doi.org/10.3390/asi1020014

Pharo, H., Sim, C., Graham, M., Gross, J., & Hayne, H. (2011). Risky business: executive function, personality, and reckless behavior during adolescence and emerging adulthood. *Behavioral Neuroscience*, *125*(6), 970–978. https://doi.org/10.1037/a0025768

Phillips, L. A., Diefenbach, M. A., Kronish, I. M., Negron, R. M., & Horowitz, C. R. (2014). The necessity-concerns framework: a multidimensional theory benefits from multidimensional analysis. *Annals of Behavioral Medicine*, *48*(1), 7–16. https://doi.org/10.1007/s12160-013-9579-2

Rand, C. S., & Sevick, M. A. (2000). Ethics in adherence promotion and monitoring. *Controlled Clinical Trials*, *21*(5, Supplement 1), S241–S247. https://doi.org/10.1016/S0197-2456(00)00085-4

Robinson, L., Arden, M. A., Dawson, S., Walters, S. J., Wildman, M. J., & Stevenson, M. (2022). A machine-learning assisted review of the use of habit formation in medication adherence interventions for long-term conditions. *Health Psychology Review*, 1–23. https://doi.org/10.1080/17437199.2022.2034516

Rosbach, M., & Andersen, J. S. (2017). Patient-experienced burden of treatment in patients with multimorbidity – a systematic review of qualitative data. *PLoS ONE*, *12*(6), e0179916. https://doi.org/10.1371/journal.pone.0179916

Sabaté, E. (2003). *Adherence to long-term therapies: Evidence for action*. World Health Organization. http://www.who.int/chronic_conditions/en/adherence_report.pdf

Sackett, D., Gibson, E., Taylor, D. W., Haynes, R. B., Hackett, B., Roberts, R., & Johnson, A. (1975). Randomised clinical trial of strategies for improving medication compliance in primary hypertension. *The Lancet*, *305*(7918), 1205–1207. https://doi.org/10.1016/S0140-6736(75)92192-3

Schoenwald, S. K., & Garland, A. F. (2013). A review of treatment adherence measurement methods. *Psychological Assessment*, *25*, 146–156. https://doi.org/10.1037/a0029715

Sinnott, C., & Bradley, C. P. (2015). Multimorbidity or polypharmacy: Two sides of the same coin? *Journal of Comorbidity*, *5*, 29–31. https://doi.org/10.15256/joc.2015.5.51

Stewart, S. J. F., Moon, Z., & Horne, R. (2023b). Medication nonadherence: health impact, prevalence, correlates and interventions. *Psychology & Health*, *38*, 726–765. https://doi.org/10.1080/08870446.2022.2144923

Stirratt, M. J., Dunbar-Jacob, J., Crane, H. M., Simoni, J. M., Czajkowski, S., Hilliard, M. E., Aikens, J. E., Hunter, C. M., Velligan, D. I., Huntley, K., Ogedegbe, G., Rand, C. S., Schron, E., & Nilsen, W. J. (2015). Self-report measures of medication adherence behavior: Recommendations on optimal use. *Translational Behavioral Medicine*, *5*(4), 470–482. https://doi.org/10.1007/s13142-015-0315-2

Thakkar, J., Kurup, R., Laba, T. L., Santo, K., Thiagalingam, A., Rodgers, A., … & Chow, C. K. (2016). Mobile telephone text messaging for medication adherence in chronic disease: a meta-analysis. *JAMA Internal Medicine*, *176*(3), 340–349. https://doi.org/10.1001/jamainternmed.2015.7667

Valin, M., Meunier, J., St-Arnaud, A., & Rousseau, J. (2006, August). Video surveillance of medication intake. In *2006 international conference of the IEEE engineering in medicine and biology society*, 6396–6399. https://doi.org/10.3390/asi1020014

Vrijens, B., De Geest, S., Hughes, D. A., Przemyslaw, K., Demonceau, J., Ruppar, T., … ABC Project Team. (2012). A new taxonomy for describing and defining adherence to medications. *British Journal of Clinical Pharmacology*, *73*(5), 691–705. https://doi.org/10.1111/j.1365-2125.2012.04167.x

Vrijens, B., Vincze, G., Kristanto, P., Urquhart, J., & Burnier, M. (2008). Adherence to prescribed antihypertensive drug treatments: longitudinal study of electronically compiled dosing histories. *BMJ*, *336*(7653), 1114–1117. https://doi.org/10.1136/bmj.39553.670231.25

Walsh, C. A., Bennett, K. E., Wallace, E., & Cahir, C. (2020). Identifying adherence patterns across multiple medications and their association with health outcomes in older community-dwelling adults with multimorbidity. *Value in Health*, *23*(8), 1063–1071. https://doi.org/10.1016/j.jval.2020.03.016

SECTION 4

Interpersonal Relations and Health

16

INTERPERSONAL RELATIONSHIPS AND HEALTH

Mariët Hagedoorn and Noa Vilchinsky

Introduction

John was a 60-year-old retired accountant who had always lived a sedentary lifestyle. He enjoyed spending most of his days reading and watching television, rarely engaging in physical activity. Despite his wife's frequent suggestions to start exercising, he always found excuses to avoid it. One afternoon, while sitting in his armchair watching TV, John suddenly felt a sharp pain in his chest that radiated to his left arm. He knew something was wrong but hesitated to call his wife, Sarah, who was out running errands. He thought he could handle it himself and didn't want to bother her. But the pain persisted, and John started feeling dizzy and short of breath. He realised that he was having a heart attack and quickly called Sarah, who immediately rushed home and called an ambulance. During the ride to the hospital, Sarah held John's hand tightly, offering him emotional support and reassurance. Upon arrival at the hospital, John was taken to the emergency room, where the medical team took over. Sarah stayed by his side, waiting anxiously for updates and asking questions to better understand John's condition. After John was stabilised and moved to the cardiac care unit, Sarah spent most of her time at the hospital, keeping John company and providing him with emotional support. She brought him his favourite books, crossword puzzles, and magazines to keep him entertained and distracted him from his health condition. Throughout his recovery, John was able to rely on Sarah and his family for support. They played a crucial role in his rehabilitation by accompanying him to all of his appointments, helping him to adhere to his rehabilitation plan, and encouraging him to stay positive and motivated. This was not always easy for Sarah because taking care of John in combination with her work was quite stressful. Nevertheless, the

DOI: 10.4324/9781003318026-20

experience brought John and Sarah closer together, as they both realised how much they relied on each other but also their family members and the medical staff in managing their health. John and Sarah had much trust in the medical staff. The physician took the time to explain John's condition, the consequences, and the lifestyle changes needed, but also to answer their questions and to carefully listen to their worries and concerns. John started taking his health seriously, implementing lifestyle changes such as regular exercise and a healthier diet, again with Sarah's support and encouragement. John gradually started to feel better and healthier, but he and Sarah worried about their intimate relationship. They could not enjoy their sexual life as before because they feared that sexual activity could cause another heart attack. Their physician advised counselling, which helped to resume a satisfying sexual relationship. Though John's health condition had a considerable impact on their lives, their relationship grew stronger, and they both felt grateful for each other's presence in their lives.

This common story, based on our patients' testimonies, illustrates how coping with illness, from its inception and beyond, is intertwined with interpersonal relationships. "No man is an island", and most of us cope with illnesses within countless social circles and different interpersonal relationships, ranging from our closest family members to our extended family, friends, peers, co-workers, employers, and health-care professionals. Therefore, to understand how an individual copes with illness, we must understand how these relationships may contribute to and hinder a person's coping efforts and health outcomes. This book section will elaborate on three types of relationships – that is, the connection with an intimate partner (Chapters 17 and 18), the bond with an informal caregiver (Chapter 19), and the interaction with health-care professionals (Chapter 20). Trust in relationships is established early on in life through attachment processes. John and Sarah showed much trust in their relationships and relied on each other and their close ones for support, but what happens if one is low in trust and does not want, or does not feel able, to rely on others? Chapter 17 focuses on the role of attachment in romantic couples dealing with health issues. John and Sarah coped as a couple rather than as two individuals, also with sexual concerns as a consequence of John's condition. What impact may illness have on sexuality, and how should patients deal with this? Chapter 18 focuses on dyadic coping with sexual challenges that patients and their partners may experience. Sarah did not hesitate to take care of John, but at times this was stressful. Why do people (not) take care of their loved ones with an illness, and how does this influence their relationship? Chapter 19 addresses the caregiving relationship in the context of illness. John and Sarah had a good relationship with the medical staff. Chapter 20 describes the importance of interpersonal interactions between patients and their health-care professionals for dealing with illness and how to establish a good relationship. Many theories have been developed to further our understanding of the complex effects of interpersonal relationships on people's lives and specifically on their adjustment to illnesses and health issues. We will next describe a number of these theories to lay the foundation for the chapters in this book section.

Attachment Theory

"A child seeks his attachment figure when he is tired, hungry, ill or alarmed."
(John Bowlby, 1969, p. 307)

According to attachment theory, we are predisposed to turn to a relevant attachment figure to seek reassurance and help in regulating our emotions when we are in distress (Bowlby, 1969). Our attachment patterns that are established during childhood are also influential in our later relationships (Mikulincer & Shaver, 2016) with our intimate partners, as well as family caregivers and health-care professionals. Early experiences with attachment figures, who are usually our parents or primary caregivers, shape our attachment orientation. During infancy, when children are not yet regulated emotionally, their attachment system is automatically activated for the purpose of bringing and keeping their attachment figure close and gaining their support. Children whose parents are supportive in a responsive and adequate way learn that support is available and, over time, develop a sense of safety in their relationships. In other words, they develop a secure attachment orientation. However, when the parents fail to offer the needed support, children learn over the course of time that support is not usually available or helpful and tend to develop less-adaptive strategies to regulate their own emotions (Mikulincer & Shaver, 2019). These strategies usually take the shape of two main insecure attachment orientations – that is, attachment anxiety and attachment avoidance (Mikulincer & Shaver, 2018). The attachment systems of people who are high in attachment anxiety tend to hyper-activate in times of threat. These individuals are preoccupied with relational cues due to a lack of consistency in the caregiving they received as children; they therefore tend to focus on cues of rejection and abandonment. Conversely, the attachment systems of people who are high in attachment avoidance tend to deactivate in the face of threat. These individuals tend to rely only on themselves, having learned that support from others is not to be expected. For the same reason, they tend to inflate their own self-views and shy away from emotional intimacy. Securely attached individuals tend to have healthier and more satisfying relationships, while those who are less securely attached may struggle with intimacy and have poorer health outcomes (Bowlby, 1969).

In line with attachment theory, research has shown that more securely attached individuals perceived support to be more available to them and felt more satisfaction with the support they received (McLeod, Berry, Hodgson, & Wearden, 2020). Specifically, more securely attached individuals were found to provide more effective caregiving, while highly anxiously attached individuals showed more compulsive and controlling forms of caregiving, and individuals high on avoidance attachment showed more unresponsive and controlling forms of caregiving (Feeney & Collins, 2001). With respect to relationships with health-care professionals, it has been shown that patients who were more securely attached reported more trust in and satisfaction with their physician than patients who were less insecurely attached (Holwerda et al., 2013).

Thus, when confronted with illness, peoples' attachment orientations are considered to play a crucial role in their adaptation process. Several chapters in this section refer to attachment theory, either in the context of relationships between intimate partners (Chapter 17), caregivers and care recipients (Chapter 19), or health-care professionals and patients (Chapter 20). In Chapter 17, there is a central role for attachment theory. More specifically, in this chapter, Paula R. Pietromonaco and Nickola C. Overall describe how dyadic attachment processes may contribute to adjustment of couples coping with illness. Drawing on their own work and the work of others, they provide an overview of the effects of individuals' own and their partners' romantic attachment security/insecurity on relational, psychological, and physical well-being of both partners. Specific attention is paid to the potential behavioural and physiological pathways underlying these effects. The authors also discuss future directions and practical applications of the knowledge.

Dyadic Coping

The dyadic coping framework describes how members of a couple manage stress and cope with challenges together rather than as individuals (e.g., Berg & Upchurch, 2007b; Bodenmann, 1995; DeLongis & O'Brien, 1990; Revenson, Kayser & Bodenmann, 2005). There are several different dyadic coping models and approaches that all focus on interpersonal processes, including within-couple stress communication, responding to each other's distress and coping behaviours, and collaboration with couples (for an overview, see Falconier & Kuhn, 2019b). What these models and approaches have in common is that they focus on the dyad (i.e., the couple) rather than the individual and examine outcomes of the dyadic coping processes for both members of the couple and their relationship. The basis of dyadic coping approaches is that a threat, such as an illness diagnosis, has an impact on both members of the couple and is often considered a shared rather than a personal problem. Effective dyadic coping includes strategies such as collaboration, joint problem-solving, and mutual responsiveness, while ineffective dyadic coping includes withdrawal, criticising, and protective buffering of one or both partners. In line with this, research has shown that strategies such as joint problem-solving are associated with better individual and relationship outcomes, including lower levels of stress, improved mental health, and higher relationship satisfaction. In contrast, strategies such as withdrawal and protective buffering were related to negative outcomes in both partners (e.g., Berg & Upchurch, 2007b; Falconier & Kuhn, 2019).

Communication plays a key role in dyadic coping. Partners need to know each other's worries and needs, for example, to be able to provide adequate support to their anxious partner or to decide on treatment options and care planning together. Research findings do not conclusively show that self-disclosure is beneficial in terms of decreasing depressed mood, as it depends, among others, on the partner's responsiveness (e.g., showing understanding and validation) and personal characteristics (e.g., attachment orientation and personal need to share emotions). Research did show that avoiding communication (e.g., protective buffering and holding back) was associated with worse emotional and relational well-being (Hasson-Ohayon et al., 2022).

Overall, dyadic coping models and approaches highlight the importance of a shared approach to coping with stress and illness within couples. By working together and providing mutual support, couples can better manage stress, find solutions for challenges and problems, and maintain healthy relationships. After an illness diagnosis, dealing with sexual challenges is one dyadic coping task that couples are often confronted with. Chapter 18 by Chiara Acquati illustrates the consequences of several prevalent illnesses on sexuality, intimacy, and well-being of couples. She also highlights interpersonal processes and dyadic coping strategies that contribute to sexual well-being and presents assessment models and psychological interventions that have been developed to address these issues.

Caregiving and Relationships

A substantial number of people confronted with illness or disability need more than occasional social support to deal with the consequences of their condition. In these situations, family members often take on the role of informal caregivers. These family members provide care and support that is above and beyond what is typical within the particular relationship, and they often do so over an extended period of time (Revenson et al., 2016b). As a consequence, the caregiver and the care recipient may feel that their relationship is out of balance. Equity theory posits that relationships are based on a cost-benefit analysis, where individuals seek balance (i.e., equity) between their investments and benefits in the relationship as compared to the investments and benefits of their partner (VanYperen & Buunk, 1990; Walster & Berscheid, 1973). For example, benefits can include companionship, emotional support, status, and material resources, while investments may include time, effort, and emotional strain. An inequitable relationship is theorised to cause distress and relationship dissatisfaction. Although partners (cq. caregivers) seem to understand and accept that patients are less able to reciprocate their investments in the relationship (Kuijer, Buunk, & Ybema, 2001), research showed that patients who felt that they underinvested in their relationship reported more depressive symptoms and burden (Beattie et al., 2017; Ybema et al., 2001) and caregivers of patients who felt underbenefit in their relationship did report more burden (Beattie et al., 2017). Collaborative dyadic coping may be a solution to reduce the potential negative consequences of unidirectional support.

Traditional caregiver models (e.g., the stress-coping model of Lazarus and Folkman, 1984; the caregiver stress process model of Pearlin et al., 1990; the caregiver stress and appraisal model of Yates et al., 1999) have an individual focus, conceptualising caregiving as a potential stressor that may result in perceived burden and distress in caregivers depending on their coping resources and strategies. Building on these caregiver models and dyadic coping models, Revenson et al. (2016b) have suggested an integrative framework for the caregiving process that conceptualises caregiving as a dyadic interpersonal interaction between the caregiver and the care recipient in a dynamic, sociocultural context that develops over time.

In Chapter 19, Val Morrison provides a comprehensive overview of caregiving and relationships. After describing the background and context of caregiving, she provides an overview of motives and willingness to provide care to a close one with an illness or disability. Why do people provide care, and what factors play a role in the willingness to provide care? Next, the chapter focuses on relational influences on caregiving, and influences of caregiving on relationships.

Patient-Provider Relationship

In the illness context, not only is the relationship between patients and their family/informal caregivers important for their health and well-being but the relationships with health-care professionals also play a crucial role. Literature reviews have shown that communication with one's health-care provider is key in making treatment choices, adherence to treatment, and psychosocial adaptation of patients (Lie et al., 2022; Zolnierek & Dimatteo, 2009). Patients need information, for example, about their symptoms, their treatment options, and the potential side effects of treatment. What could be the consequences of their illness and its treatment for daily life, for example, in terms of cognitive functioning, fatigue, and sexual functioning and intimacy (see also Chapter 18)? To make shared decisions, doctors need to know about the needs, values, goals, and preferences of their patients. Discussing serious illness with the health-care professional can be quite upsetting for patients and families, and may also be stressful for doctors if they do not feel competent in dealing with the emotions and fears of patients and families and/or their own emotions during such conversations. Yet, being able and encouraged to express emotions during a consultation may promote trust towards the health-care professional and facilitate understanding and decision-making in patients (Street et al., 2009). Patients appear to be more confident to share information if they perceive their doctor to communicate with empathy (Broadbridge et al., 2023). In other words, health-care professionals need to establish a relationship with their patients based on trust and communicate in an empathic way to promote information sharing and shared decision-making.

In Chapter 20, Arnstein Finset describes what is known about communication processes between patients and health-care professionals and how these can be optimised to promote health and well-being, for example, via understanding medical information, meeting psychosocial needs, and encouraging adaptive self-management.

Conclusion

In this chapter, we have stressed the importance of relationships in dealing with illness and introduced a number of theories and approaches that have guided research in this area. Relationships and social support have been extensively studied in the context of psychology and health. This research field started from an individual approach, examining perceived or received support in relation to well-being. Individuals who perceive or receive more support when confronted with illness generally show less distress and anxiety (e.g., Helgeson & Cohen, 1996) and better illness self-management (e.g., Gallant, 2003). These findings are important but provide limited insight into the dynamics of the exchange of support between individuals. Therefore, in contemporary studies, we see more focus on other relevant issues, such as the psycho-neurological predisposition towards bonding and attachment, the support and coping processes and effects occurring at the dyadic level rather than the individual level, and the contribution of caregivers and health-care professionals to patients' coping. As outlined earlier, the different chapters in this section focus on theories and empirical findings concerning these multifaceted issues while also describing future directions, practical implications, and interventions.

Further Reading

Berg, C. A., & Upchurch, R. (2007). A developmental-contextual model of couples with chronic illness across the adult life span. *Psychological Bulletin*, 133(6), 920–954. doi:10.1037/0033-2909.133.6.920

Falconier, M. K., & Kuhn, R. (2019). Dyadic coping in couples: A conceptual integration and a review of the empirical literature. *Frontiers in Psychology*, *10*. doi:10.3389/fpsyg.2019.00571

Revenson, T. A., Griva, K. G., Luszczynska, A, Morrison, V., Panagopoulou, E., Vilchinsky, N., & Hagedoorn, M. (2016). *Caregiving in the illness context*. Basingstoke: Palgrave Macmillan. doi:10.1057/9781137558985.0006

References

Beattie, S., Lebel, S., Petricone, D., Wilson, K. G., Harris, C., Devins, G., Huebsch, L., & Tay, J. (2017). Balancing give and take between patients and their spousal caregivers in hematopoietic stem cell transplantation. *Psycho-Oncology*, *26*, 2224–2231. doi:10.1002/pon.4340

Berg, C. A., & Upchurch, R. (2007b). A developmental-contextual model of couples with chronic illness across the adult life span. *Psychological Bulletin*, *133*(6), 920–954. doi:10.1037/0033-2909.133.6.920

Bodenmann, G. (1995). A systemic-transactional conceptualization of stress and coping in couples. *Swiss Journal of Psychology*, *54*(2), 34–4.

Bowlby, J. (1969). *Attachment and loss: Vol. I: Attachment* (2nd ed.). Basic Books. (Original work published 1969).

Broadbridge, E., Greene, K., Venetis, M. K., Lee, L. E., Banerjee, S. C., de Meritens, A. B., Catona, D., & Devine, K. A. (2023). The influence of perceived provider empathic communication on disclosure decision-making. *Health Communication*. doi:10.1080/10410236.2023.2243409

DeLongis, A., & O'Brien, T. (1990). An interpersonal framework for stress and coping: An application to the families of Alzheimer's patients. In M. A. P. Stephens, J. H. Crowther, S. E. Hobfoll, & D. L. Tennenbaum (Eds.), *Stress and coping in later-life families* (pp. 221–239). Hemisphere Publishing Corp.

Falconier, M. K., & Kuhn, R. (2019b). Dyadic coping in couples: A conceptual integration and a review of the empirical literature. *Frontiers in Psychology*, *10*. doi:10.3389/fpsyg.2019.00571

Feeney, B. C., & Collins, N. L. (2001). Predictors of caregiving in adult intimate relationships: An attachment theoretical perspective. *Journal of Personality and Social Psychology*, *80*(6), 972–994. doi:10.1037/0022-3514.80.6.972

Gallant, M. P. (2003). The influence of social support on chronic illness self-management: A review and directions for research. *Health Education and Behavior*, *30*(2), 170–195. doi:10.1177/1090198102251030

Hasson-Ohayon, I., Goldzweig, G., Braun, M., & Hagedoorn, M. (2022). Beyond "being open about it": A systematic review on cancer related communication within couples. *Clinical Psychology Review, 96*, 102176.

Helgeson, V. S., & Cohen S. (1996). Social support and adjustment to cancer: Reconciling descriptive, correlational and intervention research. *Health Psychology, 15*(2), 135–148. doi:10.1037/0278-6133.15.2.135

Holwerda, N., Sanderman, R., Pool, G., Hinnen, C., Langendijk, J. A., Bemelman, W. A., Hagedoorn, M., & Sprangers, M. A. G. (2013). Do patients trust their physician? The role of attachment style in the patient-physician relationship within one year after cancer diagnosis. *Acta Oncologica, 52*(1), 110–117. doi:10.3109/0284186X.2012.689856

Kuijer, R., Buunk, B., & Ybema, J. (2001). Are equity concerns important in the intimate relationship when one partner of a couple has cancer? *Social Psychology Quarterly, 64*(3), 267–282. doi:10.2307309011 6

Lazarus, R. S., & Folkman, S. (1984). *Stress, appraisal, and coping*. New York: Springer.

Lie, H. C., Juvet, L. K., Street, R. L., Jr., Gulbrandsen, P., Mellblom, A. V., Brembo, E. A., … Menichetti, J. (2022). Effects of physicians' information giving on patient outcomes: A systematic review. *Journal of General Internal Medicine, 37*(3), 651–663. doi:10.1007/s11606-021-07044-5

McLeod, S., Berry, K., Hodgson, C., & Wearden, A. (2020). Attachment and social support in romantic dyads: A systematic review. *Journal of Clinical Psychology, 76*(1), 59–101. doi:10.1002/jclp.22868

Mikulincer, M., & Shaver, P. (2016). *Attachment in Adulthood*. Guilford Press.

Mikulincer, M., & Shaver, P. R. (2018). Attachment theory as a framework for studying relationship dynamics and functioning. In *The Cambridge handbook of personal relationships* (pp. 175–185). Cambridge University Press. doi:10.1017/9781316417867.015

Mikulincer, M., & Shaver, P. R. (2019). Attachment orientations and emotion regulation. *Current Opinion in Psychology, 25*, 6–10. doi:10.1016/j.copsyc.2018.02.006

Pearlin, L. I., Mullan, J. T., Semple, S. J., & Skaff, M. M. (1990). Caregiving and the stress process: An overview of concepts and their measures. *The Gerontologist, 30*(5), 583–594. doi:10.1093/geront/30.5/583

Revenson, T. A., Griva, K. G., Luszczynska, A, Morrison, V., Panagopoulou, E., Vilchinsky, N., & Hagedoorn, M. (2016b). *Caregiving in the illness context*. Basingstoke: Palgrave Macmillan. doi:10.1057/9781137558985.0006

Revenson, T. A., Kayser, K., & Bodenmann, G. (Eds.) (2005). *Couples coping with stress: Emerging perspectives on dyadic coping*. American Psychological Association. doi:10.1037/11031-000

Street, R. L., Makoul, G., Arora, N. K., & Epstein, R. M. (2009). How does communication heal? Pathways linking clinician–patient communication to health outcomes. Patient *Education and Counseling, 74*(3), 295–301. doi:10.1016/j.pec.2008.11.015

VanYperen, N., & Buunk, B. (1990). A longitudinal study of equity and satisfaction in intimate relationships. *European Journal of Social Psychology 20*(4), 287–309. doi:10.1002/ejsp.2420200403

Walster, E., & Berscheid, E. (1973). New directions in equity research. *Journal of Personality and Social Psychology, 25*(2), 151–176. doi:10.1037/h0033967

Yates, M. E., Tennstedt, S., & Chang, B. A. (1999). Contributors to and mediators of psychological well-being for informal caregivers. *The Journals of Gerontology Series B: Psychological Sciences and Social Sciences, 54*(1), 12–22. doi:10.1093/geronb/54B.1.12P

Ybema, J., Kuijer, R., Buunk, B., DeJong, G., & Sanderman, R. (2001). Depression and perceptions of inequity among couples facing cancer. *Personality and Social Psychology Bulletin, 27*(1), 3–13. doi:10.1177/0146167201271001

Zolnierek, K. B. H., & Dimatteo, M. R. (2009). Physician communication and patient adherence to treatment. A meta-analysis. *Medical Care, 47*(8), 826–834. doi:10.1097/MLR.0B013E31819A5ACC

17

ATTACHMENT INSECURITY SHAPES PHYSIOLOGICAL AND BEHAVIOURAL RESPONSES TO STRESS

Implications for Couples Coping with Illness

Paula R. Pietromonaco and Nickola C. Overall

Introduction

High-quality close relationships predict better health and quality of life among those with a serious illness such as heart disease or cancer (Umberson & Montez, 2010). Poor marital quality, in contrast, is associated with risks for heart disease (e.g., coronary artery calcification) and worse health (e.g., increased mortality risk, slower wound healing; Robles et al., 2014), and contributes to disease as much as well-known risk factors (e.g., smoking, BMI, exercise; Holt-Lunstad et al., 2010). As emphasised by adult attachment theory, the links between relationship quality and health outcomes likely arise because romantic partners play a central role in regulating responses to stress (Mikulincer & Shaver, 2017), including within the context of chronic illness. Moreover, chronic illness impacts not only patients but also their romantic partners (Helgeson et al., 2018; Revenson & DeLongis, 2011). The current chapter evaluates how dyadic attachment processes may contribute to adjustment of couples coping with illness. A theoretical framework is presented to outline the effects of individuals' own and their partners' romantic attachment insecurity on both patients with chronic illness and their caregiving partners, and evidence is reviewed from research on couples in general and available research within the illness context. The final discussion highlights key directions for future research applying an attachment perspective to understand couples' adjustment when coping with illness.

 DOI: 10.4324/9781003318026-21

Theoretical Framework

Attachment theory is a broad framework for understanding why humans form close bonds with each other (e.g., Bowlby, 1969, 1973). Bowlby's theory originally focused on understanding bonds between infants and their caregivers, but groundbreaking extensions highlight parallels in the bonds between infants and caregivers and romantic partners (Hazan & Shaver, 1987; Mikulincer & Shaver, 2017). Just as infants turn to their caregivers for comfort and reassurance when they are distressed (Bowlby, 1973; Sroufe & Waters, 1977), adult romantic partners may turn to each other for help with managing and regulating their distress (Mikulincer & Shaver, 2017; Pietromonaco & Beck, 2015). Threatening situations activate the attachment system, which typically motivates people to seek comfort and support from attachment figures (e.g., romantic partner; Mikulincer & Shaver, 2017). Whether and how people seek or give care varies depending on attachment security/insecurity, which evolves from day-to-day experiences with attachment figures from childhood through adulthood (see Pietromonaco & Beck, 2015). People higher in *anxious attachment* worry that romantic partners will be unavailable, resulting in hyperactivation of the attachment system in threatening situations (i.e., heightened distress, desire for physical proximity, reassurance seeking). In contrast, people higher in *avoidance* expect that partners will be non-responsive and thus avoid depending on others, resulting in hypoactivation in threatening contexts (i.e., downplaying distress to avoid dependence, distancing from the partner, and excessive self-reliance). People higher in attachment security (low in both anxiety and avoidance) expect partners will be responsive, rely on partners when needed, and flexibly cope within threatening contexts.

Attachment security/insecurity shapes individuals' own and their partner's behaviour and physiological responses to stress and therefore has considerable relevance for understanding couples facing chronic illness (Pietromonaco et al., 2013). Figure 17.1 illustrates these dyadic processes for individuals and their partners (i.e., spouses, cohabiting partners, dating partners). Individuals' own attachment security/insecurity can shape their behavioural and physiological responses (Figure 17.1, Path A), and these variables can contribute to their adjustment and coping (e.g., psychological well-being, physical symptoms; Path B). Individuals will also be affected by their partner's attachment security/insecurity, which will influence individuals' behaviour and physiological responses within couples' interactions (Paths C), and in turn, individuals' adjustment and coping (Paths B). Other paths (e.g., Path D) are possible, but we focus on paths linked to individuals' own and their partner's attachment security/insecurity.

Attachment Security/Insecurity and Behavioural Responses to Threat

As Figure 17.1 illustrates, attachment security vs. insecurity is associated with adaptive (e.g., effective problem-solving, responsive support) vs. maladaptive (e.g., hostility, distancing) behaviour patterns that have implications for the

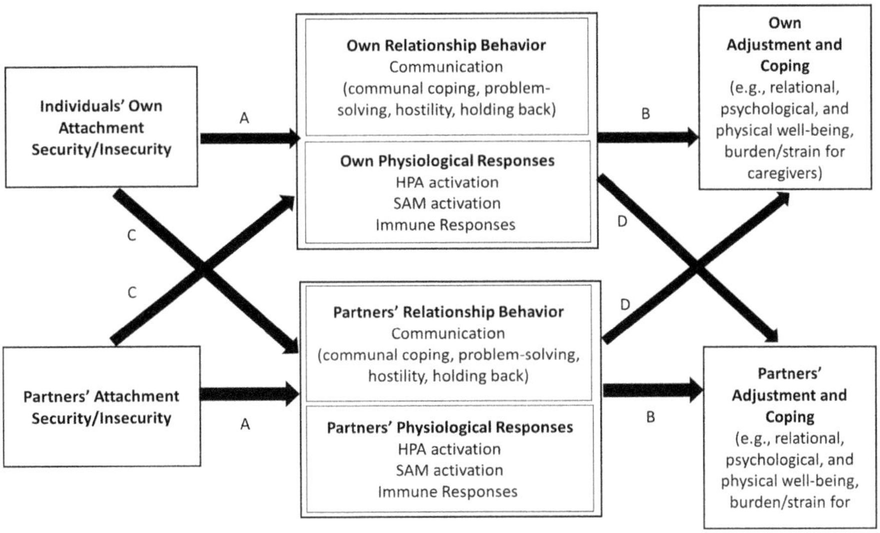

Figure 17.1 The effects of individuals' own and their partners' attachment security/insecurity on behaviour, physiological responses, and adjustment and coping.

Note: Possible paths that do not include attachment security/insecurity (e.g., between individuals' and partners' coping or individuals' behaviour and physiological responses) are not shown. HPA = hypothalamic-pituitary-adrenal; SAM = sympathetic-adrenal-medullary

psychological and physical well-being of couples' coping with illness. Across studies of couples in general as well as couples coping with illness, the findings generally indicate that both individuals' own and partners' attachment anxiety and avoidance likely promote problematic relationship behaviour (e.g., more hostility, poorer problem-solving), which in turn, undermines adjustment and coping.

Effect of Own Attachment on Own Behaviour and Adjustment (Paths A and B)

Attachment anxiety and avoidance disrupt relationship functioning via maladaptive behaviour patterns arising under stress (Paths A and B; Overall et al., 2022b). Likely due to emotional reactivity, attachment anxiety promotes destructive communication (e.g., amplified negative emotional expressions), impaired problem-solving, and poorer caregiving and careseeking (Jayamaha et al., 2017; Overall et al., 2014; Simpson et al., 1996). Likely due to avoidance of dependence, attachment avoidance is associated with less effective support, and withdrawal and hostility during conflict (Beck et al., 2014; Girme et al., 2015; Overall et al., 2013, 2015; Pietromonaco & Barrett, 1997). These processes undermine relationship quality (Overall et al., 2013, 2015) and contribute to poorer coping within stressful interactions (Path B; Mikulincer & Shaver, 2017).

Behavioural processes observed among couples in general are evident in couples coping with chronic illness and linked to their well-being (Crangle et al., 2020; Crangle & Hart, 2017; Karantzas & Gillath, 2017b; Porter et al., 2012). Both patients' and their partners' own attachment security/insecurity have been associated with poorer communication (Path A). In couples coping with cancer, both patients and partners higher in attachment anxiety evidenced more observer-coded negative affect and negative approach behaviour (e.g., blame, contempt) during cancer-related discussions, and individuals higher in avoidance showed more negative approach behaviour and less positive affect (Ramos et al., 2023). Among women with breast cancer (but not their partners), attachment anxiety predicted more overt criticism observed as participants talked about their partner and relationship (Favez et al., 2017).

These behavioural difficulties undermine relationship quality as well as poorer adjustment and coping (Path B). In couples coping with multiple sclerosis, both patients and partners higher in attachment anxiety or avoidance self-reported greater hostility during conflict and, in turn, lower relationship quality (Crangle & Hart, 2017). In couples coping with ovarian cancer, patients and partners higher in attachment anxiety or avoidance showed poorer dyadic coping (e.g., self-reported less effective problem-solving and collaboration) and, in turn, lower social well-being (Crangle et al., 2020). Furthermore, attachment anxiety and avoidance were associated with both greater self-reported holding back and disclosure during cancer-related discussions and, in turn, poorer physical well-being (Ramos et al., 2020). Among couples coping with lung cancer, patients' and partners' own higher attachment anxiety and particularly avoidance also predicted poorer psychological adjustment (e.g., anxiety symptoms, depression) and lower relationship quality (Porter et al., 2012). Finally, patients higher in avoidance reported lower relationship quality and greater distress when engaging in communal coping (e.g., viewing and discussing diabetes as a joint problem; Van Vleet & Helgeson, 2019), likely because they desire self-reliance and emotional distance.

Attachment anxiety and avoidance also disrupt support provision and relationship functioning for individuals in the caregiving role (Paths A and B). Caregivers' own higher attachment anxiety was associated with greater compulsive caregiving (i.e., overprotection, overinvolvement; Braun et al., 2012) as evident for couples in general (Feeney & Collins, 2001; Julal & Carnelley, 2012) and couples coping with type 1 diabetes (Helgeson et al., 2022). Anxious individuals' desire for excessive closeness may lead to overinvolvement in managing patients' illness, which may pose a risk for caregivers' emotional health, such as when more anxious partners of individuals diagnosed with ovarian cancer evidenced poorer dyadic coping behaviours and, in turn, lower social well-being (Crangle et al., 2020). By contrast, among couples facing metastatic cancer, caregivers higher in attachment avoidance evidenced less sensitive caregiving and greater discomfort with physical closeness during caregiving (Braun et al., 2012) and more difficulty providing emotional care (Kim & Carver, 2007).

Studies not assessing behaviour have found associations between caregivers' attachment insecurity and caregivers' adjustment, but as suggested by other work reviewed here (e.g., Crangle et al., 2020; Ramos et al., 2020), this link is likely mediated by their behaviour (Paths A and B). Caregivers higher in attachment anxiety or avoidance reported greater burden caring for their patients (e.g., spouse, relative), and for avoidant individuals, this burden was more pronounced when physically closer to the patient (Bei et al., 2022). Furthermore, anxiously attached caregivers of patients with cardiac disease who perceived greater caregiving burden experienced increased depressive symptoms over time (Vilchinsky et al., 2015), and more avoidant caregivers experienced greater strain from caregiving, more anger and depression, and lower marital quality (Porter et al., 2012).

Effect of Partner's Attachment on Individual's Behaviour and Adjustment (Paths C and D)

The partner's attachment insecurity also affects individuals' relationship behaviour (Path C), which in turn can impact individuals' adjustment and coping (Paths B). Individuals with anxiously attached spouses must manage excessive reassurance seeking and destructive behaviours, which leads to lower satisfaction and undermines individuals' ability to communicate effectively, resolve problems, and be responsive to their anxiously attached partner's needs (Carnelley et al., 1996; Overall et al., 2014). Individuals with avoidantly attached partners must contend with distancing and withdrawal, contributing to difficulties with communicating and problem-solving, as well as lower relationship satisfaction (Beck et al., 2013; Girme et al., 2015; Overall et al., 2013, 2015). Similarly, in patients coping with chronic illness, partners' higher attachment anxiety has been associated with individuals' poorer self-reported dyadic coping behaviours (e.g., poorer problem-solving, less collaboration) in patients with ovarian cancer and their spouses (Crangle et al., 2020) and, in turn, poorer social and functional well-being. Also, partner's higher attachment anxiety is associated with individuals' greater self-reported hostility during conflict and, in turn, lower relationship quality in patients with multiple sclerosis and their spouses (Crangle & Hart, 2017). Other work has shown that patients coping with cancer evidenced poorer physical well-being when their insecurely attached (anxious or avoidant) spouse self-reported either more holding back or disclosure during discussions related to cancer over the past week (Paths A and D; Ramos et al., 2020), and caregiving spouses' attachment anxiety or avoidance has been associated with poorer patient adjustment and well-being (Porter et al., 2012). Finally, patient and partner outcomes may be worse when both couple members are insecurely attached. Patients with lung cancer and their spouses showed poorer marital and psychological adjustment when both partners were insecurely (vs. securely) attached (Porter et al., 2012). Additionally, more anxiously attached patients with Alzheimer's disease experienced more physical and psychological symptoms, especially when their partner was also anxiously attached (Monin et al., 2013) and likely struggling to manage their own distress and provide care.

Summary

Both individuals' own as well as their partners' attachment security/insecurity impact behaviour and adjustment. Individuals' own attachment anxiety or avoidance is linked to more maladaptive behaviour, poorer adjustment, and, for caregivers, greater burden and strain (Paths A and B). Having a more insecurely attached partner also is associated with individuals' more destructive behaviour, and lower relational and psychological well-being for both patients and spouses (Paths C and D), although having an insecurely attached partner increases risk for poorer adjustment and well-being particularly for patients. For instance, a patient with a chronic illness who is high in attachment anxiety may excessively seek reassurance and support while also displaying greater hostility during conflict, making it difficult for their partners to respond in ways that will be reassuring and comforting and increasing the likelihood that their partners will express hostility in return.

Attachment theory suggests that anxiety and avoidance should be linked to distinct behaviours (Mikulincer & Shaver, 2017): attachment anxiety should evoke behaviours reflecting protest or excessive reassurance seeking, whereas avoidance should evoke behaviours promoting emotional distance and autonomy. Few behavioural patterns observed in the studies reviewed were unique to attachment anxiety or avoidance, but the same observed behaviour may be driven by different concerns. For example, hostility/blaming may reflect attempts to solicit the partner's attention and protest against unsatiated support needs for anxiously attached individuals but reflect attempts to distance from the partner and maintain autonomy for avoidantly attached individuals. Methodologies allowing for finer-grained distinctions among behaviours are needed.

Attachment Security/Insecurity and Physiological Responses to Threat

Physiological responses provide a window into less conscious, attachment-related affect regulation processes and are particularly important in the context of couples coping with illness because they have implications for emotional health and regulating health-relevant behaviour (Pietromonaco et al., 2015; Pietromonaco & Collins, 2017; Pietromonaco & Beck, 2019b). Few studies have examined links between attachment and health-related physiological responses among couples coping with illness, but research on couples in general suggests how these processes might apply in an illness context.

Effect of Own Attachment on Own Physiological Outcomes (Path A)

Most work examining romantic attachment and physiological responses has assessed cortisol levels, which reflect activity in the hypothalamic-pituitary-adrenal (HPA)—a major biological system activated in response to stress (Pietromonaco et al., 2015; Pietromonaco & Beck, 2019b; Pietromonaco &

Powers, 2015). Cortisol responses impact important health indicators such as inflammation (DeSantis et al., 2012), coronary artery calcification (Hamer et al., 2012), and depression (Ge et al., 2016). Consistent with anxious attachment triggering hyperactivation, greater attachment anxiety is associated with greater cortisol reactivity, or slower recovery, in response to stressful situations (Beck et al., 2013, 2023; Brooks et al., 2011; Meuwly et al., 2012; Powers et al., 2006), as well as atypical (less healthy) diurnal cortisol slopes (Jaremka, Glaser, Loving, et al., 2013; Kidd et al., 2013). Findings for attachment avoidance are more variable (Beck et al., 2013, 2023; Brooks et al., 2011; Kidd et al., 2013; Powers et al., 2006), possibly because, for less consciously controlled responses, avoidance may generate physiological hypoactivation (as typically seen for self-reported emotions) or hyperactivation. For instance, avoidant women showed greater cortisol reactivity in one study (Powers et al., 2006), but attachment avoidance was unassociated with cortisol reactivity in other studies (Brooks et al., 2011; Beck et al., 2023).

Other work has focused on the sympathetic-adrenal-medullary (SAM) system, associated with "fight-or-flight" responses (e.g., rapid heart rate) and assessed with electrodermal reactivity and cardiovascular reactivity (e.g., see Pietromonaco & Powers, 2015). When effects for SAM activation have been found for attachment anxiety, they have been consistent with hyperactivation (Feeney & Kirkpatrick, 1996; Kim, 2006). Attachment avoidance has also been associated with greater electrodermal reactivity in response to general stress (e.g., Diamond et al., 2006; Feeney & Kirkpatrick, 1996), but most findings within relational contexts are consistent with hypoactivation. Higher avoidance predicted lower electrodermal reactivity in the context of a relationship-relevant conflict discussion (Taylor et al., 2018) and dampened individuals' cardiovascular responses when suppressing (vs. expressing) emotions while discussing a distressing film with their partner (Peters et al., 2019). Similarly, avoidant individuals who reported greater stress showed cardiovascular patterns consistent with hypoactivation when discussing a relationship problem (Kim, 2006).

However, some studies have found no associations between anxiety or avoidance and SAM activation in relational contexts (Ben-Naim et al., 2013; Seedall & Wampler, 2012), which may result from contextual differences in couples' interactions. For instance, consistent with strong needs for reassurance, anxiously attached men showed greater decreases in cardiovascular arousal when receiving more emotional support during a couple interaction (Kordahji et al., 2015), and anxiously attached women showed lower electrodermal reactivity in discussions involving support for their issue (Lachmar & Seedall, 2018). Consistent with discomfort with dependence, avoidant individuals showed smaller decreases in cardiovascular arousal when receiving emotional support (Kordahji et al., 2015).

Emerging work has also shown that attachment anxiety and avoidance are associated with poorer immune functioning, which is closely tied to emotional and physical health (Jaremka, Lindgren, et al., 2013) and longitudinally predicted by marital distress (Jaremka, Glaser, Malarkey, et al., 2013). Individuals higher in attachment anxiety have shown disrupted immune responses, including fewer T-cells which facilitate adaptive immune responses (Jaremka, Glaser, Loving, et al., 2013), higher antibody titers to the Epstein-Barr virus, which reflect weaker immune control (Fagundes et al., 2014), slower wound healing (Robles et al., 2013), and a rise in Interleukin-6 (which is linked to inflammation) in patients following cardiac surgery (Kidd et al., 2014). Individuals higher in avoidance evidenced increased inflammation (indexed via interleukin-6) when they discussed a conflict with their spouse (Gouin et al., 2009), and women higher in attachment avoidance showed declines in immune functioning (indexed via natural killer cell cytotoxicity) over one-year (Picardi et al., 2013).

Effect of Partner's Attachment on Individuals' Physiological Outcomes (Path C)

Having a spouse/partner higher in anxiety or avoidance may also produce stronger physiological responses (e.g., cortisol reactivity, cardiovascular reactivity) in both patients and caregiving partners. Individuals interacting with anxiously attached spouses/partners may anticipate a greater need to reassure their partner, help regulate their heightened distress, and deal with destructive and hostile behaviour. Individuals interacting with avoidantly attached spouses/partners may anticipate the need to carefully modulate their responses (e.g., soften their responses, Overall et al., 2013) to prevent withdrawal or hostility.

Findings generally indicate that partners' attachment insecurity predicts individuals' heightened cortisol reactivity. Men with more anxious or avoidant dating partners showed greater cortisol reactivity (Powers et al., 2006), and women with more avoidant partners showed greater cortisol reactivity (Brooks et al., 2011). A study repeatedly assessing attachment insecurity and cortisol responses during early marriage illustrated that spouses' avoidance and (for wives) anxiety predict greater cortisol reactivity in anticipation of conflict discussions (Beck et al., 2023). Anxiously attached individuals specifically showed greater cortisol reactivity when their spouses were more avoidantly attached (Beck et al., 2023), perhaps because they anticipated their avoidant spouse would be insufficiently responsive during conflict.

Partners' attachment insecurity also predicts individuals' greater SAM reactivity. Individuals with more anxiously attached partners evidenced cardiovascular responses consistent with threat when anticipating discussing a distressing film (Peters et al., 2019) or a relationship disagreement (Ben-Naim et al., 2013) and greater electrodermal responses during conflict interactions (Seedall & Wampler, 2016). Findings for a partner's avoidance are less clear. Partners' greater attachment avoidance predicted individuals' greater cardiovascular threat responses when individuals were instructed to suppress their emotions while discussing a distressing film (Peters et al., 2019) but predicted lower cardiovascular reactivity during a conflict discussion, especially when individuals were instructed to suppress their emotions (Ben-Naim et al., 2013). However, paralleling findings examining greater cortisol reactivity (Beck et al., 2023), when partners were more avoidant, anxiously attached individuals showed greater electrodermal reactivity during a conflict discussion (Taylor et al., 2018).

Summary

In general, individuals' own attachment anxiety predicts heightened physiological responses to stress for cortisol, SAM-related responses, and disrupted immune functioning. Findings for individuals' own avoidance are inconsistent for cortisol reactivity but tend to show hypoactivation for SAM reactivity in relational contexts, consistent with suppressing negative emotions, along with disrupted immune functioning. Partners' attachment anxiety also predicts greater physiological reactivity (e.g., cortisol reactivity, cardiovascular reactivity), possibly because interactions with more anxious partners are more taxing (e.g., more effort is required to be responsive and to comfort anxiously attached partners). Although partners' attachment avoidance has less consistent effects, anxiously attached individuals show greater physiological reactivity to stress when their spouses/partners are more avoidant (Beck et al., 2013; Taylor et al., 2018). This pairing may be especially at risk for poorer adjustment because the two partners have opposing goals—anxious individuals' need for excessive reassurance vs. avoidant partners' need for distance—and thus may find it difficult to meet each other's needs. In the face of greater physiological reactivity, patients with chronic illnesses who are high in attachment anxiety will likely have trouble framing requests for support in ways that do not threaten their avoidant partners' need for autonomy and distrust of partners. As a result, it may be difficult for patients high in attachment anxiety to obtain the reassurance that they desire, and their partners may be more likely to feel burdened (e.g., see Overall et al., 2022b).

The effects of own and partners' attachment and health-related physiological responses have rarely been studied among patients and their partners, let alone whether attachment-related physiological responses subsequently predict adjustment. Yet stress-related physiological responses have been linked to psychological and physical well-being (Chida & Steptoe, 2010; Turner et al., 2020), and therefore, attachment-related physiological responses likely contribute to adjustment and coping in the context of illness for both patients and caregivers (Path B). Illustrating the importance of examining the effects discussed here in an illness context, one study found that when breast cancer survivors (patients) were more anxiously attached, their spouses showed less healthy (flatter) diurnal cortisol slopes (Hsiao et al., 2014).

Future Directions and Applications

Our dyadic attachment analysis reveals several key directions for future research. Research on couples coping with illness has primarily focused on links between attachment and self-reported communication patterns. Extending work to observed behaviour will provide broader assessments less affected by demand characteristics and global relationship perceptions (Heyman et al., 2014), and the potential to capture distinctions between anxious versus avoidant attachment (e.g., hostility in protest versus pushing partner away). Further work also needs to examine additional dyadic attachment processes that may shape coping, such as whether support that meets patients' attachment-related needs facilitates psychological adjustment (George-Levi et al., 2020; Vilchinsky et al., 2010). When caregivers used active engagement (e.g., asking the patient how he feels), male cardiac patients higher in attachment anxiety declined in anxiety symptoms, whereas patients lower in attachment anxiety showed increased symptoms (Vilchinsky et al., 2010). Active engagement may help meet anxious individuals' need for constant reassurance and emotional support, whereas it may be intrusive for patients who are more securely attached.

Investigating how physiological and behavioural responses to stress reciprocally influence each other will advance understanding of how attachment shapes coping and adjustment. For example, women showed elevated cortisol when their negative conflict behaviour (e.g., criticising) was followed by their husband's withdrawal (Kiecolt-Glaser et al., 1996). These combinations are likely to be magnified when couple members are insecurely attached, worsening adjustment. Additional dyadic processes also are likely to be important (e.g., coregulation; Sbarra & Hazan, 2008). For example, marital partners show similar daily cortisol levels (Saxbe & Repetti, 2010), and similarity in cortisol patterns during conflict increases over time (Laws et al., 2015). Furthermore, attachment anxiety and avoidance have been associated with couples' greater physiological correspondence (Helm et al., 2012). Amplification of synchrony between patients' and caregivers' physiological responses may contribute to why attachment insecurity risks poor coping and adjustment. Finally, health disparities associated with race/ethnicity and socioeconomic status underscore the need for research that includes more diverse samples to determine generalizability as well as variability in the dyadic processes associated with risk or resilience (e.g., Ross et al., 2019).

Dyadic attachment processes also have relevance for practitioners working with couples coping with illness. Interventions will likely promote better psychological and physical well-being when they are tailored to the specific attachment needs of the couple. For example, patients higher in attachment anxiety may benefit from interventions that emphasise reassurance and responsive support from their partners, whereas patients higher in avoidance may benefit from indirect, autonomy-sensitive support that is less likely to threaten needs for self-reliance (Overall et al., 2022b). Similarly, caregiving spouses who are securely attached may benefit from behavioural interventions designed to help them provide responsive support to patients. The same intervention, however, may be less successful when caregiving spouses are avoidant and are uncomfortable giving support.

Conclusion

Individuals' own and their partners' attachment security/insecurity shape behaviour and physiological responses and, in turn, adjustment and coping. When individuals or their partners evidence greater attachment anxiety or avoidance, individuals behave more poorly in relationship interactions and show poorer adjustment. Additionally, individuals' and their partners' attachment anxiety is associated with greater physiological reactivity to stress, which over time may contribute to poorer health and well-being. Our application of these established processes to the illness context reveals that additional work is needed to understand the important role of attachment in couples coping with illness. Advancing understanding regarding how attachment security/insecurity shapes couples' behaviour and physiological responses to illness-related stress will also provide an empirical foundation for designing tailored interventions for patient-caregiver pairs that address different forms of attachment insecurity.

Further Reading

Karantzas, G. C., & Gillath, O. (2017). Stress and wellbeing during chronic illness and partner death in later-life: The role of social support. *Current Opinion in Psychology*, *13*, 75–80. https://doi.org/10.1016/j.copsyc.2016.05.009

Overall, N. C., Pietromonaco, P. R., & Simpson, J. A. (2022). Buffering and spillover of adult attachment insecurity in couple and family relationships. *Nature Reviews Psychology*, *1*(2), 101–111. https://doi.org/10.1038/s44159-021-00011-1

Pietromonaco, P. R., & Beck, L. A. (2019). Adult attachment and physical health. *Current Opinion in Psychology*, *25*, 115–120. https://doi.org/10.1016/j.copsyc.2018.04.004

References

Beck, L. A., Pietromonaco, P. R., DeBuse, C. J., Powers, S. I., & Sayer, A. G. (2013). Spouses' attachment pairings predict neuroendocrine, behavioral, and psychological responses to marital conflict. *Journal of Personality and Social Psychology*, *105*(3), 388–424. https://doi.org/10.1037/a0033056

Beck, L. A., Pietromonaco, P. R., DeVito, C. C., Powers, S. I., & Boyle, A. M. (2014). Congruence between spouses' perceptions and observers' ratings of responsiveness: The role of attachment avoidance. *Personality & Social Psychology Bulletin*, *40*(2), 164–174. https://doi.org/10.1177/0146167213507779

Beck, L. A., Pietromonaco, P. R., Ge, F., Carnes, N. C., Laws, H., & Powers, S. I. (2023). Spouses' attachment orientations shape physiological responses to relational stress over time. *Journal of Social and Personal Relationships*, *40*(10), 3121–3146. https://doi.org/10.1177/02654075231169305

Bei, E., Mashevich, K., Rotem-Mindali, O., Galin-Soibelman, S., Kalter-Leibovici, O., Schifter, T., & Vilchinsky, N. (2022). Extremely distant and incredibly close: Physical proximity, emotional attachment and caregiver burden. *International Journal of Environmental Research and Public Health*, *19*(14), 8722. https://doi.org/10.3390/ijerph19148722

Ben-Naim, S., Hirschberger G, Ein-Dor T, & Mikulincer M. (2013). An experimental study of emotion regulation during relationship conflict interactions: The moderating role of attachment orientations. *Emotion*, *13*(3), 506–519. https://doi.org/10.1037/a0031473

Bowlby, J. (1969). *Attachment and loss: Vol. I: Attachment* (2nd ed.). Basic Books. (Original work published 1969).

Bowlby, J. (1973). *Attachment and loss: Vol. 2. Separation: Anxiety and anger*. Basic Books.

Braun, M., Hales, S., Gilad, L., Mikulincer, M., Rydall, A., & Rodin, G. (2012). Caregiving styles and attachment orientations in couples facing advanced cancer. *Psycho-Oncology*, *21*(9), 935–943. https://doi.org/10.1002/pon.1988

Brooks, K. P., Robles, T. F., & Dunkel, S. C. (2011). Adult attachment and cortisol responses to discussions with a romantic partner. *Personal Relationships*, *18*(2), 302–320. https://doi.org/10.1111/j.1475-6811.2011.01357.x

Carnelley, K. B., Pietromonaco, P. R., & Jaffe, K. (1996). Attachment, caregiving, and relationship functioning in couples: Effects of self and partner. *Personal Relationships*, *3*(3), 257–277. https://doi.org/10.1111/j.1475-6811.1996.tb00116.x

Chida, Y., & Steptoe, A. (2010). Greater cardiovascular responses to laboratory mental stress are associated with poor subsequent cardiovascular risk status: A meta-analysis of prospective evidence. *Hypertension (Dallas, Tex.: 1979)*, *55*(4), 1026–1032. https://doi.org/10.1161/HYPERTENSIONAHA.109.146621

Crangle, C. J., & Hart, T. L. (2017). Adult attachment, hostile conflict, and relationship adjustment among couples facing multiple sclerosis. *British Journal of Health Psychology*, *22*(4), 836–853. https://doi.org/10.1111/bjhp.12258

Crangle, C. J., Torbit, L. A., Ferguson, S. E., & Hart, T. L. (2020). Dyadic coping mediates the effects of attachment on quality of life among couples facing ovarian cancer. *Journal of Behavioral Medicine*, *43*(4), 564–575. https://doi.org/10.1007/s10865-019-00096-3

DeSantis, A. S., DiezRoux, A. V., Hajat, A., Aiello, A. E., Golden, S. H., Jenny, N. S., Seeman, T. E., & Shea, S. (2012). Associations of salivary cortisol levels with inflammatory markers: The Multi-Ethnic Study of Atherosclerosis. *Psychoneuroendocrinology*, *37*(7), 1009–1018. https://doi.org/10.1016/j.psyneuen.2011.11.009

Diamond, L. M., Hicks, A. M., & Otter-Henderson, K. (2006). Physiological evidence for repressive coping among avoidantly attached adults. *Journal of Social and Personal Relationships*, *23*(2), 205–229. https://doi.org/10.1177/0265407506062470

Fagundes, C. P., Jaremka, L. M., Glaser, R., Alfano, C. M., Povoski, S. P., Lipari, A. M., Agnese, D. M., Yee, L. D., Carson, W. E. I., Farrar, W. B., Malarkey, W. B., Chen, M., & Kiecolt-Glaser, J. K. (2014). Attachment anxiety is related to Epstein–Barr virus latency. *Brain, Behavior, and Immunity*, *41*, 232–238. https://doi.org/10.1016/j.bbi.2014.04.002

Favez, N., Cairo Notari, S., Antonini, T., & Charvoz, L. (2017). Attachment and couple satisfaction as predictors of expressed emotion in women facing breast cancer and their partners in the immediate post-surgery period. *British Journal of Health Psychology*, *22*(1), 169–185. https://doi.org/10.1111/bjhp.12223

Feeney, B. C., & Collins, N. L. (2001). Predictors of caregiving in adult intimate relationships: An attachment theoretical perspective. *Journal of Personality and Social Psychology*, *80*, 972–994. https://doi.org/10.1037/0022-3514.80.6.972

Feeney, B. C., & Kirkpatrick, L. A. (1996). Effects of adult attachment and presence of romantic partners on physiological responses to stress. *Journal of Personality and Social Psychology*, *70*(2), 255–270. https://doi.org/10.1037/0022-3514.70.2.255

Ge, F., Pietromonaco, P. R., DeBuse, C. J., Powers, S. I., & Granger, D. A. (2016). Concurrent and prospective associations between HPA axis activity and depression symptoms in newlywed women. *Psychoneuroendocrinology*, *73*, 125–132. https://doi.org/10.1016/j.psyneuen.2016.07.217

George-Levi, S., Peleg, S., Vilchinsky, N., Rafaeli, E., Khaskiaa, A., Mosseri, M., & Hod, H. (2020). Attachment insecurity hinders cardiac patients' ability to receive partners' care: A longitudinal dyadic study. *Journal of Social and Personal Relationships*, *37*(5), 1494–1512. https://doi.org/10.1177/0265407519900998

Girme, Y. U., Overall, N. C., Simpson, J. A., & Fletcher, G. J. O. (2015). "All or nothing": Attachment avoidance and the curvilinear effects of partner support. *Journal of Personality and Social Psychology*, *108*(3), 450–475. https://doi.org/10.1037/a0038866

Gouin, J.-P., Glaser, R., Loving, T. J., Malarkey, W. B., Stowell, J., Houts, C., & Kiecolt-Glaser, J. K. (2009). Attachment avoidance predicts inflammatory responses to marital conflict. *Brain, Behavior, and Immunity*, *23*(7), 898–904. https://doi.org/10.1016/j.bbi.2008.09.016

Hamer, M., Endrighi, R., Venuraju, S. M., Lahiri, A., & Steptoe, A. (2012). Cortisol responses to mental stress and the progression of coronary artery calcification in healthy men and women. *PLoS ONE*, *7*(2), 1–6. https://doi.org/10.1371/journal.pone.0031356

Hazan, C., & Shaver, P. (1987). Romantic love conceptualized as an attachment process. *Journal of Personality and Social Psychology*, *52*(3), 511–524. https://doi.org/10.1037/0022-3514.52.3.511
Helgeson, V. S., Allen, N. A., Tracy, E. L., Butner, J., & Berg, C. A. (2022). Diabetes stress contagion among romantic partners: A daily diary investigation. *Journal of Behavioral Medicine*, *45*(5), 716–727. https://doi.org/10.1007/s10865-022-00337-y
Helgeson, V. S., Jakubiak, B., Van Vleet, M., & Zajdel, M. (2018). Communal coping and adjustment to chronic illness: Theory update and evidence. *Personality and Social Psychology Review*, *22*(2), 170–195. https://doi.org/10.1177/1088868317735767
Helm, J. L., Sbarra, D., & Ferrer, E. (2012). Assessing cross-partner associations in physiological responses via coupled oscillator models. *Emotion*, *12*, 748–762. https://doi.org/10.1037/a0025036
Heyman, R. E., Lorber, M. F., Eddy, J. M., & West, T. V. (2014). Behavioral observation and coding. In H. T. Reis & C. M. Judd (Eds.), *Handbook of research methods in social and personality psychology, 2nd ed* (pp. 345–372). Cambridge University Press.
Holt-Lunstad, J., Smith TB, & Layton JB. (2010). Social relationships and mortality risk: A meta-analytic review. *PLoS Medicine*, *7*, 1–20. https://doi.org/10.1371/journal.pmed.1000316
Hsiao, F.-H., Jow, G.-M., Kuo, W.-H., Huang, C.-S., Lai, Y.-M., Liu, Y.-F., & Chang, K.-J. (2014). The partner's insecure attachment, depression and psychological well-being as predictors of diurnal cortisol patterns for breast cancer survivors and their spouses. *Stress: The International Journal on the Biology of Stress*, *17*(2), 169–175. https://doi.org/10.3109/10253890.2014.880833
Jaremka, L. M., Glaser, R., Loving, T. J., Malarkey, W. B., Stowell, J. R., & Kiecolt-Glaser, J. K. (2013). Attachment anxiety is linked to alterations in cortisol production and cellular immunity. *Psychological Science*, *24*(3), 272–279. https://doi.org/10.1177/0956797612452571
Jaremka, L. M., Glaser, R., Malarkey, W. B., & Kiecolt-Glaser, J. K. (2013). Marital distress prospectively predicts poorer cellular immune function. *Psychoneuroendocrinology*, *38*(11), 2713–2719. https://doi.org/10.1016/j.psyneuen.2013.06.031
Jaremka, L. M., Lindgren, M. E., & Kiecolt-Glaser, J. K. (2013). Synergistic relationships among stress, depression, and troubled relationships: Insights from psychoneuroimmunology. *Depression and Anxiety*, *30*(4), 288–296. https://doi.org/10.1002/da.22078
Jayamaha, S. D., Girme, Y. U., & Overall, N. C. (2017). When attachment anxiety impedes support provision: The role of feeling unvalued and unappreciated. *Journal of Family Psychology*, *31*(2), 181–191. https://doi.org/10.1037/fam0000222
Julal, F. S., & Carnelley, K. B. (2012). Attachment, perceptions of care and caregiving to romantic partners and friends. *European Journal of Social Psychology*, *42*(7), 832–843. https://doi.org/10.1002/ejsp.1914
Karantzas, G. C., & Gillath, O. (2017b). Stress and wellbeing during chronic illness and partner death in later-life: The role of social support. *Current Opinion in Psychology*, *13*, 75–80. https://doi.org/10.1016/j.copsyc.2016.05.009
Kidd, T., Hamer M, & Steptoe A. (2013). Adult attachment style and cortisol responses across the day in older adults. *Psychophysiology*, *50*(9), 841–847. https://doi.org/10.1111/psyp.12075
Kidd, T., Poole L, Leigh E, Ronaldson A, Jahangiri M, & Steptoe A. (2014). Attachment anxiety predicts IL-6 and length of hospital stay in coronary artery bypass graft surgery (CABG) patients. *Journal of Psychosomatic Research*, *77*(2), 155–157. https://doi.org/10.1016/j.jpsychores.2014.06.002
Kiecolt-Glaser, J. K., Newton, T., Cacioppo, J. T., MacCallum, R. C., Glaser, R., & Malarkey, W. B. (1996). Marital conflict and endocrine function: Are men really more physiologically affected than women? *Journal of Consulting and Clinical Psychology*, *64*(2), 324–332. https://doi.org/10.1037/0022-006X.64.2.324

Kim, Y. (2006). Gender, attachment, and relationship duration on cardiovascular reactivity to stress in a laboratory study of dating couples. *Personal Relationships*, *13*(1), 103–114. https://doi.org/10.1111/j.1475-6811.2006.00107.x
Kim, Y., & Carver, C. S. (2007). Frequency and difficulty in caregiving among spouses of individuals with cancer: Effects of adult attachment and gender. *Psycho-Oncology*, *16*(8), 714–723. https://doi.org/10.1002/pon.1110
Kordahji, H., Bar-Kalifa E, & Rafaeli E. (2015). Attachment insecurity as a moderator of cardiovascular arousal effects following dyadic support. *Journal of Research in Personality*, *57*, 89–99. https://doi.org/10.1016/j.jrp.2015.04.004
Lachmar, E. M., & Seedall, R. B. (2018). Psychophysiological arousal and perceived support during couple support interactions: The role of attachment anxiety and avoidance. *American Journal of Family Therapy*, *46*(5), 525–540. https://doi.org/10.1080/01926187.2019.1571958
Laws, H. B., Sayer, A. G., Pietromonaco, P. R., & Powers, S. I. (2015). Longitudinal changes in spouses' HPA responses: Convergence in cortisol patterns during the early years of marriage. *Health Psychology*, *34*(11), 1076–1089. https://doi.org/10.1037/hea0000235
Meuwly, N., Bodenmann, G., Germann, J., Bradbury, T. N., Ditzen, B., & Heinrichs, M. (2012). Dyadic coping, insecure attachment, and cortisol stress recovery following experimentally induced stress. *Journal of Family Psychology*, *26*(6), 937–947. https://doi.org/10.1037/a0030356
Mikulincer, M., & Shaver, P. R. (2017). *Attachment in adulthood: Structure, dynamics and change* (2nd ed.). Guilford Publications.
Monin, J. K., Schulz, R., & Kershaw, T. S. (2013). Caregiving spouses' attachment orientations and the physical and psychological health of individuals with Alzheimer's disease. *Aging & Mental Health*, *17*(4), 508–516. https://doi.org/10.1080/13607863.2012.747080
Overall, N. C., Fletcher, G. J. O., Simpson, J. A., & Fillo, J. (2015). Attachment insecurity, biased perceptions of romantic partners' negative emotions, and hostile relationship behavior. *Journal of Personality and Social Psychology*, *108*(5), 730–749. https://doi.org/10.1037/a0038987
Overall, N. C., Girme, Y. U., Lemay, E. P. Jr., & Hammond, M. D. (2014). Attachment anxiety and reactions to relationship threat: The benefits and costs of inducing guilt in romantic partners. *Journal of Personality and Social Psychology*, *106*(2), 235–256. https://doi.org/10.1037/a0034371
Overall, N. C., Pietromonaco, P. R., & Simpson, J. A. (2022b). Buffering and spillover of adult attachment insecurity in couple and family relationships. *Nature Reviews Psychology*, *1*(2), 101–111. https://doi.org/10.1038/s44159-021-00011-1
Overall, N. C., Simpson, J. A., & Struthers, H. (2013). Buffering attachment-related avoidance: Softening emotional and behavioral defenses during conflict discussions. *Journal of Personality and Social Psychology*, *104*(5), 854–871. https://doi.org/10.1037/a0031798
Peters, B. J., Overall, N. C., Girme, Y. U., & Jamieson, J. P. (2019). Partners' attachment insecurity predicts greater physiological threat in anticipation of attachment-relevant interactions. *Journal of Social and Personal Relationships*, *36*(2), 469–489. https://doi.org/10.1177/0265407517734655
Picardi, A., Miglio R, Tarsitani L, Battisti F, Baldassari M, Copertaro, A., Mocchegiani, E., Cascavilla, I., & Biondi M. (2013). Attachment style and immunity: A 1-year longitudinal study. *Biological Psychology*, *92*(2), 353–358. https://doi.org/10.1016/j.biopsycho.2012.10.001
Pietromonaco, P. R., & Barrett, L. F. (1997). Working models of attachment and daily social interactions. *Journal of Personality and Social Psychology*, *73*(6), 1409–1423. https://doi.org/10.1037/0022-3514.73.6.1409

Pietromonaco, P. R., & Beck, L. A. (2015). Attachment processes in adult romantic relationships. In M. Mikulincer, P. R. Shaver, J. A. Simpson, J. F. Dovidio, M. Mikulincer, P. R. Shaver, J. A. Simpson, & J. F. Dovidio (Eds.), *APA handbook of personality and social psychology, Volume 3: Interpersonal relations* (2013-35884-002; pp. 33–64). American Psychological Association. https://doi.org/10.1037/14344-002

Pietromonaco, P. R., & Beck, L. A. (2019b). Adult attachment and physical health. *Current Opinion in Psychology, 25*, 115–120. https://doi.org/10.1016/j.copsyc.2018.04.004

Pietromonaco, P. R., & Collins, N. L. (2017). Interpersonal mechanisms linking close relationships to health. *American Psychologist, 72*(6), 531–542. https://doi.org/10.1037/amp0000129

Pietromonaco, P. R., DeVito, C. C., Ge, F., & Lembke, J. (2015). Health and attachment processes. In J. A. Simpson, W. S. Rholes, J. A. Simpson, & W. S. Rholes (Eds.), *Attachment theory and research: New directions and emerging themes* (2015-13436-011; pp. 287–318). Guilford Press.

Pietromonaco, P. R., & Powers, S. I. (2015). Attachment and Health-Related Physiological Stress Processes. *Current Opinion in Psychology, 1*, 34–39. https://doi.org/10.1016/j.copsyc.2014.12.001

Pietromonaco, P. R., Uchino, B. N., & Dunkel Schetter, C. (2013). Close relationship processes and health: Implications of attachment theory for health and disease. *Health Psychology, 32*(5), 499–513. https://doi.org/10.1037/a0029349

Porter, L., Keefe, F., Davis, D., Rumble, M., Scipio, C., & Garst, J. (2012). Attachment styles in patients with lung cancer and their spouses: Associations with patient and spouse adjustment. *Supportive Care in Cancer, 20*(10), 2459–2466. https://doi.org/10.1007/s00520-011-1367-6

Powers, S. I., Pietromonaco, P. R., Gunlicks, M., & Sayer, A. (2006). Dating couples' attachment styles and patterns of cortisol reactivity and recovery in response to a relationship conflict. *Journal of Personality and Social Psychology, 90*(4), 613–628. https://doi.org/10.1037/0022-3514.90.4.613

Ramos, K., Langer, S. L., Todd, M., Romano, J. M., Ghosh, N., Keefe, F. J., Baucom, D. H., Syrjala, K. L., & Porter, L. S. (2020). Attachment style, partner communication, and physical well-being among couples coping with cancer. *Personal Relationships, 27*(3), 526–549. https://doi.org/10.1111/pere.12330

Ramos, K., Leo, K., Porter, L. S., Romano, J. M., Baucom, B. R. W., & Langer, S. L. (2023). Attachment in couples coping with cancer: Associations with observed communication and long-term health. *International Journal of Environmental Research and Public Health, 20*(7), Article 7. https://doi.org/10.3390/ijerph20075249

Revenson, T. A., & DeLongis, A. (2011). Couples coping with chronic illness. In S. Folkman (Ed.), *The Oxford handbook of stress, health, and coping* (pp. 101–123). Oxford University Press.

Robles, T. F., Brooks, K. P., Kane HS, & Dunkel, S. C. (2013). Attachment, skin deep? Relationships between adult attachment and skin barrier recovery. *International Journal of Psychophysiology, 88*(3), 241–252. https://doi.org/10.1016/j.ijpsycho.2012.04.007

Robles, T. F., Slatcher, R. B., Trombello, J. M., & McGinn, M. M. (2014). Marital quality and health: A meta-analytic review. *Psychological Bulletin, 140*(1), 140–187. https://doi.org/10.1037/a0031859

Ross, J. M., Karney, B. R., Nguyen, T. P., & Bradbury, T. N. (2019). Communication that is maladaptive for middle-class couples is adaptive for socioeconomically disadvantaged couples. *Journal of Personality and Social Psychology, 116*(4), 582–597. https://doi.org/10.1037/pspi0000158

Saxbe, D. E., & Repetti, R. L. (2010). For better or worse? Coregulation of couples' cortisol levels and mood states. *Journal of Personality and Social Psychology, 98*(1), 92–103. https://doi.org/10.1037/a0016959

Sbarra, D. A., & Hazan, C. (2008). Coregulation, dysregulation, self-regulation: An integrative analysis and empirical agenda for understanding adult attachment, separation, loss, and recovery. *Personality and Social Psychology Review*, *12*(2), 141–167. https://doi.org/10.1177/1088868308315702

Seedall, R. B., & Wampler, K. S. (2012). Emotional congruence within couple interaction: The role of attachment avoidance. *Journal of Family Psychology*, *26*(6), 948–958. https://doi.org/10.1037/a0030479

Seedall, R. B., & Wampler, K. S. (2016). Couple emotional experience: Effects of attachment anxiety in low and high structure couple interactions. *Journal of Family Therapy*, *38*(3), 340–363. https://doi.org/10.1111/1467-6427.12113

Simpson, J. A., Rholes, W. S., & Phillips, D. (1996). Conflict in close relationships: An attachment perspective. *Journal of Personality and Social Psychology*, *71*(5), 899–914. https://doi.org/10.1037/0022-3514.71.5.899

Sroufe, L. A., & Waters, E. (1977). Attachment as an organizational construct. *Child Development*, *48*(4), 1184–1199. https://doi.org/10.2307/1128475

Taylor, N. C., Seedall, R. B., Robinson, W. D., & Bradford, K. (2018). The systemic interaction of attachment on psychophysiological arousal in couple conflict. *Journal of Marital and Family Therapy*, *44*(1), 46–60. https://doi.org/10.1111/jmft.12239

Turner, A. I., Smyth, N., Hall, S. J., Torres, S. J., Hussein, M., Jayasinghe, S. U., Ball, K., & Clow, A. J. (2020). Psychological stress reactivity and future health and disease outcomes: A systematic review of prospective evidence. *Psychoneuroendocrinology*, *114*, 104599. https://doi.org/10.1016/j.psyneuen.2020.104599

Umberson, D., & Montez, J. K. (2010). Social relationships and health: A flashpoint for health policy. *Journal of Health and Social Behavior*, *51*(Suppl), S54–S66. https://doi.org/10.1177/0022146510383501

Van Vleet, M., & Helgeson, V. S. (2019). I am a rock; I am an island: Implications of avoidant attachment for communal coping in adults with type 2 diabetes. *Journal of Social and Personal Relationships*, 1, *36*(11–12), 3711–3732. https://doi.org/10.1177/0265407519832671

Vilchinsky, N., Dekel, R., Revenson, T. A., Liberman, G., & Mosseri, M. (2015). Caregivers' burden and depressive symptoms: The moderational role of attachment orientations. *Health Psychology*, *34*(3), 262–269. https://doi.org/10.1037/hea0000121

Vilchinsky, N., Haze-Filderman, L., Leibowitz, M., Reges, O., Khaskia, A., & Mosseri, M. (2010). Spousal support and cardiac patients' distress: The moderating role of attachment orientation. *Journal of Family Psychology*, *24*(4), 508–512. https://doi.org/10.1037/a0020009

18

AN OVERVIEW OF THE IMPACT OF CHRONIC MEDICAL ILLNESS ON SEXUALITY

Chiara Acquati

Introduction

Sexuality is a central aspect of quality of life and psychological well-being of the individual, which can be negatively affected – either directly or indirectly, permanently or temporarily – by an illness. The World Health Organization has defined sexual health (WHO, 2006) as

> *a state of physical, mental, and social wellbeing in relation to sexuality. It requires a positive and respectful approach to sexuality and sexual relationships and the possibility of having pleasurable and safe sexual experiences, free of coercion, discrimination, and violence.*

Often overlooked in the context of chronic illness, there has been increasing attention to addressing illness-related sexual concerns as a result of a deeper understanding of their pervasive impact on quality of life and recognition of the complex interplay of bio-psychosocial factors that shape functioning, satisfaction, and intimacy with a partner (Basson, 2000, 2010; Katz, 2021; Buehler, 2021).

Early models of the human sexual response cycle primarily emphasised anatomical and physiological aspects. Models developed by Masters and Johnson (1966) and later Kaplan (1995) proposed a linear, sequential progression of phases related to desire, arousal, plateau, orgasm, and resolution. In contrast, Basson introduced a circular model of sexual response, which acknowledged the role of intimacy, communication, and other relationship factors for sexual motivation, response, and satisfaction (Basson, 2000, 2010). Later, Cleary and Hegarty (2011) defined the neo-theoretical framework, in which sexuality comprises sexual response, sexual self-concept, and intimate relationships. These broader conceptualisations have coincided with growing awareness of

 DOI: 10.4324/9781003318026-22

psychological and interpersonal aspects that influence the experience of sexuality in the context of illness. Verschuren et al. (2010) have proposed a conceptual framework depicting the impact of chronic disease on sexual functioning and well-being that highlights the interaction between physical, psychological, and relational factors in determining the individual's adjustment.

Considering the current and projected burden posed by chronic illness to individuals, families, and society (Hajat & Stein, 2018), improvements in treatments and symptom management, and advocacy efforts that centred sexual health as an unmet need in clinical care (Reese et al., 2017; Steinke et al., 2013; Wittmann, Mehta, McCaughan, et al., 2022), attending to sexuality and intimacy-related concerns is of critical importance. The chapter aims to illustrate the repercussions of some of the most prevalent illnesses on sexual function, sexuality, and well-being of patients, partners, and their relationships. The chapter also emphasises interpersonal processes and dyadic coping strategies that contribute to sexual well-being and presents psychological interventions that have been developed to address these issues.

Impact of Chronic Illness on Patients' and Partners' Sexuality

Cancer

Cancer remains a life-threatening disease that can result in adverse physical, psychosocial, or behavioural outcomes. Recent data indicate that cancer incidence and mortality are growing, and it has been estimated that there will be 28.4 million cases globally in 2040 (Sung et al., 2021).

Cancer-related sexual dysfunction is one of the most common and distressing consequences of the illness, which untreated persists or worsens over time (Elliott & Matthew, 2018; Reese et al., 2017; Traa, Braeken, et al., 2015). Research has predominantly emphasised sex-specific cancer types – breast, gynaecological, and prostate cancer (Grondhuis Palacios et al., 2018; Levin et al., 2010; Li et al., 2022; Oberguggenberger et al., 2017; Ussher et al., 2012; Wittmann et al., 2015; Wittmann, Mehta, Bober, et al., 2022). Recent contributions extend to mixed populations, such as colorectal, anal, and bladder cancer (Acquati et al., 2022; Martin et al., 2023; Savoie et al., 2023). More than half of female cancer survivors experience sexual issues, with variations in prevalence due to cancer type, stage of the disease, timing of assessment, instruments, and characteristics of the sample (Bober & Varela, 2012; Reese et al., 2022; van Roij et al., 2022). Changes in sexual frequency and satisfaction are linked to a variety of factors, including the physical effects of cancer treatment, such as vaginal dryness, lubrication difficulties, and dyspareunia; psychological influences, like body image concerns, decreased sexual interest; and altered relationship dynamics that may lead to avoidance of sexual activity (Congard et al., 2019; Katz, 2021; Loaring et al., 2015; Reese et al., 2022). Furthermore, breast cancer survivors have reported dissatisfaction with their post-reconstruction body image and changed breast and nipple sensitivity (Lovelace et al., 2019). When considering prostate cancer, sexual dysfunction is the most frequent side effect, affecting up to 85% of survivors (Capogrosso et al., 2019; Gupta et al., 2023). Sexual difficulties are often due to a combination of physical and psychological issues. Prostate cancer treatment can lead to erectile dysfunction, orgasm changes, and penile shortening (Capogrosso et al., 2019; Emanu et al., 2016). Reduced libido (Katz, 2021) has been linked to changes in body image, fatigue, incontinence, and discomfort. Sex-specific difficulties are frequently associated with feelings of isolation, anxiety, depression, inadequacy, decreased sexual confidence, and affected masculinity (Zhu & Wittmann, 2022). Additionally, in the case of colorectal and pelvic cancers, patients experience unique sources of distress, including bowel control or incontinence, stomas, negative body image, and sexual health issues affecting sexual satisfaction (Abelson et al., 2018; Reese et al., 2018; Zhu & Wittmann, 2022). There is consensus in the literature about worse outcomes – both in terms of sexual activity and relationship quality – experienced by patients with a permanent ostomy (Abelson et al., 2018; Acquati et al., 2022). Individuals with stomas tend to avoid intimacy with a partner due to concerns related to leakage, odour, and noises (Marques et al., 2018; Zhu & Wittmann, 2022), feeling sexually unattractive, and the majority report a negative impact on the couple relationship (Pazar et al., 2015).

Sexual dysfunction has been associated with increased psychological distress, worse quality of life, reduced self-esteem, and posttraumatic symptomatology (Acquati et al., 2022; Bober & Varela, 2012; Heyne et al., 2021; Reese et al., 2018; Wittmann, 2016). Sexual health concerns, depression, and anxiety often lead to a self-perpetuating cycle where negative thoughts lead to impaired function, loss of libido, and reduced enjoyment, which ultimately discourage sexual activity (Hyde et al., 2017; Zhu & Wittmann, 2022). While often neglected in earlier works, the impact of the disease on partners' sexuality and intimacy is also significant (Loaring et al., 2015; Ussher et al., 2013; Ussher et al., 2011; Wittmann et al., 2014), given that they are the primary support person (Acquati et al., 2023a). The dynamics of the caregiving relationship often act as obstacles, making it challenging to cope with the dual role of caregiver and sexual partner while grieving sexual losses (Canzona et al., 2019; Grondhuis Palacios et al., 2018; Levin et al., 2010; Wittmann, 2016; Wittmann et al., 2015) and facing significant supportive needs (Acquati et al., 2023b; Li et al., 2022). Elevated psychological and sexual distress are reported by partners over time (Acquati et al., 2022), while lower depressive symptoms and emotional distress were documented among couples engaging in communication patterns characterised by disclosure and active engagement (Kayser et al., 2018; Traa, Braeken, et al., 2015; Traa, De Vries, et al., 2015). Partners fear initiating sex and experience difficulties renegotiating their sexual relationship with the patient, challenges often associated with dissatisfaction with sex life (Gupta et al., 2023). While the presence of sexual dysfunction has been associated with poorer psychological well-being and quality of life (Heyne et al., 2021; Reese et al., 2018), coping with cancer-related sexual difficulties is a process that relies on the characteristics of the couple relationship. Emotional closeness, intimacy, communication, and shared coping strategies have been associated with sexual satisfaction (Manne et al., 2004; Rottmann et al., 2022; van Roij et al., 2022; Wittmann, 2016). This datum is confirmed by qualitative accounts which have highlighted that grieving and accepting sexual change, often developing realistic expectations, contributed to better adjustment (Canzona et al., 2019; Gupta et al., 2023; Wittmann, 2016; Wittmann et al., 2015). Furthermore, the ability to redefine sexual intimacy, to place greater value on sex as a medium for relational intimacy, the integration of non-penetrative practices, and open communication often become a way to nurture emotional closeness and connection (Beck et al., 2013; Reese et al., 2010).

Cardiac Illness

Cardiovascular disease (CVD) is one of the leading causes of death worldwide (Park et al., 2023; Tsao et al., 2023): it accounts for 19 million deaths (Tsao et al., 2023), and recent data estimate mortality to reach 23 million by 2030 (Tsao et al., 2023).

The physical and psychological consequences of the disease – anxiety, depression, and quality of life – negatively affect sexual functioning (Epifanio et al., 2023; Park et al., 2023; Simeone et al., 2020). People diagnosed with CDV are three times more likely to experience sexual dysfunction, with prevalence rates up to 89% (Park et al., 2023). Patients with CVD experience reduced libido, desire, and satisfaction, and they tend to avoid sexual activity (Abbasi et al., 2020). Erectile dysfunction, premature ejaculation, and anxiety related to sexual performance (Simeone et al., 2020; Thylén & Brännström, 2015) are common, while sexual difficulties reported by females include lack of interest and lubrication. Differently from men, women tend to avoid or cease engaging in sex (Assari, 2014; Lindau et al., 2012): fear of recurrence and difficulties in lifestyle adjustment prevent them from resuming sexual activities previously enjoyed (Simeone et al., 2020).

Impaired sexual function has been linked to reduced quality of life, psychological well-being, and quality of the relationship with the partner (Baert et al., 2019; Epifanio et al., 2023). The interplay between quality of life, emotional distress, and sexual health has been investigated in recent contributions (Smith, 2022; Smith & Baucom, 2017). Depressive symptoms mediated the association between sexual function and quality of life (Kriston et al., 2010), while the relationship between quality of life and sexual satisfaction was mediated by anxiety (Epifanio et al., 2023), supporting the relevance of psychological mechanisms. Elevated anxiety and decreased motivation for sex were often the result of functional limitations and worse self-reported health, while sexual satisfaction contributes to greater health-related quality of life (Reese et al., 2012).

Multiple aspects of the relationship are affected, including adjustment to the diagnosis, role changes, sexual concerns, and impaired communication (Katz, 2021; Smith, 2022). Relationship strain, reduced communication, and emotional closeness have been reported, in addition to lower sexual satisfaction (Byrne et al., 2017). Recent investigations highlight the positive impact of close relationships on CDV risk factors and survival, emphasising the importance of relationship quality for patients' and partners' well-being (Bouchard et al., 2023; Smith, 2022; Smith & Baucom, 2017). Conversely, relationship strain and dissolution have negative consequences for physical health (Smith, 2022; Smith & Baucom, 2017; Smith et al., 2012), with links to ischaemic incidents, atherosclerosis, and worse prognosis. Tulloch et al. (2020) highlighted relationship changes experienced by patients and partners, with emotional and communication disconnection, overprotection, lifestyle changes, and role adjustment being the key transitions for the dyad. However, not all changes were negative, as some participants disclosed that the experience strengthened the couple relationship (Tulloch et al., 2020). Similarly, a longitudinal study reported that most partnered patients were sexually active before and after myocardial infarction, and that satisfaction remained elevated (Thylén & Brännström, 2015).

Diabetes

Diabetes mellitus is a chronic metabolic disease which can lead to severe organ damage, complications, and adverse psychological consequences (Centers for Disease Control and Prevention, 2023). Globally, approximately 529 million people live with diabetes, and it is estimated that the disease will affect more than 1.31 billion people by 2050 (Ong et al., 2023).

Systematic reviews and meta-analyses established that approximately 38.5% of women diagnosed with type 1 diabetes report sexual dysfunction, while 52.5% of men experience erectile problems (Parmar et al., 2022; Zhang et al., 2023). Among the most common sexual health concerns there are erectile and orgasmic dysfunction for men, while women experience decreased desire, arousal, orgasm, and satisfaction compared to healthy controls (Bjerggaard et al., 2015; Parmar et al., 2022; Van Cauwenberghe et al., 2022). A study by Van Cauwenberghe et al., conducted on a large mixed sample, documented the association between sexual dysfunction and illness-related distress in both male and female respondents (Van Cauwenberghe et al., 2022). Approximately 17% of men and 47% of women diagnosed with type 2 were sexually inactive, and 57% and 42% of them were unable to fulfil their sexual needs (Bjerggaard et al., 2015). Two groups appear to be particularly vulnerable: young adults diagnosed with type I diabetes – because of the need to renegotiate illness complications, the use of insulin pumps, and sexual relationships (Santos et al., 2020) – and sexual and gender minority (SGM) groups who report elevated level of non-compliance with diabetes management guidelines (Tran et al., 2021).

Psychosocial issues, including self-esteem, attractiveness, and relationship concerns, are often associated with sexual dysfunction (Barnard et al., 2019). It has been demonstrated that severity of depressive symptoms correlates with sexual function, sexual frequency, and lower illness acceptance (Sansone et al., 2022). Partners often reported significant worry, stress, and anxiety associated with managing hypoglycaemia to the extent that they often neglected their own health and social networks (Lawton et al., 2014; Rintala et al., 2013). Many felt that diabetes affected their daily routines, with greater distress associated with episodes of hypoglycaemia, poorer glucose management, lower relationship satisfaction, and greater involvement in patient care (Polonsky et al., 2016). Partner engagement contributed to better glycemic control, diet, and exercise (Trief et al., 2017); in contrast, overprotective behaviours were associated with less frequent blood glucose measurement and dietary adherence (Johnson et al., 2015). Importantly, better emotional well-being is documented when patients perceive the illness to be a shared experience (Johnson, Anderson, Walker, et al., 2013; Johnson et al., 2015; Peyrot et al., 2018).

Studies confirm that both partners report lower levels of sexual enjoyment and satisfaction (Lister et al., 2013); however, couples' acceptance of the illness contributes to sexual (Atwood et al., 2006; Lister et al., 2013) and marital adjustment (Gillibrand & Stevenson, 2007; Pereira et al., 2016). For instance, sexual satisfaction of patients is positively associated with their own and their partners' dyadic adjustment, with greater dissatisfaction experienced by female respondents and by those who had more dysfunctional beliefs and lower dyadic adjustment (Pereira et al., 2016). Recent literature supports the relationship between sexual and dyadic functioning (Kaplan Serin et al., 2020) and has further investigated how diabetes distress, sexual function, and relationship with a partner (de Wit et al., 2020; Strom & Egede, 2012) are linked to psychological and care management outcomes (Fisher et al., 2004; Pereira et al., 2016). These associations were confirmed both cross-sectionally and prospectively: Trief et al. (2006) revealed that higher marital stress was associated with poor blood glucose control, while Roberson and Fincham (2018) identified that marital strain and poor communication contributed to a lower level of diabetes management. Furthermore, studies have underscored that although partners reported concordant appraisal of sexual relationships, the effective communication of concerns and sexual preferences was impaired (Messina et al., 2021; van Pinxteren et al., 2023).

Interpersonal Processes and Dyadic Coping

One of the most interesting developments of the application of integrative and bio-psychosocial models to the experience of couples confronted by chronic illness is the relevance assumed by interpersonal processes and dyadic coping (Bertschi et al., 2021; Brotto et al., 2016; Weitkamp et al., 2021; Wittmann et al., 2015). Consistently, research has indicated that effective communication, self and perceived partner disclosure, and partner responsiveness contribute to greater intimacy (Kim et al., 2008; Kuenzler et al., 2011; Segrin & Badger, 2014), which according to the Interpersonal Process Model of Intimacy (Manne & Badr, 2010; Manne et al., 2004) is key to supporting couples' adjustment to stress. Greater levels of intimacy and low psychological distress were observed when using mutual constructive communication (Manne et al., 2010; Manne et al., 2018). Spousal disclosure and perceived support have been associated with greater intimacy and well-being (Kayser et al., 2018; Manne & Badr, 2008; Manne et al., 2010). Conversely, withdraw, holding back, and protective buffering were linked to poorer relationship functioning, coping, and psychological well-being (Manne & Badr, 2008; Manne et al., 2015). The importance of communication for sexual health outcomes was confirmed by a meta-analysis (Mallory et al., 2019), which documented its association with diverse domains of sexual function. Similarly, Fischer et al. (2022) highlighted that difficulties in emotion regulation are related to sexual issues and dissatisfaction.

Dyadic coping describes the stress management process and coordinated strategies implemented by partners when faced with external stressors (Bodenmann, 1995, 1997). Across conceptualisations, positive individual and conjoint dyadic coping styles contribute to better marital functioning, psychological well-being, health-related quality of life, and illness management (Falconier et al., 2015; Falconier & Kuhn, 2019; Johnson, Anderson, Walker, et al., 2013). Two recent systematic reviews investigated the role of dyadic coping in the context of disability and chronic physical illness (Bertschi et al., 2021; Weitkamp et al., 2021). Dyadic coping was associated with physical, emotional, and relational outcomes (Weitkamp et al., 2021), and couples were most able to adjust to chronic health impairments when these were appraised as interpersonal experiences (Bertschi et al., 2021). Specifically, altered sexual intimacy was a result of the complex changes in the couple relationship, which affected dyadic interactions and conjoint coping (Bertschi et al., 2021). In diabetes, confidence in the intimate relationship and deriving satisfaction from caring for one's partner were associated with increased involvement in discussions about the illness and adopting a communal orientation (Johnson, Anderson, Wilcox, et al., 2013). Shared illness appraisals correlated with improved self-regulation, self-care, and overall health (Berg et al., 2020; Helgeson et al., 2019; Lee et al., 2020). In contributions focusing on type 2 diabetes, communal coping aided psychological adjustment, relationship satisfaction, and care behaviours. However, excessive overlap among partners led to perceived partner overprotection (Helgeson et al., 2017; Van Vleet et al., 2018, 2019; Zajdel et al., 2018), with differential benefits by role, sex, and race (Helgeson et al., 2020). When considering cardiac illness, less effective partner support was reported when negative or low levels of positive dyadic coping characterised the relational exchange (Rapelli et al., 2021). In cancer, perceptual congruence of dyadic coping between partners was associated with improved emotional and sexual adjustment (Acquati, 2023; Stulz et al., 2022). Couples characterised by congruent appraisals of stress communication and delegated dyadic coping tended to report marital satisfaction, while sexual adjustment was linked to similar perceptions of common dyadic coping.

Psychological Interventions in the Context of Chronic Illness

Psychoeducation and Sexual Counselling/Rehabilitation

Psychoeducational interventions have been extensively used when addressing sexual problems (DuHamel et al., 2016; Kingsberg et al., 2017; Mestre-Bach et al., 2022; Xu et al., 2023). Psychoeducation blends professionally provided psychotherapeutic and educational components (Kim et al., 2015). These interventions have shown positive results in diminishing depression and anxiety, enhancing adjustment to illness, and improving coping (Katz-Wise & Hyde, 2014; Kim et al., 2015). In the context of sexuality, the literature has also reported that psychoeducation enhances the use of vaginal dilators, intercourse, and sexual function (Katz, 2021; Sopfe et al., 2021). A meta-analysis demonstrated that sexuality-focused interventions after cancer contributed to medium to large effect size and that they were effective for cognitive and psychological outcomes and higher rates of compliance (Kim et al., 2015). Additionally, delivering interventions in a face-to-face format coupled with internet or web-based check-ins/resources led to greater effect sizes. In the context of cardiac illness, the Cardiac Health and Relationship Management and Sexuality (CHARMS) intervention was rated feasible and acceptable (Murphy et al., 2018), but no evidentiary support for sexual counselling was reported in a Cochrane Review (Byrne et al., 2016). Several chronic illnesses necessitate sexual rehabilitation (D'Eath et al., 2018; Murphy et al., 2018), which includes sex education, psychological support, introduction to the use of assistive devices, exercise, and lifestyle modification. These have been investigated in the context of cardiovascular disease, stroke, and multiple sclerosis (MS), but sources recommend additional studies given the limited number of randomised controlled trials (Auger et al., 2023; Giannopapas et al., 2023; Stratton et al., 2020). Cognitive-behavioural therapy (CBT) has been extensively applied to the treatment of sexual problems (Metz et al., 2018) because of its focus on cognitive restructuring, behavioural activation, and problem-solving. CBT helps correct misconceptions, eliminate anxiety in sexual relations, and expand sexual behaviours by integrating training related to communication skills and sexual techniques (Metz et al., 2018; Xu et al., 2023). A recent meta-analysis indicated that CBT and psychoeducation effectively increased sexual function and satisfaction among women with breast cancer (Xu et al., 2023).

Mindfulness-Based Interventions

While the value of mindfulness as a treatment modality has been demonstrated for a variety of health-related problems, recently, authors have started to apply this approach to sexual health issues (Banbury, Chandler, & Lusher, 2023; Banbury, Lusher, et al., 2023; Jaderek & Lew-Starowicz, 2019) since mindfulness can mitigate negative self-thoughts, increase well-being, and self-efficacy that are critical for satisfactory sexuality (Leavitt et al., 2019). Systematic reviews and meta-analyses support the benefits of mindfulness for erectile dysfunction, lubrication, desire, orgasm, arousal, and pain (Jaderek & Lew-Starowicz, 2019; Larraz et al., 2023; Stephenson & Kerth, 2017), with moderate effect sizes reported for desire, arousal, and pain (Banbury, Lusher, et al., 2023). In the context of chronic illness, mindfulness has been applied to individuals with cancer, MS, and diabetes (Banbury, Chandler, & Lusher, 2023; Banbury, Lusher, et al., 2023; Giannopapas et al., 2023). Bossio et al. have demonstrated the feasibility of a mindfulness-based group therapy aimed at expanding couples' sexual intimacy, with moderate improvement in sexual satisfaction and mindfulness by patients, which was accompanied by a small decrease in partners' relationship satisfaction and heightened anxiety in both (Bossio et al., 2021). Moreover, Kemerer et al. (2023) have documented improvements in sexual distress, satisfaction, and quality of life when comparing group mindfulness and group CBT versus no treatment.

Couple-Based Interventions

Accounting for the interdependence of patients' and partners' well-being translates into intervention modalities that involve the dyad. Couple-based interventions are particularly promising in the context of chronic illness as (1) patients and partners' sexual function and well-being are impacted, (2) the dyad capitalises on their reciprocal skills and competences to effectively communicate illness-related burden and renegotiate sexuality and intimacy, and (3) partners are perceived as an integral part of the process. A systematic review of interventions for couples coping with chronic illnesses conducted by Berry et al. (2017) underscored that couple-based interventions are more effective than patient-only ones. Specifically, "relationship counselling" approaches were most effective in addressing intimacy and sexual communication, except for cognitive-behavioural skills training targeting relationship or intimacy difficulties. In that case, improved sexual self-schema, intimacy, and relationship quality (Kuijer et al., 2004; Scott et al., 2004) were reported. Other reviews conducted in the context of cancer (Carroll et al., 2016; Scott & Kayser, 2009) highlighted that interventions involving partners had a more favourable impact on sexual outcomes, psychological well-being, and body image. Li and Loke (2014) further supported the positive effects of couple-based interventions on communication, sexual functioning, marital satisfaction, and quality of life, while Hu et al. (2019) highlighted that some improvements may be short-term. However, conflicting findings have been reported in more recent works: a meta-analysis by Li et al. (2020) documented a lack of significant results for sexual function and sexual self-concept of patients and partners, whether males or females. The only beneficial effect was recorded for partners' sexual relationships. Similar indications were reported in breast cancer (Li et al., 2023). These variations in findings may be due to the heterogeneity of cancer types, stage of the disease, psychosexual impairment of the dyad, and measures utilised. Additional methodological limitations include small sample size, study designs, description of the randomisation process, and limited reporting about couples who withdrew from programmes (Badr et al., 2019; Berry et al., 2017; Jonsdottir et al., 2018; Li et al., 2020).

Conclusion

The chapter offered a review of the literature related to the impact of chronic illness on sexuality, underscoring the profound and prolonged consequences for patients and partners. Emphasis was placed on the role of dyadic coping and effective communication strategies in achieving optimal outcomes, alongside an examination of current intervention approaches. As our knowledge is mostly grounded in heterosexual, non-Hispanic White samples from Western cultures, these insights may not adequately represent the experiences and needs of individuals from Black, Indigenous, and People of Colour (BIPOC) communities and SGM groups, underlining a significant need for more inclusive research focusing on equitable approaches to care. Additionally, qualitative and mixed methods studies may be utilised to further characterise patients' and partners' experiences, as well as evolving interpersonal dynamics and care transitions that may challenge sexual relationships. Evidence pertaining to the effectiveness of interventions and their integration into standard care has yielded mixed results: while psychological interventions have recently gained momentum, short-term improvements, often reported by only one partner, have been documented. These findings emphasise the need for more rigorous research efforts, including larger and more diverse samples, use of validated questionnaires, and options such as community-engaged research to breach barriers. It is essential to understand more factors contributing to positive outcomes and mechanisms leading to change. A multidisciplinary approach is urged to ensure that the evolving needs of patients, partners, and dyads can be assessed across the illness continuum and that intervention strategies – from pharmacological options, pelvic floor rehabilitation, use of lubricants, dilators, assistive devices, to psychological and therapeutic approaches – be offered in a timely and personalised manner.

Further Reading

Braybrook, D., Bristowe, K., Timmins, L., Roach, A., Day, E., Clift, P., Rose, R., Marshall, S., Johnson, K., Sleeman, K. E., & Harding, R. (2023). Communication about sexual orientation and gender between clinicians, LGBT+ people facing serious illness and their significant others: a qualitative interview study of experiences, preferences, and recommendations. *BMJ Quality & Safety*, *32*(2), 109–120. https://doi.org/10.1136/bmjqs-2022-014792

Igerc, I., & Schrems, B. (2023). Sexual well-being needs of patients with chronic illness expressed in health care: A scoping review. *Journal of Clinical Nursing*, *32*(19–20), 6832–6848. https://doi.org/10.1111/jocn.16773

O'Connor, S. R., Connaghan, J., Maguire, R., Kotronoulas, G., Flannagan, C., Jain, S., Brady, N., & McCaughan, E. (2019). Healthcare professionals perceived barriers and facilitators to discussing sexual wellbeing with patients after diagnosis of chronic illness: A mixed-methods evidence synthesis. *Patient Education and Counseling*, *102*(5), 850–863. https://doi.org/10.1016/j.pec.2018.12.015

References

Abbasi, A., Ebrahimi, H., Bagheri, H., Basirinezhad, M. H., Mirhosseini, S., & Mohammadpourhodki, R. (2020). A randomized trial of the effect of peer education on the sexual quality of life in patients with myocardial infarction. *J Complement Integr Med*, *17*(3). https://doi.org/10.1515/jcim-2019-0204

Abelson, J. S., Chait, A., Shen, M. J., Charlson, M., Dickerman, A., & Yeo, H. L. (2018). Sources of distress among patients undergoing surgery for colorectal cancer: a qualitative study. *J Surg Res*, *226*, 140–149. https://doi.org/10.1016/j.jss.2018.01.017

Acquati, C., Head, K. J., Rand, K. L., Alwine, J. S., Short, D. N., Cohee, A. A., Champion, V. L., & Draucker, C. B. (2023a). Psychosocial experiences, challenges, and recommendations for care delivery among partners of breast cancer survivors: a qualitative study. *Int J Environ Res Public Health*, *20*(4). https://doi.org/10.3390/ijerph20042786

Acquati, C., Hendren, S., Wittmann, D., Reese, J. B., Karam, E., Duby, A., Dunn, K. B., & Kayser, K. (2022). Psychological and sexual distress in rectal cancer patients and partners. *Psychooncology*, *31*(6), 920–928. https://doi.org/10.1002/pon.5880

Acquati, C., Kayser, K., Wittmann, D., Hendren, S., Reese, J.B., Karam, E., Duby, A., Dunn, K.B. (2023b). Congruence of Dyadic Coping Behaviours among Rectal Cancer Patients and Their Partners: Implications for Emotional, Relational, and Sexual Health Outcomes, International Psycho Oncology Society, Milan, Italy: IPOS 2023 Abstracts Booklet. *Journal of Psychosocial Oncology Research and Practice*, *5*(S1): e111, September 2023. | DOI: 10.1097/OR9.0000000000000111

Assari, S. (2014). Intercourse avoidance among women with coronary artery disease. *The Journal of Sexual Medicine*, *11*(7), 1709–1716. https://doi.org/10.1111/jsm.12459

Atwood, J. D., Klucinec, E., & Neaver, E. (2006). A combined-constructionist therapeutic approach to couples experiencing erectile dysfunction: Part I. *Contemporary Family Therapy*, *28*(4), 393–402. https://doi.org/10.1007/s10591-006-9017-8

Auger, L.-P., Filiatrault, J., Allegue, D. R., Vachon, B., Thomas, A., Morales, E., & Rochette, A. (2023). Sexual rehabilitation after a stroke: A multi-site qualitative study about influencing factors and strategies to improve services. *Sexuality and Disability*, *41*(3), 503–529. https://doi.org/10.1007/s11195-023-09795-x

Badr, H., Bakhshaie, J., & Chhabria, K. (2019). Dyadic interventions for cancer survivors and caregivers: State of the science and new directions. *Semin Oncol Nurs*, *35*(4), 337–341. https://doi.org/10.1016/j.soncn.2019.06.004

Baert, A., Pardaens, S., De Smedt, D., Puddu, P. E., Ciancarelli, M. C., Dawodu, A., De Sutter, J., De Bacquer, D., & Clays, E. (2019). Sexual activity in heart failure patients: Information needs and association with health-related quality of life. *International Journal of Environmental Research and Public Health*, *16*(9), 1570. https://www.mdpi.com/1660-4601/16/9/1570

Banbury, S., Chandler, C., & Lusher, J. (2023). A systematic review exploring the effectiveness of mindfulness for sexual functioning in women with cancer. *Psych*, *5*(1), 194–208. https://www.mdpi.com/2624-8611/5/1/15

Banbury, S., Lusher, J., Snuggs, S., & Chandler, C. (2023). Mindfulness-based therapies for men and women with sexual dysfunction: a systematic review and meta-analysis. *Sexual and Relationship Therapy*, *38*(4), 534–555. https://doi.org/10.1080/14681994.2021.1883578

Barnard, K. D., Naranjo, D., Johnson, N., Norton, A., Scibilia, R., Reidy, C., Tutton, S., & Meeking, D. (2019). Diabetes and female sexual health: an ongoing challenge. *Practical Diabetes*, *36*(5), 165–169. https://doi.org/10.1002/pdi.2238

Basson, R. (2000). The female sexual response: a different model. *J Sex Marital Ther*, *26*(1), 51–65. https://doi.org/10.1080/009262300278641

Basson, R. (2010). Sexual function of women with chronic illness and cancer. *Womens Health (Lond)*, *6*(3), 407–429. https://doi.org/10.2217/whe.10.23

Beck, A. M., Robinson, J. W., & Carlson, L. E. (2013). Sexual values as the key to maintaining satisfying sex after prostate cancer treatment: the physical pleasure–relational intimacy model of sexual motivation. *Archives of Sexual Behavior*, *42*(8), 1637–1647. https://doi.org/10.1007/s10508-013-0168-z

Berg, C. A., Helgeson, V. S., Tracy, E. L., Butner, J. E., Kelly, C. S., Van Vleet, M., & Litchman, M. L. (2020). Daily illness appraisal and collaboration in couples with type 1 diabetes. *Health Psychology*, *39*(8), 689.

Berry, E., Davies, M., & Dempster, M. (2017). Exploring the effectiveness of couples interventions for adults living with a chronic physical illness: a systematic review. *Patient Educ Couns*, *100*(7), 1287–1303. https://doi.org/10.1016/j.pec.2017.02.015

Bertschi, I. C., Meier, F., & Bodenmann, G. (2021). Disability as an interpersonal experience: a systematic review on dyadic challenges and dyadic coping when one partner has a chronic physical or sensory impairment. *Frontiers in psychology*, *12*, 624609.
Bjerggaard, M., Charles, M., Kristensen, E., Lauritzen, T., Sandbæk, A., & Giraldi, A. (2015). Prevalence of sexual concerns and sexual dysfunction among sexually active and inactive men and women with screen-detected type 2 diabetes. *Sex Med*, *3*(4), 302–310. https://doi.org/10.1002/sm2.91
Bober, S. L., & Varela, V. S. (2012). Sexuality in adult cancer survivors: challenges and intervention. *J Clin Oncol*, *30*(30), 3712–3719. https://doi.org/10.1200/jco.2012.41.7915
Bodenmann, G. (1995). A systemic-transactional conceptualization of stress and coping in couples. *Swiss Journal of Psychology / Schweizerische Zeitschrift für Psychologie / Revue Suisse de Psychologie*, *54*(1), 34–49.
Bodenmann, G. (1997). Dyadic coping: A systemic-transactional view of stress and coping among couples: Theory and empirical findings. *European Review of Applied Psychology / Revue Européenne de Psychologie Appliquée*, *47*(2), 137–141.
Bossio, J. A., Higano, C. S., & Brotto, L. A. (2021). Preliminary development of a mindfulness-based group therapy to expand couples' sexual intimacy after prostate cancer: a mixed methods approach. *Sex Med*, *9*(2), 100310. https://doi.org/10.1016/j.esxm.2020.100310
Bouchard, K., Gareau, A., Greenman, P. S., Lalande, K., Sztajerowska, K., & Tulloch, H. (2023). What's love got to do with it? Relationship quality appraisals and quality of life in couples facing cardiovascular disease. *Health Psychol Behav Med*, *11*(1), 2237564. https://doi.org/10.1080/21642850.2023.2237564
Brotto, L., Atallah, S., Johnson-Agbakwu, C., Rosenbaum, T., Abdo, C., Byers, E. S., Graham, C., Nobre, P., & Wylie, K. (2016). Psychological and interpersonal dimensions of sexual function and dysfunction. *The Journal of Sexual Medicine*, *13*(4), 538–571.
Byrne, M., Doherty, S., Fridlund, B. G., Mårtensson, J., Steinke, E. E., Jaarsma, T., & Devane, D. (2016). Sexual counselling for sexual problems in patients with cardiovascular disease. *Cochrane Database Syst Rev*, *2*(2), Cd010988. https://doi.org/10.1002/14651858.CD010988.pub2
Byrne, M., Murphy, P., D'Eath, M., Doherty, S., & Jaarsma, T. (2017). Association Between Sexual Problems and Relationship Satisfaction Among People With Cardiovascular Disease. *J Sex Med*, *14*(5), 666–674. https://doi.org/10.1016/j.jsxm.2017.03.252
Canzona, M. R., Fisher, C. L., & Ledford, C. J. W. (2019). Perpetuating the cycle of silence: the intersection of uncertainty and sexual health communication among couples after breast cancer treatment. *Support Care Cancer*, *27*(2), 659–668. https://doi.org/10.1007/s00520-018-4369-9
Capogrosso, P., Vertosick, E. A., Benfante, N. E., Eastham, J. A., Scardino, P. J., Vickers, A. J., & Mulhall, J. P. (2019). Are We Improving Erectile Function Recovery After Radical Prostatectomy? Analysis of Patients Treated over the Last Decade. *European Urology*, *75*(2), 221–228. https://doi.org/10.1016/j.eururo.2018.08.039
Carroll, A. J., Baron, S. R., & Carroll, R. A. (2016). Couple-based treatment for sexual problems following breast cancer: A review and synthesis of the literature. *Support Care Cancer*, *24*(8), 3651–3659. https://doi.org/10.1007/s00520-016-3218-y
Cleary, V., & Hegarty, J. (2011). Understanding sexuality in women with gynaecological cancer. *Eur J Oncol Nurs*, *15*(1), 38–45. https://doi.org/10.1016/j.ejon.2010.05.008
Congard, A., Christophe, V., Duprez, C., Baudry, A. S., Antoine, P., Lesur, A., Loustalot, C., Guillemet, C., Leclercq, M., Segura, C., Carlier, D., Lefeuvre-Plesse, C., Simon, H., Frenel, J. S., & Vanlemmens, L. (2019). The self-reported perceptions of the repercussions of the disease and its treatments on daily life for young women with breast cancer and their partners. *J Psychosoc Oncol*, *37*(1), 50–68. https://doi.org/10.1080/07347332.2018.1479326

D'Eath, M., Byrne, M., Murphy, P., Jaarsma, T., McSharry, J., Murphy, A. W., Doherty, S., Noone, C., & Casey, D. (2018). Participants' Experiences of a Sexual Counseling Intervention During Cardiac Rehabilitation: A Nested Qualitative Study Within the CHARMS Pilot Randomized Controlled Trial. *J Cardiovasc Nurs*, *33*(5), E35–e45. https://doi.org/10.1097/jcn.0000000000000482

de Wit, M., Trief, P. M., Huber, J. W., & Willaing, I. (2020). State of the art: understanding and integration of the social context in diabetes care. *Diabet Med*, *37*(3), 473–482. https://doi.org/10.1111/dme.14226

DuHamel, K., Schuler, T., Nelson, C., Philip, E., Temple, L., Schover, L., Baser, R. E., Starr, T. D., Cannon, K., Jennings, S., Jandorf, L., & Carter, J. (2016). The sexual health of female rectal and anal cancer survivors: results of a pilot randomized psycho-educational intervention trial. *J Cancer Surviv*, *10*(3), 553–563. https://doi.org/10.1007/s11764-015-0501-8

Elliott, S., & Matthew, A. (2018). Sexual Recovery Following Prostate Cancer: Recommendations From 2 Established Canadian Sexual Rehabilitation Clinics. *Sex Med Rev*, *6*(2), 279–294. https://doi.org/10.1016/j.sxmr.2017.09.001

Emanu, J. C., Avildsen, I. K., & Nelson, C. J. (2016). Erectile dysfunction after radical prostatectomy: prevalence, medical treatments, and psychosocial interventions. *Current Opinion in Supportive and Palliative Care*, *10*(1), 102–107. https://doi.org/10.1097/spc.0000000000000195

Epifanio, M. S., La Grutta, S., Alfano, P., Marcantonio, S., Piombo, M. A., Ammirata, M., Rebulla, E., Grassi, S., Leone, S., Clemenza, F., Girgenti, R., Lo Baido, R., & Di Blasi, M. (2023). Sexual Satisfaction and Quality of Life in Cardiovascular Patients: The Mediating Role of Anxiety. *Healthcare (Basel)*, *11*(3). https://doi.org/10.3390/healthcare11030290

Falconier, M. K., Jackson, J. B., Hilpert, P., & Bodenmann, G. (2015). Dyadic coping and relationship satisfaction: A meta-analysis. *Clinical Psychology Review*, *42*, 28–46. https://doi.org/10.1016/j.cpr.2015.07.002

Falconier, M. K., & Kuhn, R. (2019). Dyadic Coping in Couples: A Conceptual Integration and a Review of the Empirical Literature [Systematic Review]. *Frontiers in psychology*, *10*. https://doi.org/10.3389/fpsyg.2019.00571

Fischer, V. J., Andersson, G., Billieux, J., & Vögele, C. (2022). The Relationship Between Emotion Regulation and Sexual Function and Satisfaction: A Scoping Review. *Sex Med Rev*, *10*(2), 195–208. https://doi.org/10.1016/j.sxmr.2021.11.004

Fisher, L., Chesla, C. A., Chun, K. M., Skaff, M. M., Mullan, J. T., Kanter, R. A., & Gardiner, P. S. (2004). Patient-Appraised Couple Emotion Management and Disease Management Among Chinese American Patients With Type 2 Diabetes. *Journal of Family Psychology*, *18*(2), 302–310. https://doi.org/10.1037/0893-3200.18.2.302

Giannopapas, V., Kitsos, D., Tsogka, A., Tzartos, J. S., Paraskevas, G., Tsivgoulis, G., Voumvourakis, K., Giannopoulos, S., & Bakalidou, D. (2023). Sexual dysfunction therapeutic approaches in patients with multiple sclerosis: a systematic review. *Neurol Sci*, *44*(3), 873–880. https://doi.org/10.1007/s10072-022-06572-0

Gillibrand, R., & Stevenson, J. (2007). The role of partner relationships in the young person's adherence to the diabetes self-care regime. *Int J Behav Med*, *14*(3), 151–155. https://doi.org/10.1007/bf03000186

Grondhuis Palacios, L. A., Krouwel, E. M., den Oudsten, B. L., den Ouden, M. E. M., Kloens, G. J., van Duijn, G., Putter, H., Pelger, R. C. M., & Elzevier, H. W. (2018). Suitable sexual health care according to men with prostate cancer and their partners. *Supportive Care in Cancer*, *26*(12), 4169–4176. https://doi.org/10.1007/s00520-018-4290-2

Gupta, N., Zebib, L., Wittmann, D., Nelson, C. J., Salter, C. A., Mulhall, J. P., Byrne, N., Nolasco, T. S., & Loeb, S. (2023). Understanding the sexual health perceptions, concerns, and needs of female partners of prostate cancer survivors. *J Sex Med*, *20*(5), 651–660. https://doi.org/10.1093/jsxmed/qdad027

Hajat, C., & Stein, E. (2018). The global burden of multiple chronic conditions: A narrative review. *Prev Med Rep*, *12*, 284–293. https://doi.org/10.1016/j.pmedr.2018.10.008

Helgeson, V. S., Berg, C. A., Kelly, C. S., Van Vleet, M., Zajdel, M., Tracy, E. L., & Litchman, M. L. (2019). Patient and partner illness appraisals and health among adults with type 1 diabetes. *J Behav Med*, *42*(3), 480–492. https://doi.org/10.1007/s10865-018-0001-1

Helgeson, V. S., Jakubiak, B., Seltman, H., Hausmann, L., & Korytkowski, M. (2017). Implicit and explicit communal coping in couples with recently diagnosed type 2 diabetes. *Journal of Social and Personal Relationships*, *34*(7), 1099–1121. https://doi.org/10.1177/0265407516669604

Helgeson, V. S., Naqvi, J. B., Seltman, H., Vaughn, A. K., Korytkowski, M., Hausmann, L. R. M., & Gary-Webb, T. L. (2020). Links of communal coping to relationship and psychological health in type 2 diabetes: actor-partner interdependence models involving role, sex, and race. *Ann Behav Med*, *54*(5), 346–359. https://doi.org/10.1093/abm/kaz052

Heyne, S., Esser, P., Geue, K., Friedrich, M., & Mehnert-Theuerkauf, A. (2021). Frequency of Sexual Problems and Related Psychosocial Characteristics in Cancer Patients—Findings From an Epidemiological Multicenter Study in Germany [Original Research]. *Frontiers in psychology*, *12*. https://doi.org/10.3389/fpsyg.2021.679870

Hu, Y., Liu, T., & Li, F. (2019). Association between dyadic interventions and outcomes in cancer patients: a meta-analysis. *Support Care Cancer*, *27*(3), 745–761. https://doi.org/10.1007/s00520-018-4556-8

Hyde, M. K., Newton, R. U., Galvão, D. A., Gardiner, R. A., Occhipinti, S., Lowe, A., Wittert, G. A., & Chambers, S. K. (2017). Men's help-seeking in the first year after diagnosis of localised prostate cancer. *European Journal of Cancer Care*, *26*(2), e12497. https://doi.org/10.1111/ecc.12497

Jaderek, I., & Lew-Starowicz, M. (2019). A Systematic Review on Mindfulness Meditation-Based Interventions for Sexual Dysfunctions. *J Sex Med*, *16*(10), 1581–1596. https://doi.org/10.1016/j.jsxm.2019.07.019

Johnson, M. D., Anderson, J. R., Walker, A., Wilcox, A., Lewis, V. L., & Robbins, D. C. (2013). Common dyadic coping is indirectly related to dietary and exercise adherence via patient and partner diabetes efficacy. *J Fam Psychol*, *27*(5), 722–730. https://doi.org/10.1037/a0034006

Johnson, M. D., Anderson, J. R., Walker, A., Wilcox, A., Lewis, V. L., & Robbins, D. C. (2015). Spousal overprotection is indirectly associated with poorer dietary adherence for patients with type 2 diabetes via diabetes distress when active engagement is low. *British Journal of Health Psychology*, *20*(2), 360–373. https://doi.org/10.1111/bjhp.12105

Johnson, M. D., Anderson, J. R., Wilcox, A., Walker, A., Robbins, D. C., & Lewis, V. L. (2013). Relationship beliefs and illness appraisals are differentially associated with specific ways of coping in spouses of patients with type 2 diabetes. *Psychol Health*, *28*(12), 1442–1459. https://doi.org/10.1080/08870446.2013.822499

Jonsdottir, J. I., Jonsdottir, H., & Klinke, M. E. (2018). A systematic review of characteristics of couple-based intervention studies addressing sexuality following cancer. *J Adv Nurs*, *74*(4), 760–773. https://doi.org/10.1111/jan.13470

Kaplan, E. H. (1995). Model-based representations of human sexual behavior. Sexual Nature Sexual Culture. University of Chicago Press: Chicago, 353–370.

Kaplan Serin, E., Duman, M., & Yilmaz, S. (2020). Sexual Life Quality and Marital Adjustment in Women With and Without Diabetes. *Sexuality and Disability*, *38*(4), 625–635. https://doi.org/10.1007/s11195-020-09663-y

Katz-Wise, S. L., & Hyde, J. S. (2014). Sexuality and gender: The interplay. In *APA handbook of sexuality andpsychology, Vol. 1: Person-based approaches* (pp. 29–62). American Psychological Association. https://doi.org/10.1037/14193-002

Katz, A. (2021). *Sexuality and Illness: A Guidebook for Health Professionals* (1st ed.). Routledge. https://doi.org/10.4324/9781003145745

Kayser, K., Acquati, C., Reese, J. B., Mark, K., Wittmann, D., & Karam, E. (2018). A systematic review of dyadic studies examining relationship quality in couples facing colorectal cancer together. *Psycho-Oncology*, *27*(1), 13–21. https://doi.org/10.1002/pon.4339

Kemerer, B. M., Zdaniuk, B., Higano, C. S., Bossio, J. A., Camara Bicalho Santos, R., Flannigan, R., & Brotto, L. A. (2023). A randomized comparison of group mindfulness and group cognitive behavioral therapy vs control for couples after prostate cancer with sexual dysfunction. *J Sex Med*, *20*(3), 346–366. https://doi.org/10.1093/jsxmed/qdac038

Kim, J. H., Yang, Y., & Hwang, E. S. (2015). The Effectiveness of Psychoeducational Interventions Focused on Sexuality in Cancer. *Cancer Nurs*, *38*(5), E32–42. https://doi.org/10.1097/ncc.0000000000000212

Kim, Y., Kashy, D. A., Wellisch, D. K., Spillers, R. L., Kaw, C. K., & Smith, T. G. (2008). Quality of life in couples dealing with cancer: Dyadic and individual adjustment among breast and prostate cancer survivors and their spousal caregivers. *Annals of Behavioral Medicine*, *35*(2), 230–238. https://doi.org/10.1007/s12160-008-9026-y

Kingsberg, S. A., Althof, S., Simon, J. A., Bradford, A., Bitzer, J., Carvalho, J., Flynn, K. E., Nappi, R. E., Reese, J. B., Rezaee, R. L., Schover, L., & Shifrin, J. L. (2017). Female Sexual Dysfunction-Medical and Psychological Treatments, Committee 14. *J Sex Med*, *14*(12), 1463–1491. https://doi.org/10.1016/j.jsxm.2017.05.018

Kriston, L., Günzler, C., Agyemang, A., Bengel, J., & Berner, M. M. (2010). Effect of Sexual Function on Health-Related Quality of Life Mediated by Depressive Symptoms in Cardiac Rehabilitation. Findings of the SPARK Project in 493 Patients. *The Journal of Sexual Medicine*, *7*(6), 2044–2055. https://doi.org/10.1111/j.1743-6109.2010.01761.x

Kuenzler, A., Hodgkinson, K., Zindel, A., Bargetzi, M., & Znoj, H. J. (2011). Who cares, who bears, who benefits? Female spouses vicariously carry the burden after cancer diagnosis. *Psychol Health*, *26*(3), 337–352. https://doi.org/10.1080/08870440903418877

Kuijer, R. G., Buunk, B. P., De Jong, G. M., Ybema, J. F., & Sanderman, R. (2004). Effects of a brief intervention program for patients with cancer and their partners on feelings of inequity, relationship quality and psychological distress. *Psychooncology*, *13*(5), 321–334. https://doi.org/10.1002/pon.749

Larraz, A. M. C., Moya, A. V., & Actis, C. C. (2023). Mindfulness-Based Intervention and Sexuality: A Systematic Review. *Trends Psychiatry Psychother*. https://doi.org/10.47626/2237-6089-2021-0459

Lawton, J., Rankin, D., Elliott, J., Heller, S. R., Rogers, H. A., De Zoysa, N., & Amiel, S. (2014). Experiences, views, and support needs of family members of people with hypoglycemia unawareness: interview study. *Diabetes Care*, *37*(1), 109–115. https://doi.org/10.2337/dc13-1154

Leavitt, C. E., Lefkowitz, E. S., & Waterman, E. A. (2019). The role of sexual mindfulness in sexual wellbeing, Relational wellbeing, and self-esteem. *Journal of Sex & Marital Therapy*, *45*(6), 497–509. https://doi.org/10.1080/0092623X.2019.1572680

Lee, J., Helgeson, V., Van Vleet, M., Tracy, E., Kent de Grey, R., Zajdel, M., & Berg, C. (2020). Implications of we-talk for relationships and health among patients with type 1 diabetes and their spouses. *Journal of Social and Personal Relationships*. https://doi.org/10.1177/0265407519865613

Levin, A. O., Carpenter, K. M., Fowler, J. M., Brothers, B. M., Andersen, B. L., & Maxwell, G. L. (2010). Sexual morbidity associated with poorer psychological adjustment among gynecological cancer survivors. *Int J Gynecol Cancer*, *20*(3), 461–470. https://doi.org/10.1111/IGC.0b013e3181d24ce0

Li, M., Chan, C. W. H., Chow, K. M., Xiao, J., & Choi, K. C. (2020). A systematic review and meta-analysis of couple-based intervention on sexuality and the quality of life of cancer patients and their partners. *Support Care Cancer*, *28*(4), 1607–1630. https://doi.org/10.1007/s00520-019-05215-z

Li, M., Zhang, L., Li, N., Luo, X., Chen, J., Zhang, Y., Xiong, C., Zhao, M., Guo, Z., & Yan, J. (2023). Effects of couple-based dyadic interventions on breast cancer patients and their intimate partners: A systematic review and meta-analysis. *J Adv Nurs*, *79*(9), 3192–3213. https://doi.org/10.1111/jan.15639

Li, Q., & Loke, A. Y. (2014). A systematic review of spousal couple-based intervention studies for couples coping with cancer: direction for the development of interventions. *Psychooncology*, *23*(7), 731–739. https://doi.org/10.1002/pon.3535

Li, R., Wittmann, D., Nelson, C. J., Salter, C. A., Mulhall, J. P., Byrne, N., Nolasco, T. S., Ness, M., Gupta, N., Cassidy, C., Crisostomo-Wynne, T., & Loeb, S. (2022). Unmet Sexual Health Needs of Patients and Female Partners Following Diagnosis and Treatment for Prostate Cancer. *J Sex Med*, *19*(12), 1797–1803. https://doi.org/10.1016/j.jsxm.2022.08.195

Lindau, S. T., Abramsohn, E., Gosch, K., Wroblewski, K., Spatz, E. S., Chan, P. S., Spertus, J., & Krumholz, H. M. (2012). Patterns and Loss of Sexual Activity in the Year Following Hospitalization for Acute Myocardial Infarction (a United States National Multisite Observational Study). *American Journal of Cardiology*, *109*(10), 1439–1444. https://doi.org/10.1016/j.amjcard.2012.01.355

Lister, Z., Fox, C., & Wilson, C. M. (2013). Couples and Diabetes: A 30-Year Narrative Review of Dyadic Relational Research. *Contemporary Family Therapy*, *35*(4), 613–638. https://doi.org/10.1007/s10591-013-9250-x

Loaring, J. M., Larkin, M., Shaw, R., & Flowers, P. (2015). Renegotiating sexual intimacy in the context of altered embodiment: the experiences of women with breast cancer and their male partners following mastectomy and reconstruction. *Health Psychol*, *34*(4), 426–436. https://doi.org/10.1037/hea0000195

Lovelace, D. L., McDaniel, L. R., & Golden, D. (2019). Long-Term Effects of Breast Cancer Surgery, Treatment, and Survivor Care. *J Midwifery Womens Health*, *64*(6), 713–724. https://doi.org/10.1111/jmwh.13012

Mallory, A., Stanton, A., & Handy, A. (2019). Couples' Sexual Communication and Dimensions of Sexual Function: A Meta-Analysis. *The Journal of Sex Research*, *56*, 1–17. https://doi.org/10.1080/00224499.2019.1568375

Manne, S., & Badr, H. (2008). Intimacy and relationship processes in couples' psychosocial adaptation to cancer. *Cancer*, *112*(11 Suppl), 2541–2555. https://doi.org/10.1002/cncr.23450

Manne, S., & Badr, H. (2010). Intimacy processes and psychological distress among couples coping with head and neck or lung cancers. *Psychooncology*, *19*(9), 941–954. https://doi.org/10.1002/pon.1645

Manne, S., Badr, H., Zaider, T., Nelson, C., & Kissane, D. (2010). Cancer-related communication, relationship intimacy, and psychological distress among couples coping with localized prostate cancer. *J Cancer Surviv*, *4*(1), 74–85. https://doi.org/10.1007/s11764-009-0109-y

Manne, S., Kashy, D. A., Zaider, T., Lee, D., Kim, I. Y., Heckman, C., Penedo, F., Kissane, D., & Virtue, S. M. (2018). Interpersonal processes and intimacy among men with localized prostate cancer and their partners. *J Fam Psychol*, *32*(5), 664–675. https://doi.org/10.1037/fam0000404

Manne, S., Ostroff, J., Rini, C., Fox, K., Goldstein, L., & Grana, G. (2004). The interpersonal process model of intimacy: the role of self-disclosure, partner disclosure, and partner responsiveness in interactions between breast cancer patients and their partners. *J Fam Psychol*, *18*(4), 589–599. https://doi.org/10.1037/0893-3200.18.4.589

Manne, S. L., Kissane, D., Zaider, T., Kashy, D., Lee, D., Heckman, C., & Virtue, S. M. (2015). Holding back, intimacy, and psychological and relationship outcomes among couples coping with prostate cancer. *J Fam Psychol*, *29*(5), 708–719. https://doi.org/10.1037/fam0000096

Marques, A. D. B., Amorim, R. F., Landim, F. L. P., Moreira, T. M. M., Branco, J. G. O., Morais, P. B., & Santos, Z. (2018). Body consciousness of people with intestinal stomach: A phenomenological study. *Rev Bras Enferm*, *71*(2), 391–397. https://doi.org/10.1590/0034-7167-2016-0666

Martin, R., Renouf, T., Rigby, J., Hafeez, S., Thurairaja, R., Kumar, P., Cruickshank, S., & Van-Hemelrijck, M. (2023). Female sexual function in bladder cancer: A review of the evidence. *BJUI Compass*, *4*(1), 5–23. https://doi.org/10.1002/bco2.186

Masters, W. H., & Johnson, V. E. (1966). *Human sexual response*. Little, Brown.

Messina, R., Due-Christensen, M., Keller-Senn, A., Polek, E., Fantini, M. P., & Sturt, J. (2021). Couples living with type 1 diabetes: An integrative review of the impacts on health and wellbeing. *J Health Psychol*, *26*(3), 412–437. https://doi.org/10.1177/1359105318817356

Mestre-Bach, G., Blycker, G. R., & Potenza, M. N. (2022). Behavioral Therapies for Treating Female Sexual Dysfunctions: A State-of-the-Art Review. *J Clin Med*, *11*(10). https://doi.org/10.3390/jcm11102794

Metz, M. E., Epstein, N. B., & McCarthy, B. (2018). *Cognitive-behavioral therapy for sexual dysfunction*. Routledge/Taylor & Francis Group.

Murphy, P. J., Noone, C., D'Eath, M., Casey, D., Doherty, S., Jaarsma, T., Murphy, A. W., O'Donnell, M., Fallon, N., Gillespie, P., Jalali, A., Sharry, J. M., Newell, J., Toomey, E., Steinke, E. E., & Byrne, M. (2018). The CHARMS pilot study: a multi-method assessment of the feasibility of a sexual counselling implementation intervention in cardiac rehabilitation in Ireland. *Pilot Feasibility Stud*, *4*, 88. https://doi.org/10.1186/s40814-018-0278-4

Oberguggenberger, A., Martini, C., Huber, N., Fallowfield, L., Hubalek, M., Daniaux, M., Sperner-Unterweger, B., Holzner, B., Sztankay, M., Gamper, E., & Meraner, V. (2017). Self-reported sexual health: Breast cancer survivors compared to women from the general population – an observational study. *BMC Cancer*, *17*(1), 599. https://doi.org/10.1186/s12885-017-3580-2

Ong, K. L., Stafford, L. K., McLaughlin, S. A., Boyko, E. J., Vollset, S. E., Smith, A. E., Dalton, B. E., Duprey, J., Cruz, J. A., Hagins, H., Lindstedt, P. A., Aali, A., Abate, Y. H., Abate, M. D., Abbasian, M., Abbasi-Kangevari, Z., Abbasi-Kangevari, M., Abd ElHafeez, S., Abd-Rabu, R., … Vos, T. (2023). Global, regional, and national burden of diabetes from 1990 to 2021, with projections of prevalence to 2050: a systematic analysis for the Global Burden of Disease Study 2021. *The Lancet*, *402*(10397), 203–234. https://doi.org/10.1016/S0140-6736(23)01301-6

Park, J. J., Doo, S. W., Kwon, A., Kim, D. K., Yang, W. J., Song, Y. S., Shim, S. R., & Kim, J. H. (2023). Effects of Sexual Rehabilitation on Sexual Dysfunction in Patients with Cardiovascular Disease: A Systematic Review and Meta-Analysis. *World J Mens Health*, *41*(2), 330–341. https://doi.org/10.5534/wjmh.220124

Parmar, R. S., Verma, S., Neelkamal, Pathak, V. K., & Bhadoria, A. S. (2022). Prevalence of erectile dysfunction in Type 2 diabetes mellitus (T2DM) and its predictors among diabetic men. *J Family Med Prim Care*, *11*(7), 3875–3879. https://doi.org/10.4103/jfmpc.jfmpc_1130_21

Pazar, B., Yava, A., & Başal, Ş. (2015). Health-related quality of life in persons living with a urostomy. *J Wound Ostomy Continence Nurs*, *42*(3), 264–270. https://doi.org/10.1097/won.0000000000000110

Pereira, M. G., Marques, O., Rodrigues, Â., Santos, J., & Pedras, S. (2016). Sexual satisfaction in patients with diabetes type 2 and their partners.

Peyrot, M., Egede, L., Funnell, M., Hsu, W., Ruggiero, L., & Stuckey, H. (2018). US Ethnic Group Differences in Family Member Support for People With Diabetes in the 2nd Diabetes Attitudes, Wishes and Needs (DAWN2) Study. *Diabetes Educ*, *44*(3), 249–259. https://doi.org/10.1177/0145721718770767

Polonsky, W. H., Fisher, L., Hessler, D., & Johnson, N. (2016). Emotional Distress in the Partners of Type 1 Diabetes Adults: Worries About Hypoglycemia and Other Key Concerns. *Diabetes Technol Ther*, *18*(5), 292–297. https://doi.org/10.1089/dia.2015.0451
Centers for Disease Control and Prevention. (2023). *What is Diabetes?* Retrieved October 29, 2023 from https://www.cdc.gov/diabetes/basics/diabetes.html
Rapelli, G., Donato, S., Pagani, A. F., Parise, M., Iafrate, R., Pietrabissa, G., Giusti, E. M., Castelnuovo, G., & Bertoni, A. (2021). The Association Between Cardiac Illness-Related Distress and Partner Support: The Moderating Role of Dyadic Coping [Original Research]. *Frontiers in psychology*, *12*. https://doi.org/10.3389/fpsyg.2021.624095
Reese, J. B., Bober, S. L., & Daly, M. B. (2017). Talking about women's sexual health after cancer: Why is it so hard to move the needle? *Cancer*, *123*(24), 4757–4763. https://doi.org/10.1002/cncr.31084
Reese, J. B., Handorf, E., & Haythornthwaite, J. A. (2018). Sexual quality of life, body image distress, and psychosocial outcomes in colorectal cancer: a longitudinal study. *Support Care Cancer*, *26*(10), 3431–3440. https://doi.org/10.1007/s00520-018-4204-3
Reese, J. B., Keefe, F. J., Somers, T. J., & Abernethy, A. P. (2010). Coping with sexual concerns after cancer: the use of flexible coping. *Support Care Cancer*, *18*(7), 785–800. https://doi.org/10.1007/s00520-010-0819-8
Reese, J. B., Shelby, R. A., & Taylor, K. L. (2012). Sexual quality of life in patients undergoing coronary artery bypass graft surgery. *Psychol Health*, *27*(6), 721–736. https://doi.org/10.1080/08870446.2011.623781
Reese, J. B., Zimmaro, L. A., McIlhenny, S., Sorice, K., Porter, L. S., Zaleta, A. K., Daly, M. B., Cribb, B., & Gorman, J. R. (2022). Coping With Changes to Sex and Intimacy After a Diagnosis of Metastatic Breast Cancer: Results From a Qualitative Investigation With Patients and Partners. *Front Psychol*, *13*, 864893. https://doi.org/10.3389/fpsyg.2022.864893
Rintala, T. M., Jaatinen, P., Paavilainen, E., & Astedt-Kurki, P. (2013). Interrelation between adult persons with diabetes and their family: a systematic review of the literature. *J Fam Nurs*, *19*(1), 3–28. https://doi.org/10.1177/1074840712471899
Roberson, P. N. E., & Fincham, F. (2018). Is relationship quality linked to diabetes risk and management?: It depends on what you look at. *Fam Syst Health*, *36*(3), 315–326. https://doi.org/10.1037/fsh0000336
Rottmann, N., Larsen, P. V., Johansen, C., Hagedoorn, M., Dalton, S. O., & Hansen, D. G. (2022). Sexual activity in couples dealing with breast cancer. A cohort study of associations with patient, partner and relationship-related factors. *Frontiers in psychology*, *13*, 828422.
Sansone, A., Mollaioli, D., Ciocca, G., Limoncin, E., Colonnello, E., & Jannini, E. A. (2022). Sexual Dysfunction in Men and Women with Diabetes: A Reflection of their Complications? *Curr Diabetes Rev*, *18*(1), e030821192147. https://doi.org/10.2174/1573399817666210309104740
Santos, A. N., Pascoal, P. M., & Barros, L. (2020). Sexuality in Emerging Adults with Type 1 Diabetes Mellitus: An Exploratory Study Using Thematic Analysis. *J Sex Marital Ther*, *46*(3), 234–245. https://doi.org/10.1080/0092623x.2019.1682730
Savoie, M. B., Paciorek, A., Van Loon, K., Anwar, M., Atreya, C. E., Johnson, P. C., Kenfield, S. A., Laffan, A., Levin, A. O., Smith, J. F., Stanfield, D., Venook, A., Zhang, L., Van Blarigan, E. L., & Rowen, T. (2023). Sexual function remains persistently low in women after treatment for colorectal cancer and anal squamous cell carcinoma. *J Sex Med*, *20*(4), 439–446. https://doi.org/10.1093/jsxmed/qdac047
Scott, J. L., Halford, W. K., & Ward, B. G. (2004). United we stand? The effects of a couple-coping intervention on adjustment to early stage breast or gynecological cancer. *J Consult Clin Psychol*, *72*(6), 1122–1135. https://doi.org/10.1037/0022-006x.72.6.1122
Scott, J. L., & Kayser, K. (2009). A review of couple-based interventions for enhancing women's sexual adjustment and body image after cancer. *Cancer J*, *15*(1), 48–56. https://doi.org/10.1097/PPO.0b013e31819585df

Segrin, C., & Badger, T. A. (2014). Psychological and physical distress are interdependent in breast cancer survivors and their partners. *Psychol Health Med*, *19*(6), 716–723. https://doi.org/10.1080/13548506.2013.871304

Simeone, S., Guillari, A., Pucciarelli, G., Stile, F., Gargiulo, G., Esposito, M., Alvaro, R., & Rea, T. (2020). Sexual Health After Acute Myocardial Infarction: The Lived Experience of Women During the First-Year Post Discharge. *Sexuality and Disability*, *38*(3), 547–560. https://doi.org/10.1007/s11195-020-09627-2

Smith, T. W. (2022). Intimate Relationships and Coronary Heart Disease: Implications for Risk, Prevention, and Patient Management. *Curr Cardiol Rep*, *24*(6), 761–774. https://doi.org/10.1007/s11886-022-01695-4

Smith, T. W., & Baucom, B. R. W. (2017). Intimate relationships, individual adjustment, and coronary heart disease: Implications of overlapping associations in psychosocial risk. *Am Psychol*, *72*(6), 578–589. https://doi.org/10.1037/amp0000123

Smith, T. W., Uchino, B. N., Berg, C. A., & Florsheim, P. (2012). Marital discord and coronary artery disease: a comparison of behaviorally defined discrete groups. *J Consult Clin Psychol*, *80*(1), 87–92. https://doi.org/10.1037/a0026561

Sopfe, J., Pettigrew, J., Afghahi, A., Appiah, L. C., & Coons, H. L. (2021). Interventions to Improve Sexual Health in Women Living with and Surviving Cancer: Review and Recommendations. *Cancers*, *13*(13), 3153. https://www.mdpi.com/2072-6694/13/13/3153

Steinke, E. E., Jaarsma, T., Barnason, S. A., Byrne, M., Doherty, S., Dougherty, C. M., Fridlund, B., Kautz, D. D., Mårtensson, J., Mosack, V., & Moser, D. K. (2013). Sexual counseling for individuals with cardiovascular disease and their partners: a consensus document from the American Heart Association and the ESC Council on Cardiovascular Nursing and Allied Professions (CCNAP). *Circulation*, *128*(18), 2075–2096. https://doi.org/10.1161/CIR.0b013e31829c2e53

Stephanie Buehler, P. D. C. S. T. S. (2021). *What Every Mental Health Professional Needs to Know About Sex, Third Edition*. Springer Publishing Company. https://books.google.com/books?id=yhQ3EAAAQBAJ

Stephenson, K. R., & Kerth, J. (2017). Effects of Mindfulness-Based Therapies for Female Sexual Dysfunction: A Meta-Analytic Review. *The Journal of Sex Research*, *54*(7), 832–849. https://doi.org/10.1080/00224499.2017.1331199

Stratton, H., Sansom, J., Brown-Major, A., Anderson, P., & Ng, L. (2020). Interventions for sexual dysfunction following stroke. *Cochrane Database Syst Rev*, *5*(5), Cd011189. https://doi.org/10.1002/14651858.CD011189.pub2

Strom, J. L., & Egede, L. E. (2012). The impact of social support on outcomes in adult patients with type 2 diabetes: a systematic review. *Curr Diab Rep*, *12*(6), 769–781. https://doi.org/10.1007/s11892-012-0317-0

Stulz, A., Favez, N., & Flahault, C. (2022). Emotional and Sexual Adaptation to Colon Cancer: Perceptual Congruence of Dyadic Coping Among Couples. *Front Psychol*, *13*, 802603. https://doi.org/10.3389/fpsyg.2022.802603

Sung, H., Ferlay, J., Siegel, R. L., Laversanne, M., Soerjomataram, I., Jemal, A., & Bray, F. (2021). Global Cancer Statistics 2020: GLOBOCAN Estimates of Incidence and Mortality Worldwide for 36 Cancers in 185 Countries. *CA: A Cancer Journal for Clinicians*, *71*(3), 209–249. https://doi.org/10.3322/caac.21660

Thylén, I., & Brännström, M. (2015). Intimate relationships and sexual function in partnered patients in the year before and one year after a myocardial infarction: A longitudinal study. *Eur J Cardiovasc Nurs*, *14*(6), 468–477. https://doi.org/10.1177/1474515115571061

Traa, M. J., Braeken, J., De Vries, J., Roukema, J. A., Slooter, G. D., Crolla, R. M., Borremans, M. P., & Den Oudsten, B. L. (2015). Sexual, marital, and general life functioning in couples coping with colorectal cancer: a dyadic study across time. *Psychooncology*, *24*(9), 1181–1188. https://doi.org/10.1002/pon.3801

Traa, M. J., De Vries, J., Bodenmann, G., & Den Oudsten, B. L. (2015). Dyadic coping and relationship functioning in couples coping with cancer: a systematic review. *Br J Health Psychol*, *20*(1), 85–114. https://doi.org/10.1111/bjhp.12094
Tran, P., Tran, L., & Tran, L. (2021). Influence of sexual orientation on diabetes management in US adults with diabetes. *Diabetes Metab*, *47*(1), 101177. https://doi.org/10.1016/j.diabet.2020.07.004
Trief, P. M., Jiang, Y., Beck, R., Huckfeldt, P. J., Knight, T., Miller, K. M., & Weinstock, R. S. (2017). Adults with type 1 diabetes: Partner relationships and outcomes. *Journal of Health Psychology*, *22*(4), 446–456. https://doi.org/10.1177/1359105315605654
Trief, P. M., Morin, P. C., Izquierdo, R., Teresi, J., Starren, J., Shea, S., & Weinstock, R. S. (2006). Marital quality and diabetes outcomes: The IDEATel Project. *Families, Systems, & Health*, *24*(3), 318.
Tsao, C. W., Aday, A. W., Almarzooq, Z. I., Anderson, C. A. M., Arora, P., Avery, C. L., Baker-Smith, C. M., Beaton, A. Z., Boehme, A. K., Buxton, A. E., Commodore-Mensah, Y., Elkind, M. S. V., Evenson, K. R., Eze-Nliam, C., Fugar, S., Generoso, G., Heard, D. G., Hiremath, S., Ho, J. E., … Martin, S. S. (2023). Heart Disease and Stroke Statistics-2023 Update: A Report From the American Heart Association. *Circulation*, *147*(8), e93–e621. https://doi.org/10.1161/cir.0000000000001123
Tulloch, H., Bouchard, K., Clyde, M. J., Madrazo, L., Demidenko, N., Johnson, S., & Greenman, P. (2020). Learning a new way of living together: a qualitative study exploring the relationship changes and intervention needs of patients with cardiovascular disease and their partners. *BMJ Open*, *10*(5), e032948. https://doi.org/10.1136/bmjopen-2019-032948
Ussher, J. M., Perz, J., & Gilbert, E. (2012). Changes to sexual well-being and intimacy after breast cancer. *Cancer Nurs*, *35*(6), 456–465. https://doi.org/10.1097/NCC.0b013e3182395401
Ussher, J. M., Sandoval, M., Perz, J., Wong, W. K. T., & Butow, P. (2013). The Gendered Construction and Experience of Difficulties and Rewards in Cancer Care. *Qualitative Health Research*, *23*(7), 900–915. https://doi.org/10.1177/1049732313484197
Ussher, J. M., Tim Wong, W. K., & Perz, J. (2011). A qualitative analysis of changes in relationship dynamics and roles between people with cancer and their primary informal carer. *Health*, *15*(6), 650–667. https://doi.org/10.1177/1363459310367440
Van Cauwenberghe, J., Enzlin, P., Nefs, G., Ruige, J., Hendrieckx, C., De Block, C., & Pouwer, F. (2022). Prevalence of and risk factors for sexual dysfunctions in adults with type 1 or type 2 diabetes: Results from Diabetes MILES - Flanders. *Diabetic Medicine*, *39*(1), e14676. https://doi.org/10.1111/dme.14676
van Pinxteren, M., Delobelle, P., Levitt, N., Smith, K., Majikela-Dlangamandla, B., & McGrath, N. (2023). 'I accept his manhood is on life-support': A qualitative understanding of the impact of diabetes on sexual relationships among men and women living with type 2 diabetes and their partners in South Africa. *Diabetic Medicine*, *40*(11), e15203. https://doi.org/10.1111/dme.15203
van Roij, J., Raijmakers, N., Johnsen, A. T., Hansen, M. B., Thijs-Visser, M., & van de Poll-Franse, L. (2022). Sexual health and closeness in couples coping with advanced cancer: Results of a multicenter observational study (eQuiPe). *Palliat Med*, *36*(4), 698–707. https://doi.org/10.1177/02692163221074541
Van Vleet, M., Helgeson, V. S., Seltman, H. J., Korytkowski, M. T., & Hausmann, L. R. M. (2018). Communally coping with diabetes: An observational investigation using the actor-partner interdependence model. *J Fam Psychol*, *32*(5), 654–663. https://doi.org/10.1037/fam0000414
Van Vleet, M., Helgeson, V. S., Seltman, H. J., Korytkowski, M. T., & Hausmann, L. R. M. (2019). An examination of the communal coping process in recently diagnosed diabetes. *J Soc Pers Relat*, *36*(4), 1297–1316. https://doi.org/10.1177/0265407518761226
Verschuren, J. E., Enzlin, P., Dijkstra, P. U., Geertzen, J. H., & Dekker, R. (2010). Chronic disease and sexuality: a generic conceptual framework. *J Sex Res*, *47*(2), 153–170. https://doi.org/10.1080/00224491003658227

Weitkamp, K., Feger, F., Landolt, S. A., Roth, M., & Bodenmann, G. (2021). Dyadic coping in couples facing chronic physical illness: a systematic review. *Frontiers in psychology, 12*, 722740.

Wittmann, D. (2016). Emotional and sexual health in cancer: partner and relationship issues. *Curr Opin Support Palliat Care, 10*(1), 75–80. https://doi.org/10.1097/spc.0000000000000187

Wittmann, D., Carolan, M., Given, B., Skolarus, T., An, L., Palapattu, G., & Montie, J. (2014). Exploring the role of the partner in couples' sexual recovery after surgery for prostate cancer. *Supportive Care in Cancer: Official Journal of the Multinational Association of Supportive Care in Cancer, 22*. https://doi.org/10.1007/s00520-014-2244-x

Wittmann, D., Carolan, M., Given, B., Skolarus, T. A., Crossley, H., An, L., Palapattu, G., Clark, P., & Montie, J. E. (2015). What couples say about their recovery of sexual intimacy after prostatectomy: toward the development of a conceptual model of couples' sexual recovery after surgery for prostate cancer. *J Sex Med, 12*(2), 494–504. https://doi.org/10.1111/jsm.12732

Wittmann, D., Mehta, A., Bober, S. L., Zhu, Z., Daignault-Newton, S., Dunn, R. L., Braun, T. M., Carter, C., Duby, A., Northouse, L. L., Koontz, B. F., Glodé, L. M., Brandon, J., Bangs, R., McPhail, J., McPhail, S., Arab, L., Paich, K., Skolarus, T. A., … Pollack, C. E. (2022). TrueNTH Sexual Recovery Intervention for couples coping with prostate cancer: Randomized controlled trial results. *Cancer, 128*(7), 1513–1522. https://doi.org/10.1002/cncr.34076

Wittmann, D., Mehta, A., McCaughan, E., Faraday, M., Duby, A., Matthew, A., Incrocci, L., Burnett, A., Nelson, C. J., Elliott, S., Koontz, B. F., Bober, S. L., McLeod, D., Capogrosso, P., Yap, T., Higano, C., Loeb, S., Capellari, E., Glodé, M., … Mulhall, J. P. (2022). Guidelines for Sexual Health Care for Prostate Cancer Patients: Recommendations of an International Panel. *J Sex Med, 19*(11), 1655–1669. https://doi.org/10.1016/j.jsxm.2022.08.197

WHO (2006). *Defining Sexual Health - Report of a Technical Consultation on Sexual Health 28–31 January 2002* (Sexual Health Document Series, Issue).

Xu, J., Xue, B., Li, L., Qiao, J., Redding, Sharon R., & Ouyang, Y.-Q. (2023). Psychological interventions for sexual function and satisfaction of women with breast cancer: A systematic review and meta-analysis. *Journal of Clinical Nursing, 32*(9–10), 2282–2297. https://doi.org/10.1111/jocn.16194

Zajdel, M., Helgeson, V. S., Seltman, H. J., Korytkowski, M. T., & Hausmann, L. R. M. (2018). Daily Communal Coping in Couples With Type 2 Diabetes: Links to Mood and Self-Care. *Annals of Behavioral Medicine, 52*(3), 228–238. https://doi.org/10.1093/abm/kax047

Zhang, X., Zhu, Z., Tang, G., & Xu, H. (2023). Prevalence and predictors of sexual dysfunction in females with type 1 diabetes: a systematic review and meta-analysis. *J Sex Med, 20*(9), 1161–1171. https://doi.org/10.1093/jsxmed/qdad104

Zhu, A., & Wittmann, D. (2022). Barriers to sexual recovery in men with prostate, bladder and colorectal cancer. *Urol Oncol, 40*(9), 395–402. https://doi.org/10.1016/j.urolonc.2020.08.005

19

CAREGIVING AND RELATIONSHIPS

Val Morrison

Introduction

A substantial number of people confronted with illness or disability need more than occasional social support to deal with the consequences of their condition. In these situations, family members often take on the role of informal caregivers, whether out of love and loyalty, a desire to reciprocate, or out of a sense of necessity or obligation. Many informal caregivers provide care for a parent; others provide care for a spouse or partner or for a close friend; whatever the relationship, its quality and character can vary. What are the consequences of caregiving for caregivers, the care recipients, and the relationship between them over time? What are the unmet needs of informal caregivers, and how can society best support them?

The Context and Characteristics of Informal Family Caregiving

Population changes have resulted in estimates that three in every five of us will be required to provide care to a family member or friend at some point in our lives. Increasing life expectancy, changes in the gender distribution in the workforce, and smaller family sizes seen over recent generations place considerable demands on formal care systems and also on informal caregivers. Almost two-thirds of those aged over the retirement age will currently be living with at least one chronic health condition, many will be living with functional limitations following surgery such as knee or hip replacement that necessitate help from another person, and many will be living with mental health challenges (European Chronic Disease Alliance [ECDA], 2019). In an ageing society, these figures are increasing, whilst simultaneously, health and social care services have been experiencing downward investment (e.g., Matharu et al., 2022). The predicted decline in the availability of informal caregivers is leading to a 'care gap' expected to grow over

DOI: 10.4324/9781003318026-23

the coming decades (Pickard, 2015), which will have considerable consequences for caregivers, care recipients, families and societies.

Definitions of informal caregiving can vary across studies and across legislative, policy, and practice contexts – for example, on the basis of the hours of care provided (Bauer & Sousa-Poza, 2015; European Quality of Life Survey, 2016). When referring to 'informal caregiving', we mean the provision of usually unpaid care to a family member or friend with a chronic illness, disability, or other long-lasting health and care needs (Revenson et al., 2016). Family itself has seen a shift in definition over time, from a family understood as a 'nuclear family' of co-resident parents and children to a family that includes single-parent families, step-families, and extended families, of which not all members may live under the same roof due to employment mobility and globalisation (Bei et al., 2020, Croucher et al., 2020). Caregiving by definition includes at least two people who have a close relationship, and therefore, to understand the impact of caregiving, we need to pay attention to the caregiver, the care recipient, and their relationship.

The tasks of caregiving can be many and varied, ranging from providing emotional support and encouragement to providing practical or material help, and for many, caregiving includes personal care tasks. Some care tasks may be more familiar to the caregiver than others in the context of the person they are providing care for. For example, in the scenario of a female spouse providing care to her male partner following a stroke, carrying out the household chores, shopping, or cooking may be part of the typical spousal role, whereas helping their partner dress, feed, or bathe may not be. Gendered roles exist in most societies, and although the increased proportions of women in employment over the past few decades has led to a readjustment or sharing of household tasks, the norms and expectations with regard to caregiving still remain in the female domain, albeit becoming more socially acceptable for men (Maynard et al., 2018). The feminine role is viewed as encompassing nurturing, with a masculine role encompassing providing; hence, it is often reported that female caregivers more often help with emotional, nursing, or personal care, whereas male caregivers help with household finances or practical tasks (Maynard et al., 2018). This differential and gendered distribution of care may level out however if caregiving is present within a spousal context where both are retired (Hoffmann & Rodrigues, 2010; Zygouri et al., 2021). In addition, the nature and extent of caring tasks will vary depending on whether or not the caregiver and care recipient are co-resident. Co-resident caregivers are more likely to be engaged in personal or nursing care, whereas distance caregivers may be more engaged in emotional care or organisational and instrumental support (Bei et al., 2023). In most national surveys, for example, the Survey of Health, Ageing, and Retirement in Europe (e.g., Börsch-Supan, 2022), a significant minority of informal caregivers are spouses (20%–25%) who are (typically) co-resident with their care recipients, until for some, the care recipient enters a nursing home or other residential care. Female spouses more commonly act as solo carers, whereas male spouses more often share the caregiving of their wife partner with other family members, mainly adult children (Bertogg & Strauss, 2018). Adult children or children-in-law, mostly middle-aged, often with child dependents, make up the lion's share of caregivers (60% in the above SHARE database, for example). Where adult children share the care of an ill, disabled, or ageing parent, little is as yet known about how caregiving is shared between siblings. What we do know suggests that there is not necessarily an equal division of labour, with influences found relating to the characteristics of the individual child. As stated earlier, men and women may take on different tasks, and, more broadly, daughters typically provide more care than sons. Other influences on caregiving tasks include the individual's personality, their relationship with the care recipient (type and quality), their values and motivations, their other life roles (work, partner, children), the specific needs of the care recipient and any associated economic cost, and, finally, their geographical location (Vergauwen & Mortelmans, 2019; Bei et al., 2023).

Whilst the recorded prevalence of informal caregiving varies across the world, the contribution of informal caregiving to the sustainability of health and social care systems is unquestionable (Seddon & Robinson, 2015). In the United Kingdom (UK) alone, there are an estimated 10.6 million caregivers (Carers UK, 2022). The 2022 State of Caring survey of over 12,000 caregivers showed that whilst 26% of the caregivers are providing care full time, 41% juggle caring responsibilities with paid employment (half of those work full time). Almost half of this survey sample provided care for 90 hours or more a week, and just under a fifth of the sample had additional childcare responsibilities. In the UK, caregiver support was recently valued at around £530 million *a day* during the COVID pandemic, a time when many health and social care services were suspended.

Caregiving is not without its consequences. In the aforementioned 2022 survey (Carers UK, 2022), a fifth of the sample (> 12.000 informal caregivers) reported that their physical health was bad or very bad (21%), 30% said their mental health was bad or very bad, and over a quarter (29%) said they felt lonely often or always. In fact, psychological well-being amongst family caregivers is typically found to be lower than found amongst non-caregivers, as is their self-rated physical health (e.g., Berglund et al., 2015). There is also relatively consistent evidence that spousal caregivers experience greater negative impact of caregiving on their relationship with the care recipient than do other family members (Pinquart & Sörensen, 2011), potentially accounted for by the intensity of typically co-resident caregiving but also due to the impact on more intimate and communal relationships (e.g., Bauer & Sousa-Poza, 2015, Revenson et al., 2016).

Why Provide Informal Care?

Why do family and friends provide care for a loved one who is facing health challenges, chronic conditions, or disability? We cannot assume that all *choose* to do so! It is a central tenet of psychological theories of coping with stressful events that humans prefer choice over non-choice, a perception of control as opposed to helplessness (e.g., Deci & Ryan, 1985, self-determination theory). Yet, a national telephone survey of 1397 caregivers in the United States (US) found that 44% reported a lack of choice in taking on the role, and, furthermore, this lack of choice was more prevalent amongst educated and older caregivers (Schulz et al., 2012). Lack of choice was greatest amongst co-resident members of the family, for example, for spouses for whom 'care' is assumed to be an inherent characteristic of the relationship. However, it was also high amongst non-co-resident adult children. Greater choice was reported by those caring for other relatives or a non-relative. Less choice in taking on the role was reported by caregivers of those with long-term physical health conditions or mental health or behavioural problems. In a more recent study conducted across eight European countries and Israel (Zarzycki et al., 2024), 75% of the 946 caregivers assessed indicated that they had no choice in adopting their caregiving role. Not having a choice but acting out of perceived obligation towards family members, familism, and ethnicity have previously been shown to predict both initial and continued motivation to care (Dykstra & Fokkema, 2012; Parveen et al., 2011, 2013, 2014; Parveen and Morrison, 2012, Silverstein et al., 2006).

Many factors underlie, promote, and maintain motivations and willingness to provide informal care, as evidenced in several reviews. Firstly, although focused on cancer caregiving, Burridge et al.'s (2007) systematic review of 17 studies usefully identified four groups of willingness-to-care indicators: *demographic indicators*, including, for example, caregiver and care recipient gender and age (female, older), co-residency factors, and relationship type; *physical indicators* including the caregiver's own health, the illness characteristics of the care recipient and whether there are mobility, behavioural, or emotional issues; *social indicators* including relational factors such as care recipient responsiveness or gratitude for care, access to welfare services and support; and, finally, *psychological indicators*, such as the caregivers own mental health, feelings of attachment or relational anxiety, perceived ability to care, and perceived choice.

These broad groupings of indicators were developed further in our own extensive systematic review of qualitative studies (Zarzycki, Morrison, et al., 2022; Zarzycki, Seddon, et al., 2022) where we found evidence that cultural and societal factors (105 studies), as well as personal and relational factors (103 studies) strongly underpinned motivations and willingness to care. The ethno-cultural context of the caregiving role is underpinned by culture-specific norms, beliefs in culturally and spiritually underpinned illness causation and control, and beliefs around caregiving generated from socialisation. Societal norms and perceived expectations, such as gendered roles, norms and expectations of caregiving, and perceptions of (non) available health and social care services, further shaped caregiver motivations and willingness to provide care (Zarzycki et al., 2022). Personal factors shaping motivations and initial and sustained willingness to care included caregiver characteristics, finding meaning in the role, illness cognitions, and situational and temporal aspects of the individual caregiving context. Relationship quality is one contextual factor found to be associated with initial motivations to care (Zarzycki et al., 2022), and when poor, it is also evidenced as a factor associated with a relinquishing of the caregiver role (e.g., Knussen et al., 2005).

Several authors have identified 'resentful' caregivers, and where a sense of obligation to care or a lack of choice is also present, those caregivers may feel more burdened and consumed by caregiving (e.g., Morrison & Williams, 2020). Such resentment and feelings of being burdened can potentially lead to more controlling caregiving, and this can negatively impact the care recipients' well-being and recovery. In contrast, caregivers who are more intrinsically motivated to care and who accept their role as part of a loving relationship are less likely to experience burden or overload. What needs to be remembered also is that care recipients differ in their willingness to accept care and that this can impact the caregiver experience. A lack of insight into one's functional limitations or a lack of acceptance of limitations can mean that a caregiver's intervention, support, or advice is rejected or ignored, or found to be unhelpful, with a risk of relationship disharmony following.

Against this backdrop, and critical to this chapter, are the relational factors that underpin caregiving motivations and willingness to care both prior to, as well as during, caregiving. The chapter turns to those issues next.

Relational Influences on Caregiving

In terms of personal and relational factors, the significance of perceived and actual reciprocity, mutual appreciation, and sharing between caregiver and care recipient; the presence of affection between them; family values; and perceived caregiving obligations were highlighted in our aforementioned review (Zarzycki et al., 2022). In one of the included qualitative studies, the relationship quality reported as having pre-existed the onset of illness in a care recipient was cited as underpinning the caregiver's willingness to provide care when it was required (Williams et al., 2014). Relationship quality and interpersonal love and affection are often cited as factors contributing to motivations and willingness to care, whether the caregiver is co-located with the care recipient or caring from a distance. Feelings of love, mutual affection and bonds of *attachment* are also instrumental in maintaining the caregiving role, and the lack of such feelings can create limits on both the willingness to care and the type of care tasks performed (Sihto, 2018). Zarzycki et al. describe affection, following an interpretative phenomenological analysis of the accounts of eight caregivers, as "an embodied emotion that drove the caregiving" (Zarzycki, Seddon & Morrison, 2023, p. 73).

It is likely that relationship characteristics viewed or recorded in research at a single moment, or even at repeated moments in time, can be considered as having arisen from an individual's early attachment experience. Pietromonaco, Uchino, and Dunkel Schetter (2013) highlighted a need to more fully understand the role played by the attachments formed between a parent and a child when it came to dealing with illness or, in our context, caregiving as adults. Several studies have reported associations between secure, non-anxious, or non-avoidant attachment and finding meaning in the caregiving role, including benefit finding, and between anxious attachment and stress, distress, or burden (Kim et al., 2008; Vilchinsky et al., 2014; Hasson-Ohayon et al., 2013). Hasson-Ohayon and colleagues proposed that avoidant attachment prevented the finding of meaning in caregiving due to limiting a caregiver's social interaction or emotional investment in caregiving. (More on the contribution of attachment to interpersonal relations in the health context can be found in Chapter 17.)

Willingness, Relationship Factors, and Caregiver Outcomes

The range of influences on caregiving willingness, only some of which were identified earlier, highlights that many individual or relational factors could also potentially affect caregivers' and care recipients' well-being over time. For example, both positive and negative influences of motivations to care have been found in terms of the nature of care provided, caregiver health and well-being, and the quality of the subsequent caregiving relationship (Greenwood & Smith, 2019; Quinn et al., 2010). Some have noted that having positive relationships with one's care recipients may in fact increase the experience of negative aspects of caregiving due to the strong emotional attachment that exists (e.g., Kiecolt-Glaser & Wilson, 2017). In contrast, others have noted that having a strong emotional connection with the care recipient may help maintain caregiver psychological well-being (Fisher et al., 2011). In a large study of 1,283 dyads where one had dementia, cross-sectional data showed that self-rated relationship quality was associated with well-being and life satisfaction for both the caregiver and the care recipient individually, although there was no cross-over effect (i.e., caregiver perceptions of relationship quality were not associated with care recipient well-being and vice versa) as had been predicted (Rippon et al., 2020). Such findings have been echoed elsewhere where prospective data have been included. For example, a review of 13 studies involving heart failure patients and their caregivers, where six studies included longitudinal data, showed that indices reflecting better relationship quality and good interpersonal, dyadic communication were associated with the health and well-being of both parties (Hooker et al., 2015). Similarly, in a large longitudinal analysis of over 1,400 caregivers in a range of health conditions, the self-reported quality of the relationship with the care recipient was shown to influence the caregiver's appraisals of their own situation over time (Huo & Kim, 2023). For example, this study found that those reporting negative relationship quality at the first assessment reported greater subsequent burden at a two-year follow-up; those reporting good relationship quality at the first assessment reported greater caregiving rewards at the follow-up.

Relationship quality has also been found to influence the nature and quality of caring provided both initially and over time (e.g., Burridge et al., 2007; Morrison & Williams, 2020; Zarzycki, Seddon & Morrison, 2023). Highlighting the importance of examining caregiving relationships as dynamic and potentially changing processes, a recent weekly diary study involving a large sample of caregivers in nine countries assessed over six months found that whilst baseline relationship satisfaction did not predict variations in willingness to care (Ferraris et al., 2023), caregivers reported higher willingness to care and less burden during weeks they showed more collaborative and supportive dyadic coping strategies towards their care recipient (Ferraris et al., 2024). This highlights the importance of examining the responses to the illness and caregiving situation within a relationship rather than examining individual factors alone. These kinds of analyses of repeated measurements in intensive longitudinal design studies and data of large-scale dyadic studies offer important additions to knowledge, but we have further to go – that is, intensive longitudinal designs with a large number of dyads.

In the next section, we turn attention to the impacts of caregiving on the caregiver-care recipient relationships.

The Impact of Caregiving on Relationships

Although the majority of early literature focused primarily on the negative impacts on the caregiver, acting as a caregiver for a family member can also impact (both negatively and positively) the caregiver-care recipient relationship and the wider family. Families operate as systems, made up of component parts that can have both independent role identities outside the immediate family (e.g., teacher, factory worker), as well as perceived roles within the family (e.g., the parent, the eldest child, the baby of the family, the breadwinner, the nurturer). Early work highlighted three integrated dimensions of family system functioning, namely cohesion, adaptability and communication (Olson & Stewart, 1991), thought to be associated with better adjustment to life stressors, such as chronic illness and consequent care needs. Barnhill's early system theoretical model of health family dynamics (Barnhill, 1979, as cited in Kanervisto, Paavilainen, & Heikkilä, 2007) also highlights interaction and communication themes but adds consideration of an individual's 'role' within the family, with role reciprocity and clear generational boundaries being viewed as positive, and role conflict and diffuse generational boundaries being viewed as negative. These authors also stress the importance of identity processes, including individuation (i.e., having a clear self-concept) and mutuality (i.e., feelings of togetherness), which are considered positive processes within a family. The various themes interact – for example, to achieve mutuality, flexibility in the face of change as well as communication and individuation (clear roles), are required. The absence of family adaptability to new circumstances and the presence of poor cohesion in working together to address these changes, including poor interpersonal communication around needs or feelings, can create further obstacles to adjusting to new roles of caregiver or care recipient. There are inherent benefits to feeling part of a functional and supportive family system or social network, with a wealth of evidence as to the benefits of receiving social support at times of need. In a 'functional family', caregivers are more likely to feel that their role is fair or balanced with that of other family members, and dissatisfaction with family relationships can create emotional -and sometimes physical- distance between members that can increase caregiver, and in effect, care recipient isolation.

Bronfenbrenners' developments to his earlier bioecological systems theory (1977) highlight the importance of person-context interactions and their interconnected dynamics over time and circumstance (Bronfenbrenner, 2005). In this thinking, the relationship between a caregiver and a care recipient likely has a mutual influence, and the importance of acknowledging what is described as the 'process-person-context-time' model becomes evident when one considers findings drawn from dyadic studies. For example, studies of dyadic coping (with a range of life stressors, not solely the stress of caregiving or receiving) highlight that the transactions between parties, their collaborations over time when faced with a potential stressor, are key to more adaptive (i.e., effective) coping (Berg & Upchurch, 2007). Adaptive dyadic coping is likely facilitated by open communication and responsive behaviours within a dyad and benefits the reported well-being and perceived relationship quality of both parties (e.g., Manne et al., 2018). Although, it is worth noting that not all couples will benefit from openness and sharing of concerns due to a mismatch between one member's unwillingness to share (due to protective buffering, for example, Manne et al., 2007) and the responsiveness of the other (e.g., Dagan et al., 2014; Hagedoorn et al., 2011; Manne et al., 2014). Pointing to this two-way process, a recent 28-day diary study with 200 dyads where one was facing a cell transplant consequent to a haematological cancer reported that caregiver affect was better on days where they received more support from the care recipient. Conversely, however, care recipient affect was poorer where they experienced *receipt* of more support, and instead, they reported better affect and greater relationship satisfaction when caregiver support aided their autonomy (Kroemeke & Sobczyk-Kruszelnicka. 2022a, 2022b).

It is also worth noting here that, in addition to dyadic or familial interaction, and in addition to interacting with other members of one's social network, a significant proportion of family caregivers also have paid work outside the home. For example, Clancy and colleagues' review cites studies showing that across Organisation for Economic Co-operation and Development (OECD) countries, one in ten adults who are informal carers also had paid jobs and that one in six American employees also provided care to an ill or older family member (Clancy et al., 2020). Balancing the demands of each role can generate work-family conflict (i.e., job demands impact negatively on family roles and relationships) or family-work conflict (i.e., family caregiving demands impact negatively on the work roles and relationships). Where the needs and pressures of one domain are incompatible with the needs of the other, greater carer strain, anxiety, and depression can be the result (e.g., Kayaalp, Page, & Rospenda, 2021). The demands of caregiving can also limit a person's time and energy for paid work, which can have financial implications for the whole family, contributing to further strain within the family unit (Gordon et al., 2012). Kayaalp's findings suggest that in fact the emotional and psychological challenge of balancing the two roles is more salient to caregiver mental health than issues around the time spent on either role. However, it is notable that their large sample of working carers are carers for children and not adults with chronic physical illness or disability, which may have influenced the nature and demands of caregiving faced.

Caregivers need to be able to identify the support needs of their care recipient in order to respond to them; likewise, employers, family, and friends need to be able to identify the demands faced and any consequent support needs the caregivers might have if they are to effectively support them in their role. However, not all support needs are visible. It follows therefore that in order for others to be able to meet the support needs of another person, they need to be communicated. Caregivers need to be able to respond to both verbal and nonverbal cues from the care recipient, and these cues are more likely to be picked up on when a relationship is built on affection, empathy, and open communication. Some care recipients may find that they hide their needs from their loved ones out of a desire 'not to be a burden' or to maintain their independence (even where this may be futile) and minimise their family worrying about them; this 'protective buffering' (Coyne & Smith, 1991) can prevent the caregivers from knowing what is the appropriate care to provide. Caregivers likewise can also engage in 'protective buffering', hiding their own feelings or concerns from the care recipient and other family members, so as to shield their loved ones from their carerole related concerns or protect them from further stress or worry about the care recipient. Both caregivers and care recipients may also yield to the wishes of others so as to avoid disagreement. In this way, a lack of communication within dyadic or wider familial relationships can exacerbate a caregiver's feelings of managing alone, of isolation often reported by caregivers. Furthermore, recent reports have suggested that caregiver loneliness exacerbates the negative effects of rumination on caregiver affect, whereas social connections reduce the negative effects of rumination on their affect (Kroemeke, 2023).

In a longitudinal study of protective buffering amongst spouses/partners of women affected by breast cancer, Manne et al. (2007) highlighted the importance of *relationship satisfaction* whereby increased protective buffering over time was associated with increased distress, but only amongst couples who reported more, rather than less, relationship satisfaction. Hagedoorn and colleagues' longitudinal study of couples where one had colorectal cancer (2011) found that protective buffering of caregivers by the patient at baseline was associated with subsequently lower relationship satisfaction in caregivers, especially in those caregivers who reported at baseline that the patient had been supportive in the past. These findings suggest therefore that buffering is less beneficial where relationships are good. Perhaps the recipient of buffering feels frustration at not being told how the other person feels or what their support needs are. A caregiver who believes they are in a close and loving relationship with the care recipient but who feels they are being 'closed out' may experience reduced feelings of intimacy and togetherness, which may relate to the subsequent reports of distress.

The beliefs, feelings, expectancies, and experiences of both a caregiver and a care recipient coping with illness or disability within a family context are therefore interdependent. Studies examining such factors have tended to be dyadic in nature, with a mix of primary and secondary caregivers but with few examples addressing the wider family. The importance of a burgeoning dyadic psychology research arena such as pointed to earlier is seen in the targeting of supportive interventions seeking to reduce negative outcomes of either partner. We turn finally to briefly consider some of those interventions.

Implications for Intervention

Targeting supportive interventions at care recipients alone ignores the fact that many community-dwelling care recipients are receiving some form of support from existing family members or close friends who may themselves be in need of a supportive intervention. As shown in this chapter, adopting a caregiving role (with or without choice) carries a potential risk to the caregivers' own health outcomes. These outcomes are in part dependent on the caregiver's age and health and on the nature of the care needs they are attempting to meet, but are also influenced by their motivations, relationship quality, and the extent to which they receive support from other family or friends, or from formal services offering daycare or residential respite for example.

Dyadic or family-based interventions tend to address the communication skills of both or all members to activate effective decision-making or problem-solving (e.g., around shared care or the need for formal services) in a positive and communal manner. One example, not confined to the caregiving context, is Coping Oriented Couples Therapy. Drawing on stress and coping models applied widely in health psychology, this intervention has shown efficacy in terms of reducing depression within a marriage (Bodenmann et al., 2008), although this same intervention did not enhance reported relationship satisfaction or dyadic coping. Other examples of couples-based intervention can be found predominantly, but not solely, in the cancer literature. For example, a review of ten intervention studies conducted with dyads where one member has breast cancer reported benefits to quality of life, relationship functioning, and distress for both the women with breast cancer and their partners in the majority of studies (Brandao, Schulz & Matos, 2014). Mixed methods of delivery and varied forms and content of couples-based intervention are common, and full evaluation of the barriers and facilitators of implementation and uptake of such programmes is needed (for a review, see Badr & Krebs, 2013). This is the goal of a Couples Coping with Cancer Together Programme, which was developed for implementation with positive results first coming from a feasibility evaluation involving patients, partners, and health professionals who would deliver the programme as part of standard care (Bitz et al., 2020).

As highlighted in this chapter, caregiving is dynamic and fluctuates depending on many factors including the nature of the care recipient's health condition and the responses of the caregiver to those care needs. Evidence is growing that couple-based interventions in the context of chronic or episodic health conditions can be as effective, if not more effective, as those directly targeting the patient or the caregiver alone. Thus in concluding this chapter, we point to a need for regular and repeated assessment of caregivers' experiences and needs, and examination of the perceived impact of caregiving on the quality of the caregiver-care receiver relationship to inform the development and delivery of effective support to caregivers, care recipients, and their wider families.

Further Reading

Badr, H. (2017). New frontiers in couple-based interventions in cancer care: Refining the prescription for spousal communication. *Acta Oncologica*, *56*, 139–145. DOI: 10.1080/0284186X.2016.1266079

Mikulincer, M., Shaver, P. (2020). Applications of attachment theory and research: The blossoming of relationship science. In J. P. Forgas, W. Crano, & K. Fiedler (Eds.), *Applications of social psychology: How social psychology can contribute to the solution of real-world problems* (pp. 187–206). Routledge. DOI: 10.4324/9780367816407-10

Schulz, R., Beach, S.R., Czaja, S.J., Martire, L.M., & Monin, J.K. (2020). Family Caregiving for older adults. *Annual Review of Psychology*, *71*(1), 635–659.

References

Badr, H., & Krebs, P. (2013). A systematic review and meta-analysis of psychosocial interventions for couples coping with cancer. *Psychooncology*, 22, 1688–1704.

Barnhill, L.R. (1979). Healthy family systems. *The Family Coordinator*, 28, 94–100.

Bauer, J. M., & Sousa-Poza, A. (2015). Impacts of informal caregiving on caregiver employment, health, and family. *Journal of Population Ageing*, 8, 113–145. https://doi.org/10.1007/s12062-015-9116-0

Bei, E., Morrison, V., Zarzycki, M., & Vilchinsky, N. (2023, Early Access). Barriers, facilitators, and motives to provide distance care, and the consequences for distance caregivers: a mixed-methods systematic review. *Social Science and Medicine*, 321. https://doi.org/10.1016/j.socscimed.2023.115782

Bei, E., Rotem-Mindali, O., & Vilchinsky, N. (2020). Providing care from afar: a growing yet understudied phenomenon in the caregiving field. *Frontiers in Psychology*, 11. https://doi.org/10.3389/fpsyg.2020.00681

Berg, C.A., & Upchurch, R. (2007). A developmental-contextual model of couples coping with chronic illness across the adult life span. *Psychological Bulletin*, 133, 920–954.

Berglund, E., Lytsy, P., & Westerling, R. (2015). Health and wellbeing in informal caregivers and non-caregivers: a comparative cross-sectional study of the Swedish general population. *Health and Quality of Life Outcomes*, 13, 109. https://doi.org/10.1186/s12955-015-0309-2

Bertogg, A., & Strauss, S. (2018). Spousal care-giving arrangements in Europe: the role of gender, socio-economic status and the welfare state. *Ageing and Society*, 40, 735–58.

Bitz, C., Kent, E.E., Clark, K., & Loscalzo, M. (2020). Couples coping with cancer together: successful implementation of a caregiver program as standard of care. *Psychooncology*, 29, 902–909. https://doi.org/10.1002/pon.536

Bodenmann, G., Plancherel, B., Beach, S.R.H., Widmer, K., Gabriel, B., Meuwley, N., Charvoz, L., … Schram, E. (2008). Effects of coping-oriented couples therapy on depression: a randomized clinical trial. *Journal of Consulting and Clinical Psychology*, 76, 944–954.

Börsch-Supan, A. (2022). Survey of Health, Ageing and Retirement in Europe (SHARE) Wave 6. Release version: 8.0.0. SHARE-ERIC. Data set. https://doi.org/10.6103/SHARE.w6.800

Brandao, T., Schulz, M.S., & Matos, P.M. (2014). Psychological intervention with couples coping with breast cancer: a systematic review. *Psychology & Health*, 29, 491–516.

Bronfenbrenner, U. (1977). Toward and experimental ecology of human development. *American Psychologist*, 32, 513–531
Bronfenbrenner, U. (2005). *Making Human Beings Human: Bioecological Perspectives on Human Development*. Thousand Oaks, CA: Sage Publications.
Burridge, L., Winch, S., & Clavarino, A. (2007). Reluctance to care: a systematic review and development of a conceptual framework. *Cancer Nursing*, 30(2), E9–E19.
Carers UK (2022). State of Caring 2022; A snapshot of unpaid care in the UK, November 2022. https://www.carersuk.org/media/p4kblx5n/cukstateofcaring2022report.pdf
Clancy, R.L., Fisher, G.G., Daigle, K.L., Henle, C., McCarthy, J., & Fruhauf, C.A. (2020). Eldercare and work among informal caregivers: a multidisciplinary review and recommendations for future research. *Journal of Business and Psychology*, 35, 9–27.
Coyne, J.C., & Smith, D.A.F. (1991). Couples coping with a myocardial infarction: a contextual perspective on wives' distress. *Journal of Personality and Social Psychology*, 61, 404–12.
Croucher, K., Gilroy, R., Bevan, M., Attuyer, K. (2020). The mobilities of care in later life: exploring the relationship between caring and mobility in the lives of older people, *Ageing Society*, 41, 1788–1809.
Dagan, M., Sanderman, R., Hoff, C., Meijerink, W.J.H.J., Baas, P.C., van Haastert, M., & Hagedoorn, M. (2014). The interplay between partners' responsiveness and patients' need for emotional expression in couples coping with cancer. *Journal of Behavioral Medicine*, 37, 828–838.
Deci, E. L., & Ryan, R. M. (1985). *Intrinsic motivation and self-determination in human behavior*. New York, NY: Plenum.
Dykstra, P. A., & Fokkema, T. (2012). Norms of filial obligation in the Netherlands. *Population*, 67(1), 97–122. https://doi.org/10.3917/pope.1201.0097
European Chronic Disease Alliance (ECDA) (2019). Chronic Diseases in Europe. Retrieved from https://alliancechronicdiseases.org/wp-content/uploads/Guide-for-European-Commissioner-for-Health-Chronic-diseases-in-Europe-ECDA-2019.pdf (accessed February 25th 2023).
European Quality of Life Survey (2016). https://www.eurofound.europa.eu/publications/series/european-quality-of-life-survey-2016
Ferraris, G., Gerain, P., Zarzycki, M., Elayan, S., Morrison, V., Sanderman, R., & Hagedoorn, M. (2024, early access). The associations of dyadic coping strategies with caregiver's willingness to care and burden: a weekly diary study. *Journal of Health Psychology*. doi:10.1177/13591053231223838[VM(1]
Ferraris, G., Zarzycki, M., Gerain, P., Elayan, S., Morrison, V., Sanderman, R., & Hagedoorn, M. (2023, early access). Does willingness to care fluctuate over time? A weekly diary study among informal caregivers. *Psychology & Health*. DOI:10.1080/08870446.2023.2249538
Fisher, G.G., Franks, M.M., Plassman, B.L., Brown, S.L., Potter, G.G., Llewellyn, D., ...Langa, K.M. (2011). Caring for individuals with dementia and cognitive impairment not dementia: findings from the aging, demographics, and memory study. *Journal of the American Geriatric Society*, 59, 488–494.
Gordon JR, Pruchno RA, Wilson-Genderson M, Marcinkus MW, & Rose M (2012). Balancing caregiving and work: role conflict and role strain dynamics. *Journal of Family Issues*, 33, 662–689.
Greenwood, N., & Smith, R. (2019). Motivations for being informal carers of people living with dementia: A systematic review of qualitative literature. *BMC Geriatrics*, 19(1). https://doi.org/10.1186/s12877-019-1185-0
Hagedoorn, M., Puterman, E., Sanderman, R., Wiggers, T., Bass, P.C., van Haastert, M., & de Longis, A. (2011). Is self-disclosure in couples coping with cancer associated with improvement in depressive symptoms? *Health Psychology*, 30, 753–762.

Hasson-Ohayon, I., Goldzweig, G., Sela-Oren, T. Pizem, N., Bar-Sela, G., Wolf, I. (2013). Attachment style, social support and finding meaning among spouses of colorectal cancer patients: gender differences. *Palliative and Supportive Care*, doi:10.1017/S1478951513000242

Hoffmann, F., & Rodrigues, R. (2010). *Informal Carers: Who Takes Care of Them?, Policy Brief 4/2010*, Vienna: European Centre.

Hooker, S.A., Grigsby, M.E., Riegel, B., & Bekelman, D.B. (2015). The impact of relationship quality on health-related outcomes in heart failure patients and their informal family caregivers: An integrative review. *Journal of Cardiovascular Nursing*, 30, 552–563.

Huo, M., & Kim, K. (2023). Lasting impact of relationhips on caregiving difficulties, burden, and rewards. *Journal of Social and Personal Relationships*, 40, 1288–310.

Kanervisto, M., Paavilainen, E., & Heikkilä, J. (2007). Family dynamics in families of severe COPD patients. *Journal of Clinical Nursing*, 16, 1498–1505.

Kayaalp, A., Page, K.J., & Rospenda, K.M. (2021). Caregiver burden, work-family conflict, family-work conflict and mental health of caregivers: A mediational longitudinal study. *Work & Stress*, 35, 217–240.

Kiecolt-Glaser, J.K., & Wilson, S.J. (2017). Love-sick: how couples' relationships influence health. *Annual Review of Clinical Psychology*, 13, 421–443.

Kim, Y., Carver, C.S., Deci, E.L., & Kasser, T. (2008). Adult attachment and psychological well-being in cancer caregivers: The mediational role of spouses' motives for caregiving. *Journal of Health Psychology*, 27, S144–S154.

Knussen, C., Tolson, D., Swan, I.R.C., Stott, D.J., & Brogan, C.A. (2005). Stress proliferation in carer: the relationship between caregiving stressors and deterioration in family relationships. *Psychology & Health*, 20, 207–221.

Kroemeke, A., & Sobczyk-Kruszelnicka M. (2022a). Daily analysis of autonomy support and well-being in patient-caregiver dyads facing haematopoietic cell transplantation. *British Journal of Health Psychology*, 27, 789–801. doi:10.1111/bjhp.12573

Kroemeke, A., & Sobczyk-Kruszelnicka, M. (2022b). Daily stress and received social support in hematopoietic cell transplant patient-caregiver dyads. *Anxiety Stress & Coping*. 35, 673–686. doi:10.1080/10615806.2021.1994555

Kroemeke, A. (2023). Daily associations between loneliness and intra- and interpersonal ruminative thoughts in cancer patient-caregiver dyads. Paper presented at *the 37th Annual Conference of the European Health Psychology Society*, Bremen, September 5th.

Manne, S.L., Norton, T.R., Ostroff, J.S. Winkel, G., Fox, K., & Grana, G. (2007). Protective buffering and psychological distress among couples coping with breast cancer: the moderating role of relationship satisfaction. *Journal of Family Psychology* 21, 380–8.

Manne, S., Kashy, D.A., Zaider, T., Lee, D., Kim, I.Y., Heckman, C., Penedo, F., … Virtue, S.M. (2018). Interpersonal processes and intimacy among men with localized prostate cancer and their partners. *Journal of Family Psychology*, 32, 664–675.

Manne, S., Myers, S., Ozga, M., Kissane, D., Kashy, D., Rubin, S., … Rosenblum, N. (2014). Holding back sharing concerns, dispositional emotional expressivity, perceived unsupportive responses and distress among women newly diagnosed with gyneacological cancers. *General Hospital Psychiatry*, 1, 81–87.

Matharu, G.S., Culliford, D.J., Blom, A.W., & Judge, A. (2022). Projections for primary hip and knee replacement surgery up to the year 2060: an analysis based on data from The National Joint Registry for England, Wales, Northern Ireland and the Isle of Man. *The Annals of the Royal College of Surgeons of England*, 104, 443–448.

Maynard, K., Llagan, C., Sethi, B., & Williams, A. (2018). Gender- based analysis of working-carer men: a North American scoping review, *International Journal of Care and Caring*, 2, 27–48.

Morrison, V., & Williams K. (2020). Gaining Longitudinal Accounts of Carers' Experiences Using IPA and Photograph Elicitation. *Front. Psychol.* 11, 521382. doi:10.3389/fpsyg.2020.521382

Olson, D.H. & Stewart, K.L. (1991). Family systems and health behaviours. In H.E. Schroeder (ed.), *New Directions in Health Psychology Assessment*. New York: Hemisphere.
Parveen, S., & Morrison, V. (2012). Predicting caregiver gains: a longitudinal study. *British Journal of Health Psychology*, 17, 711–723. https://doi.org/10.1111/j.2044-8287.2012.02067.x
Parveen, S., Morrison, V., & Robinson, C. A. (2011). Ethnic variations in the caregiver role: A qualitative study. *Journal of Health Psychology*, 16, 862–872. https://doi.org/10.1177/1359105310392416
Parveen, S., Morrison, V., & Robinson, C. A. (2013). Ethnicity, familism and willingness to care: Important influences on caregiver mood? *Aging & Mental Health*, 17, 115–124. https://doi.org/10.1080/13607863.2012.717251
Parveen, S., Morrison, V., & Robinson, C. A. (2014). Does coping mediate the relationship between familism and caregiver outcomes? *Aging & Mental Health*, 18, 255–259. https://doi.org/10.1080/13607863.2013.827626
Pickard, L. (2015). A growing care gap? The supply of unpaid care for older people by their adult children in England to 2032. *Ageing and Society*, 35, 96–123. https://doi.org/10.1017/S0144686X13000512
Pietromonaco, P.R., Uchino, B. & Dunkel Schetter, C. (2013). Close relationship processes and health: implications of attachment theory for health and disease. *Health Psychology*, 32, 499–513. http://dx.doi.org/10.1037/a0029349
Pinquart, M., & Sörensen, S. (2011). Spouses, adult children, and children-in-laws as caregviers of older adults: a meta-analytic comparison. *Psychology and Aging*, 26, 1–14.
Quinn, C., Clare, L., & Woods, R. T. (2010). The impact of motivations and meanings on the wellbeing of caregivers of people with dementia: a systematic review. *International Psychogeriatrics*, 22, 43–55. https://doi.org/10.1017/S1041610209990810
Revenson, T., Griva, K., Luszczynska, A., Morrison, V., Panagopoulou, E., Vilchinsky, N., & Hagedoorn, M. (2016). *Caregiving in the illness context*. Palgrave McMillan.
Rippon, I., Quinn, C., Martyr, A., Morris, R., Nelis, S.M., Jones, I.R., … Clare, L. (2020). The impact of relationship quality on life satisfaction and well-being in dementia caregiving dyads: findings from the IDEAL study, *Aging & Mental Health*, 24, 1411–1420, https://doi.org/10.1080/13607863.2019.1617238
Schulz, R., Beach, S.R., Cook, T.B., Martire, L.M., Tomlinson, J.M., & Monin, J.K. (2012). Predictors and consequences of perceived lack of choice in becoming an informal caregiver. *Aging and Mental Health*, 16, 712–21. https://doi.org/10.1080/13607863.2011.651439
Seddon, D., & Robinson, C. (2015). Carer assessment: continuing tensions and dilemmas for social care practice. *Health & Social Care in the Community*, 23, 14–22. https://doi.org/10.1111/hsc.12115
Sihto, T. (2018). Distances and proximities of care: analysing emotio-spatial distances in informal caring. *Emotion, Space and Society*, 29, 62–68. https://doi.org/10.1016/j.emospa.2018.10.002
Silverstein, M., Gans, D., & Yang, F. M. (2006). Intergenerational support to aging parents: the role of norms and needs. *Journal of Family Issues*, 27, 1068–1084. https://doi.org/10.1177/0192513X06288120
Vergauwen, J., & Mortelmans, D. (2019). An integrative analysis of sibling influences on adult children's caregiving for parents. *Ageing & Society*, 1–25. https://doi.org/10.1017/S0144686X19001156
Vilchinsky, N., Dekel, R., Revenson, T.A. Liberman, G., & Mosseri, M. (2014). Care- givers' burden and depressive symptoms: the moderational role of attachment orientations. *Health Psychology*. https://doi.org/10.1037/hea0000121
Williams, K., Morrison, V., & Robinson, C. (2014). Exploring caregiving experiences: caregiver coping and making sense of illness. *Ageing & Mental Health*. https://doi.org/10.1080/13607863.2013.860425

Zarzycki, M., Vilchinsky, N., Bei, E., Ferraris, G., & Morrison, V. (2024). Cross-country variations in the caregiver role: evidence from the ENTWINE-iCohort study.

Zarzycki, M., Seddon, D., & Morrison, V. (2023). Informal caregiver motivations, values, challenges and gains: A photovoice and interpretative phenomenological analysis of interrelationships. *Journal of Health Psychology*, 28, 568–582. doi:10.1177/13591053221124647

Zarzycki, M., Morrison, V., Bei, E., & Seddon, D. (2022). Cultural and societal motivations for being informal caregivers: a qualitative systematic review and meta-synthesis, *Health Psychology Review*, https://doi.org/10.1080/17437199.2022.2032259

Zarzycki, M., Seddon, D., Bei, E., & Morrison, V. (2022). Why do they care? A qualitative systematic review and metasynthesis of personal and relational motivations for providing informal care. *Health Psychology Review*, https://doi.org/10.1080/17437199.2022.2058581

Zygouri, I., Cowdell, F., Ploumis, A., Gouva, M. and Mantzoukas, S. (2021). Gendered experiences of providing informal care for older people: a systematic review and thematic synthesis, *BMC Health Services Research*, 21, 730, doi:10.1186/s12913-021-06736-2.

20

PATIENT-PROVIDER RELATIONSHIPS

A Linchpin in Medical Care

Arnstein Finset

Patient-Provider Relationships – Clarifying the Problem

The task of the health-care provider is to attend to patients' symptoms and health. But the patient is *a person*, not only a carrier of a disease. To acknowledge that fact, the provider must establish a *relationship* with the patient. Thus, the practice of medical care, from general practice to the intensive care unit, may be seen as a practice of social interaction. Health-care providers demonstrate specific expertise in assessment, treatment, and care, but to implement these tasks, they also need communicative skills, such as building rapport, eliciting concerns, providing information, and handling emotional reactions. Most medical procedures require that the patient must relate to some provider, for better or worse. Without efficient communication and trustworthy relationships between patients and providers, the very foundation of the medical system would crumble, leaving it utterly incapable of fulfilling its mission – to empower people in their relentless battle against their medical afflictions.

However, even if the relevance of provider-patient relations has been recognized ever since the Hippocrates oath, the patient perspective and the relationship with patients have traditionally not been considered a part of the scientific agenda. Medicine has been dominated by a disease-oriented and rather paternalistic approach and a biomedical model of health and disease inspired by the body-mind dualism dating back to Descartes (Engel, 1977). Communication skills have been dismissed as the *art* of medicine rather than an evidence-based series of skills (Inui, 1998). As a reaction against a rather doctor-centered health care, the idea of a patient-centered medicine (Balint, 1969), and later person-centered (Ekman et al., 2011) and relationship-centered care (Inui, 1996) were launched.

Up to the 1960s, there was little, if any, research on the patient-provider relationship in medicine, at least outside psychiatry. When systematic research on patient-provider communication appeared in the 1970s, '80s, and '90s, the basic

 DOI: 10.4324/9781003318026-24

doctor-centeredness of the doctor-patient dialogue in the mainstream of modern medicine was documented in several important studies (for instance, Roter & Hall, 1987). One example is Ford et al.'s (1996) study of cancer care in Great Britain. In their analyses of 117 audio-recorded outpatient consultations, they found that clinicians tended to be quite directive, for instance, by using closed rather than open-ended questions. Patients asked few questions and were seldom given space to initiate discussion. Psychosocial issues were seldom discussed. The study attracted wide attention in cancer care in Great Britain and stimulated the development of communication skills training programs and a plea for more patient-centered communication practices (Maguire, 1999).

As more studies on provider-patient relations were conducted and published, communication skills training with an emphasis on patient-centered communication gradually became a part of the curricula in medical school and other arenas of teaching health-care providers. Over the years, an increased emphasis on the patient perspective and on the patient-provider relationship led to a plea for more active patient participation in health care, for instance, in terms of involvement in medical decision-making (Charles et al., 1997). Patient involvement and patient engagement have become important trends in health care in general, not the least reflected in the clinical encounter (Graffigna & Barello, 2022).

What has been the rationale for this shift from a strict disease-oriented medicine to an emphasis on the patient perspective and on the patient-provider relationship? Several factors have contributed to these changes. First, on an ideological level, the development reflected new ideas and ideals in society in general. In the years following World War II, ideas about human rights and humanistic values were emphasized and applied also in the development of health care. Kogan et al. examined the different definitions of patient-centered care (PCC) and found a strong ideological value base. The six most prominent values of PCC were holistic or whole-person care, respect and value, choice, dignity, self-determination, and purposeful living, all reflecting ideological trends of human rights and equality in democratic societies at large (Kogan et al., 2016).

Second, a large body of empirical evidence was gradually published, indicating that patient-centered and relationship-centered communication practices may have a significant positive impact on different outcomes. Such studies have reinforced the further development of PCC. PCC has been found to be associated with higher patient satisfaction (Salisbury et al., 2010) and adherence to treatment (Zolnierek & Dimatteo, 2009), as well as fewer complaints and malpractice claims (Tamblyn et al., 2007). Attention to communication skills may also impact health-care utilization (Bertakis & Azari, 2011). For instance, a recent review summarized interventions designed to improve communication at hospital discharge (Becker et al., 2021). The researchers found that a communication intervention at discharge was significantly associated with fewer hospital readmissions. Finally, a number of studies have also demonstrated positive associations between the communication behavior of health-care providers and patients and specific health outcomes, such as reduced symptoms (Di Blasi et al., 2001), hypertension (Kaplan et al., 1989), and metabolic complications (Del Canale et al., 2012).

Moreover, evidence shows that some individuals are particularly sensitive to the impact of the patient-provider relationship. Research on attachment orientations may serve as an example. When sick or in pain, patients may seek a caring figure, not only a provider of pills and procedures. However, people differ in their ability to relate to others, partly depending on their attachment orientation (see Chapter 16 in this volume). Recent research suggests that patients high on insecure attachment may be particularly sensitive to provider communication styles (Palmer Kelly et al., 2019). A person-centered approach may therefore be helpful for vulnerable individuals. For instance, Brenk-Franz et al. (2017) found that the quality of the patient-provider relationship mediated the effect of attachment on self-management in patients with multiple chronic conditions. A more person-centered communication approach adapted to the attachment orientations of the vulnerable patient was associated with a better outcome.

In this chapter, we will describe and discuss the encounter between patients and health-care providers based on the research literature over the last 50 or so years. Our emphasis will be on the patient-*physician* relationship, both because it has been more extensively studied than patient relations to other health-care providers and because of the central position of the physician in health care. Terms such as 'clinical encounter', 'consultation', and 'medical interview' will be applied interchangeably. Examples of how to handle specific tasks during the encounter are presented in the text and in separate boxes.[1]

A Suggested Model of Efficient/Useful Consultation

Over the last 40 years, several models have been suggested to characterize the encounter between patient and provider in health care. Gulbrandsen and Finset (2019) have recently suggested a model for the consultation inspired by the Four Habits Model (Stein et al., 2010) and other sources in the patient-centered tradition. According to their model, the provider should entertain two perspectives simultaneously throughout the consultation: collect and provide information about the medical condition, which is the reason for the encounter, and attend to the patient as a person in an interpersonal relationship. A slightly adjusted version of the model will form the basic structure of this chapter (Figure 20.1).

Beginning the Consultation

Establishing Rapport and Eliciting Patient Concerns

Research attention has been directed to three different aspects of the opening of the consultation: establishing rapport, eliciting patient concerns, and setting an agenda (Stein et al., 2005, 2010). The first minute of the consultation is important for establishing rapport. A friendly greeting and a few informal remarks may make the patient feel at ease. Hall et al. (2009) showed that rapport between medical students and patients during the first minute of the talk was significantly related to rapport later on in the consultation. An emphasis on establishing

Stages	Person and relationship	Health condition
Beginning	Establish rapport Elicit concerns	Negotiate an agenda
Information gathering	Explore patient perspective Acknowledge emotions and show empathy	Explore symptoms and medical history Perform physical examination
Sharing information and decisions, summarizing, closing	Secure patient understanding Involve patient in decisions	Share information Provide lifestyle counseling Summarize and close

Figure 20.1 Model of the medical consultation. (Adapted from Gulbrandsen & Finset, 2019).

Skreddersydde samtaler – en veileder i medinsinsk kommunikasjon ([Tailored conversations – a primer in medical communication] Oslo: Gyldendal).

rapport and getting a good start has also been found to be associated with increased patient satisfaction (Wallace et al., 2009).

In most cases, establishing rapport and eliciting concerns occur in parallel. Robinson and Heritage (2006) found that approximately 90% of all primary care visits started with one of two types of opening statements – that is, an open-ended question such as, "What can I do for you?", or a closed-ended question indicating prior knowledge or assumption of what the patient's problems would be, such as, "I understand that you're having some leg problems?" They found that patients were significantly more satisfied with the open-ended version.

After the opening statement, patients present their concerns and reasons for the appointment. Several studies have shown that a large portion (75% to 80%) of patients' first statements are being interrupted by the doctor before the patient has spontaneously stopped talking (Rhodes et al. 2004, Beckman & Frankel, 1984). In a recent review, the mean time to interruption was 18 seconds (Coyle et al., 2022). As there is often much valuable information in the patients' first expressions of their concerns, a good rule of thumb, efficient as well as respectful, is therefore to let the patients present their initial concerns uninterrupted.

Negotiating an Agenda

A third aspect of the beginning of the consultation is agenda setting: identifying patient talk topics, identifying clinician talk topics, agreement of shared priorities, establishing conversational focus in collaboration with the patient (Gobat et al., 2015). Several studies indicate that agenda setting is often neglected in medical consultations. Studies have shown that there is less risk that patients will bring up new concerns toward the end of the visit in consultations where the doctor has elicited patient concerns up front and set an agenda early in the consultation (White et al., 1994). If the provider and patient fail to negotiate an agenda, there is an increased risk that common ground is not reached (Dyche & Swiderski, 2005). In some studies, physicians were trained to plan the consultation together with patients. In the intervention groups, consultation duration did not increase, and patients reported more satisfaction with the consultation (Mauksch et al., 2008).

Information Gathering

Explore Symptoms and Medical History

Information gathering is, in many cases, the main content of the consultation, up to 80% of the time in some studies. Particular attention has been given to two aspects of the explorations of symptoms and medical history: open versus closed questions and active listening. As mentioned earlier, early studies indicated that doctors most often used closed questions in medical interviews. Too much use of closed questions may narrow the attention of the patient and provider to the agenda of the provider rather than the patient. Open questions are important in the early phase of the interview, whereas closed questions may be useful in the investigation of specific symptoms. The use of open questions has been found to predict how much medical information would come up during the interview (Takemura et al., 2005).

Active listening in the clinical encounter is understood as a communication style in which the clinician actively facilitates the patient's talk, especially in the case of sensitive topics. Eide et al. applied sequence analysis to a study of consultations in cancer care in Norway and found that the best way to elicit patient concerns was to take a small pause to open up for more talk about the concern (Eide et al., 2003).

Physical Examination

A physical examination is common in many clinical encounters, not only with a physician but also in dental consultations, physical therapy sessions, etc., and should be regarded as part of the patient-provider relationship. Verbal communication is most often limited to small comments during the examination itself (Cleland et al., 2013). In a study of respiratory infections, Heritage et al. (2010) studied the effect of positive comments during the physical exam compared to comments on findings indicating disease. In the latter case, it was more difficult to convince the patient that antibiotics were unnecessary. The findings indicate that patients are perceptive to signals from the doctor during the exam, and physician talk during the exam influences patient expectations. Findings such as these indicate that during the physical examination, doctors should concentrate on the exam as such and give information about the findings after the exam is finished.

Exploring the Patient Perspective

The information-gathering phase will often be concentrated on the medical condition of the patient. However, when asked, patients also emphasize the importance of relating to their own understanding of their situation (Zeh et al., 2021) and tend to be more satisfied with doctors who show interest in the patient's own perspective on their condition (Tallman et al., 2007). See Box 20.1 for examples of questions related to the patient perspective.

For the health-care provider, knowledge about the patient's own understanding of their medical condition may give important input on how the provider may best inform the patient. Moreover, patients' own understanding of their condition has been found to be important for adherence to treatment recommendations (Miller, 2016). Stewart et al. found that active exploration of the patient's own perspective was associated with an experience of a shared understanding between the patient and the physician, which was related to better self-reported health (Stewart et al., 2000).

The patient perspective does not only include the patient's understanding of the medical condition, but also contextual factors such as loss of social support or financial hardship. Lack of attention to such issues may have a profound negative impact on patients (Weiner et al., 2020). Based on audio recordings of real-life consultations, Weiner et al. (2013) investigated the extent to which contextual issues were adequately addressed. They found that contextual 'red flags' were more likely to be resolved or improved if contextual issues had been identified during the consultation.

An important aspect of exploring the patient perspective is to consider the family and other significant social relationships, as family members may represent valuable resources for patients both in terms of emotional support and as informal carers. Therefore, interviewing families is an essential skill for physicians and other health-care providers. Family members are often present as a

Box 20.1 Interviewing about the Patient Perspective – Examples

What are your own thoughts about your condition?
What do you think is the cause of your condition?
Do you have any worries about your condition?
What are the consequences of your condition in your daily life?
What is the impact of your condition on your family?
What is most important for you in your present condition?
What do you expect that we can do for you?

third party in medical consultations. However, in research as well as in communication skills training, the role of family members has often been ignored (Campbell et al., 2002). One exception is an interview study by Andrades et al. (2013) among relatives who had accompanied patients in medical consultations. They found that companions tended to remain passive and did not contribute to the physician-patient relationship. To promote better practices in involving family members in the consultation, a team of Australian researchers developed guidelines for involving families in medical consultations in cancer care (Laidsaar-Powell et al., 2018a). In some cases, family relations may be difficult, with negative consequences for the patient. Laidsaar-Powell et al. (2018b) therefore developed a special set of guidelines explaining how to handle challenging situations, such as relating to dominant, controlling, or coercive family members.

Acknowledging Emotions and Showing Empathy

The patient perspective will often include an emotional expression. In the model illustrated in Figure 4.2, emotional talk is linked to the information-gathering phase of the consultation. However, emotions may arise in any phase of the clinical encounter. Three major topics have been studied: patient expressions of emotion, provider responses to patient emotions, and positive effects of empathic behavior.

Patient Expression of Emotion

Patients often express emotions in clinical encounters. In a recent summary of 77 research articles, Ruben et al. (2021) found that emotional codes represented 28% of clinician talk and 30% of patient talk. The Verona Coding Definitions of Emotional Sequences (VR-CoDES), a coding system of emotional behavior in clinical encounters, makes a distinction between cues, defined as a verbal or non-verbal hint that suggests an underlying unpleasant emotion but lacks clarity, and concerns, defined as a clear and unambiguous expression of an unpleasant current emotion (Zimmermann et al., 2011). In all published studies so far, cues are far more common than concerns (Del Piccolo et al., 2017). Thus, care providers are advised to pay attention to cues for emotional uneasiness, no less than to explicit emotional concerns.

Provider Responses to Patient's Emotions

How do providers respond to patients' cues and concerns? The VR-CoDES defines two dimensions of provider responses: the degree to which the provider gives room for further disclosure and the extent to which the response is explicit or not (Del Piccolo et al., 2011). Typically, an expression of emotion from the patient may have both a medical aspect and an emotional one. For instance, if the patient says, "I worry about the surgery I am about to have", the clinician may respond explicitly to the emotion ("What is your main worry?") or give room to further disclosure in a non-explicit way by making a brief pause or a nod, indicating that the patient may go on. The clinician may also seemingly ignore the emotion but pick up on the medical aspect ("This surgery is a rather simple procedure") or ignore the patient's point completely and continue with an unrelated question.

From a clinical point of view, there is consensus about the importance of acknowledging patients' emotions in clinical encounters and giving room for the expression of their emotions. However, research findings indicate that several factors influence whether or not the clinician actually gives room for further disclosure. If the clinician elicited the cue or concern, and the patient expressed the emotion more explicitly, then the clinician is more likely to provide room for more talk about the emotional concern. Moreover, dependent on the context, nurses appear to be more receptive to patients' emotions than physicians. In a study of cancer care in Norway, all three factors (i.e., initiation, explicitness, and profession) had an impact on the responsivity of the clinician (Finset et al., 2013). If the emotion was rather vague and self-initiated in a consultation with a physician, less than 15% of the emotional expressions were picked up. On the other hand, 85% of more explicit emotions elicited by the provider were detected in consultations with nurses.

Responding to emotions may be challenging for many providers. The patient's story may sometimes elicit difficult emotions in the provider. In communication skills training, awareness of one's own emotions is an important element in teaching providers to handle patients' emotions (Stein et al. 2010).

Effects of Empathic Provider Behavior

In the literature on emotional communication in clinical encounters, the behavior of providers is often described in terms of empathy. There are several definitions of empathy. A distinction is often made between cognitive empathy, the provider's ability to observe an expression of emotion from the patient, and the emotional aspect, the provider's own emotional response to the patient's expression. Empathy may be seen as a sequence, starting with the patient's expression of emotion, followed by the perception (cognitive aspect), vicarious experience (emotional aspect), and empathic response by the clinician (Finset & Ørnes, 2017). Thus, showing empathy is not simply a question of expressing empathic utterances. Empathic responses to patient emotions require a genuine interest on the part of the provider and openness to being moved by the patient's emotions. Still, attention to how empathy may be expressed verbally is important. See Box 20.2 for examples of empathic responses.

Several studies have examined the effect of empathic behavior on the part of the clinician, most often based on the patient's subjective experience. Neumann et al. (2012) summarized a number of studies on different aspects of empathy and its association with different variables. The researchers concluded that the provider would get more information from the patient about symptoms and concerns and also more precise diagnostic information by applying an empathic

Box 20.2 Examples of Empathic Responses

Acknowledgment *(Example: That must be tough for you.)*
Naming *(Example: You say that you are afraid?)*
Observing *(Example: I can see that this affects you emotionally)*
Legitimizing *(Example: It is quite natural to respond like that.)*
Support *(Example: I would like to help you...)*
Partnership *(Example: Let us see if we together...)*
Praise *(Example: how brave of you to bring this up.)*

communication style. They found that empathic communication is associated with patient satisfaction and adherence, better coping with disease, better health-related quality of life, and less depression. Derksen et al. (2013) reported similar findings in a review article on empathy in general practice. Also, in a large study of 21.000 patients with diabetes in Italy, Del Canale et al. (2012) found that patients with a general practitioner with high scores on empathic communication had significantly lower occurrence of metabolic complications than those whose general practitioner had lower scores.

Sharing Information and Decisions, Summarizing, and Closing

Sharing Information and Securing Understanding

Giving information is a crucial aspect of the clinical encounter. However, there is evidence that in many medical consultations, the time allotted to information provision is rather brief and often less than advised. Manalastas et al. (2021) analyzed the structure of 78 consultations in primary care. On average, 79% of the time was occupied by gathering information, whereas sharing information and decisions comprised only 14% of the consultation time. Under time pressure, information sharing may sometimes be performed too hastily, shortcutting important aspects of information giving, such as checking what the patient knows and believes and securing patient understanding. See Box 20.3 for a list of rules on how to provide information in medical encounters.

A number of studies, both observational studies and controlled interventions, have shown effects of information sharing on several outcome variables, including patient adherence to medical advice and treatment. A review article on the effect of provider-patient communication concluded that there is a 19% higher risk of non-adherence among patients whose physician communicates poorly than among patients whose physician communicates well (Zolnierek & Dimatteo, 2009). A large part of the effect is related to information providing.

The effect of information provision on health outcomes has also been reported in several studies. One of the most well-known and cited examples is a study from Boston, Massachusetts, from the late 1980s (Kaplan et al., 1989). They

Box 20.3 How to Provide Information in Medical Encounters

Check the patient's knowledge and understanding
Use simple language, avoid medical jargon
Prioritize, select the most important information, avoid unnecessary detail
Portion the information, include pauses between each chunk of information
Provide structure
Present important information with confidence
Be attentive to the patient's reaction, adapt information giving to the patient
Encourage patient to ask questions, create a dialogue, avoid long monologues
Check patient understanding, for instance, by teach-back techniques
Supplement oral information with visualizations and written summaries

found that information giving was one of the communication variables most strongly and consistently related to self-reported recovery from symptoms, use of health-care services, and certain physiological measures such as blood sugar level for patients with diabetes and blood pressure.

A recent article reviewed randomized controlled studies aimed to test the effect of information giving on recall and recognition, behavioral outcomes, and physical health outcomes (Lie et al., 2022). The authors concluded that using deliberate communication strategies to frame information can be quite effective in improving patients' outcomes, such as providing structure, persuasions, and visualizations.

Involving Patients in Decision-Making

Health-care providers, particularly physicians, have traditionally held the primary responsibility for making decisions regarding treatment. Making decisions is a major function of the medical interview. It is not limited to one important decision about treatment, sometimes referred to as the index decision. On the contrary, decisions are made throughout the consultation. In a study of 372 videotaped encounters in a general hospital setting, consultations, on average, contained 13.4 decisions per encounter (Ofstad et al., 2018). In the last 20 years, there has been an increased interest in involving the patient more in decision-making (Elwyn et al., 2012). This appears to be a logical consequence of a patient-centered attitude to the patient-doctor relationship. See Box 20.4.

Still, there is evidence that shared decision-making (SDM) is only to a limited extent implemented in standard medical care. Alsulamy et al. (2020) have reviewed the literature on barriers and facilitators to shared decisions. They concluded that a perceived lack of time was the most important perceived barrier. However, a recent review reported variability in the association between the use of SDM and consultation duration, showing that applying SDM does not necessarily lead to longer consultations (Veenendaal et al., 2023).

Box 20.4 Four Steps in the Process of Shared Decision-Making

The professional informs the patient that a decision is to be made and that the patient's opinion is important;

The professional explains the options and the pros and cons of each relevant option.

The professional and patient discuss the patient's preferences; the professional supports the patient in deliberation.

The professional and patient discuss patient's decisional role preference, make or defer the decision, and discuss possible follow-up.

Source: Stiggelbout, Pieterse, & De Haes, 2015

Providing Lifestyle Counseling

For many patients, the medical consultation goes beyond information gathering and information provision. For patients with chronic conditions, lifestyle counseling may be part of the consultation. However, communication to promote coping is often missing from medical consultations. For instance, Lundeby et al. (2015) showed that tailored communication skills training can improve physicians' emphasis on assessment of patient personal resources and coping strategies.

Several different communication strategies have been developed in lifestyle counseling. The most well-known example is probably motivational interviewing. Motivational interviewing was originally designed to motivate patients with drug abuse problems to change behavior. Patients might experience ambivalence when it comes to adopting lifestyle changes recommended by health-care providers. The approach of motivational interviewing is to avoid moralism but rather roll with the resistance and allow the patients to express both positive and negative aspects of making lifestyle changes. It has proved to be an effective communication approach to lifestyle changes in several chronic conditions (Copeland et al., 2015).

Summarizing and Closing

Concluding an interaction can pose challenges within the patient-provider dynamic. Research into the structure of clinical encounters often reveals that the closing phase tends to be brief, although there are noteworthy exceptions to this trend. An illustrative example is the "by-the-way" scenario. If the provider has not adequately addressed all of the patient's concerns, the patient might introduce a new issue on the way out, saying, "By the way, I just wondered…" This is sometimes referred to as the "doorknob phenomenon" (Kowalski et al., 2018), which may be mitigated through effective initial engagement and agenda setting (Gobat et al., 2015).

Conclusions

Taken together, the studies reviewed in the present chapter have confirmed the importance of patient-provider relations in health care. Some studies indicate that a transition from a paternalistic, doctor-centered communication style to more person-centered relationships moves slowly. A Dutch study investigating changes in communication behavior from 1986 to 2002 did not find a development toward more patient-centered practices (Bensing et al., 2006). We do not know whether this is true also for the last 20 years. However, communication skills training programs over the years have become more common in medical schools and in health-care education in general. Hopefully, the future will gradually bring more emphasis in health care on patient's perspective and involvement.

In the title of the chapter, we suggested that the patient-provider relationship is a linchpin of medical care. A linchpin is a fastener used to prevent a wheel or other part from sliding off the axle. The metaphor emphasizes the important role of the relationship between patient and provider in making health care available. In the future, some of the tasks handled by human health-care providers today may be handled by robots and other digital tools. However, human providers will still have important roles in future health care, not the least to secure that patients are being understood and respected as human beings, not merely as impersonal carriers of disease.

Note

1 Sources for the boxes include Fortin et al., 2019; Gulbrandsen & Finset, 2019; Kurtz & Silverman, 1996; and Stein, et al., 2010).

Further Reading

Fortin, A. H., Dwamena, F., Frankel, R., Lepisto, B. L., & Smith, R. C. (2019). *Smith's patient-centered interviewing. An evidence based method.* New York: McGraw Hill Education.

Schwartz, R, Hall, J.H., & Osterberg, L.G. (2021). *Emotion in the clinical encounter*. New York: McGraw Hill.

Chou, C. L., & Coley, L. (2017). *Communication Rx: Transforming healthcare through relationship-centered communication*. New York: McGraw Hill.

References

Alsulamy, N., Lee, A., Thokala, P., & Alessa, T. (2020). What Influences the Implementation of Shared Decision Making: An Umbrella Review. *Patient Educ Couns*, 103, 2400–2407s .

Andrades, M., Kausar, S., & Ambreen, A. (2013). Role and Influence of the Patient's Companion in Family Medicine Consultations: "The Patient's Perspective". *J Family Med Prim Care*, *2*(3), 283–287.

Balint, E. (1969). The possibilities of patient-centered medicine. *J R Coll Gen Pract*, *17*(82), 269–276.

Becker, C., Zumbrunn, S., Beck, K., Vincent, A., Loretz, N., Müller, J., ... Hunziker, S. (2021). Interventions to Improve Communication at Hospital Discharge and Rates of Readmission: A Systematic Review and Meta-analysis. *JAMA Netw Open*, *4*(8), e2119346.

Beckman, H. B., & Frankel, R. M. (1984). The effect of physician behavior on the collection of data. *Ann Intern Med, 101*(5), 692–696.
Bensing, J. M., Tromp, F., van Dulmen, S., van den Brink-Muinen, A., Verheul, W., & Schellevis, F. G. (2006). Shifts in doctor-patient communication between 1986 and 2002: a study of videotaped general practice consultations with hypertension patients. *BMC Fam Pract, 7*, 62.
Bertakis, K. D., & Azari, R. (2011). Determinants and outcomes of patient-centered care. *Patient Educ Couns, 85*(1), 46–52.
Brenk-Franz, K., Strauß, B., Tiesler, F., Fleischhauer, C., Schneider, N., & Gensichen, J. (2017). Patient-provider relationship as mediator between adult attachment and self-management in primary care patients with multiple chronic conditions. *J Psychosom Res, 97*, 131–135.
Campbell, T. L., McDaniel, S. H., Cole-Kelly, K., Hepworth, J., & Lorenz, A. (2002). Family interviewing: a review of the literature in primary care. *Fam Med, 34*(5), 312–318.
Charles, C., Gafni, A., & Whelan, T. (1997). Shared decision-making in the medical encounter: what does it mean? (or it takes at least two to tango). *Soc Sci Med, 44*(5), 681–692.
Cleland, J., de la Croix, A., Cotton, P., Coull, S., & Skelton, J. (2013). Student-patient communication during physical examination. *Clin Teach, 10*(2), 84–87.
Copeland, L., McNamara, R., Kelson, M., & Simpson, S. (2015). Mechanisms of change within motivational interviewing in relation to health behaviors outcomes: a systematic review. *Patient Educ Couns, 98*(4), 401–411.
Coyle, A. C., Yen, R. W., & Elwyn, G. (2022). Interrupted opening statements in clinical encounters: A scoping review. *Patient Educ Couns, 105*(8), 2653–2663.
Del Canale, S., Louis, D. Z., Maio, V., Wang, X., Rossi, G., Hojat, M., & Gonnella, J. S. (2012). The relationship between physician empathy and disease complications: an empirical study of primary care physicians and their diabetic patients in Parma, Italy. *Acad Med, 87*(9), 1243–1249.
Del Piccolo, L., de Haes, H., Heaven, C., Jansen, J., Verheul, W., Bensing, J., … Finset, A. (2011). Development of the Verona coding definitions of emotional sequences to code health providers' responses (VR-CoDES-P) to patient cues and concerns. *Patient Educ Couns, 82*(2), 149–155.
Del Piccolo, L., Finset, A., Mellblom, A. V., Figueiredo-Braga, M., Korsvold, L., Zhou, Y., … Humphris, G. (2017). Verona Coding Definitions of Emotional Sequences (VR-CoDES): Conceptual framework and future directions. *Patient Educ Couns, 100*(12), 2303–2311. doi:10.1016/j.pec.2017.06.026
Derksen, F., Bensing, J., & Lagro-Janssen, A. (2013). Effectiveness of empathy in general practice: A systematic review. *Br J Gen Pract, 63*(606), e76-e84.
Di Blasi, Z., Harkness, E., Ernst, E., Georgiou, A., & Kleijnen, J. (2001). Influence of context effects on health outcomes: a systematic review. *Lancet, 357*(9258), 757–762.
Dyche, L., & Swiderski, D. (2005). The effect of physician solicitation approaches on ability to identify patient concerns. *J Gen Intern Med, 20*(3), 267–270. doi: 10.1111/j.1525-1497.2005.40266.x
Eide, H., Graugaard, P., Holgersen, K., & Finset, A. (2003). Physician communication in different phases of a consultation at an oncology outpatient clinic related to patient satisfaction. *Patient Educ Couns, 51*(3), 259–266. doi: 10.1016/s0738-3991(02)00225-2
Ekman, I., Swedberg, K., Taft, C., Lindseth, A., Norberg, A., Brink, E., … Sunnerhagen, K. S. (2011). Person-centered care--ready for prime time. *Eur J Cardiovasc Nurs, 10*(4), 248–251.
Elwyn, G., Frosch, D., Thomson, R., Joseph-Williams, N., Lloyd, A., Kinnersley, P., … Barry, M. (2012). Shared decision making: a model for clinical practice. *J Gen Intern Med*, 27(10), 1361–1367. doi: 10.1007/s11606-012-2077-6
Engel, G. L. (1977). The need for a new medical model: a challenge for biomedicine. *Science, 196*(4286), 129–136.

Finset, A., Heyn, L., & Ruland, C. (2013). Patterns in clinicians' responses to patient emotion in cancer care. *Patient Educ Couns*, *93*(1), 80–85.

Finset, A., & Ørnes, K. (2017). Empathy in the Clinician-Patient Relationship: The Role of Reciprocal Adjustments and Processes of Synchrony. *J Patient Exp*, *4*(2), 64–68.

Ford, S., Fallowfield, L., & Lewis, S. (1996). Doctor-patient interactions in oncology. *Soc Sci Med*, *42*(11), 1511–1519.

Fortin, A. H., Dwamena, F., Frankel, R., Lepisto, B. L., & Smith, R. C. (2019b). *Smith*s patient-centered interviewing. An evidence.based method.* New York: McGraw Hill Education

Gobat, N., Kinnersley, P., Gregory, J. W., & Robling, M. (2015). What is agenda setting in the clinical encounter? Consensus from literature review and expert consultation. *Patient Educ Couns*, *98*(7), 822–829.

Graffigna, G., & Barello, S. (2022). How does patient engagement work in a real-world setting? Recommendations, caveats, and challenges from a psychosocial perspective. *Patient Educ Couns*, *105*(12), 3567–3573. doi: 10.1016/j.pec.2022.08.009

Gulbrandsen, P., & Finset, A. (2019). *Skreddersydde samtaler - en veileder i medinsinsk kommunikasjon [Tailored conversations - a primer in medical communication].* Oslo: Gyldendal.

Hall, J. A., Roter, D. L., Blanch, D. C., & Frankel, R. M. (2009). Observer-rated rapport in interactions between medical students and standardized patients. *Patient Educ Couns*, *76*(3), 323–327. doi: 10.1016/j.pec.2009.05.009

Heritage, J., Elliott, M. N., Stivers, T., Richardson, A., & Mangione-Smith, R. (2010). Reducing inappropriate antibiotics prescribing: the role of online commentary on physical examination findings. *Patient Educ Couns*, *81*(1), 119–125.

Inui, T. S. (1996). What are the sciences of relationship-centered primary care. *J Fam Pract*, *42*(2), 171–177.

Inui, T. S. (1998). Establishing the doctor-patient relationship: science, art, or competence? *Schweiz Med Wochenschr*, *128*(7), 225–230.

Kaplan, S. H., Greenfield, S., & Ware, J. E., Jr. (1989). Assessing the effects of physician-patient interactions on the outcomes of chronic disease. *Med Care*, *27*(3 Suppl), S110–127. doi: 10.1097/00005650-198903001-00010

Kogan, A. C., Wilber, K., & Mosqueda, L. (2016). Person-centered care for older adults with chronic conditions and functional impairment: A systematic literature review. *J Am Geriatr Soc*, *64*(1), e1–7. doi: 10.1111/jgs.13873

Kowalski, C. P., McQuillan, D. B., Chawla, N., Lyles, C., Altschuler, A., Uratsu, C. S., … Grant, R. W. (2018). 'The Hand on the Doorknob': Visit agenda setting by complex patients and their primary care physicians. *J Am Board Fam Med*, *31*(1), 29–37. doi:10.3122/jabfm.2018.01.170167

Kurtz, S. M., & Silverman, J. D. (1996). The Calgary-Cambridge Referenced Observation Guides: an aid to defining the curriculum and organizing the teaching in communication training programmes. *Med Educ*, *30*(2), 83–89.

Laidsaar-Powell, R., Butow, P., Boyle, F., & Juraskova, I. (2018a). Facilitating collaborative and effective family involvement in the cancer setting: Guidelines for clinicians (TRIO Guidelines-1). *Patient Educ Couns*, *101*(6), 970–982.

Laidsaar-Powell, R., Butow, P., Boyle, F., & Juraskova, I. (2018b). Managing challenging interactions with family caregivers in the cancer setting: Guidelines for clinicians (TRIO Guidelines-2). *Patient Educ Couns*, *101*(6), 983–994.

Lie, H. C., Juvet, L. K., Street, R. L., Jr., Gulbrandsen, P., Mellblom, A. V., Brembo, E. A., … Menichetti, J. (2022). Effects of Physicians' Information Giving on Patient Outcomes: a Systematic Review. *J Gen Intern Med*, *37*(3), 651–663.

Lundeby, T., Gulbrandsen, P., & Finset, A. (2015). The Expanded Four Habits Model-A teachable consultation model for encounters with patients in emotional distress. *Patient Educ Couns*, *98*(5), 598–603.

Maguire, P. (1999). Improving communication with cancer patients. *Eur J Cancer*, *35*(14), 2058–2065.
Manalastas, G., Noble, L. M., Viney, R., & Griffin, A. E. (2021). What does the structure of a medical consultation look like? A new method for visualising doctor-patient communication. *Patient Educ Couns*, *104*(6), 1387–1397.
Mauksch, L. B., Dugdale, D. C., Dodson, S., & Epstein, R. (2008). Relationship, communication, and efficiency in the medical encounter: creating a clinical model from a literature review. *Arch Intern Med*, *168*(13), 1387–1395.
Miller, T. A. (2016). Health literacy and adherence to medical treatment in chronic and acute illness: A meta-analysis. *Patient Educ Couns*, *99*(7), 1079–1086.
Neumann, M., Scheffer, C., Tauschel, D., Lutz, G., Wirtz, M., & Edelhäuser, F. (2012). Physician empathy: definition, outcome-relevance and its measurement in patient care and medical education. *GMS Zeitschrift für medizinische Ausbildung*, *29*(1).
Ofstad, E. H., Frich, J. C., Schei, E., Frankel, R. M., Šaltytė Benth, J., & Gulbrandsen, P. (2018). Clinical decisions presented to patients in hospital encounters: a cross-sectional study using a novel taxonomy. *BMJ Open*, *8*(1), e018042.
Palmer Kelly, E., Tsilimigras, D. I., Hyer, J. M., & Pawlik, T. M. (2019). Understanding the use of attachment theory applied to the patient-provider relationship in cancer care: Recommendations for future research and clinical practice. *Surg Oncol*, *31*, 101–110.
Rhodes, K. V., Vieth, T., He, T., Miller, A., Howes, D. S., Bailey, O., … Levinson, W. (2004). Resuscitating the physician-patient relationship: emergency department communication in an academic medical center. *Ann Emerg Med*, *44*(3), 262–267.
Robinson, J. D., & Heritage, J. (2006). Physicians' opening questions and patients' satisfaction. *Patient Educ Couns*, *60*(3), 279–285.
Roter, D. L., & Hall, J. A. (1987). Physicians' interviewing styles and medical information obtained from patients. *Journal of General Internal Medicine*, *2*, 325–329. https://link.springer.com/article/10.1007/BF02596168
Ruben, M.A., Stosic, M.D., Roter, D.L. (2021). Emotion dialogue in the medical encounter: When and how often does it happen? In R. Schwartz, J.A. Hall, L.G. Osterberg (Eds.), *Emotion in the clinical encounter*, pp. 83–109. New York: McGrawHill
Salisbury, C., Wallace, M., & Montgomery, A. A. (2010). Patients' experience and satisfaction in primary care: secondary analysis using multilevel modelling. *Bmj*, *341*, c5004.
Stein, T., Frankel, R. M., & Krupat, E. (2005). Enhancing clinician communication skills in a large healthcare organization: a longitudinal case study. *Patient Educ Couns*, *58*(1), 4–12.
Stiggelbout, A. M., Pieterse, A. H., & De Haes, J. C. (2015). Shared decision making: Concepts, evidence, and practice. *Patient Educ Couns*, *98*(10), 1172–1179.
Stein, T., Krupat, E., & Frankel, R. (2010). Talking with patients using the Four Habits Model: Kaiser Permanente.
Stewart, M., Brown, J. B., Donner, A., McWhinney, I. R., Oates, J., Weston, W. W., & Jordan, J. (2000). The impact of patient-centered care on outcomes. Journal of Family Practice, *49*(9), 796–804.
Takemura, Y., Sakurai, Y., Yokoya, S., Otaki, J., Matsuoka, T., Ban, N., … Tsuda, T. (2005). Open-ended questions: are they really beneficial for gathering medical information from patients? *Tohoku J Exp Med*, *206*(2), 151–154.
Tallman, K., Janisse, T., Frankel, R. M., Sung, S. H., Krupat, E., & Hsu, J. T. (2007). Communication practices of physicians with high patient-satisfaction ratings. *Perm J*, *11*(1), 19–29.
Tamblyn, R., Abrahamowicz, M., Dauphinee, D., Wenghofer, E., Jacques, A., Klass, D., … Hanley, J. A. (2007). Physician scores on a national clinical skills examination as predictors of complaints to medical regulatory authorities. *Jama*, *298*(9), 993–1001.
Veenendaal, H. V., Chernova, G., Bouman, C. M., Etten-Jamaludin, F. S. V., Dieren, S. V., & Ubbink, D. T. (2023). Shared decision-making and the duration of medical consultations: A systematic review and meta-analysis. *Patient Educ Couns*, *107*, 107561.

Wallace, L. S., Cassada, D. C., Ergen, W. F., & Goldman, M. H. (2009). Setting the stage: Surgery patients' expectations for greetings during routine office visits. *J Surg Res*, *157*(1), 91–95.

Weiner, S., Schwartz, A., Altman, L., Ball, S., Bartle, B., Binns-Calvey, A., … Wopat, M. (2020). Evaluation of a Patient-Collected Audio Audit and Feedback Quality Improvement Program on Clinician Attention to Patient Life Context and Health Care Costs in the Veterans Affairs Health Care System. *JAMA Netw Open*, *3*(7), e209644.

Weiner, S. J., Schwartz, A., Sharma, G., Binns-Calvey, A., Ashley, N., Kelly, B., … Harris, I. (2013). Patient-centered decision making and health care outcomes: an observational study. *Ann Intern Med*, *158*(8), 573–579.

White, J., Levinson, W., & Roter, D. (1994). "Oh, by the way …": the closing moments of the medical visit. *J Gen Intern Med*, *9*(1), 24–28. doi: 10.1007/bf02599139

Zeh, S., Christalle, E., Zill, J. M., Härter, M., Block, A., & Scholl, I. (2021). What do patients expect? Assessing patient-centredness from the patients' perspective: an interview study. *BMJ Open*, *11*(7), e047810. doi: 10.1136/bmjopen-2020-047810

Zimmermann, C., Del Piccolo, L., Bensing, J., Bergvik, S., De Haes, H., Eide, H., … Finset, A. (2011). Coding patient emotional cues and concerns in medical consultations: The Verona coding definitions of emotional sequences (VR-CoDES). *Patient Educ Couns*, *82*(2), 141–148.

Zolnierek, K. B., & Dimatteo, M. R. (2009). Physician communication and patient adherence to treatment: a meta-analysis. *Med Care*, *47*(8), 826–834.

SECTION 5

Chronic Diseases

21
INTRODUCTION TO CHRONIC DISEASES

Konstadina Griva and Stanton P. Newman

Introduction

The biggest challenge facing healthcare is the category of conditions that are termed chronic diseases. These are sometimes referred to as 'noncommunicable diseases' (NCDs). Conditions are considered chronic if they last one year or more and either require ongoing medical attention, limit activities/daily living, or both (National Center for Chronic Disease Prevention and Health Promotion, 2022). Chronic illnesses have a variable trajectory, and an individual's condition may deteriorate, enter remission, or fluctuate, but their defining characteristic is that they persist. Typically, they have only a limited potential for a cure, and much of healthcare focuses on treating and managing the symptoms. The possibility of cures or treatments that halt the progression of the chronic disease is increasing with the advent of new treatments (e.g., biologics in rheumatology). Chronic diseases are also often managed by a variety of behaviours executed by the patient as opposed to the physician, such as taking medication, monitoring diet, exercising, and following up with healthcare professionals. These behaviours are expected to control or inhibit disease progression and to minimise disease side effects and disruptions to daily living.

Chronic diseases encompass a diverse group of disorders that may affect various parts of the body, organs, or body systems and may include physical and mental disorders. They are often the result of a combination of genetic, physiological, environmental, and (modifiable) behaviours/lifestyle factors. The lifestyle or behavioural causes of chronic disease are important, as they are modifiable and major risk factors and include smoking, poor nutrition, being overweight or obese, excessive alcohol consumption, and insufficient physical activity (The Institute for Health Metrics and Evaluation, 2020). The identification and evidence regarding these causal factors informed the implementation of national and global NCDs surveillance and prevention programmes in recent decades.

DOI: 10.4324/9781003318026-26

Despite these programmes, rates of NCDs remain high, with growing numbers of young adults developing NCDs such as early-onset diabetes mellitus, which have an excess risk and more "aggressive phenotype" (Magliano et al., 2020; Sattar et al., 2019).

Besides individual behaviours, environmental factors (i.e., air pollution, water contamination, etc.) and the cascade of climatic changes caused by global warming are major contributors to poor health and NCDs (Guo et al., 2018). Although these are potentially modifiable factors, they require societal cohesion and agreement for an appropriate response which has proved to be more elusive to achieve. The impact of environmental factors is not evenly distributed across the globe. Climate-related health risks disproportionally affect the most vulnerable and disadvantaged populations and regions. Both behavioural and environmental risks sit on the complex background of a wide range of social determinants of health, as well as the known inequalities in these determinants.

The most prevalent chronic diseases are cardiovascular diseases, such as heart attacks and stroke, cancer, diabetes, and chronic respiratory diseases, such as chronic obstructive pulmonary disease and asthma. These four groups of diseases account for over 80% of all premature NCD deaths (i.e., mortality occurring before the average life expectancy). The number of individuals affected by NCDs is rising steadily, and NCDs account for more than 74% of deaths globally, with a disproportionate impact in low- and middle-income countries where more than three-quarters of global NCD deaths occur (World Health Organization, 2023b).

One reason that chronic disease poses such a challenge to healthcare is the sheer number of individuals who have these conditions. Precise numbers are difficult to determine, as they rely on diagnosis and health infrastructures, which differ widely in different countries. One study of OECD countries used self-report of having a long-term condition and found that one in three individuals reported living with chronic conditions (OECD, 2021). It is important that this study found both country differences and socio-economic gradients where the poorest individuals were more likely to report having a chronic condition. Rates of NCDs in the main increase with age such that the absolute burden of NCDs is significantly influenced by the size and age structure of a nation's population.

While depression is often excluded from an overview of NCDs, in any consideration of the overall number of individuals with chronic disease, it is important to note that 280 million individuals in the world are estimated by WHO to suffer from depression (World Health Organization, 2023a). In addition, depression is a major cause of suicide which is the fourth leading cause of death in 15- to 29-year-olds.

Chronic conditions are not only the major cause of death but also disability in the world. The sum of disability and premature death is referred to as the 'burden of disease' and can be measured by a metric called 'Disability Adjusted Life Years' (DALYs). One DALY is equivalent to one lost year of healthy living either through disability or premature death. The figure for 2019 indicates that cardiovascular disease resulted in over 350 million DALYs in contrast to cancers, which resulted in approximately 250 million (Roser et al., 2021).

The impact of the number of individuals with chronic disease and the need for ongoing healthcare and support results in an enormous financial burden on families and society. For example, the overall US costs of chronic disease are projected to accumulate by 2030 to more than $42 trillion, with medical outlays and productivity losses (work absenteeism, presenteeism, permanent withdrawal from the workforce, and job interruption) costing $8,600 per person (Partnership to Fight Chronic Disease, n.d.). In an era of scarce resources and competing priorities, an understanding of productivity loss due to NCDs' mortality has led to an increased focus on NCDs. While exact estimates may vary according to the methodology used, evidence is consistent that indirect costs of NCDs are staggering (ranging from $19,000 per (CVD) cardiovascular death in the European Union (Leal et al., 2006) to $288,000 per cancer death in the United States (Ekwueme et al., 2011). These costs are likely to increase further due to demographic shifts and changing labour force profiles.

The socio-economic costs associated with NCDs make prevention and control of NCDs a major development imperative for all nations. The 2030 Agenda for Sustainable Development recognises NCDs as a major challenge for sustainable development and therefore set a target to reduce by one-third premature mortality (NCDs) between 2015 and 2030 (target 3.4; United Nations, n.d.), yet most countries, especially in those with low resources, have made little progress in achieving this goal. The COVID-19 pandemic has upended national programmes and aggravated clinical outcomes for individuals with NCDs. People with chronic diseases have been disproportionately affected, with higher incidence of severe COVID-19 (i.e., higher complication rates when infected) and disruptions in services and care leading to excess mortality (Ezzati et al., 2022; Guan et al., 2020).

While survival has been a critical issue more recently the focus has shifted from lifespan (adding years to life) to health span and adding 'life' to years. The amazing pace and wider availability of medical innovation and early detection have transformed many NCDs (i.e., HIV, cancer, cardiovascular disease) and/or end-stage conditions, such as chronic kidney disease, from acute or life-limiting illnesses to chronic conditions that can be effectively managed with treatment protocols comprising medical/pharmacological interventions and lifestyle modifications. The reductions in mortality coupled with reductions in fertility have led to an ageing population globally with the net result of an overall increase in rates of NCDs. As more individuals are affected by NCDs and are now living longer with their condition(s), there is an urgency *for* interventions which focus on enhancing quality of life and assisting individuals to self-manage their condition. The journey through a chronic condition is of particular interest to health psychology in that, in most cases, they have a significant impact on the individual's life. The person who has the disease has not only to deal with their symptoms and adjust to the treatment of what are often complex regimens but also, in many cases, to adjust to a reduction in activities, including employment. In addition, many of these conditions are controllable and preventable, and through alterations in lifestyle, such as stopping smoking, increasing exercise, and improving diet. In many cases, individuals with a chronic condition are supported by friends, family, and caring professionals. This is not simple, as it requires significant adjustments to relationships, as having others assist with what are often very personal issues frequently impinges on self-identity and esteem. For the carers, performing a role for which they have had little training and for which they often have to sacrifice their own ambitions frequently creates a significant burden on their mental health.

While it is customary to begin chapters or articles on outcomes in NCDs with the statement that these have seldom been investigated and/or "that little is known about this outcomes in this condition", the proliferation of research over the last decades means that this is no longer true or the case for most NCDs and that more and more is now known about adaptation and interventions for various NCDs populations than has been previously recognised. The breadth of issues and research involved in NCDs is enormous and poses a daunting task to attempt to cover in a volume such as this.

Our approach to organising the wealth of existing information has been to focus on key issues relevant to NCDs as opposed to chapters on specific NCDs and to bring examples as needed to highlight the evidence across NCDs. Many of the prevalent chronic conditions, though unique in their own attributes and demands, share common challenges associated with their management. These include dealing with symptoms and disability; monitoring physical indicators; managing complex medication regimens; maintaining proper levels of nutrition, diet, and exercise; adjusting to the psychological and social demands, including difficult lifestyle adjustments; and engaging in effective interactions with healthcare providers.

However, even the selection of possible topics we present is limited. We note at the outset that several topics, including social support and caregivers, theories of how people think about their condition (Illness cognitions), behaviour change interventions, and specific lifespan groups such as the elderly and children, amongst others, are not covered in this section. Some are discussed in other sections of the textbook.

We have also chosen to predominantly synthesise the evidence from chronic physical diseases rather than mental health conditions, yet this is not intended to imply that mental health disorders are less important or do not pose a significant challenge to manage and treat appropriately. It is important to recognise that mental health is closely intertwined with poor physical health. NCDS are usually accompanied by emotional sequelae that adversely impact outcomes. Depression, for instance, a highly prevalent comorbidity in NCDs, can worsen the outcome of physical health problems (both overall health and disease specific) or increase the risk for the development of NCDs. As such, screening guidelines for depression are widely used in working with people with physical health conditions (e.g., National Institute for Health and Care Excellence (NICE) in the United Kingdom and the US Preventive Services Task Force; Siu et al., 2016).

For this section, we have assembled a group of international experts who are at the forefront of the field to write the relevant chapters in this section that consider important concepts and issues that transcend specific chronic conditions, and we summarise these here:

Chapter 22 – "Coping with Symptoms and Treatments" (Frederick H. F. Chan and Konstadina Griva)

NCDs are associated with many symptoms, including pain, fatigue, and neurocognitive difficulties, to name a few. These may be related to the disease and/or its treatment. They can persist over time, and there are often no evidence-based treatment options to alleviate or eliminate them. The opening chapter in this section discusses in detail the symptomatic burden and profile related to NCDs, including pain, fatigue, and cognitive dysfunction and some relevant interventions that have been developed. While it is tempting to consider each of these symptoms in isolation and also to separate physical and emotional symptoms (see Chapter 21), it is important to highlight that these (emotional and physical) co-occur and are related to each other, which results in a complex picture for individuals with chronic conditions.

Chapter 23 – "The Psychosocial Impact of Chronic Disease" (Evangelos C. Karademas and Yael Benyamini)

Successful adaptation to chronic diseases requires assimilation and accommodation of physical impairments/decline and symptoms, treatment regime(s), rearrangement of life goals, valued activities or priorities, and regulation of emotional aspects of the journey with NCD. Adaptation and disease management extend beyond the physical symptoms to include broader emotional experiences of people with NCDs and the range of contextual factors influencing these experiences. The literature on adjustment to chronic disease has become increasingly sophisticated. This chapter provides a selective overview of the emotional/psychosocial issues in NCDs. These are rarely present in isolation (as clear and distinct entities). They often feature a cascade of negative emotions that span across a broad range of different chronic diseases. It is also important that in some cases, individuals appear to derive some psychological benefits from dealing with the adversity that the chronic disease presents with the result that they appear well-adjusted and in positive mood (Shelley E. Taylor, 1983).

Chapter 24 – "Adherence and Self-Management" (Rui She)

The management of NCDS requires demanding self-management behaviours, such as taking multiple medications or following other treatment requirements (e.g., dialysis, rehabilitation programmes), as well as various dietary, fluid, or exercise recommendations. Disease outcomes depend on how effectively individuals can implement and sustain these complex self-management skills in daily life. The chapter provides a selective overview of the conceptual evolution of adherence and self-management, including prevalence, impact, and drivers of nonadherence in various NCDs. It also outlines the relevant theoretical frameworks and evidence-based interventions that have been shown to be efficacious and cost-effective in the promotion and facilitation of self-management, with improvements in patients' knowledge, skills, and motivation leading to improved biomedical, behavioural, and psychosocial outcomes.

Chapter 25 – "The Role of Technology in Chronic Disease" (Elizabeth Broadbent and Kate Loveys)

As with most activities in the world today, the introduction of technologies to healthcare and the management of chronic disease has and continues to have a major impact on the delivery of care. These technologies have the capacity to increase the delivery of early signs and symptoms of a condition to the healthcare system. This in turn enables a more rapid response with the potential of reducing both mortality and morbidity by early intervention. It also has the potential to provide reassurance to individuals with chronic disease and their families that their health is being monitored. The introduction of technology also has the potential to reduce costs, although increased surveillance may result in increased costs. The closing chapter addresses the new 'digital health' approaches for disease management in the context of NCDs and how these digital systems are reconfiguring disease management at all levels of healthcare.

Further Reading

GBD 2019 Viewpoint Collaborators. Five insights from the Global Burden of Disease Study 2019. *Lancet*. 2020;396(10258):1135–1159. doi: 10.1016/S0140-6736(20)31404-5

NCD Countdown 2030 collaborators. NCD Countdown 2030: pathways to achieving Sustainable Development Goal target 3.4. *Lancet*. 2020;396(10255):918-934. doi: 10.1016/S0140-6736(20)31761-X

Prince, M., Patel, V., Saxena, S., Maj, M., Maselko, J., Phillips, M. R., Rahman, A. No health without mental health. *Lancet*. 2007;370(9590):859–77. doi: 10.1016/S0140-6736(07)61238-0

WHO on health topic "Non Communicable diseases" that has wealth data reports and publications on this topic across countries. https://www.who.int/health-topics/noncommunicable-diseases#tab=tab_1

References

Ekwueme, D. U., Guy, G. P., Li, C., Rim, S. H., Parelkar, P., & Chen, S. C. (2011). The health burden and economic costs of cutaneous melanoma mortality by race/ethnicity-United States, 2000 to 2006. *Journal of the American Academy of Dermatology*, *65*(5 Suppl 1), S133.e1–S133.e12. https://doi.org/10.1016/J.JAAD.2011.04.036

Ezzati, M., Kontis, V., Bennett, J. E., Parks, R. M., Rashid, T., Pearson-Stuttard, J., Asaria, P., Zhou, B., Guillot, M., Mathers, C. D., Khang, Y. H., & McKee, M. (2022). Lessons learned and lessons missed: Impact of the coronavirus disease 2019 (COVID-19) pandemic on all-cause mortality in 40 industrialised countries and US states prior to mass vaccination. *Wellcome Open Research*, *6*. https://doi.org/10.12688/WELLCOMEOPENRES.17253.2

Guan, W., Ni, Z., Hu, Y., Liang, W., Ou, C., He, J., Liu, L., Shan, H., Lei, C., Hui, D. S. C., Du, B., Li, L., Zeng, G., Yuen, K.-Y., Chen, R., Tang, C., Wang, T., Chen, P., Xiang, J., … Zhong, N. (2020). Clinical Characteristics of Coronavirus Disease 2019 in China. *New England Journal of Medicine*, *382*(18), 1708–1720. https://doi.org/10.1056/NEJMOA2002032/SUPPL_FILE/NEJMOA2002032_DISCLOSURES.PDF

Guo, C., Zhang, Z., Lau, A. K. H., Lin, C. Q., Chuang, Y. C., Chan, J., Jiang, W. K., Tam, T., Yeoh, E. K., Chan, T. C., Chang, L. Y., & Lao, X. Q. (2018). Effect of long-term exposure to fine particulate matter on lung function decline and risk of chronic obstructive pulmonary disease in Taiwan: a longitudinal, cohort study. *The Lancet. Planetary Health*, *2*(3), e114–e125. https://doi.org/10.1016/S2542-5196(18)30028-7

Leal, J., Luengo-Fernández, R., Gray, A., Petersen, S., & Rayner, M. (2006). Economic burden of cardiovascular diseases in the enlarged European Union. *European Heart Journal*, *27*(13), 1610–1619. https://doi.org/10.1093/EURHEARTJ/EHI733

Magliano, D. J., Sacre, J. W., Harding, J. L., Gregg, E. W., Zimmet, P. Z., & Shaw, J. E. (2020). Young-onset type 2 diabetes mellitus – implications for morbidity and mortality. *Nature Reviews. Endocrinology*, *16*(6), 321–331. https://doi.org/10.1038/S41574-020-0334-Z

National Center for Chronic Disease Prevention and Health Promotion. (2022). *About chronic diseases*. https://www.cdc.gov/chronicdisease/about/index.htm

OECD. (2021). Chronic conditions. In *Health at a Glance 2021: OECD Indicators*. OECD Publishing. https://doi.org/10.1787/908b2da3-en

Partnership to Fight Chronic Disease. (n.d.). *What is the cost of chronic disease on America?* Retrieved November 7, 2023, from https://www.fightchronicdisease.org/sites/default/files/pfcd_blocks/PFCD_US.FactSheet_FINAL1%20%282%29.pdf

Roser, M., Ritchie, H., & Spooner, F. (2021). *Burden of disease*. Our World in Data. https://ourworldindata.org/burden-of-disease

Sattar, N., Rawshani, A., Franzén, S., Rawshani, A., Svensson, A. M., Rosengren, A., Mcguire, D. K., Eliasson, B., & Gudbjörnsdottir, S. (2019). Age at Diagnosis of Type 2 Diabetes Mellitus and Associations With Cardiovascular and Mortality Risks. *Circulation*, *139*(19), 2228–2237. https://doi.org/10.1161/CIRCULATIONAHA.118.037885

Siu, A. L., Bibbins-Domingo, K., Grossman, D. C., Baumann, L. C., Davidson, K. W., Ebell, M., García, F. A. R., Gillman, M., Herzstein, J., Kemper, A. R., Krist, A. H., Kurth, A. E., Owens, D. K., Phillips, W. R., Phipps, M. G., & Pignone, M. P. (2016). Screening for Depression in Adults: US Preventive Services Task Force Recommendation Statement. *JAMA*, *315*(4), 380–387. https://doi.org/10.1001/JAMA.2015.18392

Taylor, S. E. (1983). Adjustment to threathening events: a theory of cognitive adaptation. *American Psychologist*, *38*(11), 1161–1173.

The Institute for Health Metrics and Evaluation. (2020, October 15). *The Lancet: Latest global disease estimates reveal perfect storm of rising chronic diseases and public health failures fuelling COVID-19 pandemic*. https://www.healthdata.org/news-events/newsroom/news-releases/lancet-latest-global-disease-estimates-reveal-perfect-storm

United Nations. (n.d.). *Goal 3: Ensure healthy lives and promote well-being for all at all ages*. Retrieved November 7, 2023, from https://www.un.org/sustainabledevelopment/health/

World Health Organization. (2023a, March 31). *Depressive disorder (depression)*. https://www.who.int/news-room/fact-sheets/detail/depression

World Health Organization. (2023b, September 16). *Noncommunicable diseases*. https://www.who.int/news-room/fact-sheets/detail/noncommunicable-diseases

22

COPING WITH SYMPTOMS AND TREATMENTS

Frederick H. F. Chan, Stanton P. Newman, and Konstadina Griva

Introduction

The presence of many chronic diseases and associated symptoms, as well as the treatments and medical regimen that they necessitate, are accompanied by substantial burden on the individual. People living with these chronic diseases experience symptoms (e.g., pain, fatigue, nausea) that affect their functional capacity and quality of life. These symptoms may be directly caused by the pathophysiology of the disease itself or may be a result of treatments and can vary widely across individuals depending on many factors. Symptoms may not be disease-specific, such as fatigue, but accompany a wide range of chronic conditions. Symptoms are the subjective experience reported by patients (e.g., pain) that may reflect a condition or disease and should be differentiated from signs (e.g., high blood pressure), which are objective evidence of disease.

The subjective report of symptoms typically forms the basis of most clinical encounters. In particular, the initial help-seeking consultation is usually driven by symptom experience which may also drive an individual to request a diagnosis, further testing, and medication. Beliefs and perceptions about symptoms also influence responses to chronic disease and related treatments. People with diabetes or asthma, for example, manage their condition by monitoring symptoms and making decisions related to medication intake and treatment(s). Experience of medication side effects may increase the likelihood of non-adherence, whereas in conditions such as asthma, lack of symptoms may discourage adherence to preventative medication.

This chapter provides a selective overview of common symptoms experienced in chronic diseases, theories conceptualising symptom experience, available tools for measuring symptoms, implications of symptoms for patient outcomes, and strategies for managing these symptoms.

DOI: 10.4324/9781003318026-27

Concepts and Definitions

In the context of chronic diseases, symptoms may be a result of the disease itself, comorbidities, medical procedures, or treatment, including medication (Cleeland, 2007). Various terminologies have been used to describe the experience of symptoms, and these are often mapped onto prevalence, severity, and impact of symptoms. Conceptual models of symptom experience outline the sequence or phases of this experience, including the production and occurrence of symptoms, individuals' perception and beliefs about the symptoms, the expression and consequences of symptoms, and individuals' coping behaviours in response to symptoms (Armstrong, 2003; Fu et al., 2007). Symptom experience is defined as the "perception of the frequency, intensity, distress, and meaning of symptoms as they are produced and expressed" (Armstrong, 2003). Symptom experience is an individual's perception and response to symptom occurrence and distress (Fu et al., 2004). Symptom occurrence involves two aspects of symptoms: frequency (i.e., number of times an individual experiences a symptom within a given timeframe) and duration (i.e., persistence of a symptom) (Fu et al., 2004). The occurrence of symptoms may then result in symptom distress, which refers to the extent of physical, emotional, and mental suffering or discomfort reported by individuals in response to symptoms (Fu et al., 2004, 2007).

A related concept is symptom burden, which refers to the "subjective, quantifiable prevalence, frequency, and severity of symptoms that place a physiologic burden on patients and may produce multiple negative physical, psychological, and emotional patient responses" (Gapstur, 2007). Put another way, symptom burden is the summary expression of the severity and impact of symptoms imposed on individuals with a certain disease or receiving certain treatments (Cleeland, 2007; Gapstur, 2007). Understanding symptom burden in chronic disease is crucial because of the potential impact of symptom burden on the individuals' mental health, functional status, quality of life, and survival (Armstrong, 2003). The experience of symptoms and the burden that they produce are also important determinants of how patients cope with or respond to their illness (Fu et al., 2007; Leventhal et al., 1984).

Despite some discrepancies in how researchers conceptualise symptom burden and related terms, there is a general consensus that symptom burden is dynamic and multidimensional (Gapstur, 2007). It is dynamic because symptoms may intensify or lessen over the course of disease and treatment trajectories, and their frequency and severity may vary depending on multiple factors, including demographic aspects of the patients (e.g., age, gender) and psychological characteristics (e.g., personality, mood). It is multidimensional because symptom burden is concerned not only with patients' perceived frequency and severity of their symptoms but also the meaning or interpretation that they assign to the symptoms, the distress that symptoms create, and the consequences or impact on their daily lives.

It is worth noting that some symptoms commonly seen in chronic diseases may also be considered an integral part of the disease itself. For example, chronic pain, defined as pain that persists or recurs for longer than three months, constitutes a diagnostic entity by itself, whereas in the context of other diseases such as cancer, pain could be a symptom caused by the tumour or a side effect caused by chemotherapy, in which case it is referred to as chronic secondary pain or cancer-related pain (Treede et al., 2019). A related phenomenon is the depressive symptoms which are prevalent in various chronic diseases. If the depressive symptoms reach a certain level, they may be considered major depressive disorder.

The complex aetiology of many chronic diseases and mechanisms of their treatments result in the fact that individual symptoms seldom occur in isolation. In cancer research, it has been reported that, on average, patients experience 11 to 13 concurrent symptoms (Fan et al., 2007). These co-occurring symptoms may or may not be interrelated, but there is growing evidence that common biological mechanisms may be contributors to several symptoms that follow the same time course (Cleeland, 2007).

It is not uncommon for symptoms to co-occur in clusters, defined as two or more symptoms that co-occur in a non-random fashion; are related to one another through a common aetiology or mechanism, shared variance, or a common outcome; and are distinct from other symptom clusters (Dodd et al., 2001). The concept and identification of symptom clusters have gained considerable traction in recent research. Current symptom management approaches have also evolved to move from focusing on a single symptom to exploring symptom clusters. The number of symptoms within clusters and their composition, intensity, and durations vary, and there are many different patterns of co-occurring symptoms. For example, a pain-fatigue-insomnia-depression cluster is common in many cancer patients and survivors (Li, 2021) with complex synergistic effects, interactions, and temporal associations. Pain could compromise sleep, which can increase fatigue and then collectively exacerbate depression. In the context of chronic kidney disease, several distinct symptom clusters have also been identified, including uraemic (e.g., nausea, shortness of breath), neuromuscular (e.g., numbness in extremities, sore muscles, cramps), and skin (e.g., itching, dry skin) clusters, which were found to be associated with depression and poorer quality of life (Amro et al., 2014). In addition to identifying symptom clusters by examining correlations among symptoms in patients with a certain type of chronic disease, recent work has focused on mapping variability in how individuals experience symptom clusters.

Theoretical Models

There are several models to conceptualise and map symptoms experience. These may have some overlapping components but also may have a different focus on aspects of symptom experience.

The symptoms experience model summarises three categories of factors that influence symptom production and symptom perception (i.e., antecedents) (Armstrong, 2003). These include demographic (e.g., age, gender), disease-related (e.g., type and stage of disease, type of treatment, comorbidity), and individual characteristics (e.g., health knowledge, past experience, personality). The experience of each symptom can be described in terms of frequency, intensity, perceived physical or mental distress caused by the symptoms, and situational and existential meaning that individuals attribute to the symptoms (Armstrong, 2003). Situational meaning refers to the perceived impact of symptoms on patients' daily life (e.g., inability to exercise due to pain), whereas existential meaning refers to patients' sense of vulnerability and mortality as a result of symptom perception (e.g., breathlessness as a reminder of impending mortality; Armstrong, 2003). In some cases, symptoms may have a positive meaning, for example, when the intensity of symptoms reminds the patient that the treatment is effective. The symptoms experience model further describes potential consequences of symptoms, which include changes in quality of life, mood, functional status, and survival.

The Common-Sense Model of Self-Regulation (or Common-Sense Model, CSM) (Leventhal et al., 1984) has made a major contribution to research on chronic disease. This dynamic model describes the perceptual/cognitive, emotional, and behavioural processes involved in interpreting and managing health threats (Leventhal et al., 2016). Symptoms are critical in self-regulation. The experience of symptoms drives an individual to make sense of or assign meaning to the problem, which generates cognitive and emotional representations of the symptom/illness (Leventhal et al., 1984). The cognitive processes address questions such as, "What is it" (identity, referring to assigned label or symptoms), "What is the cause of the illness/symptom" (perceived causes), "How long is it likely to last" (timeline for illness and symptom that could be acute, chronic, or episodic), "What is the impact on life" (perceived consequences), and "Can it be cured or minimised" (control/cure that can include personal control and treatment control or effectiveness; Leventhal et al., 1984; Weinman et al., 1996)? The overall "illness coherence" (i.e., how well an individual feels they understand the condition) has been proposed as a meta-cognition that reflects how patients evaluate the coherence or usefulness of their symptoms/illness representations (Moss-Morris et al., 2002). Emotional representation is the extent to which patients are emotionally influenced by the illness/symptoms (e.g., fear, distress, anger). Cognitive and emotional representations may interact with each other and are dynamic throughout the course of disease and treatment (Weinman et al., 1996). Following the formation of these representations, patients may adopt coping behaviours (e.g., taking medications), which are then evaluated in the appraisal stage, where individuals determine whether or not to continue the coping strategies (Broadbent et al., 2006; Horne & Weinman, 2002; Leventhal et al., 1984). Finally, the appraisal result could feed into the formation of updated representations (e.g., "my pain can be controlled by medication") (Broadbent et al., 2006). The hypotheses of CSM have been further confirmed by empirical research which showed associations between the dimensions of cognitive/emotional representations and important outcomes, including psychological and social well-being, role performance, vitality, and overall quality of life (Brooke & Lusher, 2012; Hagger & Orbell, 2003).

More recently, an integrative model of symptom and illness representations has been proposed. The Symptom and Illness Attitude Model (SIAM) was developed based on various theories and aims to optimise the assessment of illness/symptom representations and identify variables moderating the relationships between these representations and affective or behavioural consequences (Petersen et al., 2011). This model defines symptom perception as "the sum of a number of interactions between beliefs and affective evaluations" (Petersen et al., 2011). In other words, whether an individual interprets a sensation or experience as a pathological symptom not only depends on their beliefs about the symptom (e.g., intensity, quality) but also their affective evaluation of the beliefs. For example, an individual who experiences mild breathlessness (i.e., weak belief) but considers this sensation as extremely negative (i.e., strong negative evaluation) can have catastrophising interpretations of the symptom. The SIAM also suggests that symptom representations are not the sole contributors to comorbid affective disorders or behavioural intentions (Petersen et al., 2011). Other salient representations; competing beliefs, attitudes, or norms; and contextual information should also be taken into account.

Measurement

Various methods and questionnaires have been developed to assess symptoms experience. Self-report measures typically require individuals to recall symptom occurrence, their intensity, and/or "bother" over a recent period of time, with some covering a range of symptoms most pertinent to the condition (e.g., Symptom Distress Scale; Fu et al., 2007) and others focusing on specific symptoms (e.g., Chalder Fatigue Scale; Cella & Chalder, 2010).

Given their multidimensionality, assessment of symptoms may include sensory qualities and intensity, location (e.g., number of pain sites), and timing (i.e., frequency and duration), as well as cognitive and emotional aspects such as the associated distress, meaning, and impact on daily functioning or quality of life (Barsevick et al., 2006). There are a multitude of tools and measurement approaches, each with strengths and limitations that need to be carefully considered in relation to the purpose of assessment and/or the specific research objectives or population of interest. The majority of available assessment tools either measure multiple dimensions of one symptom (e.g., pain duration and intensity) or measure one dimension of multiple symptoms (e.g., frequency or bother of symptoms).

Some measures focus on the cognitive and affective aspects of a certain symptom. The Pain Catastrophising Scale and the Fatigue Catastrophising Scale both assess catastrophising thoughts in relation to pain or fatigue (e.g., "I keep thinking about how much it hurts") (Jacobsen et al., 2004; Sullivan et al., 1995). The Fear of Pain Questionnaire assesses individuals' fear or anxiety about their pain, which may not be occurring at the time (McNeil & Rainwater, 1998). These measures may not directly reflect individuals' current symptom experience but provide an overall evaluation of the impact of a person's symptoms.

Given that retrospective recall may be influenced by response bias (i.e., peak-end heuristics; symptom reports disproportionately influenced by the most intense ("peak") and the most recent part of the experience ("end") closest to the reporting time), methods of assessment that avoid these difficulties have been suggested. For example, measuring symptoms as a dynamic process in real-time using methodologies such as ecological momentary assessment offers advantages in that retrospective biases are avoided, but they have a high burden of completion (May et al., 2018).

Some symptoms could also be assessed with objective methods. Measures secondary to the pain sensation, such as facial expressions of pain, and pain behaviours, such as rubbing and sighing (Keefe & Block, 1982; Prkachin et al., 2002), despite modification by personal and cultural display norms, have been shown to be reliable indicators of pain. The observation of these non-verbal behaviours may be labour intensive but may be especially helpful for assessing individuals with cognitive impairments or those unable to complete self-report questionnaires. Physiological markers such as pupil reflexes have also been suggested as potential objective pain assessment tools (Cowen et al., 2015).

Epidemiology

Patients with chronic diseases experience multiple symptoms on a daily basis. For instance, in patients with end-stage renal disease receiving haemodialysis treatment, one study found that 22 out of 47 symptoms queried were experienced at least "a little of the time" (Curtin et al., 2002), and another study reported an average of nine symptoms (e.g., fatigue, itching, pain, dry skin) at any given time (Weisbord et al., 2005). The frequency and severity of symptoms differ across diseases. For example, while fatigue was found to be the most severe symptom in cancer patients in one study (Cleeland et al., 2013), diabetes patients appeared to report pain more commonly than fatigue (Sudore et al., 2012), and patients with heart failure tended to report dyspnoea more frequently (Khan et al., 2015).

A large body of research has investigated the epidemiology of individual symptoms in different disease contexts. Pain, defined as "an unpleasant sensory and emotional experience associated with, or resembling that associated with, actual or potential tissue damage" (Raja et al., 2020), is widespread across diseases. Pain has been commonly reported in cancer (33 to 66% depending on stage and treatment; van den Beuken-van Everdingen et al., 2007, 2016), diabetes (41.8% for acute pain and 39.7% for chronic pain; Sudore et al., 2012), and chronic kidney disease (over 58% considering all stages; Davison et al., 2014; 82% to 92% in those receiving haemodialysis treatment; Brkovic et al., 2016). Although pain is not a signature symptom in chronic heart failure, where fatigue and shortness of breath are more common, studies still reported high pain prevalence in these patients, ranging from 23% to 85% (Alemzadeh-Ansari et al., 2017). It is of note that pain itself is considered to be a chronic disease if the pain persists or recurs for more than three months (Treede et al., 2019). It was estimated that 10% of the global population experience chronic pain and that one in ten adults is newly diagnosed with chronic pain each year (Goldberg & McGee, 2011).

Fatigue, described as the subjective sense of weakness, lack of energy, and tiredness (either physical or mental) that is not relieved by rest, is a common and debilitating symptom across many chronic disease conditions (Goërtz et al., 2021). Individuals with one or more chronic conditions are more likely to experience chronic and severe fatigue compared to those without any chronic condition (Goërtz et al., 2021). Studies on specific disease populations have found high rates of fatigue, with 49%–52% in cancer (Al Maqbali et al., 2021; Ma et al., 2020), 65.6% in multiple sclerosis (Weiland et al., 2015), 69%–88% in heart failure (Fini & Cruz, 2009), and 44% and 50% in type 1 and type 2 diabetes, respectively (Romadlon et al., 2022). In chronic kidney disease, fatigue is considered a core outcome by the "Standardised Outcomes in Nephrology (SONG)" Initiative (SONG Initiative, 2017), and its prevalence ranges from 60% to as high as 97% in patients receiving long-term renal replacement therapies (Jhamb et al., 2008).

While widely researched in the dementia and Alzheimer's disease literature, subjective cognitive complaints are gaining traction in other chronic disease contexts. Cognitive complaints (e.g., forgetfulness, difficulty concentrating) refer to the self-experienced changes in cognitive ability or difficulties in everyday cognitive performance. These complaints are highly common in individuals with diabetes, heart disease, cancer, and kidney disease (Chan, Goh, et al., 2022; Chan, Newman, et al., 2022; Hill et al., 2021; Pullens et al., 2010) and may be a result of the disease itself or its treatments, such as chemotherapy and dialysis (Chan, Goh, et al., 2022; Kim et al., 2022).

There is growing research interest in the clustering and fluctuating nature of symptoms. Using a novel natural language processing approach to analyse electronic health records, a study identified five distinct symptom clusters, including cognitive (e.g., confusion), cardiovascular (e.g., shortness of breath), mental health (e.g., depression), gastrointestinal (e.g., nausea), and a cluster with pain and other symptoms (Koleck et al., 2021). The cognitive cluster was common among cancer, diabetes, and heart failure, whereas the pain and other symptom clusters were shared among chronic obstructive pulmonary disease, diabetes, and cancer. The cardiovascular cluster was only found in heart failure and diabetes, whereas chronic obstructive pulmonary disease patients had a unique mental health cluster, and cancer patients had a unique gastrointestinal cluster (Koleck et al., 2021). Using ecological momentary assessments, studies have shown substantial diurnal fluctuations in pain intensity across time and individuals (Pagé et al., 2022). Using prospective designs, some studies identified individual variability in longitudinal symptom trajectories (e.g., persistent high symptoms, deterioration, recovery) that were associated with differential health outcomes (Chan et al., 2023; Ng et al., 2015). Future attempts such as these can advance our current understanding of symptoms experience, which is largely based on cross-sectional observations of individual symptoms.

It is noteworthy that in many circumstances, symptoms persist for a long time, even after cessation of treatments. Cancer survivors frequently report symptoms such as fatigue and sleep disturbance, with more than 30% perceiving these symptoms as severe as patients undergoing active treatments (Wu & Harden,

2015). The possibility of cancer recurrence also triggers unique psychological symptoms at the survivorship phase, such as fear of recurrence (Sharpe et al., 2017). In other contexts, such as contraction of COVID-19 and admission to intensive care units, the disease or treatment per se may be short term, but symptoms can persist into long-term survivorship. A significant percentage of COVID-19 survivors reported fatigue, dyspnoea, memory loss, concentration difficulties, and insomnia one-year post-infection (Han et al., 2022). Intensive care survivors reported pain, fatigue, sleep disturbance, and depression and anxiety three months after discharge with no significant improvement at one year (Langerud et al., 2018).

It is beyond the scope of the current chapter to review all common symptoms in various chronic diseases. Most prior work has focused on pain, fatigue, sleep disturbance, and psychological/emotional distress. Some symptoms such as cognitive complaints, nausea, lack of appetite, and itching have received less attention but are also important determinants for patient outcomes and hence require further study.

Associated or Precipitative Factors

Theoretical frameworks outline a range of factors that may contribute to the occurrence, perception, and experience of symptoms, including sociodemographic, clinical, and psychosocial parameters. Certain sociodemographic factors, including unemployment, singleness, lower socioeconomic status, and lower educational level, have been linked to higher symptom burden (Cai et al., 2022; Chen et al., 2021; Wu & Harden, 2015). Clinical factors such as the type and stages or severity of disease and treatment also contribute to differential symptoms experience. For instance, pain and fatigue are more prevalent in patients with advanced-stage cancers and those receiving active treatment in comparison to patients with localised cancer and those who completed treatment (Al Maqbali et al., 2021; Ma et al., 2020; van den Beuken-van Everdingen et al., 2007).

Psychosocial (mood, beliefs, personality) and cognitive factors are also highly pertinent in symptom perception and interpretations. Individuals may hold different beliefs about their symptoms, and these may be influenced by personality traits. Neuroticism, for example, has been associated with higher symptom reporting because individuals high in neuroticism may be more self-focused and attentive to physical sensations and are more likely to attribute benign sensations to a negative underlying cause (Feldman et al., 1999). By contrast, individuals high in resilience (i.e., ability to face adversity) and optimism tend to report fewer symptoms (Ruiz-Rodríguez et al., 2022). Cognitive bias may also interact with psychosocial processes. Patients with high anxiety/negative affect may exhibit attentional bias or hypervigilance towards threat cues, such as unpleasant bodily sensations, which may inflate symptom reports (Merckelbach et al., 2019). Attentional bias towards pain-related information has been proposed to underlie the development and maintenance of chronic pain (Vlaeyen & Linton, 2000). Patients with depression may also have negative memory bias (i.e., tendency to memorise and recall negative memories), which can increase the reporting of past symptoms (Merckelbach et al., 2019). More recently, patients' expectations have received a lot of attention in context of symptoms experienced. The nocebo effect is defined as "the experience of adverse events or unpleasant symptoms in response to an inert medication or procedure" (Faasse & Petrie, 2013) and is often mediated through negative emotions and cognitive bias (Aslaksen & Lyby, 2015). When patients are expecting symptoms resulting from their illness or side effects as the result of treatments, their attention is focused on these symptoms, which increases the likelihood that they detect and report these symptoms (Faasse & Petrie, 2013).

Symptoms and Other Outcomes

The way individuals perceive and experience symptoms related to chronic disease and treatments affect physical, psychological, and behavioural outcomes, ranging from clinical prognosis to daily functioning, adherence, and quality of life. Studies and reviews have concluded that symptoms have a negative impact on functional capacity and quality of life (Chen et al., 2021; Dodd et al., 2001; Li, 2021; Wu & Harden, 2015). Longitudinal studies that assessed baseline symptom report and survival for up to two years have found that the frequency/severity and distress of various symptoms or symptom clusters (e.g., shortness of breath, fatigue, confusion, pain-fatigue-sleep cluster) were independent predictors of mortality (Li, 2021; Reuben et al., 1988; Trajkovic-Vidakovic et al., 2012). Importantly, the effect of symptoms on mortality may be mediated through a behavioural pathway. Cleeland (2007) suggested that symptoms caused by treatments may delay the initiation of treatment or result in early treatment termination, which may be one reason why symptoms are associated with mortality. Although dialysis is a life-maintaining treatment in patients with kidney failure, the experience and expectation of pain due to dialysis are a common reason for shortened or missed dialysis sessions (Zhang et al., 2020). Some patients regret their decision to initiate dialysis, and some withdraw from dialysis if their pain becomes too severe. Suboptimal adherence to treatments for long-term conditions may in turn lead to increased risk of death. In dialysis patients, studies have shown that skipping one or more haemodialysis sessions in a month was associated with a 25% increase in mortality over two years (Clark et al., 2014).

It is important to note however that the relationship between symptoms and adherence is not linear, and in some circumstances, the presence of symptoms resulting from a disease can in fact increase the level of adherence if the treatment is considered effective in managing the particular symptom (Kardas et al., 2013). This suggests that patients' beliefs may play an important role in determining how they respond to their symptoms. Horne and Weinman (2002) found that patients who have more doubts about the necessity of medications, those with more concerns about the adverse effects, and those who perceive the consequences of illness more negatively were more likely to be non-adherent. Individuals who experience pain, especially those who have high fear of pain, may engage in avoidance behaviours (e.g., avoiding exercise) as a coping strategy to reduce movement-related pain and prevent injury. However, in the long term, pain avoidance behaviour may contribute to increased fear of pain and pain catastrophising, which further exacerbates chronic pain (Vlaeyen & Linton, 2000).

Management of Symptoms

The theory of symptom management defines symptom management strategies as "efforts to avert, delay, or minimise the symptom experience" (Bender et al., 2008). The subjective experience of symptoms, together with the influence of personal, environmental, and health-related factors, prompt an individual to initiate one or more management strategies, which may change the status of symptoms through three pathways: (1) reducing the frequency of symptom occurrence, (2) mitigating the severity or intensity of symptoms, and (3) relieving the distress caused by the symptoms (Bender et al., 2008).

In symptom research and clinical practice, symptom management strategies are broadly categorised into pharmacological and non-pharmacological interventions. Pharmacological interventions include conventional medications (e.g., antidepressants, opioids) and dietary supplements (e.g., vitamins). Non-pharmacological strategies may include physical (e.g., exercise, physical therapy), psychological (e.g., cognitive behavioural therapy, psychoeducation, relaxation), behavioural (sleep hygiene, diet), and complementary and alternative approaches (e.g., acupuncture, aromatherapy).

To date, the majority of symptom management strategies focus on addressing one individual symptom (e.g., analgesics to reduce pain in chronic pain patients (Knopp-Sihota et al., 2022); erythropoietin-stimulating agents to alleviate fatigue in chronic kidney disease patients (Metzger et al., 2021)). Health-care providers typically provide management recommendations according to single-symptom clinical guidelines (Kwekkeboom et al., 2020). As a result, patients who report multiple symptoms are likely to receive information on each individual symptom and are recommended various medications and self-management strategies that target each symptom (Kwekkeboom et al., 2020). This adds to the already very high symptom and treatment burdens of chronic disease patients. Patients and their families are required to opt for symptom management strategies among the various recommendations for each symptom and to implement and adhere to these strategies once initiated. This approach makes the experience of chronic disease and its associated symptoms and treatments even more burdensome. Another problem with the focus on single-symptom management is that it neglects potential interactions between different symptoms and management strategies. An intervention effective in alleviating one symptom may exacerbate another symptom. For example, opioid analgesics are commonly used for pain management but can exacerbate symptoms such as fatigue and constipation (Barsevick et al., 2006).

Kwekkeboom et al. (2020) carried out a review of clinical guidelines to identify symptom management strategies recommended across at least two cancer symptoms. They identified 167 treatment strategies, of which 88 (including 41 pharmacological and 47 non-pharmacological strategies) were recommended or considered potentially beneficial for at least two symptoms according to clinical guidelines (Kwekkeboom et al., 2020). Five strategies were recommended for nine or more symptoms. These include exercise, psychoeducation, antidepressants, acupuncture/acupressure, and relaxation (Kwekkeboom et al., 2020). For instance, psychoeducation has been recommended for anorexia, anxiety, cognitive impairment, constipation, depression, dyspnoea, fatigue, pain, and sleep-wake disturbances, and is potentially beneficial for diarrhoea, nausea, and vomiting. The authors of this review called for a paradigm shift from single- to multi-symptom management, selecting strategies that may alleviate multiple symptoms at the same time, which may be more efficient, more cost-effective, and less burdensome (Kwekkeboom et al., 2020).

A challenge to the management of chronic disease and associated symptoms is the nocebo effect. From an ethical and legal standpoint, informed consent is essential for any intervention adopted. However, by providing information about the potential side effects of a treatment, health-care providers can induce nocebo effects. Experimental studies have found that providing individuals with threatening information about upcoming pain would increase their experienced pain intensity and distress in a later pain task (Todd et al., 2016). In real-world contexts, even reading medication labels or simply verbal suggestions may increase side-effect reporting (Faasse & Petrie, 2013). This nocebo effect can in turn increase symptom and treatment burden, contribute to treatment non-adherence, and may result in patients choosing alternative but less effective strategies that are perceived to have less or no adverse effects (Faasse & Petrie, 2013). It is therefore important for health-care providers to recognise the effect of patient expectations and nocebo effects during symptom management practice. Although strategies to reduce nocebo effects remain understudied and have not yet translated into clinical settings, some methods have shown opportunities to be integrated into future practice. For instance, informing patients about the nocebo effect has been shown to be able to reduce side effect reporting (Pan et al., 2019) and alter patients' information needs towards desiring less information about the side effects (Nestoriuc et al., 2021). Information framing that uses non-threatening language and places more focus on treatment information on positive outcomes and patients' ability to cope with mild symptoms may also be effective strategies to reduce nocebo effects (Faasse & Petrie, 2013).

Conclusions

Patients with chronic diseases experience high symptom and treatment burdens that may increase mortality and hospitalisation risks, compromise functional performance and quality of life, and affect psychological and social well-being. This chapter provided an overview of common symptoms in chronic disease, theoretical models describing symptoms experience, methods of symptom measurement, influencing factors and consequences of symptoms, as well as management of symptoms. Despite the amount of research conducted on this topic, our knowledge of the aetiology of various symptoms, the interaction between symptoms, and strategies to assess and manage symptoms remain limited. Advancing our understanding of symptoms experienced in chronic diseases is crucial because this would allow for high-quality patient-centred care.

Some critical gaps are evident. In particular, prior research and current clinical practice focus mainly on individual symptoms. Symptoms are typically studied in isolation, and studies rarely consider the existence of symptom clusters and interactions among various symptoms. Current practice is also predominantly based on single-symptom guidelines without taking into account the effect of a certain symptom management strategy on other co-occurring symptoms. There is a need to shift towards a multi-symptom focus in both research and practice that would provide deeper insights into the complex aetiology of multiple symptoms and enable more efficient, more cost-effective, and less burdensome management strategies. This is particularly the case for multimorbid patients with a number of co-occurring chronic diseases where some treatments and management strategies for individual symptoms may be in conflict. In addition, previous research mainly focused on symptoms such as pain, fatigue, sleep disturbance, and depression. Other symptoms (e.g., cognitive complaints, nausea, itching) in various disease contexts are less well understood and warrant further study.

Further Reading

Rask, M. T., Frostholm, L., Hansen, S. H., Petersen, M. W., Ørnbøl, E., & Rosendal, M. (2023, January 24). Self-help interventions for persistent physical symptoms: a systematic review of behaviour change components and their potential effects. *Health Psychology Review*, 1–42. https://doi.org/10.1080/17437199.2022.2163917

Stone, A. A., Schneider, S., & Smyth, J. M. (2023, May 9). Evaluation of Pressing Issues in Ecological Momentary Assessment. *Annual Review of Clinical Psychology*, *19*(1), 107–131. https://doi.org/10.1146/annurev-clinpsy-080921-083128

Mendoza-Quispe, D., Perez-Leon, S., Alarcon-Ruiz, C. A., Gaspar, A., Cuba-Fuentes, M. S., Zunt, J. R., Montori, V. M., Bazo-Alvarez, J. C., & Miranda, J. J. (2023, July). Scoping review of measures of treatment burden in patients with multimorbidity: advancements and current gaps. *Journal of Clinical Epidemiology*, *159*, 92–105. https://doi.org/10.1016/j.jclinepi.2023.05.013

References

Al Maqbali, M., Al Sinani, M., Al Naamani, Z., Al Badi, K., & Tanash, M. I. (2021). Prevalence of Fatigue in Patients With Cancer: A Systematic Review and Meta-Analysis. *Journal of Pain and Symptom Management*, *61*(1), 167–189.e14. https://doi.org/10.1016/j.jpainsymman.2020.07.037

Alemzadeh-Ansari, M. J., Ansari-Ramandi, M. M., & Naderi, N. (2017). Chronic pain in chronic heart failure: A review article. *Journal of Tehran University Heart Center*, *12*(2), 49–56.

Amro, A., Waldum, B., Dammen, T., Miaskowski, C., & Os, I. (2014). Symptom clusters in patients on dialysis and their association with quality-of-life outcomes. *Journal of Renal Care*, *40*(1), 23–33. https://doi.org/10.1111/jorc.12051

Armstrong, T. S. (2003). Symptoms experience: a concept analysis. *Oncology Nursing Forum*, *30*(4), 601–606. https://doi.org/10.1188/03.ONF.601-606

Aslaksen, P. M., & Lyby, P. S. (2015). Fear of pain potentiates nocebo hyperalgesia. *Journal of Pain Research*, *8*, 703–710. https://doi.org/10.2147/JPR.S91923

Barsevick, A. M., Whitmer, K., Nail, L. M., Beck, S. L., & Dudley, W. N. (2006). Symptom cluster research: Conceptual, design, measurement, and analysis issues. *Journal of Pain and Symptom Management*, *31*(1), 85–95. https://doi.org/10.1016/j.jpainsymman.2005.05.015

Bender, M. S., Janson, S. L., Franck, L. S., & Lee, K. A. (2008). Theory of Symptom Management. In M. J. Smith & P. R. Liehr (Eds.), *Middle Range Theory for Nursing* (4th Edition, pp. 145–158). Springer.

Brkovic, T., Burilovic, E., & Puljak, L. (2016). Prevalence and severity of pain in adult end-stage renal disease patients on chronic intermittent hemodialysis: a systematic review. *Patient Preference and Adherence*, *10*, 1131–1150. https://doi.org/10.2147/PPA.S103927

Broadbent, E., Petrie, K. J., Main, J., & Weinman, J. (2006). The Brief Illness Perception Questionnaire. *Journal of Psychosomatic Research*, *60*, 631–637. https://doi.org/10.1016/j.jpsychores.2005.10.020

Brooke, J., & Lusher, J. (2012). The components of the common sense model of self-regulation revisited: a systematic review and meta-analysis. In B. S. Savic, S. H. Touzery, K. S. Savic, & J. Zurc (Eds.), *5th International Scientific Conference Quality Health Care Treatment in the Framework of Education, Research and Multi Professional Collaboration - Towards the Health of Individuals and the Society: Proceedings of Lectures with Peer Review* (p. Vol. 5, pp. 91–99). College of Nursing Jesenice.

Cai, T., Huang, Y., Huang, Q., Xia, H., & Yuan, C. (2022). Symptom trajectories in patients with breast cancer: An integrative review. *International Journal of Nursing Sciences*, *9*, 120–128. https://doi.org/10.1016/j.ijnss.2021.12.011

Cella, M., & Chalder, T. (2010). Measuring fatigue in clinical and community settings. *Journal of Psychosomatic Research*, *69*, 17–22. https://doi.org/10.1016/j.jpsychores.2009.10.007

Chan, F. H. F., Goh, Z. Z. S., Zhu, X., Tudor Car, L., Newman, S., Khan, B. A., & Griva, K. (2022). Subjective cognitive complaints in end-stage renal disease: a systematic review and meta-analysis. *Health Psychology Review*.

Chan, F. H. F., Newman, S., Khan, B. A., & Griva, K. (2022). The role of subjective cognitive complaints in self-management among haemodialysis patients: a cross-sectional study. *BMC Nephrology*, *23*, 363. https://doi.org/10.1186/s12882-022-02994-2

Chan, F. H. F., Newman, S., Khan, B. A., & Griva, K. (2023). Prevalence and trajectories of subjective cognitive complaints and implications for patient outcomes: a prospective study of haemodialysis patients. *British Journal of Health Psychology*.

Chen, F., Leng, Y., Zhang, L., Xu, J., Zhang, D., Qin, Y., Li, J., & Zheng, Y. (2021). The Correlation of Symptom Clusters and Functional Performance in Adult Acute Leukemia Patients under Chemotherapy. *Cancer Nursing*, *44*(5), E287–E295. https://doi.org/10.1097/NCC.0000000000000816

Clark, S., Farrington, K., & Chilcot, J. (2014). Nonadherence in dialysis patients: Prevalence, measurement, outcome, and psychological determinants. *Seminars in Dialysis*, *27*(1), 42–49. https://doi.org/10.1111/sdi.12159

Cleeland, C. S. (2007). Symptom burden: multiple symptoms and their impact as patient-reported outcomes. *Journal of the National Cancer Institute. Monographs*, *77030*(37), 16–21. https://doi.org/10.1093/jncimonographs/lgm005

Cleeland, C. S., Zhao, F., Chang, V. T., Sloan, J. A., O'Mara, A. M., Gilman, P. B., Weiss, M., Mendoza, T. R., Lee, J. W., & Fisch, M. J. (2013). The symptom burden of cancer: Evidence for a core set of cancer-related and treatment-related symptoms from the Eastern Cooperative Oncology Group Symptom Outcomes and Practice Patterns study. *Cancer*, *119*(24), 4333–4340. https://doi.org/10.1002/cncr.28376

Cowen, R., Stasiowska, M. K., Laycock, H., & Bantel, C. (2015). Assessing pain objectively: The use of physiological markers. *Anaesthesia*, *70*, 828–847. https://doi.org/10.1111/anae.13018

Curtin, R. B., Bultman, D. C., Thomas-Hawkins, C., Walters, B. A. J., & Schatell, D. (2002). Hemodialysis patients' symptom experiences: effects on physical and mental functioning. *Nephrology Nursing Journal*, *29*(6), 562–574.

Davison, S. N., Koncicki, H., & Brennan, F. (2014). Pain in chronic kidney disease: A scoping review. *Seminars in Dialysis*, *27*(2), 188–204. https://doi.org/10.1111/sdi.12196

Dodd, M. J., Miaskowski, C., & Paul, S. M. (2001). Symptom Clusters and Their Effect on the Functional Status of Patients With Cancer. *Oncology Nursing Forum*, *28*(3), 465–470.

Faasse, K., & Petrie, K. J. (2013). The nocebo effect: Patient expectations and medication side effects. *Postgraduate Medical Journal*, *89*, 540–546. https://doi.org/10.1136/postgradmedj-2012-131730

Fan, G., Filipczak, L., & Chow, E. (2007). Symptom clusters in cancer patients: a review of the literature. *Current Oncology*, *14*(5), 173–179. https://doi.org/10.3747/co.2007.145

Feldman, P. J., Cohen, S., Doyle, W. J., Skoner, D. P., & Gwaltney, J. M. (1999). The impact of personality on the reporting of unfounded symptoms and illness. *Journal of Personality and Social Psychology*, *77*(2), 370–378. https://doi.org/10.1037/0022-3514.77.2.370

Fini, A., & de Cruz, D. A. L. M. da. (2009). Characteristics of fatigue in heart failure patients: a literature review. *Revista Latino-Americana de Enfermagem*, *17*(4), 557–565. https://doi.org/10.1590/s0104-11692009000400019

Fu, M. R., LeMone, P., & McDaniel, R. W. (2004). An integrated approach to an analysis of symptom management in patients with cancer. *Oncology Nursing Forum*, *31*(1), 65–70. https://doi.org/10.1188/04.ONF.65-70

Fu, M. R., McDaniel, R. W., & Rhodes, V. A. (2007). Measuring symptom occurrence and symptom distress: Development of the symptom experience index. *Journal of Advanced Nursing*, *59*(6), 623–634. https://doi.org/10.1111/j.1365-2648.2007.04335.x

Gapstur, R. L. (2007). Symptom burden: A concept analysis and implications for oncology nurses. *Oncology Nursing Forum*, *34*(3), 673–680. https://doi.org/10.1188/07.ONF.673-680

Goërtz, Y. M. J., Braamse, A. M. J., Spruit, M. A., Janssen, D. J. A., Ebadi, Z., Van Herck, M., Burtin, C., Peters, J. B., Sprangers, M. A. G., Lamers, F., Twisk, J. W. R., Thong, M. S. Y., Vercoulen, J. H., Geerlings, S. E., Vaes, A. W., Beijers, R. J. H. C. G., van Beers, M., Schols, A. M. W. J., Rosmalen, J. G. M., & Knoop, H. (2021). Fatigue in patients with chronic disease: results from the population-based Lifelines Cohort Study. *Scientific Reports*, *11*, 20977. https://doi.org/10.1038/s41598-021-00337-z

Goldberg, D. S., & McGee, S. J. (2011). Pain as a global public health priority. *BMC Public Health*, *11*, 770. https://doi.org/10.1186/1471-2458-11-770

Hagger, M. S., & Orbell, S. (2003). A meta-analytic review of the common-sense model of illness representations. *Psychology and Health*, *18*(2), 141–184. https://doi.org/10.1080/0887044031000081321

Han, Q., Zheng, B., Daines, L., & Sheikh, A. (2022). Long-Term Sequelae of COVID-19: A Systematic Review and Meta-Analysis of One-Year Follow-Up Studies on Post-COVID Symptoms. *Pathogens*, *11*, 269.

Hill, N. L., Bhargava, S., Brown, M. J., Kim, H., Bhang, I., Mullin, K., Phillips, K., & Mogle, J. (2021). Cognitive complaints in age-related chronic conditions: A systematic review. *PLoS ONE*, *16*(7), e0253795. https://doi.org/10.1371/journal.pone.0253795

Horne, R., & Weinman, J. (2002). Self-regulation and self-management in asthma: Exploring the role of illness perceptions and treatment beliefs in explaining non-adherence to preventer medication. *Psychology and Health*, *17*(1), 17–32. https://doi.org/10.1080/08870440290001502

Jacobsen, P. B., Andrykowski, M. A., & Thors, C. L. (2004). Relationship of Catastrophizing to Fatigue among Women Receiving Treatment for Breast Cancer. *Journal of Consulting and Clinical Psychology*, *72*(2), 355–361. https://doi.org/10.1037/0022-006X.72.2.355

Jhamb, M., Weisbord, S. D., Steel, J. L., & Unruh, M. (2008). Fatigue in Patients Receiving Maintenance Dialysis: A Review of Definitions, Measures, and Contributing Factors. *American Journal of Kidney Diseases*, *52*(2), 353–365. https://doi.org/10.1053/j.ajkd.2008.05.005

Kardas, P., Lewek, P., & Matyjaszczyk, M. (2013). Determinants of patient adherence: A review of systematic reviews. *Frontiers in Pharmacology*, *4*, 91. https://doi.org/10.3389/fphar.2013.00091

Keefe, F. J., & Block, A. R. (1982). Development of an observation method for assessing pain behavior in chronic low back pain patients. *Behavior Therapy*, *13*, 363–375. https://doi.org/10.1016/S0005-7894(82)80001-4

Khan, R. F., Feder, S., Goldstein, N. E., & Chaudhry, S. I. (2015). Symptom burden among patients who were hospitalized for heart failure. *JAMA Internal Medicine*, *175*(10), 1713–1715. https://doi.org/10.1001/jamainternmed.2015.3871

Kim, H.-J., Jung, S.-O., Kim, E., & Abraham, I. (2022). Association of chemotherapy and subjective cognitive impairment in breast cancer patients: Meta-analysis of longitudinal prospective cohort studies. *European Journal of Oncology Nursing*, *57*, 102099. https://doi.org/10.1016/j.ejon.2022.102099

Knopp-Sihota, J. A., MacGregor, T., Reeves, J. T. H., Kennedy, M., & Saleem, A. (2022). Management of Chronic Pain in Long-Term Care: A Systematic Review and Meta-Analysis. *Journal of the American Medical Directors Association*, *23*, 1507–1516. https://doi.org/10.1016/j.jamda.2022.04.008

Koleck, T. A., Topaz, M., Tatonetti, N. P., George, M., Miaskowski, C., Smaldone, A., & Bakken, S. (2021). Characterizing shared and distinct symptom clusters in common chronic conditions through natural language processing of nursing notes. *Research in Nursing and Health*, *44*(6), 906–919. https://doi.org/10.1002/nur.22190

Kwekkeboom, K. L., Wieben, A., Stevens, J., Tostrud, L., & Montgomery, K. (2020). Guideline-recommended symptom management strategies that cross over two or more cancer symptoms. *Oncology Nursing Forum*, *47*(5), 498–511. https://doi.org/10.1188/20.ONF.498-511

Langerud, A. K., Rustøen, T., Småstuen, M. C., Kongsgaard, U., & Stubhaug, A. (2018). Intensive care survivor-reported symptoms: a longitudinal study of survivors' symptoms. *Nursing in Critical Care*, *23*, 48–54. https://doi.org/10.1111/nicc.12330

Leventhal, H., Nerenz, D. R., & Steele, D. J. (1984). Illness Representations and Coping with Health Threats. In A. Baum, S. E. Taylor, & J. E. Singer (Eds.), *Handbook of Psychology and Health, Volume IV: Social Psychological Aspects of Health* (pp. 219–252). Erlbaum.

Leventhal, H., Phillips, L. A., & Burns, E. (2016). The Common-Sense Model of Self-Regulation (CSM): a dynamic framework for understanding illness self-management. *Journal of Behavioral Medicine*, *39*, 935–946. https://doi.org/10.1007/s10865-016-9782-2

Li, G. (2021). A Review of the Research on Symptom Clusters in Cancer Survivors. *Open Journal of Nursing*, *11*, 423–434. https://doi.org/10.4236/ojn.2021.116036

Ma, Y., He, B., Jiang, M., Yang, Y., Wang, C., Huang, C., & Han, L. (2020). Prevalence and risk factors of cancer-related fatigue: A systematic review and meta-analysis. *International Journal of Nursing Studies*, *111*, 103707. https://doi.org/10.1016/j.ijnurstu.2020.103707

May, M., Junghaenel, D. U., Ono, M., Stone, A. A., & Schneider, S. (2018). Ecological Momentary Assessment Methodology in Chronic Pain Research: A Systematic Review. *Journal of Pain*, *19*(7), 699–716. https://doi.org/10.1016/j.jpain.2018.01.006

McNeil, D. W., & Rainwater, A. J. (1998). Development of the Fear of Pain Questionnaire—III. *Journal of Behavioral Medicine*, *21*(4), 389–410.

Merckelbach, H., Dandachi-FitzGerald, B., van Helvoort, D., Jelicic, M., & Otgaar, H. (2019). When Patients Overreport Symptoms: More Than Just Malingering. *Current Directions in Psychological Science*, *28*(3), 321–326. https://doi.org/10.1177/0963721419837681

Metzger, M., Abdel-Rahman, E. M., Boykin, H., & Song, M. K. (2021). A Narrative Review of Management Strategies for Common Symptoms in Advanced CKD. *Kidney International Reports*, *6*, 894–904. https://doi.org/10.1016/j.ekir.2021.01.038

Moss-Morris, R., Weinman, J., Petrie, K., Horne, R., Cameron, L., & Buick, D. (2002). The revised Illness Perception Questionnaire (IPQ-R). *Psychology and Health*, *17*(1), 1–16. https://doi.org/10.1080/08870440290001494

Nestoriuc, Y., Pan, Y., Kinitz, T., Weik, E., & Shedden-Mora, M. C. (2021). Informing About the Nocebo Effect Affects Patients' Need for Information About Antidepressants—An Experimental Online Study. *Frontiers in Psychiatry*, *12*, 587122. https://doi.org/10.3389/fpsyt.2021.587122

Ng, H. J., Tan, W. J., Mooppil, N., Newman, S., & Griva, K. (2015). Prevalence and patterns of depression and anxiety in hemodialysis patients: A 12-month prospective study on incident and prevalent populations. *British Journal of Health Psychology*, *20*, 374–395. https://doi.org/10.1111/bjhp.12106

Pagé, M. G., Gauvin, L., Sylvestre, M. P., Nitulescu, R., Dyachenko, A., & Choinière, M. (2022). An Ecological Momentary Assessment Study of Pain Intensity Variability: Ascertaining Extent, Predictors, and Associations With Quality of Life, Interference and Health Care Utilization Among Individuals Living With Chronic Low Back Pain. *Journal of Pain*, *23*(7), 1151–1166. https://doi.org/10.1016/j.jpain.2022.01.001

Pan, Y., Kinitz, T., Stapic, M., & Nestoriuc, Y. (2019). Minimizing Drug Adverse Events by Informing About the Nocebo Effect—An Experimental Study. *Frontiers in Psychiatry*, *10*, 504. https://doi.org/10.3389/fpsyt.2019.00504

Petersen, S., van den Berg, R. A., Janssens, T., & Van den Bergh, O. (2011). Illness and symptom perception: A theoretical approach towards an integrative measurement model. *Clinical Psychology Review*, *31*, 428–439. https://doi.org/10.1016/j.cpr.2010.11.002

Prkachin, K. M., Hughes, E., Schultz, I., Joy, P., & Hunt, D. (2002). Real-time assessment of pain behavior during clinical assessment of low back pain patients. *Pain*, *95*, 23–30. https://doi.org/10.1016/S0304-3959(01)00369-4

Pullens, M. J. J., De Vries, J., & Roukema, J. A. (2010). Subjective cognitive dysfunction in breast cancer patients: A systematic review. *Psycho-Oncology*, *19*, 1127–1138. https://doi.org/10.1002/pon.1673

Raja, S. N., Carr, D. B., Cohen, M., Finnerup, N. B., Flor, H., Gibson, S., Keefe, F. J., Mogil, J. S., Ringkamp, M., Sluka, K. A., Song, X., Stevens, B., Sullivan, M. D., Tutelman, P. R., Ushida, T., & Vader, K. (2020). The revised International Association for the Study of Pain definition of pain: concepts, challenges, and compromises. *Pain*, *00*(00), 1–7. https://doi.org/10.1097/j.pain.0000000000001939

Reuben, D. B., Mor, V., & Hiris, J. (1988). Clinical symptoms and length of survival in patients with terminal cancer. *Archives of Internal Medicine*, *148*(7), 1586–1591.

Romadlon, D. S., Hasan, F., Wiratama, B. S., & Chiu, H. Y. (2022). Prevalence and risk factors of fatigue in type 1 and type 2 diabetes: A systematic review and meta-analysis. *Journal of Nursing Scholarship*, *54*, 546–553. https://doi.org/10.1111/jnu.12763

Ruiz-Rodríguez, I., Hombrados-Mendieta, I., Melguizo-Garín, A., & Martos-Méndez, M. J. (2022). The Importance of Social Support, Optimism and Resilience on the Quality of Life of Cancer Patients. *Frontiers in Psychology*, *13*, 833176. https://doi.org/10.3389/fpsyg.2022.833176

Sharpe, L., Thewes, B., & Butow, P. (2017). Current directions in research and treatment of fear of cancer recurrence. *Current Opinion in Supportive and Palliative Care*, *11*(3), 191–196. https://doi.org/10.1097/SPC.0000000000000288

SONG Initiative. (2017). *The SONG Handbook for establishing and implementing core outcomes in clinical trials across the spectrum of chronic kidney disease* (1st ed., Issue June). songinitiative.org/reports-and-publications/

Sudore, R. L., Karter, A. J., Huang, E. S., Moffet, H. H., Laiteerapong, N., Schenker, Y., Adams, A., Whitmer, R. A., Liu, J. Y., Miao, Y., John, P. M., & Schillinger, D. (2012). Symptom burden of adults with type 2 diabetes across the disease course: diabetes & aging study. *Journal of General Internal Medicine*, *27*(12), 1674–1681. https://doi.org/10.1007/s11606-012-2132-3

Sullivan, M. J. L., Bishop, S. R., & Pivik, J. (1995). The pain catastrophising scale: development and validation. *Psychological Assessment*, *7*(4), 524–532.

Todd, J., Sharpe, L., Colagiuri, B., & Khatibi, A. (2016). The effect of threat on cognitive biases and pain outcomes: An eye-tracking study. *European Journal of Pain*, *20*, 1357–1368. https://doi.org/10.1002/ejp.887

Trajkovic-Vidakovic, M., de Graeff, A., Voest, E. E., & Teunissen, S. C. C. M. (2012). Symptoms tell it all: A systematic review of the value of symptom assessment to predict survival in advanced cancer patients. *Critical Reviews in Oncology/Hematology*, *84*, 130–148. https://doi.org/10.1016/j.critrevonc.2012.02.011

Treede, R.-D., Rief, W., Barke, A., Aziz, Q., Bennett, M., Benoliel, R., Cohen, M., Evers, S., Finnerup, N., First, M., Giamberardino, M. A., Kaasa, S., Korwisi, B., Kosek, E., Lavand, P., Nicholas, M., Perrot, S., Scholz, J., Schug, S., … Wang, S.-J. (2019). Chronic pain as a symptom or a disease: the IASP Classification of Chronic Pain for the International Classification of Diseases (ICD-11). *Pain*, *160*(1), 19–27. https://doi.org/10.1097/j.pain.0000000000001390

van den Beuken-van Everdingen, M. H. J., de Rijke, J. M., Kessels, A. G., Schouten, H. C., van Kleef, M., & Patijn, J. (2007). Prevalence of pain in patients with cancer: A systematic review of the past 40 years. *Annals of Oncology*, *18*, 1437–1449. https://doi.org/10.1093/annonc/mdm056

van den Beuken-van Everdingen, M. H. J., Hochstenbach, L. M. J., Joosten, E. A. J., Tjan-Heijnen, V. C. G., & Janssen, D. J. A. (2016). Update on Prevalence of Pain in Patients with Cancer: Systematic Review and Meta-Analysis. *Journal of Pain and Symptom Management*, *51*(6), 1070–1090.e9. https://doi.org/10.1016/j.jpainsymman.2015.12.340

Vlaeyen, J. W. S., & Linton, S. J. (2000). Fear-avoidance and its consequences in chronic musculoskeletal pain: a state of the art. *Pain*, *85*, 317–332. papers3://publication/uuid/327BB4B4-2761-41DB-903F-9BA66D0042CF

Weiland, T. J., Jelinek, G. A., Marck, C. H., Hadgkiss, E. J., Van Der Meer, D. M., Pereira, N. G., & Taylor, K. L. (2015). Clinically significant fatigue: Prevalence and associated factors in an international sample of adults with multiple sclerosis recruited via the internet. *PLoS ONE*, *10*(2), e0115541. https://doi.org/10.1371/journal.pone.0115541

Weinman, J., Petrie, K. J., Moss-Morris, R., & Horne, R. (1996). The illness perception questionnaire: A new method for assessing the cognitive representation of illness. *Psychology and Health*, *11*, 431–445. https://doi.org/10.1080/08870449608400270

Weisbord, S. D., Fried, L. F., Arnold, R. M., Fine, M. J., Levenson, D. J., Peterson, R. A., & Switzer, G. E. (2005). Prevalence, severity, and importance of physical and emotional symptoms in chronic hemodialysis patients. *Journal of the American Society of Nephrology*, *16*(8), 2487–2494. https://doi.org/10.1681/ASN.2005020157

Wu, H. S., & Harden, J. K. (2015). Symptom Burden and quality of life in survivorship: A review of the literature. *Cancer Nursing*, *38*(1), E29–E54. https://doi.org/10.1097/NCC.0000000000000135

Zhang, K., Hannan, E., Scholes-Robertson, N., Baumgart, A., Guha, C., Kerklaan, J., Hanson, C. S., Craig, J. C., Davison, S. N., Hecking, M., & Tong, A. (2020). Patients' perspectives of pain in dialysis: systematic review and thematic synthesis of qualitative studies. *Pain*, *161*(9), 1983–1994. https://doi.org/10.1097/j.pain.0000000000001931

23

THE PSYCHOSOCIAL IMPACT OF CHRONIC DISEASE

Evangelos C. Karademas and Yael Benyamini

Introduction

Chronic diseases typically have a major impact on patients' lives and well-being despite the significant differences among diseases (e.g., regarding progression, severity of symptoms, medical treatment). Medical care and treatment have been continuously improving, resulting in better patient quality of life nowadays than in the past (e.g., Mokhtari-Hessari & Montazeri, 2020). Nevertheless, chronic conditions continue to cause a wide range of physical symptoms and difficulties and several functional limitations or impairments and often demand the extensive use of patient resources in order to adapt (de Ridder et al., 2008). Therefore, the possibility of a severe psychological health problem is significantly elevated in chronic patients in comparison to the general population. In this chapter, we will present an overview of the psychological impact of chronic illness.

The Psychological Impact of Chronic Illness

The impact of the stress and difficulties that accompany chronic illness is often manifested in the development of psychological symptoms, such as anxiety and depression. Of course, such symptoms are also present in the general population. As a measure of comparison, it is estimated that 8.4% of adults in the United States of America (USA) have suffered at least one major depressive episode (https://www.nimh.nih.gov/health/statistics/major-depression), and the prevalence of anxiety disorders in the United Kingdom (UK) general population is about 17% (https://commonslibrary.parliament.uk/research-briefings/sn06988/).

The prevalence of such symptoms is even higher among certain chronic patient populations. It should be noted, however, that the vast majority of existing studies focus on a single chronic medical condition. It is estimated that almost 25% of chronic patients (especially older patients and those with low socioeconomic

 DOI: 10.4324/9781003318026-28

status) have multimorbidity, that is, the co-existence of two or more chronic conditions (Barnett et al., 2012). Multimorbidity has been linked to increased risk of psychological health difficulties, even higher than in patients suffering from a single chronic illness (e.g., Castro-de-Araujo et al., 2022). Still, studies that focus on multimorbid patients' adaptation are rare.

Depression and Anxiety

Depression is common among people with chronic illness. Overall, patients with more severe symptoms or a poorer prognosis, patients with lower socioeconomic status, and women are more likely to report depression or anxiety (e.g., Guglielmo et al., 2018).

Thombs et al. (2006) reported that about 20% of patients with myocardial infarction may also be diagnosed with major depression up to one year after the event. Also, it is estimated that about 15% of cancer patients have suffered at least one major depression episode at some point after diagnosis (Mitchell et al., 2011). A Swedish cohort study with thousands of cancer patients showed that the possibility of a mental health problem (e.g., depression, anxiety) peaked during the first week after diagnosis (Hazards Ratio = 6.7; 95%CI 6.1–7.4), rapidly decreased thereafter but remained somewhat elevated even years after diagnosis (Hazards Ratio = 1.1; CI 1.1–1.2; Lu et al., 2016). This pattern was clear for all types of cancer but was stronger for those with poor prognosis. Blevins et al. (2020) found that the adults with type 2 diabetes are 20% to 120% more likely to report depressive symptoms compared to adults without diabetes.

Chronic patients often suffer from anxiety. The prevalence of an anxiety disorder is about 20% higher in persons with type 2 diabetes than in healthy controls (Azloubi et al., 2018). About 10%–25% of the people living with HIV/AIDS (Brandt et al., 2017) and 9%–11% of cancer patients seem to suffer from an anxiety disorder (Mitchell et al., 2011). Data from the US National Health Interview Survey showed that 22.5% of patients with rheumatoid arthritis report symptoms of anxiety (31.2% in patients with comorbid chronic pain; Guglielmo et al., 2018).

Although almost all studies show that the rate of anxiety and depression is higher among chronic patients than people without a chronic condition, the exact figures should be interpreted with caution, as they are highly dependent on the way that symptoms were assessed. For example, Thombs et al. (2006) found that when depressive symptoms were assessed with the Beck Depression Inventory, the prevalence of depression in cardiovascular patients was estimated at about 31%, but when the Hospital Anxiety and Depression Scale (HADS) was used, the prevalence was half.

Post-Traumatic Stress Symptoms (PTSS)

PTSS are also frequent after a severe illness diagnosis, particularly if it may be life-threatening, probably as a result of the intense stress (caused by events such as diagnosis or treatment side effects) in combination with a sense of low personal control over the situation. It is estimated that about 12%–13% of cardiac patients suffer from PTSS, although there is a huge heterogeneity in the estimates across studies as a result of the different measures used (Vilchinsky et al., 2017). Also, more than 30% of cancer patients may suffer from PTSS, from the time of diagnosis to several months later (e.g., Unseld et al., 2019).

Likewise, PTSS are very frequent in people living with HIV/AIDS. Ayano et al. (2020) reported a pooled prevalence of about 33% (25% when a diagnostic instrument was used instead of a screening one), while Tang et al. (2020) reported a pooled prevalence of 28%. Both studies highlighted the significant heterogeneity in the methods and the screening/diagnostic instruments used in the available studies.

Stigma

Many chronic patients feel stigmatized, and this feeling is greater in diseases that are more visible (e.g., when using a wheelchair), when patients are perceived to defy societal/moral norms (e.g., people living with HIV/AIDS), or to lack self-control (e.g., in obesity), or when the disease is perceived as transmittable (Pachankis et al., 2018). For example, several recent studies on cancer patients (e.g., Bédard et al., 2022; Fujisama et al., 2020) found that > 60% of them reported some type of stigma (e.g., self-blame, experiences related to care). Younger and low-income patients, as well as patients with breast, urinary, or gynecological cancer, reported more perceived stigma (Fujisama et al., 2020).

Stigma is also a major burden for many people living with HIV/AIDS. MacLean and Wetherall (2021) reviewed the studies conducted in South Africa and reported that 22%–43% reported a type of stigma, while 44%–88% reported the presence of at least one stigmatizing experience. Stigma is also a major problem for people with HIV/AIDS in other countries, like the USA (e.g., Babel et al., 2021).

Self and Identity in Chronic Disease

The psychological reactions to chronic diseases may reach far beyond the emotional symptoms described earlier. Bury (1982) described chronic disease as a disruptive event which brings people close to suffering and even the threat of death, shatters personal assumptions, affects relationships, and thus can profoundly affect one's biography and self-concept. Charmaz (1983) described the experience of loss of self among persons with chronic diseases, who often suffer from restricted lives, experience social isolation, and feel that they are discredited and that they burden others. These effects on self and identity may be further complicated when the disease involves high uncertainty (Nanton et al., 2016). Visible effects of the disease or treatment can further undermine self-perceptions (Versluis et al., 2022). Even in concealable diseases, internalized stigma can make it difficult to maintain a positive sense of self (O'Donnell & Habenicht, 2022).

The transition to patienthood can lead to a struggle to preserve one's self-worth and pre-illness identity (Nanton et al., 2016). Incorporating the illness into one's identity may be key to accepting the situation, affirming identity, and finding ways to thrive within the limitations involved (Bogart, 2015). The initial identity crisis can lead to despair, particularly if the bodily effects of the disease threaten one's career or relationships, yet over time, many patients find ways to resiliency (Miller et al., 2022). Some even turn the limitation into an opportunity for growth.

Trajectories of Change Over Time

Several studies have examined the ways that psychological symptoms progress over time. Despite the different methodologies employed and the time periods examined, most studies revealed a steady pattern of three to five classes of change over time (e.g., Deschênes et al., 2018; Helgeson et al., 2004; Peter et al., 2020). These classes typically include a rather stable good psychological response (i.e., very few symptoms), a chronically poor response (i.e., high distress levels across time), an initially poor but gradually improving response, and an initially good but deteriorating over time psychological response. Overall, more than 50% of the patients across diseases seem to respond well over time, whereas about 15%–20% seem to report a stably poor or deteriorating psychological response over time.

In addition, many patients experience a prolonged fear of illness recurrence. Fear of recurrence is the most common psychological concern for cancer survivors, which remains with many of them for years after the end of treatment and significantly impacts well-being, social relationships, and occupational life (Simard et al., 2013). Fear of illness progression and recurrence, as well as fear of dying, have also been reported by patients suffering from several other diseases, including cardiovascular diseases, diabetes, and autoimmune disorders (e.g., Sharpe et al., 2022).

The Impact of Psychological Response on the Progression of Illness

The co-existence of a chronic physical condition and severe psychological difficulty is not rare. The direction of their relationship, however, is less clear. Although, so far, we have examined the impact of a disease on psychological well-being, it is also likely for an existing psychological problem to cause physical problems and impact the progression of illness.

Fan et al. (2014), who prospectively examined in a meta-analytic study the role of depression as a predictor of subsequent mortality, found that the pooled hazard ratio of cardiovascular mortality in patients with major depression symptoms is 2.19 (95%CI 1.46–3.29). Krantz et al. (2022) reviewed evidence which suggests that post-traumatic stress disorder (PTSD) is a significant risk factor for the development of cardiovascular disease. There is also evidence that depression is not just a result of type 2 diabetes but rather that the two have reciprocal interactions such that each contributes to or complicates the other (Renn et al., 2011). Similarly, there is a strong bidirectional relationship between pain and depression (the "pain/depression dyad"; e.g., Khan et al., 2020).

There are multiple pathways which link medical diseases to psychological difficulties in a bidirectional way. Genetic, metabolic, immune, stress-related nervous and hormone activation, and environmental- and health behavior-related factors seem to be involved in this complicated process (Khan et al., 2020; Krantz et al., 2022).

The Impact of Illness on the Psychological Well-Being of the Patient's Family/Partner

Patients' partners and families are significantly affected by illness, as they, too, are faced with many challenges from the time of diagnosis and throughout the course of illness. Family members and partners have to deal with the impact of illness on patient functioning, and they often share patients' concerns and worries (e.g., Dobbie & Mellor, 2008). In addition, their daily life is disrupted, and they have to undertake new responsibilities, especially if they also act as the main caregiver of the patient; they are likely to face financial, social, and occupational strain as a result of caring for the patient; their relationships within the family change; and they may feel that their old life is lost (Adelman et al., 2014).

As a result, family members and partners may experience high levels of distress, depression, and anxiety, lower levels of quality of life, as well as physical symptoms and difficulties. The impact of disease on caregivers may be so severe that the total welfare costs for these persons (e.g., costs for medication) are significantly higher compared to non-caregiver controls (Løppenthin et al., 2017), and they even are a high-risk group for suicide (O'Dwyer et al., 2021).

In turn, the psychological distress and diminished quality of life experienced by family caregivers impact patient well-being. There is evidence that caregivers' psychological symptoms exacerbate patients' symptoms (and vice versa, in a continuous loop; Streck et al., 2020). Also, lower levels of partner well-being may contribute to the worsening of patient symptoms and illness progression (e.g., Randall et al., 2009). Hence, a disease exerts its impact on patients' psychological and physical health directly, as well as indirectly through its effects on their family members' well-being.

Positive Psychological Impact of Chronic Disease

Chronic disease often leads to significant physical and psychological distress and can shatter basic assumptions about oneself and the world, as described earlier. Nevertheless, the majority of patients show resilience and manage to employ positive coping strategies. Can the illness experience go even further and foster positive changes in life? Research provides ample evidence showing that alongside the struggle with the stress and distress brought about by the disease, many people also find benefits, new strengths, or a new view of their priorities and meaning in life.

The most extensive conceptualization of positive psychological impacts of traumatic events, chronic diseases included, has been proposed by Tedeschi and

Calhoun (1995). They subsumed many related constructs under the term post-traumatic growth (PTG), proposing that it spans five major domains: greater appreciation of life and reprioritization, stronger relationships with others, feelings of greater personal strength, recognition of new possibilities in life, and spiritual development. Qualitative research further supported the prevalence of these positive sequelae of chronic disease, with added emphasis on existential re-evaluation and a new awareness of the body, particularly in life-threatening diseases (Hefferon et al., 2009).

Much of this research has focused on cancer patients and cancer survivors. A scoping review of studies of patients with cancer in different body sites provided evidence of PTG, which mapped onto the five PTG domains (Menger et al., 2021). Under new possibilities, many studies identified health behavior changes. An integrative review provided evidence for PTG among women with breast cancer, manifested in a new perception of self, relatedness to others, a new life philosophy, and spiritual and religious growth. PTG was also studied in other chronic diseases, such as cardiac diseases (Lee et al., 2022), HIV/AIDS (Sawyer et al., 2010), and inflammatory bowel diseases (Hamama-Raz et al., 2020).

PTG does not necessarily occur as a result of a trauma, nor does it provide a remedy for distress. In fact, higher levels of growth are often found alongside higher levels of distress. For example, a meta-analysis reported a small but robust positive relationship between PTG and PTSD among cancer patients, which was stronger among those with advanced cancer (Marziliano et al., 2020). Among cardiac outpatients, several facets of PTG were found to be associated with PTSD (Magid et al., 2019). However, growth has often been shown to provide benefits to adaptation to disease by moderating its negative effects. For example, PTG moderated the effect of post-traumatic stress on quality of life in adults with life-threatening disease (Martz et al., 2018).

Moderators of the Psychological Impact of Chronic Illness

Multiple factors have been found to moderate the impact of illness on patients' psychological well-being. These include a range of broad (e.g., the socioeconomic status), interpersonal, and personal factors. Although the impact of these factors is exerted through their constant interactions with each other and within the broader personal, social, and illness context, a full description of this process lies beyond the scope of this chapter. Here, we will refer to several main moderators, some of which facilitate adaptation to illness and prevent the development of severe psychological difficulties, whereas others expose patients to greater risk for mental health problems.

Broader Context Factors

Lower *socioeconomic status* is strongly linked to worse health, higher levels of stress, fewer resources to effectively cope with it, and higher levels of psychological burden (Gallo & Matthews, 2003). Low education and poverty create a disadvantageous context for patients, giving rise to feelings of helplessness/hopelessness and depression (Revenson & Hoyt, 2016). Psychological adjustment to chronic illness is also harder for *minorities*, as they are likely to experience discrimination and exclusion. These difficulties are further exacerbated in certain *racial/ethnic* groups (e.g., African American and Latina patients), possibly as a result of their coping behaviors (e.g., less use of approach coping) or their mistrust toward the health-care system (Helgeson & Zajdel, 2017; Stanton et al., 2007).

With respect to *gender*, female patients are likely to report more psychological symptoms than males (e.g., Hagedoorn et al., 2008). This may be the result of the commonly documented gender differences in the rates of reported negative emotions (which are more prevalent among women) but also of the differences between males and females as far as gender roles and stereotypes are concerned. For example, both women and men may experience negative emotions following a negative diagnosis; the source of these reactions may, however, greatly differ by gender. Men may find the disease more disruptive to their identity if they are unable to provide for their families and find themselves dependent on others, while women may find it more difficult to continue to carry out family responsibilities (e.g., Emslie, 2005).

Patient-Related Factors

Patient *personality* (e.g., trait conscientiousness and neuroticism) seems to impact adaptation to illness and psychological well-being (e.g., Rassart et al., 2015). Also, dispositional *optimism* and *self-efficacy* beliefs have consistently been negatively related to anxiety, depression, and other psychological difficulties across a variety of diagnoses (e.g., Chirico et al., 2017; Rasmussen et al., 2006).

Equally important is the role of *social support* as a major protective factor for well-being. For example, it has been related to less anxiety and depression symptoms (Gonzalez-Saenz de Tejada et al., 2017), higher levels of PTG in cancer patients (Ma et al., 2022), and better mood in type 2 diabetes (Helgeson et al., 2016).

Factors Related to the Patient/Illness Interaction

Two of the most important factors concerning patient/illness interaction are illness perceptions and coping with illness. *Illness perceptions* or *representations* refer to the ways that patients (or partners, caregivers, etc.) understand and mentally represent an illness. One of the most well-known relevant theories is the Common Sense Model (CSM; Leventhal et al., 1980). According to this model, illness representations are clustered into cognitive (i.e., representations about the identity, cause, consequences, controllability, and timeline of illness) as well as emotional themes. Representations are a significant predictor of patient psychological health. Consequences, emotional representations, and identity are typically associated with poorer psychological well-being, whereas a sense of control over the situation is associated with better outcomes (Hagger et al., 2017).

Coping with illness refers to the cognitive, emotional, behavioral, and interpersonal efforts of the patient to deal with illness, its impact, treatment, and demands so as to regain as meaningful/controllable and as happy a life as possible. Several coping behaviors have been related to patient adjustment. Avoidance has been linked to reports of poorer psychological health across several diseases (e.g., Livneh, 2019), whereas approach coping behaviors (e.g., problem-solving) have been associated with better mood and lower levels of anxiety and depression (e.g., Roesch et al., 2005).

Theories of Psychological Adaptation to Disease

Several theories have tried to capture the ways that illness impacts patients' psychological well-being. One of the first relevant theories (Moos & Schaefer, 1984) emphasized the adaptive tasks that patients have to accomplish when confronted with an illness. Managing symptoms and developing functional relationships with health professionals, as well as preserving a sense of control over the situation, good social relationships, and a positive self-image are some of the tasks that patients need to fulfill. Patients perceive each task in diverse ways depending on personal and illness-related factors. The theory of cognitive adaptation to illness (Taylor, 1983) puts a similar emphasis on tasks. According to this theory, a severe event may disrupt a patient's sense of control and impact core beliefs (e.g., the belief in a just world). To adapt to the new reality, the person has to perform certain tasks – namely, to search for meaning in their experience, restore a sense of mastery, and promote self-esteem. Failure to fulfill these tasks may lead to significant psychological difficulties.

Most of the theories underscore the role of cognitive evaluations and coping. Lazarus and Folkman's (1984) transactional theory of stress underlines the importance of personal cognitive appraisals and coping strategies. The cognitive evaluations of the situation (e.g., what are the available resources) determine the problem- and/or emotion-focused coping strategies that the person will employ to deal with the condition. Choosing situation-fitting strategies may ensure better psychological adaptation (Finkelstein-Fox & Park, 2019).

Leventhal's CSM (Leventhal et al., 1980) is probably the most widely used theoretical model to describe adaptation to illness. As described earlier, according to the CSM, patients develop cognitive and emotional representations of the illness and each potential treatment option. Representations are guided by the activation of illness prototypes which incorporate personal experience, knowledge, and beliefs about the disease. Based on their representations, patients develop action plans and behave in specific ways so as to manage symptoms and regulate emotions. These, in turn, affect their physical and psychological well-being.

A new overarching theory which builds on the CSM has recently been proposed by Carroll et al. (2022). The transdiagnostic theoretical model of adjustment to long-term physical conditions highlights the factors that generate distress in chronic illness. It posits that illness disrupts personal equilibrium. In order for patients to regain their balance and achieve good adjustment, they have to develop accurate representations of illness and symptoms, establish responses that are appropriate to the situation, and be able to assess and adapt their coping mechanisms. Several generic (e.g., inter- and intra-personal, and environmental factors, like personality, socioeconomic status, cognitive bias, general self-efficacy, social support) and illness-specific variables (e.g., ongoing illness stressors, illness perceptions, health behaviors) affect the entire process. According to the model, considering these factors in assessment and intervention is key for facilitating patients' adaptation.

Still, psychological adaptation to illness is not only a matter of self-regulation of the patient but also of the ways in which close persons (e.g., partners) affect the situation. Thus, dyadic regulation/coping theories, like the Developmental Contextual Model, are also important for understanding and predicting the psychological impact of illness (Falconier & Kuhn, 2019; Weitkamp et al., 2021).

Psychosocial Interventions to Mitigate the Psychological Impact of Chronic Disease

The extensive knowledge of interventions to improve individuals' mental health and well-being serves as a basis for interventions tailored to patients with chronic diseases. Interventions for this population are covered in detail in Chapter 27 of this volume, so here we only note the important characteristics of interventions aimed at mitigating the negative psychosocial impact of chronic disease:

- *The aims of the intervention* – is it only to improve psychological health, or is it aimed at improving disease prognosis? While positive psychological assets have been linked to physical health, lasting changes may require lifestyle changes (Park et al., 2016). However, it is important to remember that improving psychological health and quality of life are worthwhile aims in themselves.
- *Targeted constructs and pathways* – different interventions targeted constructs such as resilience (Kim et al., 2019), self-efficacy (Merluzzi et al., 2019), or patient activation (Lin et al., 2020).
- *Means and techniques* – many novel interventions in this area draw from positive psychology (Brown et al., 2019) and, in general, from a holistic view of human beings by using arts or music (Köhler et al., 2020) and physical activity (Beland et al., 2020), and by administering interventions using digital technology (Sassevile et al., 2021; White et al., 2022).
- *Generic versus disease-specific, age-specific, etc.* – not every intervention fits the needs of all patients with any disease. There is more knowledge about interventions to reduce depression and anxiety in patients with cancer or cardiac disease than there is on other diseases or outcomes.
- *Level of intervention* – most interventions have focused on the individual level, with less attention to interventions at the level of the family (Gilliss et al., 2019), the health-care system, or society (particularly as related to reducing stigma; Relf et al., 2021).

In general, despite the amount of research testing specific interventions, much work is still needed on systematic reporting and evaluation of such interventions, in view of theories and while taking into account the perspectives of various stakeholders, in order to facilitate wide dissemination (Liu et al., 2019).

Conclusion

Chronic physical conditions are a major source of distress for patients and their families and may significantly impair their quality of life, probably no less than the physical symptoms and limitations. Consequently, the possibility of temporary or even long-term psychological disorders is high in chronic patients, and their effects should not be overlooked. Yet, growth alongside coping with chronic disease is also prevalent. Although growth does not in itself counter the negative psychological impact of the disease, over time, it may mitigate its effect on quality of life and may provide a different pathway for positive coping. Several theories and many studies have attempted to describe the critical factors that may increase or decrease the risk of psychological difficulties in this population. This is certainly an evolving effort. There are also many effective interventions, but more research is needed on the critical elements of these interventions and the best ways to adapt them to individuals and diseases.

Further Reading

Bonino, S. (2021). *Coping with chronic illness theories, issues and lived experiences*. Routledge.

Guillemin, F., Leplege, A., Briancon, S., Spitz, E., & Coste, J. (2018). *Perceived health and adaptation in chronic disease*. Routledge.

Marini, I., Fleming, A., & Bishop, M. (2023). *The psychological and social impact of chronic illness and disability* (8th ed.) Springer.

References

Adelman, R.D., Tmanova, L.L., Delgado, D., Dion, S., & Lachs, M.S. (2014). Caregiver burden: a clinical review. *JAMA*, *311*(10), 1052–1060. https://doi.org/10.1001/jama.2014.304

Alzoubi, A., Abunaser, R., Khassawneh, A., Alfaqih, M., Khasawneh, A., & Abdo, N. (2018). The bidirectional relationship between diabetes and depression: a literature review. *Korean Journal of Family Medicine*, *39*(3), 137–146. https://doi.org/10.4082/kjfm.2018.39.3.137

Ayano, G., Duko, B., & Bedaso, A. (2020). The prevalence of post-traumatic stress disorder among people living with HIV/AIDS: a systematic review and meta-analysis. *The Psychiatric Quarterly*, *91*(4), 1317–1332. https://doi.org/10.1007/s11126-020-09849-9

Babel, R.A., Wang, P., Alessi, E.J., Raymond, H.F., & Wei, C. (2021). Stigma, HIV risk, and access to HIV prevention and treatment services among men who have sex with men in the United States: a scoping review. *AIDS and Behavior*, *25*(11), 3574–3604. https://doi.org/10.1007/s10461-021-03262-4

Barnett, K., Mercer, S. W., Norbury, M., Watt, G., Wyke, S., & Guthrie, B. (2012). Epidemiology of multimorbidity and implications for health care, research, and medical education: a cross-sectional study. *The Lancet*, *380*(9836), 37–43. https://doi.org/10.1016/S0140-6736(12)60240-2

Bédard, S., Sasewich, H., Culling, J., Turner, S. R., Pellizzari, J., Johnson, S., & Bédard, E.L.R. (2022). Stigma in early-stage lung cancer. *Annals of Behavioral Medicine*, *56*(12), 1272–1283. https://doi.org/10.1093/abm/kaac021

Béland, M., Lavoie, K.L., Briand, S., White, U.J., Gemme, C., & Bacon, S.L. (2020). Aerobic exercise alleviates depressive symptoms in patients with a major non-communicable chronic disease: a systematic review and meta-analysis. *British Journal of Sports Medicine*, *54*(5), 272–278. https://doi.org/10.1136/bjsports-2018-099360

Blevins, L., Gonzalez, J.S., & Wagner, J. (2020). Depression and anxiety in adults with diabetes. In A.M. Delamater & D.G. Marrero (Eds.), *Behavioral diabetes. Social ecological perspectives for pediatric and adult populations* (pp. 329–352). Springer.

Bogart, K.R. (2015). Disability identity predicts lower anxiety and depression in multiple sclerosis. *Rehabilitation Psychology*, *60*, 105–109. https://doi.org/10.1037/rep0000029

Brandt, C., Zvolensky, M.J., Woods, S.P., Gonzalez, A., Safren, S.A., & 'Cleirigh, C.M. (2017). Anxiety symptoms and disorders among adults living with HIV and AIDS: a critical review and integrative synthesis of the empirical literature. *Clinical Psychology Review*, *51*, 164–184. https://doi.org/10.1016/j.cpr.2016.11.005

Brown, L., Ospina, J.P., Celano, C.M., & Huffman, J.C. (2019). The effects of positive psychological interventions on medical patients' anxiety: a meta-analysis. *Psychosomatic Medicine*, *81*(7), 595–602. https://doi.org/10.1097/psy.0000000000000722

Bury, M. (1982), Chronic illness as biographical disruption. *Sociology of Health & Illness*, *4*, 167–182. https://doi.org/10.1111/1467-9566.ep11339939

Carroll, S., Moon, Z., Hudson, J., Hulme, K., & Moss-Morris, R. (2022). An evidence-based theory of psychological adjustment to long-term physical health conditions: Applications in clinical practice. *Psychosomatic Medicine*, *84*(5), 547–559. https://doi.org/10.1097/PSY.0000000000001076

Castro-de-Araujo, L., Cortes, F., de Siqueira Filha, N. T., Rodrigues, E., Machado, D.B., de Araujo, J., Lewis, G., Denaxas, S., & Barreto, M.L. (2022). Patterns of multimorbidity and some psychiatric disorders: a systematic review of the literature. *Frontiers in Psychology*, *13*, 940978. https://doi.org/10.3389/fpsyg.2022.940978

Charmaz, K. (1983). Loss of self: a fundamental form of suffering in the chronically ill. *Sociology of Health & Illness*, *5*(2), 168–195. https://doi.org/10.1111/1467-9566.ep10491512

Chirico, A., Lucidi, F., Merluzzi, T., Alivernini, F., De Laurentiis, M., Botti, G., & Giordano, A., (2017). A meta-analytic review of the relationship of cancer coping self-efficacy with distress and quality of life. *Oncotarget*, 8, 36800–36811. https://doi.org/10.18632/oncotarget.15758

Deschênes, S.S., Burns, R.J., & Schmitz, N. (2018). Trajectories of anxiety symptoms and associations with incident cardiovascular disease in adults with type 2 diabetes. *Journal of Psychosomatic Research*, *104*, 95–100. https://doi.org/10.1016/j.jpsychores.2017.11.015

de Ridder, D., Geenen, R., Kuijer, R., & van Middendorp, H. (2008). Psychological adjustment to chronic disease. *Lancet*, *372*(9634), 246–255. https://doi.org/10.1016/S0140-6736(08)61078-8

Dobbie, M., & Mellor, D. (2008). Chronic illness and its impact: considerations for psychologists. *Psychology, Health & Medicine*, *13*(5), 583–590. https://doi.org/10.1080/13548500801983041

Emslie C. (2005). Women, men and coronary heart disease: a review of the qualitative literature. *Journal of Advanced Nursing*, *51*(4), 382–395. https://doi.org/10.1111/j.1365-2648.2005.03509.x

Falconier, M.K., & Kuhn, R. (2019). Dyadic coping in couples: A conceptual integration and a review of the empirical literature. *Frontiers in Psychology*, *10*, 571. https://doi.org/10.3389/fpsyg.2019.00571

Fan, H., Yu, W., Zhang, Q., Cao, H., Li, J., Wang, J., Shao, Y., & Hu, X. (2014). Depression after heart failure and risk of cardiovascular and all-cause mortality: a meta-analysis. *Preventive Medicine*, *63*, 36–42. https://doi.org/10.1016/j.ypmed.2014.03.007

Finkelstein-Fox, L., & Park, C.L. (2019). Control-coping goodness-of-fit and chronic illness: a systematic review of the literature. *Health Psychology Review*, *13*(2), 137–162. https://doi.org/10.1080/17437199.2018.1560229

Fujisawa, D., Umezawa, S., Fujimori, M., & Miyashita, M. (2020). Prevalence and associated factors of perceived cancer-related stigma in Japanese cancer survivors. *Japanese Journal of Clinical Oncology*, *50*(11), 1325–1329. https://doi.org/10.1093/jjco/hyaa135

Gallo, L.C., & Matthews, K.A. (2003). Understanding the association between socioeconomic status and physical health: do negative emotions play a role? *Psychological Bulletin*, *129*(1), 10–51. https://doi.org/10.1037/0033-2909.129.1.10

Gilliss, C.L., Pan, W., & Davis, L.L. (2019). Family involvement in adult chronic disease care: reviewing the systematic reviews. *Journal of Family Nursing*, *25*(1), 3–27. https://doi.org/10.1177/1074840718822365

Gonzalez-Saenz de Tejada, M., Bilbao, A., Baré, M., Briones, E., Sarasqueta, C., Quintana, J.M., Escobar, A., & CARESS-CCR Group (2017). Association between social support, functional status, and change in health-related quality of life and changes in anxiety and depression in colorectal cancer patients. *Psycho-oncology*, *26*(9), 1263–1269. https://doi.org/10.1002/pon.4303

Guglielmo, D., Hootman, J.M., Boring, M.A., Murphy, L.B., Theis, K.A., Croft, J.B., Barbour, K.E., Katz, P.P., & Helmick, C.G. (2018). Symptoms of anxiety and depression among adults with arthritis – United States, 2015-2017. MMWR. *Morbidity and Mortality Weekly Report*, *67*(39), 1081–1087. https://doi.org/10.15585/mmwr.mm6739a2

Hagedoorn, M., Sanderman, R., Bolks, H. N., Tuinstra, J., & Coyne, J.C. (2008). Distress in couples coping with cancer: A meta-analysis and critical review of role and gender effects. *Psychological Bulletin*, *134*(1), 1–30. https://doi.org/10.1037/0033-2909.134.1.1

Hagger, M. S., Koch, S., Chatzisarantis, N.L.D., & Orbell, S. (2017). The common-sense model of self-regulation: Meta-analysis and test of a process model. *Psychological Bulletin*, *143*, 1117–1154. doi: 10.1037/bul0000118

Hamama-Raz, Y., Nativ, S., & Hamama, L. (2020). Post-traumatic growth in inflammatory bowel disease patients: The role of illness cognitions and physical quality of life. *Journal of Crohn's and Colitis*, *15*(6), 1060–1067. https://doi.org/10.1093/ecco-jcc/jjaa247

Hefferon, K., Grealy, M., & Mutrie, N. (2009). Post-traumatic growth and life threatening physical illness: A systematic review of the qualitative literature. *British Journal of Health Psychology*, *14*(2), 343–378. https://doi.org/10.1348/135910708X332936

Helgeson, V.S., & Zajdel, M. (2017). Adjusting to Chronic Health Conditions. *Annual Review of Psychology*, *68*, 545–571. https://doi.org/10.1146/annurev-psych-010416-044014

Helgeson, V.S., Mascatelli, K., Seltman, H., Korytkowski, M., & Hausmann, L.R. (2016). Implications of supportive and unsupportive behavior for couples with newly diagnosed diabetes. *Health Psychology*, *35*(10), 1047–1058. https://doi.org/10.1037/hea0000388

Helgeson, V.S., Snyder, P., & Seltman, H. (2004). Psychological and physical adjustment to breast cancer over 4 years: identifying distinct trajectories of change. *Health Psychology*, 23(1), 3–15. https://doi.org/10.1037/0278-6133.23.1.3

Khan, W.U., Michelini, G., & Battaglia, M. (2020). Twin studies of the covariation of pain with depression and anxiety: A systematic review and re-evaluation of critical needs. *Neuroscience and Biobehavioral Reviews*, *111*, 135–148. https://doi.org/10.1016/j.neubiorev.2020.01.015

Kim, G.M., Lim, J.Y., Kim, E.J., & Park, S.-M. (2019). Resilience of patients with chronic diseases: a systematic review. *Health & Social Care in the Community*, *27*(4), 797-807. https://doi.org/10.1111/hsc.12620

Köhler, F., Martin, Z.-S., Hertrampf, R.-S., Gäbel, C., Kessler, J., Ditzen, B., & Warth, M. (2020). Music therapy in the psychosocial treatment of adult cancer patients: a systematic review and meta-analysis [Systematic Review]. *Frontiers in Psychology*, *11*. https://doi.org/10.3389/fpsyg.2020.00651

Krantz, D.S., Shank, L.M., & Goodie, J.L. (2022). Post-traumatic stress disorder (PTSD) as a systemic disorder: PATHWAYS to cardiovascular disease. *Health Psychology*, *41*(10), 651–662. https://doi.org/10.1037/hea0001127

Lazarus, R.S., & Folkman, S. (1984). *Stress, appraisal, and coping*. Springer.

Lee, S.Y., Park, C.L., & Laflash, S. (2022). Perceived posttraumatic growth in cardiac patients: a systematic scoping review. *Journal of Traumatic Stress*, *35*(3), 791–803. https://doi.org/10.1002/jts.22799

Leventhal, H., Meyer, D., & Nerenz, D.R. (1980). The common sense representation of illness danger. In S. Rachman (Ed.), *Contributions to medical psychology* (vol. 2, pp. 17–30). Pargamon.

Lin, M.-Y., Weng, W.-S., Apriliyasary, R.W., van Truong, P., & Tsai, P.-S. (2020). Effects of patient activation intervention on chronic diseases: a meta-analysis. *Journal of Nursing Research*, *28*(5), e116. https://doi.org/10.1097/jnr.0000000000000387

Liu, H., Mohammed, A., Shanthosh, J., News, M., Laba, T.-L., Hackett, M. L., Peiris, D., & Jan, S. (2019). Process evaluations of primary care interventions addressing chronic disease: a systematic review. *BMJ Open*, *9*(8), e025127. https://doi.org/10.1136/bmjopen-2018-025127

Livneh H. (2019). The use of generic avoidant coping scales for psychosocial adaptation to chronic illness and disability: a systematic review. *Health Psychology Open*, *6*(2), 2055102919891396. https://doi.org/10.1177/2055102919891396

Løppenthin, K., Esbensen, B.A., Østergaard, M., Ibsen, R., Kjellberg, J., & Jennum, P. (2017). Welfare costs in patients with rheumatoid arthritis and their partners compared with matched controls: a register-based study. *Clinical Rheumatology*, *36*(3), 517–525. https://doi.org/10.1007/s10067-016-3446-z

Lu, D., Andersson, T.M., Fall, K., Hultman, C.M., Czene, K., Valdimarsdóttir, U., & Fang, F. (2016). Clinical diagnosis of mental disorders immediately before and after cancer diagnosis: a nationwide matched cohort study in Sweden. *JAMA Oncology*, *2*(9), 1188–1196. https://doi.org/10.1001/jamaoncol.2016.0483

Ma, X., Wan, X., & Chen, C. (2022). The correlation between posttraumatic growth and social support in people with breast cancer: A meta-analysis. *Frontiers in Psychology*, *13*, 1060150. https://doi.org/10.3389/fpsyg.2022.1060150

MacLean, J.R., & Wetherall, K. (2021). The association between HIV-stigma and depressive symptoms among people living with HIV/AIDS: A systematic review of studies conducted in South Africa. *Journal of Affective Disorders*, *287*, 125–137. https://doi.org/10.1016/j.jad.2021.03.027

Magid, K., El-Gabalawy, R., Maran, A., & Serber, E.R. (2019). An examination of the association between post-traumatic growth and stress symptomatology in cardiac outpatients. *Journal of Clinical Psychology in Medical Settings*, *26*(3), 271–281. https://doi.org/10.1007/s10880-018-9585-4

Martz, E., Livneh, H., Southwick, S.M., & Pietrzak, R.H. (2018). Posttraumatic growth moderates the effect of posttraumatic stress on quality of life in U.S. military veterans with life-threatening illness or injury. *Journal of Psychosomatic Research*, *109*, 1–8. https://doi.org/10.1016/j.jpsychores.2018.03.004

Marziliano, A., Tuman, M., & Moyer, A. (2020). The relationship between post-traumatic stress and post-traumatic growth in cancer patients and survivors: a systematic review and meta-analysis. *Psycho-oncology*, *29*(4), 604–616. https://doi.org/10.1002/pon.5314

Menger, F., Mohammed Halim, N.A., Rimmer, B., & Sharp, L. (2021). Post-traumatic growth after cancer: a scoping review of qualitative research. *Supportive Care in Cancer*, *29*(11), 7013–7027. https://doi.org/10.1007/s00520-021-06253-2

Merluzzi, T.V., Pustejovsky, J.E., Philip, E.J., Sohl, S.J., Berendsen, M., & Salsman, J.M. (2019). Interventions to enhance self-efficacy in cancer patients: A meta-analysis of randomized controlled trials. *Psychooncology*, *28*(9), 1781–1790. https://doi.org/10.1002/pon.5148

Miller, V.J., Nahar, S., Praetorius, R., & Rivedal, J. (2022). The art of living with chronic health conditions. *Illness, Crisis & Loss*, *30*(1), 51–67. https://doi.org/10.1177/1054137319857088
Mitchell, A.J., Chan, M., Bhatti, H., Halton, M., Grassi, L., Johansen, C., & Meader, N. (2011). Prevalence of depression, anxiety, and adjustment disorder in oncological, haematological, and palliative-care settings: a meta-analysis of 94 interview-based studies. *The Lancet. Oncology*, *12*(2), 160–174. https://doi.org/10.1016/S1470-2045(11)70002-X
Mokhtari-Hessari, P., & Montazeri, A. (2020). Health-related quality of life in breast cancer patients: review of reviews from 2008 to 2018. *Health and Quality of Life Outcomes*, *18*(1), 338. https://doi.org/10.1186/s12955-020-01591-x
Moos, J.H., & Schaefer, J.A. (1984). The crisis of physical illness: An overview and conceptual approach. In R.H. Moos (Ed.), *Coping with physical illness: New perspectives* (pp. 3–25). Plenum.
Nanton, V., Munday, D., Dale, J., Mason, B., Kendall, M., & Murray, S. (2016). The threatened self: Considerations of time, place, and uncertainty in advanced illness. *British Journal of Health Psychology*, *21*(2), 351–373. https://doi.org/10.1111/bjhp.12172
O'Donnell, A.T., & Habenicht, A.E. (2022). Stigma is associated with illness self-concept in individuals with concealable chronic illnesses. *British Journal of Health Psychology*, *27*(1), 136–158. https://doi.org/10.1111/bjhp.12534
O'Dwyer, S.T., Janssens, A., Sansom, A., Biddle, L., Mars, B., Slater, T., Moran, P., Stallard, P., Melluish, J., Reakes, L., Walker, A., Andrewartha, C., & Hastings, R.P. (2021). Suicidality in family caregivers of people with long-term illnesses and disabilities: a scoping review. *Comprehensive Psychiatry*, *110*, 152261. https://doi.org/10.1016/j.comppsych.2021.152261
Pachankis, J.E., Hatzenbuehler, M.L., Wang, K., Burton, C.L., Crawford, F.W., Phelan, J.C., & Link, B.G. (2018). The burden of stigma on health and well-being: A taxonomy of concealment, course, disruptiveness, aesthetics, origin, and peril across 93 stigmas. *Personality & Social Psychology Bulletin*, *44*(4), 451–474. https://doi.org/10.1177/0146167217741313
Park, N., Peterson, C., Szvarca, D., Vander Molen, R.J., Kim, E.S., & Collon, K. (2016). Positive psychology and physical health: research and applications. *American Journal of Lifestyle Medicine*, *10*(3), 200–206. https://doi.org/10.1177/1559827614550277
Peter, R.S., Meyer, M.L., Mons, U., Schöttker, B., Keller, F., Schmucker, R., Koenig, W., Brenner, H., & Rothenbacher, D. (2020). Long-term trajectories of anxiety and depression in patients with stable coronary heart disease and risk of subsequent cardiovascular events. *Depression and Anxiety*, *37*(8), 784–792. https://doi.org/10.1002/da.23011
Randall, G., Molloy, G.J., & Steptoe, A. (2009). The impact of an acute cardiac event on the partners of patients: A systematic review. *Health Psychology Review*, *3*(1), 1–84. https://doi.org/10.1080/17437190902984919
Rasmussen, H.N., Wrosch, C., Scheier, M.F., & Carver, C.S. (2006). Self-regulation processes and health: the importance of optimism and goal adjustment. *Journal of Personality*, *74*(6), 1721–1747. https://doi.org/10.1111/j.1467-6494.2006.00426.x
Rassart, J., Luyckx, K., Berg, C.A., Bijttebier, P., Moons, P., & Weets, I. (2015). Psychosocial functioning and glycemic control in emerging adults with Type 1 diabetes: A 5-year follow-up study. *Health Psychology*, *34*(11), 1058–1065. https://doi.org/10.1037/hea0000212
Relf, M.V., Holzemer, W., Holt, L., Nyblade, L., & Ellis Caiola, C. (2021). A review of the state of the science of HIV and stigma: context, conceptualization, measurement, interventions, gaps, and future priorities. *Journal of the Association of Nurses in AIDS Care*, *32*(3), 392–407. https://doi.org/10.1097/jnc.0000000000000237
Renn, B.N., Feliciano, L., & Segal, D.L. (2011). The bidirectional relationship of depression and diabetes: a systematic review. *Clinical Psychology Review*, *31*(8), 1239–1246. https://doi.org/10.1016/j.cpr.2011.08.001

Revenson, T.A., & Hoyt, M.A. (2016). Chronic illness and mental health. In H.S. Friedman (Ed.), *Encyclopedia of mental health* (2nd Ed; pp. 284–292). Academic Press. https://doi.org/10.1016/B978-0-12-397045-9.00151-8

Roesch, S. C., Adams, L., Hines, A., Palmores, A., Vyas, P., Tran, C., Pekin, S., & Vaughn, A. A. (2005). Coping with prostate cancer: a meta-analytic review. *Journal of Behavioral Medicine*, *28*(3), 281–293. https://doi.org/10.1007/s10865-005-4664-z

Sasseville, M., LeBlanc, A., Boucher, M., Dugas, M., Mbemba, G., Tchuente, J., Chouinard, M.-C., Beaulieu, M., Beaudet, N., Skidmore, B., Cholette, P., Aspiros, C., Larouche, A., Chabot, G., & Gagnon, M.-P. (2021). Digital health interventions for the management of mental health in people with chronic diseases: a rapid review. *BMJ Open*, *11*(4), e044437. https://doi.org/10.1136/bmjopen-2020-044437

Sawyer, A., Ayers, S., & Field, A.P. (2010). Posttraumatic growth and adjustment among individuals with cancer or HIV/AIDS: a meta-analysis. *Clinical Psychology Review*, *30*(4), 436–447. https://doi.org/10.1016/j.cpr.2010.02.004

Sharpe, L., Michalowski, M., Richmond, B., Menzies, R.E., & Shaw, J. (2022). Fear of progression in chronic illnesses other than cancer: a systematic review and meta-analysis of a transdiagnostic construct. *Health Psychology Review*, 1–20. Advance online publication. https://doi.org/10.1080/17437199.2022.2039744

Simard, S., Thewes, B., Humphris, G., Dixon, M., Hayden, C., Mireskandari, S., & Ozakinci, G. (2013). Fear of cancer recurrence in adult cancer survivors: A systematic review of quantitative studies. *Journal of Cancer Survivorship: Research and Practice*, *7*(3), 300–322. https://doi.org/10.1007/s11764-013-0272-z

Stanton, A.L., Revenson, T.A., & Tennen, H. (2007). Health psychology: psychological adjustment to chronic disease. *Annual Review of Psychology*, *58*, 565–592. https://doi.org/10.1146/annurev.psych.58.110405.085615

Streck, B.P., Wardell, D.W., LoBiondo-Wood, G., & Beauchamp, J. (2020). Interdependence of physical and psychological morbidity among patients with cancer and family caregivers: Review of the literature. *Psycho-oncology*, *29*(6), 974–989. https://doi.org/10.1002/pon.5382

Tang, C., Goldsamt, L., Meng, J., Xiao, X., Zhang, L., Williams, A.B., & Wang, H. (2020). Global estimate of the prevalence of post-traumatic stress disorder among adults living with HIV: a systematic review and meta-analysis. *BMJ Open*, *10*(4), e032435. https://doi.org/10.1136/bmjopen-2019-032435

Taylor, S.E. (1983). Adjustment to threatening events: A theory of cognitive adaptation. *American Psychologist*, *38*(11), 1161–1173. https://doi.org/10.1037/0003-066X.38.11.1161

Tedeschi, R.G., & Calhoun, L.G. (1995). *Trauma and transformation: Growing in the aftermath of suffering*. Sage.

Thombs, B.D., Bass, E.B., Ford, D.E., Stewart, K.J., Tsilidis, K.K., Patel, U., Fauerbach, J.A., Bush, D.E., & Ziegelstein, R.C. (2006). Prevalence of depression in survivors of acute myocardial infarction. *Journal of General Internal Medicine*, *21*(1), 30–38. https://doi.org/10.1111/j.1525-1497.2005.00269.x

Unseld, M., Krammer, K., Lubowitzki, S., Jachs, M., Baumann, L., Vyssoki, B., Riedel, J., Puhr, H., Zehentgruber, S., Prager, G., Masel, E. K., Preusser, M., Jaeger, U., & Gaiger, A. (2019). Screening for post-traumatic stress disorders in 1017 cancer patients and correlation with anxiety, depression, and distress. *Psycho-oncology*, *28*(12), 2382–2388. https://doi.org/10.1002/pon.5239

Versluis, A., Alphen, K. V., Dercksen, W., Haas, H., Kaptein, A. A., & Hurk, C. V. D. (2022). Looking bad: Female patients drawing their representation of chemotherapy-induced alopecia. *Journal of Health Psychology*, *27*(13), 3013–3027. https://doi.org/10.1177/13591053221075503

Vilchinsky, N., Ginzburg, K., Fait, K., & Foa, E.B. (2017). Cardiac-disease-induced PTSD (CDI-PTSD): a systematic review. *Clinical Psychology Review*, *55*, 92–106. https://doi.org/10.1016/j.cpr.2017.04.009

Weitkamp, K., Feger, F., Landolt, S. A., Roth, M., & Bodenmann, G. (2021). Dyadic coping in couples facing chronic physical illness: a systematic review. *Frontiers in Psychology*, *12*, 722740. https://doi.org/10.3389/fpsyg.2021.722740

White, V., Linardon, J., Stone, J.E., Holmes-Truscott, E., Olive, L., Mikocka-Walus, A., Hendrieckx, C., Evans, S., & Speight, J. (2022). Online psychological interventions to reduce symptoms of depression, anxiety, and general distress in those with chronic health conditions: a systematic review and meta-analysis of randomized controlled trials. *Psychological Medicine*, *52*(3), 548–573. https://doi.org/10.1017/S0033291720002251

24

SELF-MANAGEMENT AND ADHERENCE IN THE CONTEXT OF CHRONIC DISEASES

Rui She and Konstadina Griva

Introduction

The increasing life expectancy and population aging have resulted in a dramatic rise in the number of individuals affected by chronic diseases. Currently, 50% of people live with at least one chronic disease, and approximately one-third have multiple conditions (Bamm et al., 2013; OECD, 2019). Chronic diseases, such as cardiovascular diseases, cancer, chronic respiratory diseases, and diabetes, account for 74% of mortality globally, with 41 million deaths annually (World Health Organization, 2022). Chronic diseases impose an enormous and growing burden on individuals, families, and society, as well as on health-care systems. It is estimated that chronic diseases consume more than 60% of health-care spending (Leroy et al., 2014; Wolff et al., 2002). Therefore, effective management of chronic diseases is imperative to address the increasing numbers of patients and escalating costs.

A core response of the health-care system to this challenge requires moving toward more patient-centered and collaborative care from the traditional disease-centered approach. Chronic disease self-management is one of the key components and requires an integrated approach with the active involvement of the patient, family, and health-care professional. Self-management is designed to empower patients by providing them with the knowledge, resources, and skills required to adhere to long-term preventive or therapeutic regimens and effectively manage their conditions. When patients are more informed, involved, and empowered, they engage more effectively with their health-care providers and take a proactive role in making day-to-day decisions about the management of their illness. The self-management approach holds particular significance for individuals with chronic diseases, as the patients bear the responsibility for their daily care over the prolonged course of chronic illness.

 DOI: 10.4324/9781003318026-29

Chronic Disease Self-Management

Concept and Definition

The term 'self-management' was first used by Thomas Creer in the 1970s to denote the active participation of patients in their treatment and has evolved beyond the practice of merely providing information and increasing patient knowledge. Grady and Gough defined self-management as the day-to-day management of chronic conditions by individuals over the course of an illness. Corbin and Strauss further expanded upon this definition by illustrating three sets of tasks for living with a chronic illness: medical (e.g., treatment adherence), role (e.g., creating new meaning behaviors or life roles), and emotional management (e.g., psychological adjustment) (Corbin & Strauss, 1988). As self-management is often based on the patient's perceived problems, six central self-management skills have been proposed, including problem-solving, decision-making, resource utilization, formation of patient-provider partnerships, action planning, and self-tailoring (Lorig & Holman, 2003). It is important to note that self-management goes beyond adherence to treatment guidelines; it incorporates the management of symptoms, lifestyle changes, and psychosocial and spiritual consequences of illness, with the support of family, community, and health-care professionals. Udlis further delineates five dimensions of self-management: knowledge, resources, adherence to a plan, active participation, and informed decision-making (Udlis, 2011).

More recently, self-management has been described as a dynamic, interactive, and daily process in which individuals engage to manage a chronic illness (Schulman-Green et al., 2012). This perspective includes processes such as focusing on illness needs (e.g., learning about condition and health needs, taking ownership of health needs), activating available resources (e.g., health care, psychological, and spiritual resources), and adapting to life with a chronic illness (e.g., processing emotions, adjusting, and integrating illness into daily life) (Schulman-Green et al., 2012). These processes of self-management have greater specificity than previous conceptualizations and may be used to guide intervention development. It is worth noting that the relative importance of self-management processes may differ for each patient based on their trajectory of chronic illness, personal beliefs, and related concerns. Therefore, a holistic model of care that recognizes the need for individualized approaches is highly recommended.

Overview of Self-Management Interventions

Self-management interventions (SMIs) are supportive interventions systematically provided by health-care professionals, peers, or laypersons to enhance patients' skills and confidence in managing chronic diseases. Extensive research has shown that SMIs can provide benefits for participants in terms of knowledge, self-management behaviors, treatment adherence, self-efficacy, and improved health status when compared to standard care for a variety of conditions (Barlow et al., 2002; Ha Dinh et al., 2016). Additionally, these programs have contributed to reductions in hospitalizations, readmission rates, days in hospital, outpatient visits, health-care utilization, and costs. However, it is important to acknowledge that there is considerable variability in SMIs, including differences in the components used, delivery, targeted outcomes, measurement tools, adopted techniques, evaluation, and use of theoretical frameworks. Consequently, caution should be made when utilizing techniques like meta-analysis to determine the effectiveness of SMIs across different studies.

Key components of SMIs that have been widely used include (1) provision of knowledge and information about chronic conditions; (2) psychological strategies to support people adjusting to life with a chronic condition; (3) strategies to support treatment adherence; (4) practical support for physical care tailored to the specific condition, including action plans, support for daily activities, and disease-specific training; (5) social support as appropriate; and (6) access to health-care and supportive services (Barlow et al., 2002; Taylor et al., 2014b). In a meta-review of 77 systematic reviews on SMIs, lifestyle advice was found to be the most frequently employed component (72%), followed by psychological strategies (69%) and information (49%). The least utilized self-management components were supportive care resources and co-operation with health-care professionals (Vernooij et al., 2016). Positive results were observed in 58% of interventions based solely on patient activation techniques (e.g., reminders, diaries, action plans, health monitoring, problem-solving), 67% when in combination with information, and 57% when combined with information and collaboration with health-care providers.

SMIs for patients with chronic diseases encompass a variety of techniques aimed at improving self-management behaviors and outcomes. These techniques include patient education, behavioral skills, goal setting, psychosocial support, symptom monitoring, and eliciting support from health-care providers. While certain techniques, such as providing information and professional support, can be applicable across all chronic conditions, others are more specific to particular conditions or contexts. For example, in the management of asthma, the provision of action plans to facilitate timely self-management during attacks can be highly beneficial (Shahaj et al., 2019). Conversely, individuals living with stable but disabling conditions like stroke, progressive neurological disease, and inflammatory arthropathies may require more emphasis on therapy, rehabilitation, and psychosocial support. By tailoring the interventions to the specific needs of each condition, SMIs can be more effective in improving patient outcomes.

Commonly evaluated outcomes in SMIs include clinical assessments, self-reported symptoms, psychosocial outcomes (e.g., quality of life), functional status (e.g., activities of daily life), and patients' treatment adherence and satisfaction (Lu et al., 2014; Newman et al., 2004b). Many studies assess multiple outcomes, which could dilute the overall effectiveness if outcomes are not specifically targeted or distal to intervention elements and/or processes are included. To accurately evaluate an SMI, it is important to align the outcomes measured with the intended targets for change (Newman et al., 2004b). The SMI needs to be directed to the specific challenges associated with a particular condition. For example, self-management in asthma primarily focuses on acquiring the skills needed to manage medication and symptoms, while existing SMIs for dementia tend to concentrate almost exclusively on the psychological well-being of patients with dementia (Veld et al., 2020).

When developing SMIs for patients with chronic diseases, several factors should be considered. First, it is essential to take into account the characteristics of the disease, including available treatment options, disease duration, developmental trajectory or prognosis, and its impact on daily life. Second, the intervention should be tailored to the individual patient by considering their priorities, preferences, health literacy, cultural and linguistic issues, and perceived health concerns to maximize its effectiveness. Additionally, the feasibility of implementing SMIs within the health-care setting, the available resources, and relevant stakeholders should be considered to increase the acceptability and sustainability of interventions.

Adherence: Concept, Measurements, and Determinants

Adherence is closely linked to chronic disease management, as it is pivotal for the effectiveness of prescribed therapies and disease outcomes (Gebremichael et al., 2019; Morgado et al., 2010). However, treatment nonadherence remains a major issue and challenge for health-care services. The average rate of medication nonadherence across different chronic diseases ranges from 50% to 79%, and the prevalence is even higher for nonadherence to dietary restrictions, prescribed exercise, or lifestyle modification (DiMatteo et al., 2002; Peh et al., 2021). Low adherence can lead to negative outcomes, such as increased adverse drug events, reduced quality of life, patient and physician frustrations, and increased morbidity and mortality (Ulrik et al., 2006; Vrijens et al., 2008). Treatment nonadherence not only affects the patients and their families but also has a significant impact on the health-care system with prolonged care services and increased health-care costs (Iuga & McGuire, 2014; McGrady & Hommel, 2013). These findings underscore the urgent need for a better understanding of the determinants of adherence to inform the development of SMIs.

Definition of Adherence

There are at least three terms commonly used in adherence research. Compliance describes "the extent to which the patient's behavior coincides with medical or healthcare advice" (Sackett et al., 1978). Since the 1990s, the term 'compliance' has been gradually replaced by 'adherence', as compliance implies a lack of autonomy and passivity on the patient's part, while adherence emphasizes a shared agreement between health-care professionals and patients in developing a treatment plan (Chakrabarti, 2014). Adherence has been defined by the World Health Organization (WHO) as "the degree to which the person's behavior-taking medication, following a diet, and/or executing lifestyle changes, corresponds with the agreed recommendations from a health care provider" (World

Health Organization, 2003). 'Concordance' is a more recent term, emphasizing the patient-prescriber relationship and interaction, and the degree to which the prescription represents a shared decision (Bell et al., 2007). However, the concept and measurement of concordance lack clarity.

An assumption underlying these three concepts is that the prescription from health-care providers is appropriate; hence, all terms refer back in varying degrees to the act of prescribing (Horne et al., 2005). Overall, a clear and refined conceptualization of adherence is important to ensure consistency and standardization in measuring patients' adherence levels.

Operationalization and Measurement of Adherence

An accurate assessment of adherence is necessary for providing better evidence of the consequences and predictors of adherence, for effective and efficient treatment planning, and for a valid analysis of treatment efficacy. In an attempt to achieve greater accuracy in measurement, various tools have been developed for a wide range of diseases (Anghel et al., 2019; Lam & Fresco, 2015).

Adherence can be operationalized as a continuous or dichotomous outcome. The levels of adherence can be calculated as the overall percentage of doses taken, the concentration of the drug/metabolite, or the score of adherence scales. A dichotomous measure of adherence requires a cutoff value to distinguish adherence and nonadherence. In medication adherence, it is typically considered adherent if an individual takes between 80% and 120% of prescribed medications over a given period (Morrison et al., 2015). For self-reported scales, a predetermined cutoff value is often used to classify adherence and nonadherence (e.g., Morisky Medication Adherence Scale). However, the dichotomous measurement of adherence has been criticized for the arbitrary selection of a cutoff point, which may lack a biological or pharmacological basis (Farmer, 1999). In practice, the categorization into good and bad adherence can be considered to be conceptually poorly related to medication response as it maps poorly onto the dose-response phenomenon, which is a continuous function.

Generally, methods of the measurements of adherence can be classified as direct or indirect, or be labeled as subjective or objective (Anghel et al., 2019). Direct methods involve the assessment of drug concentrations or metabolite levels in body fluids and direct observation of the patient's adherence behavior. Although direct measures are considered more accurate and can provide physical evidence to prove the patient has taken the prescription, there are drawbacks regarding their use. Indirect methods are more commonly used in adherence research, including pill counts, electronic monitoring devices, the use of electronic health records, and self-reported measures. Table 24.1 provides a brief overview of the available methods for measuring treatment adherence.

Although there is no "gold standard" for measuring adherence, each has advantages and disadvantages that should be taken into consideration when choosing an appropriate method in any evaluation of adherence. Subjective measures generally offer a higher cost-effectiveness ratio, are often utilized in

Table 24.1 Measurement of adherence

Methods of Assessment	*Parameter Used*	*Advantages*	*Disadvantages*
Direct			
Measurement of drug/metabolite levels	Concentration of the drug/ metabolite in body fluids	Valid and objective	Costly, invasive, individual variation in drug pharmacokinetics, generally unsuitable for psychiatric patients and those under multidrug regimes
Direct observation	Patient's adherence behavior observed by health-care workers	Accurate for hospitalized or institutionalized patients	Impractical for large-scale implementation; Subject to bias from the patient (e.g., white-coat adherence)
Indirect			
Pill counts	Ratio of the number of doses taken to the number of doses received between two appointments	Simple; low cost; mostly used in clinical trials	No evidence of ingested medication; inability to identify adherence pattern; unfeasible for non-discrete dosages; potential underestimation (medication refill by patients)
Secondary database analysis (e.g., prescription refill data, insurance claims, registries)	Medication possession ratio (MPR), Multiple Interval Measure of Medication Acquisition (CMA)	Easy to use; inexpensive; non-invasive; allow for population-based analysis; patients not aware that they are being monitored	No proof of actual intake of medicine; possibility of overestimation

(*Continued*)

Table 24.1 (Continued)

Methods of Assessment	*Parameter Used*	*Advantages*	*Disadvantages*
Self-reported (questionnaires and scales, patient-kept diaries, patient interviews)	A value that is interpreted based on the measurement tool	Easy to use; inexpensive	Overestimate adherence Subjective, influenced by recall or reporting bias
Electronic monitoring devices (e.g., Medication Event Monitoring System)	Overall percentage of doses taken; Dosing regime	Objective; additional information on degree and pattern of adherence; often used as a reference standard for validating adherence measurement	High cost; equipment issues; patient aware of the evaluation; no evidence of medication ingestion

clinical settings, and are useful to identify barriers or facilitators of adherence and predict nonadherence. Self-reported assessments are preferable in resource-limited clinical settings; however, for low-literacy populations, interviews should be used instead of questionnaires. On the other hand, objective measures provide a more precise and accurate estimation of the actual behavior and are typically used in research. Objective measures, such as pill counts and electronic monitoring devices, may have higher accuracy but should be balanced with considerations of manpower and cost. Importantly, whatever the approach to measuring adherence, the strategies employed should meet basic psychometric standards of acceptable reliability and validity.

The current state of the art in measuring adherence behavior involves a multimethod approach that integrates feasible self-reports and objective measures (World Health Organization, 2003). A meta-analysis of patient adherence and medical outcomes suggested that research should use measures that are continuous instead of dichotomous, use more than one measure of adherence, and include self-report (DiMatteo et al., 2002). Lastly, while existing research has primarily focused on medication adherence, further investigation should be conducted to understand adherence to other health behaviors, such as lifestyle advice and rehabilitation therapy, as these self-management behaviors significantly impact patients' health and well-being.

Determinants of Adherence

An understanding of the determinants of adherence is critical in designing effective interventions to promote adherence. Adherence is a complex phenomenon that is not solely the responsibility of patients; it is influenced by various factors related to the patients themselves, the nature of the disease and its treatments, and the health-care system (DiMatteo et al., 2002; Kardas et al., 2013; World Health Organization, 2003; Shahin et al., 2019).

Patient-Related Factors

Sociodemographic Factors. There are mixed findings about the associations between sociodemographic factors and adherence. Some factors (e.g., age) showed differential association with adherence across conditions, necessitating separate evaluations for each condition. Generally, poor socioeconomic and sociodemographic status, including low income, poverty, lower education levels, financial constraints, unemployment, lack of social support networks, unstable living conditions, living alone, and family dysfunction, have negative effects on adherence. Patients facing these challenges may have limited access to necessary health care and other resources and may have competing priorities for disease treatment.

Health Knowledge, Health Beliefs, and Cognitive Factors. Health knowledge, literacy, beliefs, and attitudes about the disease and treatment have significant impacts on patients' adherence behavior, including knowledge and skill in managing the disease symptoms and treatment, perceived need for treatment, perceived effect of treatment, negative/positive beliefs and attitudes toward the disease and treatment, perceived risk related to the disease, perceived confidence in performing illness-management behaviors, concerns about the adverse effect of treatment, motivation to treatment adherence, and illness representations (patients' beliefs and expectations about an illness or somatic symptom). Many of the factors align with constructs in the established models such as the Health Belief Model (HBM), Theory of Planned Behavior (TPB), and Common-Sense Model of Self-regulation (CSM).

- The HBM proposes that an individual's health behavior is determined by their perception of disease severity, susceptibility to the disease, perceived benefits and barriers to that behavior, self-efficacy, and cue to action. HBM has been used in understanding adherence behavior in various chronic diseases and to inform the development of interventions to improve adherence (Jones et al., 2014a; Kamran et al., 2014).
- The TPB suggests that attitude, subjective norm, and perceived behavioral control together shape an individual's behavioral intentions, which is the most proximal predictor of behavior. Meta-analyses have indicated that TPB is an appropriate framework for understanding adherence behaviors, with all three core components of TPB significantly influencing adherence intention, particularly perceived behavior control (Rich et al., 2015).

- The CSM posits that individuals develop cognitive and emotional representations of their diseases, which can influence the formation of coping behaviors and expectations of physical and emotional outcomes (Leventhal et al., 2016). Illness representations have been associated with medication adherence (Shahin et al., 2019). Specifically, patients who experienced fewer symptoms and less emotional responses and perceived their illness as more chronic, more controllable, and less consequences on life were more likely to adhere to treatment. However, a meta-analysis of 23 studies found a weak association between different illness representations and adherence, suggesting that the CSM may not be the most appropriate model to use in predictive studies of adherence (Brandes & Mullan, 2014).

Other Cognitive and Emotional Factors. Cognitive deficits, low attention and working memory, forgetfulness, perceived disease stigma, and coping styles have also been found to be associated with treatment adherence. Negative psychological status (e.g., lack of self-worth, distress, depression, hopelessness, anxieties over the complexity of the drug regimen) could also have an aversive impact on adherence.

Condition-Related Factors

Condition-related factors refer to specific illness-related demands faced by patients, which can be further categorized into three areas: disease control (i.e., symptoms, complications, severity, and acute events), disease characteristics (i.e., time since diagnosis, prognosis, complexity, complications), and patient-specific (i.e., comorbidities, medical history, previous treatment experience, and self-perceived health) (Peh et al., 2021). These factors can potentially impact adherence through their influence on patients' risk perception, the importance of following treatment to avoid negative health consequences, and the priority placed on adherence.

Treatment-Related Factors

Most treatment-related factors are associated with treatment effects (i.e., effectiveness, side effects, risk, and benefits), treatment regimen (i.e., complexity, dosing, type, pill burden, frequency, clarity of label instruction, concomitant medications, physical properties of drugs, flexibility of medication plan, and interference in routine), and cost of treatment (Kardas et al., 2013; Peh et al., 2021). For instance, poly-medication, high dosage frequency, complex regimen, poor taste of the drug, and large tablet size might lead to underuse of prescription. It is suggested that unique attributes of specific diseases and therapies do not supersede the common factors affecting adherence but rather modify their influence (World Health Organization, 2003). To be most effective, adherence interventions should be customized according to the individual patient's requirements. By considering these treatment-related factors and tailoring interventions accordingly, health-care providers can help improve adherence rates and ultimately enhance patient outcomes.

Health Care–Related Factors

Health care–related factors can be broadly divided into health-care provider–related and health-care system–related. Health-care provider characteristics include good relationships and communication, ability to relate to the patient, provision of information, collaborative decision-making, race equality, trust in providers, adequate length of consultations, positive attitude toward the patients, and high quality of health-care services are more likely to motivate the patients regarding regimen adherence. Health-care-system-related factors include accessibility and affordability to health-care services, continuity of care, adequate medical facilities, regulation processes (e.g., waiting time), health insurance coverage (where appropriate), prescription coverage, regular community support, follow-up visits, and efficient medication distribution systems. In some systems, cost is an important health-care issue, which can have a significant impact on patient adherence, especially on missing appointments or treatments.

Key Questions in Self-Management Interventions

SMIs for patients with chronic diseases often involve multicomponent and complex approaches. These interventions aim to enhance participants' self-management skills and confidence while taking into account the challenges of living with a chronic condition. Consequently, the multicomponent SMI is often recommended as a comprehensive "package" of self-management practices (Barlow et al., 2002). However, the use of multicomponent approaches can make it challenging to determine the specific mechanisms that lead to improvements in health outcomes. Understanding the more effective components of these interventions is further complicated by the use of indirect comparisons, where different interventions are often compared to usual care rather than directly against one another. Additionally, the methodologies of SMIs vary significantly, making it difficult to identify factors that wield a specific influence on effectiveness.

To provide a synthesis of current systematic review literature on SMIs, many meta-reviews have been conducted. For example, a meta-review on asthma concluded that effective self-management involves patient education, action plans, and regular professional review (Pinnock et al., 2017). Similarly, a meta-review on diabetes self-management suggested that while no single approach appeared optimally effective, effective programs tended to be multicomponent and provide adequate contact time (Captieux et al., 2018). Another meta-review regarding stroke SMIs highlighted the varying needs for self-management support across the trajectory of recovery, the usefulness of goal setting and action planning, the importance of good patient-professional communication, and the need for emotional support (Pearce et al., 2015). Wilson's meta-review on interventions targeting self-regulation to improve medication adherence found that self-monitoring, personalized feedback on adherence, or SMIs demonstrated small-to-medium effect sizes, while other components, including goal setting, barrier identification, problem-solving, and stress management showed little evidence of improving adherence (Wilson et al., 2020).

It is important to note that the findings of these meta-reviews are not consistent across different chronic conditions and targeted outcomes. To gain a more comprehensive understanding of SMIs, meta-regression techniques are increasingly employed to explore outcome variations across trials and assess the association between intervention-specific characteristics and better outcomes. Table 24.2 presents an overview of SMI studies that have utilized meta-regression techniques to investigate factors affecting intervention effectiveness. The findings provide preliminary evidence that (1) integration of behavioral change techniques (BCTs) in SMIs may increase the intervention efficacy (El-Gayar et al., 2021; Fan & Sidani, 2009); (2) specific BCTs such as self-monitoring, action planning, problem-solving, goal setting, and active involvement of participants may be particularly effective (Denford et al., 2014; El-Gayar et al., 2021; Kebede et al., 2018; Parry et al., 2018); (3) SMIs in collaboration with health-care professionals may enhance the effectiveness of interventions in improving health outcomes (Odgers-Jewell et al., 2017; Parry et al., 2018); (4) SMIs may be more effective in younger patients compared to older patients (Hou et al., 2018; Miles et al., 2011; Nkhoma et al., 2021; Tao & Or, 2013); and (5) longer intervention duration may be associated with a greater intervention effect size (Jonkman, Westland, et al., 2016b; Kebede et al., 2018; Mannucci et al., 2022) although nonsignificant or negative findings are also reported (El-Gayar et al., 2021; Peng et al., 2019; Van Truong et al., 2021). A more detailed discussion on SMI components and mode of delivery is provided next.

Components of Self-Management Interventions

Behavioral Change Techniques

One important component of SMIs is the use of BCTs to improve self-management behaviors and health outcomes. BCTs are observable, replicable, and irreducible components of the interventions that lead to causal processes meant to regulate behavior. Studies have shown that when combined with patient education, the use of behavioral strategies can improve treatment adherence by an average of 25% (Burkhart & Dunbar-Jacob, 2002). Interventions focusing on behavioral issues also show a larger intervention effect size in self-care behaviors and metabolic outcomes than other types of SMIs (e.g., educational, psychological, or mixed) (Fan & Sidani, 2009).

Although many studies have attempted to identify the most effective BCTs, the findings are not consistent. For instance, the meta-analysis on the efficacy of BCTs in mHealth for the self-management of diabetes showed that the most frequently applied BCTs were self-monitoring of behaviors, feedback on the outcome of behavior, instruction on how to perform the behavior, and credible sources. However, among all BCTs, action planning and self-monitoring of outcomes seem to be the most effective ones (EI-Gayar et al., 2021). In contrast, other meta-regression studies have indicated a higher efficacy in interventions employing goal setting (Parry et al., 2018), active involvement of participants

Table 24.2 Summary of factors affecting the effectiveness of SMIs based on meta-regression literature

Author & Year	*Condition (Patients)*	*Number of Studies*	*Sample Size*	*Mean Age (SD)*	*Intervention*	*Main Findings of Subgroup Analysis and Meta-regression*
Mannucci et al. (2022)	Type 2 diabetes	14 trials	NR	60.8	Educational programs	– Longer trial duration, higher baseline mean age and duration of diabetes, and lower baseline HbA1c were correlated with greater efficacy of group-based programs in reducing HbA1c. – No significant difference in efficacy of glycemic control between group-based and individual programs.
Othman et al. (2021)	Type 2 diabetes	142 trials	25,511	NR	Diabetes self-management education	– Meta-regression analyses demonstrated that skills-related attributes had an estimated effect suggesting improvement in knowledge and that information-related attributes had an estimated effect suggesting improvement in quality of life. – Skill- and information-related attributes did not have an estimated effect, suggesting improvement in physical activity or in HbA1c.

El-Gayar, Ofori, and Nawar (2021)	Diabetes	21 trials	1,920	51.2	BCTs in mHealth for self-management of diabetes	– Interventions that used behavior theory for developing mHealth apps were not statistically different from those that did not. – Intervention duration was not significant in the meta-regression. – Increased use of behavior change techniques may result in slightly higher HbA1c reduction. – Among all BCTs, the most effective ones appear to be 'action planning' and 'self-monitoring' of outcome(s) of behavior.
Van Truong et al. (2021)	Hypertension	12 trials	2,714	60–79	SMI	– SMI significantly decreased blood pressure and increased self-efficacy and medication adherence in older adult patients with hypertension, with no significant effect on body mass index. – No significant association between the effect size of blood pressure and sex distribution/age, settings, type of interventions. – SMI of shorter than six months duration had a larger effect size for blood pressure than did those implementing interventions for six months or longer.

(Continued)

Table 24.2 (Continued)

Author & Year	*Condition (Patients)*	*Number of Studies*	*Sample Size*	*Mean Age (SD)*	*Intervention*	*Main Findings of Subgroup Analysis and Meta-regression*
Nkhoma et al. (2021)	Diabetes	39 trials	6,861	51.6	Digital health-led diabetes self-management education and support	**Significant**: – The higher the mean baseline HbA1c, the more significant the reduction at follow-up. – The higher the mean study age, the smaller the reduction in HbA1c. – Using mobile applications and patient portals had a better impact on glycemic control than other tools. **Nonsignificant**: Frequency, intervention content, ethnicity, risk of bias, design, tailored, attrition rate, blinding, hypertension, sample size, gender ratio
Hodkinson et al. (2020)	Asthma	105 trials	27,767	NR	SMI to reduce health-care use and improve quality of life	– Multidisciplinary case management and regularly supported self-management were most effective at reducing health-care use in patients with symptoms of severe asthma at baseline.
Peng et al. (2019)	Chronic kidney disease (CKD)	19 trials	2,540	55–75	SMI	– Though this review did not find evidence of specific contributors (age, treatment duration, and diabetic kidney disease) to heterogeneity, these effects might have differed according to baseline CKD stage, race, or the prevalence of disease.

Aggarwal et al. (2019)	Chronic orofacial pain	14 trials	NR	NR	SMI	**Significant**: – Packages of physical and psychosocial self-regulation and education appear beneficial. **Nonsignificant**: – Meta-regression showed nonsignificant effects for biofeedback on long-term pain and depression.
Parry et al. (2018)	Women with cardiac pain	57 trials	13,047	62.8 (8.8)	SMI	– SMI for cardiac pain were more effective if they included a greater proportion of women, goal setting, and collaboration/support from health-care providers.
Kebede et al. (2018)	Type 2 diabetes	21 trials	3,787	NR	Digital interventions	**Significant**: – Interventions with a baseline HbA1c level above 7.5% and employing the BCTs 'problem-solving' and 'self-monitoring outcomes of behavior' had a higher effect size in reduced HbA1c levels. – Interventions with a three- to four-month duration and a six- to eight-month duration displayed significant associations with the effect size, indicating that 6 to 8 months of intervention duration resulted in a pronounced reduction of HbA1c levels. **Nonsignificant**: Mode of delivery and theory-based intervention did not have an impact on the intervention's effectiveness.

(Continued)

Table 24.2 (Continued)

Author & Year	*Condition (Patients)*	*Number of Studies*	*Sample Size*	*Mean Age (SD)*	*Intervention*	*Main Findings of Subgroup Analysis and Meta-regression*
Hou et al. (2018)	Diabetes	21 trials	1,550	35.3 (type 1 diabetes); 55.2 (type 2 diabetes)	Mobile phone applications and self-management	– A significant association between baseline HbA1c levels and effect size. – Studies with younger participants may report larger effect size compared with trials with older participants. – A significant dose-response relationship between health-care professionals (HCP) feedback and effect size: no HCP feedback, a mean reduction of 0.24%; low frequency, a mean reduction of 0.33%; and high frequency, a mean reduction of 1.12%.
Newham et al. (2017)	COPD	66 trials	3,518	65.6	SMI to improve health-related quality of life (HRQL)	**HRQL was significantly improved in**: – COPD patients with severe symptoms but not patients with moderate symptoms; – SMIs delivered by a single practitioner but not for multidisciplinary interventions; – multiple-session interventions but not for single-session SMI; – both individual and group-based SMIs; and – SMIs targeting mental health alongside symptom management were more effective than those focusing on symptom management alone. **Nonsignificant**: – No significant association between the number of BCTs used and intervention effectiveness for improving HRQL.

Odgers-Jewell et al. (2017)	Type 2 diabetes	47 trials	8,533	60	Group-based self-management education	**Significant**: – Greater reductions in HbA1c occurred in group-based education compared with controls at 6–10 months, 12–14 months, 18 months, and 36–48 months, but not at 24 months. – Group-based interventions facilitated by a single discipline, multidisciplinary teams, or health professionals with peer supporters were more effective at improving HbA1c than peer-led interventions. – Physician-, dietitian- and nurse-led group-based education interventions were equally effective at improving HbA1c. **Nonsignificant**: – None of these study variables and intervention characteristics (i.e., theoretical model, discipline(s) of educator(s), educator training, materials provided, delivery in primary care, both groups HbA1c $< 7\%$ at baseline, intervention length, contact time, number of participants, number of sessions, and the inclusion of family and friends) explained significant portions of heterogeneity among the studies.

(*Continued*)

Table 24.2 (Continued)

Author & Year	*Condition (Patients)*	*Number of Studies*	*Sample Size*	*Mean Age (SD)*	*Intervention*	*Main Findings of Subgroup Analysis and Meta-regression*
Jonkman et al. (2016a)	COPD	14 trials	3,282	68.1	SMI	**Significant**: – Favorable effects on some outcomes for more planned contacts and longer duration of interventions, interventions with peer contact, without log keeping, without problem-solving, and without support allocation (univariable analyses) – In multivariable analyses, only the effect of duration on all-cause hospitalization remained. **Nonsignificant**: – Other characteristics are not consistently associated with differential effects of SMI across clinically relevant outcomes.
Jonkman et al. (2016b)	Chronic illnesses	47 trials	10,596	44.6 to 69.3	SMI	– SMI showed positive effects on HRQL at six months for patients. – Meta-regression showed counterintuitive negative effects of standardized training of interventionists and peer interaction on HRQL at six months. – No components were identified that favorably affected HRQoL.

Jonkman, Westland et al. (2016c)	Patients with heart failure	32 trials	5,624	69.7 (12.4)	SMI	– Longer intervention duration reduced mortality risk, risk of HF-related hospitalization, and HF-related hospitalization at six months. – Interventions comprising standardized training of interventionists, peer contact, log keeping, or goal-setting skills appeared less effective than interventions without these characteristics.
Rich et al. (2015)	Chronic illnesses	27 trials	NR	NR	SMI based on the TPB or theory of reasoned action	– Theoretically consistent patterns of effects among the attitude, subjective norm, perceived behavioral control, intention and behavior constructs were found with small-to-medium effect sizes. Effect sizes were invariant across behavior and measurement type.
Ferguson, Swan, and Smaldone (2015)	Hispanic adults with type 2 diabetes	13 trials	2,784	48 to 70	Diabetes Self-management Education in Conjunction with Primary Care	– A greater reduction in A1C in studies where Diabetes Self-Management Education (DSME) design and/or provider type was multimodal, culturally tailored, and had low subject attrition. – No significant differences in effect sizes for study duration or intervention contact time.

(*Continued*)

Table 24.2 (Continued)

Author & Year	*Condition (Patients)*	*Number of Studies*	*Sample Size*	*Mean Age (SD)*	*Intervention*	*Main Findings of Subgroup Analysis and Meta-regression*
Tu, Xu, and Du (2015)	Inflammatory bowel disease	15 trials	2,049	NR	SMI	– Distance or remote SMIs demonstrated a larger effect size than SMI delivered face-to-face. – No evidence for a positive effect associated with specific component (materials given to patients, provider of intervention, structed or tailored information, provision drug management, symptom management, management of psychological consequences, lifestyle) of SMI in adult patients with inflammatory bowel disease in general.
Pal et al. (2014)	Type 2 diabetes	16 trials	3,578	46 to 67	Computer-based diabetes SMI	– The effect size on glycemic control was larger in the mobile phone subgroup compared to interventions delivered using home-based computers.
Ricci-Cabello et al. (2014)	Ethnic minority groups with type 2 diabetes	20 trials	3,094	NR	Diabetes self-management educational programs targeted to racial/ethnic minority groups	– Larger intervention effect sizes were observed in SMI delivered face-to-face than those supported by telecommunication, delivered individually than those delivered in a group format, as well as in those involving peer educators, including cognitive reframing techniques, and a lower number of teaching methods. – No statistically significant differences were observed for the total duration of the intervention, the number of sessions included, the duration of each session, the total number of hours of intervention, or its intensity (number of hours per month).

Denford et al. (2014)	Asthma	38 trials	7,883	NR	Behavior Change Techniques in Asthma Self-Care Interventions	– Active involvement of participants is associated with increased intervention effectiveness, but the use of stress management techniques may be counter-productive. – Existing recommendations about the 'optimal' content of asthma self-care interventions were tested but were not supported by the data.
Bolen et al. (2014)	Type 2 Diabetes	138 trials	33,124	59	Patient activation interventions (PAIs)	– Higher baseline HbA1c, pharmacist-led interventions, and longer follow-up were associated with larger HbA1c improvements. – No intervention strategy outperformed any other in adjusted meta-regression. – Interventions had no effect on hypoglycemia (evidence: low) or short-term mortality (evidence: moderate).
Tao and Or (2013)	Diabetes	52 trials	6,489	8.5 to 70.8	Self-management health information technology on glycaemic control	– Larger treatment effects in the younger age group compared with those in the older age group – Larger intervention effects were observed when the technology is a web-based application, when a mechanism for patients' health data entry is provided (manual or automatic), and when the technology is operated in the home or without location restrictions.

(*Continued*)

Table 24.2 (Continued)

Author & Year	*Condition (Patients)*	*Number of Studies*	*Sample Size*	*Mean Age (SD)*	*Intervention*	*Main Findings of Subgroup Analysis and Meta-regression*
Miles et al. (2011)	Musculoskeletal pain	16 trials	4,047	NR	SMI	**Significant**: – SMI were more effective in studies with a greater proportion of female subjects for outcomes of general mental health and global health status and younger samples for outcomes of physical/functional capability and self-efficacy. **Nonsignificant**: – Gender was not associated with effect size for pain intensity, physical/functional capability, self-efficacy, and depression. – Age was not associated with different effect sizes for other outcomes.
Bray et al. (2010)	Blood pressure	25 trials	NR	47 to 77	Self-monitoring of blood pressure	**Significant**: – Where self-monitoring was accompanied by an additional co-intervention, participants were more likely to meet target blood pressure compared to where there was none. – Other factors, including follow-up period, age, and gender, had no impact on intervention effect sizes.

Minet et al. (2010)	Type 2 diabetes	47 trials	7,677	50.3 to 72.6	Self-care management intervention	**Significant**: – Sample size and follow-up period were identified to have significant effect on the effect size in favor of small studies and short follow-up. **Nonsignificant**: – For type of intervention and duration of intervention, there was a nonsignificant effect on effect size in favor of educational techniques and short interventions.
Michie et al. (2009)	Adults	122 trials	44,747	NR	Behavior change interventions designed to promote physical activity and healthy eating	– The technique, 'self-monitoring', explained the greatest amount of among-study heterogeneity. – Interventions that combined self-monitoring with at least one other technique derived from control theory were significantly more effective than the other interventions.

(*Continued*)

Table 24.2 (Continued)

Author & Year	*Condition (Patients)*	*Number of Studies*	*Sample Size*	*Mean Age (SD)*	*Intervention*	*Main Findings of Subgroup Analysis and Meta-regression*
Fan and Sidani (2009)	Diabetes	50 trials	From 29 to 1139	56.4 (6.2)	DSME Intervention	**Significant**: – Larger effect sizes were found for behavioral types of interventions than for other types (e.g., educational, psychological, or mixed) for self-care behaviors and metabolic outcomes. – Larger effect sizes were found for mixed teaching methods for outcomes of knowledge and metabolic control compared to didactic or interactive teaching methods. In contrast, the effect size for self-care behavior was the largest for interactive teaching methods. – Larger effect sizes were found for mixed formats for knowledge and metabolic control outcomes. For self-care behaviors, one-on-one education produced a larger effect than group/mixed formats. – Educational interventions that covered multiple or mixed topics yielded consistently larger effect sizes for knowledge and metabolic control outcomes than those addressing a single topic. Focus on one topic had a greater effect size for self-management behaviors.

						– Effect sizes for knowledge and metabolic control outcomes were larger with an increase in the number of sessions offered and total contact hours and with booster sessions. – Interventions with a long duration (≥ 24 weeks) produced larger effects for all three outcomes. **Nonsignificant**: – No consistent pattern was evident across outcome variables based on strategies used to deliver education. – Mixed strategies were not more effective than individual strategies.
Bhogal, Zemek, and Ducharme (2006)	Asthma in children	4 trials	355	School-aged children	Written action plan	**Significant**: – Children assigned to symptom-based action plans had a significantly lower risk of exacerbations requiring an acute care visit and intended more frequently to continue using their plans after the study. Children assigned to peak flow-based action plans experienced a greater reduction in the number of symptomatic days per week. **Nonsignificant**: – There were no significant group differences in the rate of exacerbation requiring oral steroids or admission, school absenteeism, lung function, symptom score, quality of life, and withdrawals.

(*Continued*)

Table 24.2 (Continued)

Author & Year	*Condition (Patients)*	*Number of Studies*	*Sample Size*	*Mean Age (SD)*	*Intervention*	*Main Findings of Subgroup Analysis and Meta-regression*
Chodosh et al. (2005)	Chronic disease (diabetes, osteoarthritis, and hypertension)	53 trials	NR	NR	Chronic Disease Self-Management Programs	– None of the strategies (the RE-AIM or the Essential Elements of SMIs classification schemes, stratification by baseline severity, or assessment of effectiveness according to intermediate variables) yielded results that robustly supported any of these elements as important predictors of the effectiveness of self-management programs.
Ellis et al. (2004)	Diabetes	21 trials	2,439	24.6 to 67.2	Diabetes patient education	**Significant**: – Interventions that included a face-to-face delivery, cognitive reframing teaching method, and exercise content were more likely to improve glycemic control.
Norris et al. (2002)	Type 2 diabetes	31 studies	3,731	55 (35–67)	Self-Management Education	**Significant**: – HbA1c decreased more with additional contact time between participant and educator.

Note: BCTs, behavior change techniques; HbA1c, glycated hemoglobin; NR, not reported

(Denford et al., 2014), and problem-solving (Kebede et al., 2018). Further research is needed to accurately assess the relative efficacy of different BCTs and account for the heterogeneity of findings on the most efficacious BCTs.

Action Planning

Action planning helps patients adapt to changes in their condition by facilitating appropriate actions and behaviors. Action planning has been successfully used in the management of various chronic diseases, including asthma, diabetes, chronic obstructive pulmonary disease, cardiovascular disease, and opioid overdose (Hermana et al., 2023). For instance, asthma patients are often instructed to create and follow written action plans, which enable them to promptly identify and seek appropriate emergency treatment during acute exacerbations. Action planning has been shown to be particularly useful for patients with multiple chronic conditions, as it helps to tackle the complexity of multimorbidity (Miller et al., 2020).

Research has demonstrated the efficacy of action planning in different disease contexts (Amirova et al., 2021; Canacott et al., 2019; Howcroft et al., 2016). For instance, a review focusing on asthma concluded that action plans incorporating two to four action points, including recommendations on increasing inhaled corticosteroids and initiating oral corticosteroids, consistently reduced admissions and acute and emergency attendances (Gibson & Powell, 2004). To ensure the maximum efficacy of action planning, it is crucial to involve patients in the development and review of action plans with patients, personalize them to accommodate clinical variation, and consider cultural and social beliefs. Education and regular follow-up also enhance the effectiveness of action planning (Barrecheguren & Bourbeau, 2018; Kouri et al., 2019; Ring et al., 2011). In addition, a meta-analysis evaluating the impact of action planning on physical activity found that the interventions delivered by health-care providers were more effective (Lin et al., 2022).

Collaboration with Health-Care Professionals

Collaboration with health-care professionals is another important component of SMIs. Although it is less frequently used in comparison to other components, involving health-care professionals can improve the efficacy of interventions. For example, pharmacist-led interventions and longer follow-ups have been associated with greater improvements in glycated hemoglobin levels in individuals with diabetes (Bolen et al., 2014). Additionally, studies have shown that SMIs that incorporate input from health-care professionals are more effective in managing chronic musculoskeletal pain (Carnes et al., 2012). In addition, several systematic reviews on asthma have shown the combined effectiveness of self-management education and routine clinical assessments (Moullec et al., 2012; Pinnock et al., 2017). They suggest that self-management support is most successful when incorporated into a proactive asthma management program or embedded within organizational procedures. Researchers and policymakers should consider how to integrate self-management support into health-care routines in a feasible and cost-effective approach.

Mode of Delivery

SMIs can be delivered through various approaches: small-group meetings, individual, mHealth technologies, printed materials, and interventions delivered by health-care providers (e.g., nurses, pharmacists, and physicians), as well as interventions led by laypeople.

Efficacy of Technology-Related Self-Management Interventions

In recent years, there has been a growing focus on utilizing technology in SMIs for patients with chronic diseases, and the feasibility of integrating technology has been demonstrated. A meta-review incorporating 11 systematic reviews indicated that mobile phone text messaging significantly enhanced adherence to appointments and antiretroviral therapy, short-term smoking cessation, and some clinical and behavioral outcomes (Jones et al., 2014b). Meta-analyses have also shown that mHealth-supported interventions were effective in reducing pain and disability among patients with osteoporosis (Alhussein & Hadjileontiadis, 2022), improving HbA1c and diabetes knowledge in patients with diabetes (Nkhoma et al., 2021), and reducing blood pressure in hypertensive patients (McLean et al., 2016). However, there were conflicting findings regarding the benefits of different forms of technological support and their relative efficacy compared to the traditional approach. For instance, in the case of diabetes self-management, the use of technology to facilitate self-management support demonstrated a similar effect to conventional in-person methods (Captieux et al., 2018), while other studies have found that the effect size on glycaemic control was larger in interventions delivered through mobile phone apps or patient portals in comparison to other digital tools (Nkhoma et al., 2021; Pal et al., 2014).

Telehealth's Role in Self-Management Support for Chronic Diseases

Telehealth has the potential to facilitate self-management support for patients with chronic diseases in several ways. First, telehealth has the potential to redefine and expand existing relationships by partially taking on the role traditionally held by health-care professionals. Visualization of symptoms and feedback through technology can enhance patients' knowledge, motivation, sense of empowerment, and engagement with their support network. Successful telehealth interventions are those that can seamlessly integrate into patients' daily lives and health-care routines while being user-friendly, compatible with their existing environment and skills, and minimally disruptive to their lives and routines (Vassilev et al., 2015). It is important to note that digital SMIs do not replace traditional self-management but rather enhance patients' access to quality health care (Taylor et al., 2014b). Considering the cost-effectiveness and scalability of telehealth interventions, further research is needed to identify the mechanisms that contribute to the normalization of technologies and determine the optimal application of technology in patients' everyday lives.

Group-Based versus Individual Self-Management Interventions

Evidence on the effectiveness of group versus individual delivery of SMIs is limited due to other differences in studies that confound any clear comparison. One study specifically compared group and individual SMIs in diabetes and found that the group-based interventions resulted in greater improvements in blood glucose levels at a six-month follow-up, but no significant differences were observed for other outcomes (Newman et al., 2004b). In another review focusing on migraine or tension-type headaches, interventions conducted in groups showed larger effects compared to one-to-one delivery (Probyn et al., 2017). However, other studies have reported that individually delivered, face-to-face interventions had larger effect sizes in diabetes SMIs compared to group interventions (Ferguson et al., 2015; Ricci-Cabello et al., 2014). There is, therefore, no conclusive evidence on the relative efficacy of SMIs delivered in group versus individual format in the extant literature. Future research should identify the advantages and disadvantages of different intervention delivery modes to facilitate the optimal implementation of SMIs.

Sustainability of Self-Management Interventions

Chronic diseases often require ongoing management and self-care. Sustainability in SMIs ensures consistent and continuous support for patients with chronic diseases and enables patients to develop and maintain healthy habits, leading to better long-term health outcomes. However, some studies reported little evidence of the sustainability of SMIs in the long term (Francis et al., 2007; McLean et al., 2016). Several key factors may influence the sustainability of SMIs. At the organizational level, the integration of SMIs within health-care systems and existing care structures may enhance the sustainability of SMIs (Jordan et al., 2008). Effective communication and collaboration between health-care professionals and relevant stakeholders are crucial to ensure the ongoing support and implementation of these interventions.

At the individual level, SMIs that can be integrated into patients' daily lives and routines are more likely to be sustained (Audulv, 2013; Qama et al., 2022). It should be noted that the integration of self-management requirements in a daily routine could be affected by patients' ability to apply disease knowledge in different contexts and understand the disease symptoms and trajectory. Moreover, the involvement of patients and their families as active partners in the planning, implementation, and evaluation of SMIs also contributes to their sustainability. Engaging patients in decision-making processes and tailoring interventions to their preferences and needs can enhance their long-term commitment and adherence. More research is needed to identify and incorporate elements of program scalability, sustainability, and cost-effectiveness.

Summary

Prevalent chronic diseases pose a significant global public health challenge, and chronic disease self-management has emerged as a crucial aspect of addressing this issue. The current evidence for effectiveness suggests that chronic disease self-management can yield important benefits to patients and health-care systems, including improvements in health outcomes, quality of life, and reductions in the utilization of health-care resources. Additional research is needed, however, regarding how best to intervene and support chronic disease self-management and adherence in ways that are feasible, acceptable, impactful, and cost-effective. Identifying the most effective components of SMIs and methods by which self-management programs can be delivered and scaled for use at the population level should continue to be a priority. Future research synthesis should address whether these changes, alone and in combination with other approaches, produce meaningful and sustained changes in disease management and health improvement.

Acknowledgment

This work is supported by the Health and Medical Research Fund (HMRF) - Research Fellowship Scheme, Health Bureau, the Government of the Hong Kong SAR (Ref. 08220257).

Further Reading

Taylor, SJ, Pinnock, H, Epiphaniou, E, Pearce, G, Parke, HL, Schwappach, A, Purushotham, N, Jacob, S, Griffiths, CJ, Greenhalgh, T & Sheikh, A 2014, 'A rapid synthesis of the evidence on interventions supporting self-management for people with long-term conditions. (PRISMS Practical systematic RevIew of Self-Management Support for long-term conditions)', *Health Services and Delivery Research*, *2*(53). 1–580. https://doi.org/10.3310/hsdr02530

World Health Organization. (2003). *Adherence to long-term therapies: Evidence for action*. World Health Organization.

Newman, S., Steed, L., & Mulligan, K. (2004). Self-management interventions for chronic illness. *The Lancet*, *364*(9444), 1523–1537.

References

Aggarwal, V. R., Fu, Y., Main, C. J., & Wu, J. (2019). The effectiveness of self-management interventions in adults with chronic orofacial pain: A systematic review, meta-analysis and meta-regression. *European Journal of Pain*, *23*(5), 849–865. https://doi.org/10.1002/ejp.1358

Alhussein, G., & Hadjileontiadis, L. (2022). Digital Health Technologies for Long-term Self-management of Osteoporosis: Systematic Review and Meta-analysis. *JMIR Mhealth Uhealth*, *10*(4). https://doi.org/10.2196/32557

Amirova, A., Fteropoulli, T., Williams, P., & Haddad, M. (2021). Efficacy of interventions to increase physical activity for people with heart failure: A meta-analysis. *Open Heart*, *8*(1). https://doi.org/10.1136/openhrt-2021-001687

Anghel, L. A., Farcas, A. M., & Oprean, R. N. (2019). An overview of the common methods used to measure treatment adherence. *Medicine and Pharmacy Reports*, *92*(2), 117–122. https://doi.org/10.15386/mpr-1201

Audulv, Å. (2013). The over time development of chronic illness self-management patterns: A longitudinal qualitative study. *Medicine and Pharmacy Reports*, *13*(1), 452. https://doi.org/10.1186/1471-2458-13-452

Bamm, E. L., Rosenbaum, P., & Wilkins, S. (2013). Is Health Related Quality Of Life of people living with chronic conditions related to patient satisfaction with care? *Disability and Rehabilitation*, *35*(9), 766–774. https://doi.org/10.3109/09638288.2012.707746

Barlow, J., Wright, C., Sheasby, J., Turner, A., & Hainsworth, J. (2002). Self-management approaches for people with chronic conditions: A review. *Patient Education and Counseling*, *48*(2), 177–187. https://doi.org/10.1016/S0738-3991(02)00032-0

Barrecheguren, M., & Bourbeau, J. (2018). Self-management strategies in chronic obstructive pulmonary disease: A first step toward personalized medicine. *Current Opinion in Pulmonary Medicine*, *24*(2), 191–198. https://doi.org/10.1097/MCP.0000000000000460

Bell, J. S., Airaksinen, M. S., Lyles, A., Chen, T. F., & Aslani, P. (2007). Concordance is not synonymous with compliance or adherence. *British Journal of Clinical Pharmacology*, *64*(5), 710–711; author reply 711–713. https://doi.org/10.1111/j.1365 2125.2007.02971_1.x

Bhogal, S., Zemek, R., & Ducharme, F. M. (2006). Written action plans for asthma in children. *Cochrane Database Syst Rev* (3), Cd005306. https://doi.org/10.1002/14651858.CD005306.pub2

Bolen, S. D., Chandar, A., Falck-Ytter, C., Tyler, C., Perzynski, A. T., Gertz, A. M., Sage, P., Lewis, S., Cobabe, M., Ye, Y., Menegay, M., & Windish, D. M. (2014). Effectiveness and safety of patient activation interventions for adults with Type 2 Diabetes: Systematic review, meta-analysis, and meta-regression. *Journal of General Internal Medicine*, *29*(8), 1166–1176. https://doi.org/10.1007/s11606-014-2855-4

Brandes, K., & Mullan, B. (2014). Can the common-sense model predict adherence in chronically ill patients? A meta-analysis. *Health Psychology Review*, *8*(2), 129–153.

Bray, E. P., Holder, R., Mant, J., & McManus, R. J. (2010). Does self-monitoring reduce blood pressure? Meta-analysis with meta-regression of randomized controlled trials. *Annals of Medicine*, *42*(5), 371–386. https://doi.org/10.3109/07853890.2010.489567

Burkhart, P., & Dunbar-Jacob, J. (2002). Adherence research in the pediatric and adolescent populations: A decade in review. In L. L. Hayman, M. M. Mahon, J. R. Turner (Eds.), *Chronic illness in children: An evidence-based approach*. New York, Springer, 199–229.

Canacott, L., Moghaddam, N., & Tickle, A. (2019). Is the Wellness Recovery Action Plan (WRAP) Efficacious for improving personal and clinical recovery outcomes? A systematic review and meta-analysis. *Psychiatric Rehabilitation Journal*, *42*(4), 372–381. https://doi.org/10.1037/prj0000368

Captieux, M., Pearce, G., Parke, H. L., Epiphaniou, E., Wild, S., Taylor, S. J. C., & Pinnock, H. (2018). Supported self-management for people with type 2 diabetes: A meta-review of quantitative systematic reviews. *BMJ Open*, 8(12), e024262. https://doi.org/10.1136/bmjopen-2018-024262

Carnes, D., Homer, K. E., Miles, C. L., Pincus, T., Underwood, M., Rahman, A., & Taylor, S. J. C. (2012). Effective delivery styles and content for self-management interventions for chronic musculoskeletal pain a systematic literature review. *Clinical Journal of Pain*, *28*(4), 344–354. https://doi.org/10.1097/AJP.0b013e31822ed2f3

Chakrabarti, S. (2014). What's in a name? Compliance, adherence and concordance in chronic psychiatric disorders. *World Journal of Psychiatry*, *4*(2), 30–36. https://doi.org/10.5498/wjp.v4.i2.30

Chodosh, J., Morton, S. C., Mojica, W., Maglione, M., Suttorp, M. J., Hilton, L., Rhodes, S., & Shekelle, P. (2005). Meta-analysis: Chronic disease self-management programs for older adults. *Annals of Internal Medicine*, *143*(6), 427–438.

Corbin, J. M., & Strauss, A. (1988). *Unending work and care: Managing chronic illness at home*. Jossey-bass.
Denford, S., Taylor, R. S., Campbell, J. L., & Greaves, C. J. (2014). Effective behavior change techniques in asthma self-care interventions: Systematic review and meta-regression. *Health Psychology*, *33*(7), 577.
DiMatteo, M. R., Giordani, P. J., Lepper, H. S., & Croghan, T. W. (2002). Patient adherence and medical treatment outcomes a meta-analysis. *Medical Care*, 794–811. https://doi.org/10.1097/00005650-200209000-00009
El-Gayar, O., Ofori, M., & Nawar, N. (2021). On the efficacy of behavior change techniques in mHealth for self-management of diabetes: A meta-analysis. *Journal of Biomedical Informatics*, *119*, 103839. https://doi.org/10.1016/j.jbi.2021.103839
Ellis, S. E., Speroff, T., Dittus, R. S., Brown, A., Pichert, J. W., & Elasy, T. A. (2004). Diabetes patient education: A meta-analysis and meta-regression. *Patient Education and Counseling*, *52*(1), 97–105. https://doi.org/10.1016/s0738-3991(03)00016-8
Fan, L., & Sidani, S. (2009). Effectiveness of Diabetes Self-management Education Intervention Elements: A Meta-analysis. *Canadian Journal of Diabetes*, *33*(1), 18–26. https://doi.org/10.1016/S1499-2671(09)31005-9
Farmer, K. C. (1999). Methods for measuring and monitoring medication regimen adherence in clinical trials and clinical practice. *Clinical Therapeutics*, *21*(6), 1074–1090.
Ferguson, S., Swan, M., & Smaldone, A. (2015). Does diabetes self-management education in conjunction with primary care improve glycemic control in hispanic patients?: A systematic review and meta-analysis. *Diabetes Educator*, *41*(4), 472–484. https://doi.org/10.1177/0145721715584404
Francis, C. F., Feyer, A. M., & Smith, B. J. (2007). Implementing chronic disease self-management in community settings: Lessons from Australian demonstration projects. *Australian Health Review*, 31(4), 499–509. https://doi.org/10.1071/AH070499
Gebremichael, G. B., Berhe, K. K., & Zemichael, T. M. (2019). Uncontrolled hypertension and associated factors among adult hypertensive patients in Ayder comprehensive specialized hospital, Tigray, Ethiopia, 2018. *BMC Cardiovascular Disorders*, 19(1), 121. https://doi.org/10.1186/s12872-019-1091-6
Gibson, P. G., & Powell, H. (2004). Written action plans for asthma: An evidence-based review of the key components. *Thorax*, 59(2), 94–99. https://doi.org/10.1136/thorax.2003.011858
Ha Dinh, T. T., Bonner, A., Clark, R., Ramsbotham, J., & Hines, S. (2016). The effectiveness of the teach-back method on adherence and self-management in health education for people with chronic disease: A systematic review. *JBI Evidence Synthesis*, 14(1). https://journals.lww.com/jbisrir/Fulltext/2016/01000/The_effectiveness_of_the_teach_back_method_on.14.aspx
Hermana, S. T., Detyniecki, K., O'Hara, K., Penovich, P., Rao, V. R., Tatum, W., Long, L. C. T., Stern, J. M., Carrazana, E., & Rabinowicz, A. L. (2023). Written seizure action plans for adult patients with epilepsy: Distilling insights from emergency action plans for other chronic conditions. *Epilepsy & Behavior*, 140, Article 109002. https://doi.org/10.1016/j.yebeh.2022.109002
Hodkinson, A., Bower, P., Grigoroglou, C., Zghebi, S. S., Pinnock, H., Kontopantelis, E., & Panagioti, M. (2020). Self-management interventions to reduce healthcare use and improve quality of life among patients with asthma: Systematic review and network meta-analysis. *BMJ: British Medical Journal*, 370. https://doi.org/10.1136/bmj.m2521
Horne, R., Weinman, J., Barber, N., Elliott, R., Morgan, M., Cribb, A., & Kellar, I. (2005). *Concordance, adherence and compliance in medicine taking*. London: NCCSDO, 2005(40), 6.
Hou, C., Xu, Q., Diao, S., Hewitt, J., Li, J., & Carter, B. (2018). Mobile phone applications and self-management of diabetes: A systematic review with meta-analysis, meta-regression of 21 randomized trials and GRADE. *Diabetes, Obesity and Metabolism*, 20(8), 2009–2013. https://doi.org/10.1111/dom.13307

Howcroft, M., Walters, E. H., Wood-Baker, R., & Walters, J. A. (2016). Action plans with brief patient education for exacerbations in chronic obstructive pulmonary disease. *Cochrane Database of Systematic Reviews*, 12(12), Cd005074. https://doi.org/10.1002/14651858.CD005074.pub4

Iuga, A. O., & McGuire, M. J. (2014). Adherence and health care costs. *Risk Management and Healthcare Policy*, 7, 35–44. https://doi.org/10.2147/RMHP.S19801

Jones, C. J., Smith, H., & Llewellyn, C. (2014a). Evaluating the effectiveness of health belief model interventions in improving adherence: A systematic review. *Health Psychology Review*, 8(3), 253–269.

Jones, K. R., Lekhak, N., & Kaewluang, N. (2014b). Using mobile phones and short message service to deliver self-management interventions for chronic conditions: A meta-review. *Worldviews on Evidence-Based Nursing*, 11(2), 81–88. https://doi.org/10.1111/wvn.12030

Jonkman, N. H., Schuurmans, M. J., Groenwold, R. H. H., Hoes, A. W., & Trappenburg, J. C. A. (2016a). Identifying components of self-management interventions that improve health-related quality of life in chronically ill patients: Systematic review and meta-regression analysis. *Patient Education and Counseling*, *99*(7), 1087–1098. https://doi.org/10.1016/j.pec.2016.01.022

Jonkman, N. H., Westland, H., Groenwold, R. H., Ågren, S., Anguita, M., Blue, L., Bruggink-André de la Porte, P. W., DeWalt, D. A., Hebert, P. L., Heisler, M., Jaarsma, T., Kempen, G. I., Leventhal, M. E., Lok, D. J., Mårtensson, J., Muñiz, J., Otsu, H., Peters-Klimm, F., Rich, M. W., Riegel, B., … Hoes, A. W. (2016b). What are effective program characteristics of self-management interventions in patients with heart failure? An individual patient data meta-analysis. *Journal of Cardiac Failure*, 22(11), 861–871.

Jonkman, N. H., Westland, H., Trappenburg, J. C., Groenwold, R. H., Bischoff, E. W., Bourbeau, J., Bucknall, C. E., Coultas, D., Effing, T. W., Epton, M., Gallefoss, F., Garcia-Aymerich, J., Lloyd, S. M., Monninkhof, E. M., Nguyen, H. Q., van der Palen, J., Rice, K. L., Sedeno, M., Taylor, S. J., Troosters, T., … Schuurmans, M. J. (2016c). Characteristics of effective self-management interventions in patients with COPD: Individual patient data meta-analysis. *European Respiratory Journal*, 48(1), 55–68. https://doi.org/10.1183/13993003.01860-2015

Jordan, J. E., Briggs, A. M., Brand, C. A., & Osborne, R. H. (2008). Enhancing patient engagement in chronic disease self-management support initiatives in Australia: The need for an integrated approach. *Medical Journal of Australia*, *189*, S9–S13.

Kamran, A., Ahari, S. S., Biria, M., Malpour, A., & Heydari, H. (2014). Determinants of patient's adherence to hypertension medications: Application of health belief model among rural patients. *Annals of Medical and Health Sciences Research*, *4*(6), 922–927.

Kardas, P., Lewek, P., & Matyjaszczyk, M. (2013). Determinants of patient adherence: A review of systematic reviews. *Frontiers in Pharmacology*, *4*, 91.

Kebede, M. M., Zeeb, H., Peters, M., Heise, T. L., & Pischke, C. R. (2018). Effectiveness of digital interventions for improving glycemic control in persons with poorly controlled type 2 diabetes: A systematic review, meta-analysis, and meta-regression analysis. *Diabetes Technology & Therapeutics*, *20*(11), 767–782. https://doi.org/10.1089/dia.2018.0216

Kouri, A., Kaplan, A., Boulet, L. P., & Gupta, S. (2019). New evidence-based tool to guide the creation of asthma action plans for adults. *Canadian Family Physician*, *65*(2), 103–106. https://www.cfp.ca/content/cfp/65/2/103.full.pdf

Lam, W. Y., & Fresco, P. (2015). Medication adherence measures: An overview. *BioMed Research International*, *2015*, 217047. https://doi.org/10.1155/2015/217047

Leroy, L., Bayliss, E., Domino, M., Miller, B. F., Rust, G., Gerteis, J., Miller, T., & Network, A. M. R. (2014). The agency for healthcare research and quality multiple chronic conditions research network: Overview of research contributions and future priorities. *Medical Care*, *52*(Suppl 3), S15–22. https://doi.org/10.1097/MLR.0000000000000095

Leventhal, H., Phillips, L. A., & Burns, E. (2016). The Common-Sense Model of Self-Regulation (CSM): A dynamic framework for understanding illness self-management. *Journal of Behavioral Medicine*, *39*(6), 935–946. https://doi.org/10.1007/s10865-016-9782-2

Lin, H., Yu, P., Yang, M., Wu, D., Wang, Z., An, J. Y., Duan, H. L., & Deng, N. (2022). Making specific plan improves physical activity and healthy eating for community-dwelling patients with chronic conditions: A systematic review and meta-analysis. *Frontiers in Public Health*, *10*, Article 721223. https://doi.org/10.3389/fpubh.2022.721223

Lorig, K. R., & Holman, H. R. (2003). Self-management education: History, definition, outcomes, and mechanisms. *Annals of Behavioral Medicine*, *26*(1), 1–7.

Lu, Y., Li, Z., & Arthur, D. (2014). Mapping publication status and exploring hotspots in a research field: Chronic disease self-management. *Journal of Advanced Nursing*, *70*(8), 1837–1844. https://doi.org/10.1111/jan.12344

Mannucci, E., Giaccari, A., Gallo, M., Bonifazi, A., Belén, Á. D. P., Masini, M. L., Trento, M., & Monami, M. (2022). Self-management in patients with type 2 diabetes: Group-based versus individual education. A systematic review with meta-analysis of randomized trails. *Nutrition, Metabolism and Cardiovascular Diseases*, *32*(2), 330–336. https://doi.org/10.1016/j.numecd.2021.10.005

McGrady, M. E., & Hommel, K. A. (2013). Medication adherence and health care utilization in pediatric chronic illness: A systematic review. *Pediatrics*, *132*(4), 730–740. https://doi.org/10.1542/peds.2013-1451

McLean, G., Band, R., Saunderson, K., Hanlon, P., Murray, E., Little, P., McManus, R. J., Yardley, L., Mair, F. S., & Co-Investigators, D. (2016). Digital interventions to promote self-management in adults with hypertension systematic review and meta-analysis. *Journal of Hypertension*, 34(4), 600–612. https://doi.org/10.1097/HJH.0000000000000859

Michie, S., Abraham, C., Whittington, C., McAteer, J., & Gupta, S. (2009). Effective techniques in healthy eating and physical activity interventions: A meta-regression. *Health Psychology*, 28(6), 690–701. https://doi.org/10.1037/a0016136

Miles, C. L., Pincus, T., Carnes, D., Homer, K. E., Taylor, S. J. C., Bremner, S. A., Rahman, A., & Underwood, M. (2011). Can we identify how programmes aimed at promoting self-management in musculoskeletal pain work and who benefits? A systematic review of sub-group analysis within RCTs. *European Journal of Pain*, 15(8), 775.e771–775.e711. https://doi.org/10.1016/j.ejpain.2011.01.016

Miller, J. J., Pozehl, B. J., Alonso, W., Schmaderer, M., & Eisenhauer, C. (2020). Intervention components targeting self-management in individuals with multiple chronic conditions: An integrative review. *Western Journal of Nursing Research*, 42(11), 948–962. https://doi.org/10.1177/0193945920902146

Minet, L., Møller, S., Vach, W., Wagner, L., & Henriksen, J. E. (2010). Mediating the effect of self-care management intervention in type 2 diabetes: A meta-analysis of 47 randomised controlled trials. *Patient Education and Counseling*, *80*(1), 29–41. https://doi.org/10.1016/j.pec.2009.09.033

Morgado, M., Rolo, S., Macedo, A. F., Pereira, L., & Castelo-Branco, M. J. (2010). Predictors of uncontrolled hypertension and antihypertensive medication nonadherence. *Journal of Clinical Hypertension*, 12(4), 276–281. https://doi.org/10.1111/j.1751-7176.2009.00210.x

Morrison, A., Stauffer, M. E., & Kaufman, A. S. (2015). Defining medication adherence in individual patients. *Patient Preference and Adherence*, 9, 893–897. https://doi.org/10.2147/PPA.S86249

Moullec, G., Gour-Provencal, G., Bacon, S. L., Campbell, T. S., & Lavoie, K. L. (2012). Efficacy of interventions to improve adherence to inhaled corticosteroids in adult asthmatics: Impact of using components of the chronic care model. *Respiratory Medicine*, 106(9), 1211–1225. https://doi.org/10.1016/j.rmed.2012.06.001

Newham, J. J., Presseau, J., Heslop-Marshall, K., Russell, S., Ogunbayo, O. J., Netts, P., Hanratty, B., & Kaner, E. (2017). Features of self-management interventions for people with COPD associated with improved health-related quality of life and reduced emergency department visits: A systematic review and meta-analysis. *International Journal of Chronic Obstructive Pulmonary Disease*, *12*, 1705–1720. https://doi.org/10.2147/COPD.S133317

Newman, S., Steed, L., & Mulligan, K. (2004b). Self-management interventions for chronic illness. *The Lancet*, *364*(9444), 1523–1537. https://doi.org/10.1016/S0140-6736(04)17277-2

Nkhoma, D. E., Soko, C. J., Bowrin, P., Manga, Y. B., Greenfield, D., Househ, M., Li, Y. C., & Iqbal, U. (2021). Digital interventions self-management education for type 1 and 2 diabetes: A systematic review and meta-analysis. *Computer Methods and Programs in Biomedicine*, *210*. https://doi.org/10.1016/j.cmpb.2021.106370

Norris, S. L., Lau, J., Smith, S. J., Schmid, C. H., & Engelgau, M. M. (2002). Self-management education for adults with type 2 diabetes - A meta-analysis of the effect on glycemic control. *Diabetes Care*, *25*(7), 1159–1171. https://doi.org/10.2337/diacare.25.7.1159

Odgers-Jewell, K., Ball, L. E., Kelly, J. T., Isenring, E. A., Reidlinger, D. P., & Thomas, R. (2017). Effectiveness of group-based self-management education for individuals with Type 2 diabetes: A systematic review with meta-analyses and meta-regression. *Diabetic Medicine*, 34(8), 1027–1039. https://doi.org/10.1111/dme.13340

OECD. (2019). *Chronic disease morbidity*. doi:https://doi.org/10.1787/5101558

Othman, M. M., Khudadad, H., Dughmosh, R., Syed, A., Clark, J., Furuya-Kanamori, L., Abou-Samra, A.-B., & Doi, S. A. R. (2021). Towards a better understanding of self-management interventions in type 2 diabetes: A meta-regression analysis. *Primary Care Diabetes*, 15(6), 985–994. https://doi.org/10.1016/j.pcd.2021.06.006

Pal, K., Eastwood, S. V., Michie, S., Farmer, A., Barnard, M. L., Peacock, R., Wood, B., Edwards, P., & Murray, E. (2014). Computer-Based Interventions to Improve Self-management in Adults With Type 2 Diabetes: A Systematic Review and Meta-analysis. *Diabetes Care*, 37(6), 1759–1766. https://doi.org/10.2337/dc13-1386

Parry, M., Bjørnnes, A. K., Victor, J. C., Ayala, A. P., Lenton, E., Clarke, H., Harvey, P., Lalloo, C.,McFetridge-Durdle, J., McGillion, M. H., Price, J., Stinson, J., & Watt-Watson, J. (2018). Self-Management Interventions for Women With Cardiac Pain: A Systematic Review and Meta-analysis. *Canadian Journal of Cardiology*, *34*(4), 458–467. https://doi.org/10.1016/j.cjca.2017.12.011

Pearce, G., Pinnock, H., Epiphaniou, E., Parke, H. L., Heavey, E., Griffiths, C. J., Greenhalgh, T., Sheikh, A., & Taylor, S. J. (2015). Experiences of self-management support following a stroke: A meta-review of qualitative systematic reviews. *PLoS One*, 10(12), e0141803. https://doi.org/10.1371/journal.pone.0141803

Peh, K. Q. E., Kwan, Y. H., Goh, H., Ramchandani, H., Phang, J. K., Lim, Z. Y., Loh, D. H. F., Ostbye, T., Blalock, D. V., Yoon, S., Bosworth, H. B., Low, L. L., & Thumboo, J. (2021). An adaptable framework for factors contributing to medication adherence: Results from a systematic review of 102 conceptual frameworks. *Journal of General Internal Medicine*, 36(9), 2784–2795. https://doi.org/10.1007/s11606-021-06648-1

Peng, S., He, J., Huang, J., Lun, L., Zeng, J., Zeng, S., Zhang, L., Liu, X., & Wu, Y. (2019). Self-management interventions for chronic kidney disease: A systematic review and meta-analysis. *BMC Nephrology*, 20(1), 142. https://doi.org/10.1186/s12882-019-1309-y

Pinnock, H., Parke, H. L., Panagioti, M., Daines, L., Pearce, G., Epiphaniou, E., Bower, P., Sheikh, A., Griffiths, C. J., Taylor, S. J. C., Grp, P., & Grp, R. (2017). Systematic meta-review of supported self-management for asthma: A healthcare perspective. *BMC Medicine*, 15, 64. https://doi.org/10.1186/s12916-017-0823-7

Probyn, K., Bowers, H., Mistry, D., Caldwell, F., Underwood, M., Patel, S., Sandhu, H. K., Matharu, M., Pincus, T., & CHESS team. (2017). Non-pharmacological self-management for people living with migraine or tension-type headache: A systematic review including analysis of intervention components. *BMJ Open*, 7(8), e016670. https://doi.org/10.1136/bmjopen-2017-016670

Qama, E., Rubinelli, S., & Diviani, N. (2022). Factors influencing the integration of self-management in daily life routines in chronic conditions: A scoping review of qualitative evidence. *BMJ Open*, 12(12), Article e066647. https://doi.org/10.1136/bmjopen-2022-066647

Ricci-Cabello, I., Ruiz-Perez, I., Rojas-Garcia, A., Pastor, G., Rodriguez-Barranco, M., & Goncalves, D. C. (2014). Characteristics and effectiveness of diabetes self-management educational programs targeted to racial/ethnic minority groups: A systematic review, meta-analysis and meta-regression. *BMC Endocrine Disorders*, 14, Article 60. https://doi.org/10.1186/1472-6823-14-60

Rich, A., Brandes, K., Mullan, B., & Hagger, M. S. (2015). Theory of planned behavior and adherence in chronic illness: A meta-analysis. *Journal of Behavioral Medicine*, 38(4), 673–688. https://doi.org/10.1007/s10865-015-9644-3

Ring, N., Jepson, R., Hoskins, G., Wilson, C., Pinnock, H., Sheikh, A., & Wyke, S. (2011). Understanding what helps or hinders asthma action plan use: A systematic review and synthesis of the qualitative literature. *Patient Education and Counseling*, 85(2), E131–E143. https://doi.org/10.1016/j.pec.2011.01.025

Sackett, D. L., Haynes, R. B., Gibson, E. S., Taylor, D. W., Roberts, R. S., & Johnson, A. L. (1978). Patient compliance with antihypertensive regimens. *Patient Education and Counseling*, 1(1), 18–21. https://doi.org/10.1016/s0738-3991(78)80033-0

Schulman-Green, D., Jaser, S., Martin, F., Alonzo, A., Grey, M., McCorkle, R., Redeker, N. S., Reynolds, N., & Whittemore, R. (2012). Processes of self-management in chronic illness. *Journal of Nursing Scholarship*, *44*(2), 136–144.

Shahaj, O., Denneny, D., Schwappach, A., Pearce, G., Epiphaniou, E., Parke, H. L., Taylor, S. J. C., & Pinnock, H. (2019). Supporting self-management for people with hypertension: A meta-review of quantitative and qualitative systematic reviews. *Journal of Hypertension*, *37*(2), 264–279. https://doi.org/10.1097/hjh.0000000000001867

Shahin, W., Kennedy, G. A., & Stupans, I. (2019). The impact of personal and cultural beliefs on medication adherence of patients with chronic illnesses: A systematic review. *Patient Preference and Adherence*, 1019–1035.

Tao, D., & Or, C. K. L. (2013). Effects of self-management health information technology on glycaemic control for patients with diabetes: A meta-analysis of randomized controlled trials. *Journal of Telemedicine and Telecare*, *19*(3), 133–143. https://doi.org/10.1177/1357633X13479701

Taylor, S., Pinnock, H., Epiphanou, E., Pearce, G., Parke, H., Schwappach, A., et al. (2014b). A rapid synthesis of the evidence on interventions supporting self-management for people with long-term conditions (PRISMS Practical systematic Review of Self-Management Support for long-term conditions). *Health and Social Care Delivery Research*, 2(53).

Tu, W., Xu, G., & Du, S. (2015). Structure and content components of self-management interventions that improve health-related quality of life in people with inflammatory bowel disease: A systematic review, meta-analysis and meta-regression. *Journal of Clinical Nursing*, *24*(19–20), 2695–2709. https://doi.org/10.1111/jocn.12851

Udlis, K. A. (2011). Self-management in chronic illness: Concept and dimensional analysis. *Journal of Nursing and Healthcare of Chronic Illness*, *3*(2), 130–139.

Ulrik, C. S., Backer, V., Søes-Petersen, U., Lange, P., Harving, H., & Plaschke, P. P. (2006). The patient's perspective: Adherence or non-adherence to asthma controller therapy? *The Journal of Asthma: Official Journal of the Association for the Care of Asthma*, *43*(9), 701–704. https://doi.org/10.1080/02770900600925569

Van Truong, P., Wulan Apriliyasari, R., Lin, M.-Y., Chiu, H.-Y., & Tsai, P.-S. (2021). Effects of self-management programs on blood pressure, self-efficacy, medication adherence and body mass index in older adults with hypertension: Meta-analysis of randomized controlled trials. *International Journal of Nursing Practice*, *27*(2), e12920. https://doi.org/10.1111/ijn.12920

Vassilev, I., Rowsell, A., Pope, C., Kennedy, A., O'Cathain, A., Salisbury, C., & Rogers, A. (2015). Assessing the implementability of telehealth interventions for self-management support: A realist review. *Implementation Science*, *10*, 59. https://doi.org/10.1186/s13012-015-0238-9

Veld, J., Verkaik, R., van Meijel, B., & Francke, A. L. (2020). A systematic meta-review of self-management support for people with dementia. *Dementia-International Journal of Social Research and Practice*, *19*(2), 253–269. https://doi.org/10.1177/1471301218772894

Vernooij, R. W., Willson, M., & Gagliardi, A. R. (2016). Characterizing patient-oriented tools that could be packaged with guidelines to promote self-management and guideline adoption: A meta-review. *Implementation Science*, *11*, 52. https://doi.org/10.1186/s13012-016-0419-1

Vrijens, B., Vincze, G., Kristanto, P., Urquhart, J., & Burnier, M. (2008). Adherence to prescribed antihypertensive drug treatments: Longitudinal study of electronically compiled dosing histories. *BMJ*: *British Medical Journal*, *336*(7653), 1114–1117. https://doi.org/10.1136/bmj.39553.670231.25

World Health Organization. (2003). *Adherence to long-term therapies: Evidence for action*. World Health Organization.

World Health Organization. (2022). *Noncommunicable diseases*. https://www.who.int/news-room/fact-sheets/detail/noncommunicable-diseases

Wilson, T. E., Hennessy, E. A., Falzon, L., Boyd, R., Kronish, I. M., & Birk, J. L. (2020). Effectiveness of interventions targeting self-regulation to improve adherence to chronic disease medications: A meta-review of meta-analyses. *Health Psychology Review*, *14*(1), 66–85. https://doi.org/10.1080/17437199.2019.1706615

Wolff, J. L., Starfield, B., & Anderson, G. (2002). Prevalence, expenditures, and complications of multiple chronic conditions in the elderly. *Archives of Internal Medicine*, *162*(20), 2269–2276. https://doi.org/10.1001/archinte.162.20.2269

25

THE ROLE OF TECHNOLOGY IN CHRONIC ILLNESS

Elizabeth Broadbent and Kate Loveys

Chapter Outline

The first section describes the recent rise in the use of technology for managing chronic conditions and documents contributing factors to this increase. Section 2 describes different types of telehealth systems, including video conferencing and web-based portals. Section 3 describes ways in which connected devices can assist with assessment, diagnosis, and intervention delivery by combining sensors with transmitters, algorithms, actuators, and the cloud (on-demand data storage). Section 4 goes on to describe different platforms over which automated self-management interventions for chronic illness can be provided and outlines the evidence for their acceptability and efficacy. Section 5 discusses the advantages, disadvantages, and limitations of using technology for managing chronic illness. Finally, conclusions are presented in Section 6.

Section 1 The Rapid Rise in Technologies for Chronic Illness

Being diagnosed with a chronic illness can come as a shock. Individuals must learn how to manage their illness and live with its potential consequences over the long term. Many patients with chronic illness experience disease-specific distress or general anxiety and depression at higher rates than the general population. It is important to treat distress, depression, or anxiety, not least because they can interfere with effective coping behaviours, such as monitoring symptoms of disease, taking regular tests, seeking medical care, adhering to recommended treatments, and changing health behaviours.

Psychological therapies have been shown to be effective in improving mental health and disease outcomes, but not all patients have access to such treatments.

DOI: 10.4324/9781003318026-30

Barriers to care include distance, cost, and a paucity of trained health-care professionals. Technologies can help reduce some of these barriers by enabling patients to more easily access treatment for both psychological distress and for the chronic illness itself. As this chapter will outline, technologies can help patients monitor their health, allow them to attend health services remotely, and increase access to disease-specific information and effective treatments in a cost-effective and convenient manner.

Three major drivers have contributed to the rapid increase in the use of remote health-care technologies. First, the ageing population has resulted in an increased prevalence of chronic illness, resulting in health-care demands that cannot be met using traditional delivery methods. Face-to-face services struggle to cope, resulting in long waiting lists and infrequent appointments. Second, advances in technology, including the invention and widespread adoption of the internet, smartphones, sensors, and algorithms, have enabled the development of new forms of devices for health monitoring and treatment delivery. And, third, the 2019 coronavirus pandemic and isolation measures forced service providers to provide remote care.

A multitude of overlapping terms have arisen to refer to health technologies. There is yet to be a consensus of definitions, so they are often used interchangeably. The terms ehealth and digital health are used as umbrella terms for the use of health technology. Ehealth (electronic health) was first introduced by marketing and subsequently adopted by academics to refer to the delivery of health-care services through the internet and related technologies (Eysenbach, 2001), and "the use of information and communication technologies in support of health" (WHO, 2022). 'Digital health' is a more recent term that covers much the same ground, with the potential to also include genomics (Scott and Mars, 2019). 'Telehealth' is an older term which has also been used to cover many different technologies. Telehealth has been defined as "the delivery of healthcare from a distance using information communication technology, which enables the provision of synchronous and asynchronous consultations between patients and clinicians" (Snoswell et al., 2021). Mhealth (mobile health) is a sub-discipline that focuses on the use of mobile phone applications to collect health data for interventions to improve care (Cameron et al., 2017). The internet of healthy things refers to networked health devices that consist of sensors and processing abilities to collect and share data with other networked things over the internet (Maskeliūnas et al., 2019). In this chapter, we use telehealth as an umbrella term and more specific terms where appropriate.

Section 2 Telehealth Systems

Telehealth enables interactions between providers and patients through various modalities, including real-time video conferencing, telephone, email, text messaging, web-based portals, or remote monitoring. It can increase access to care for people in rural or isolated communities. Telehealth is used in many specialties, including cardiovascular disease, endocrinology, psychology/psychiatry, dermatology, neurology, nephrology, ophthalmology, obstetrics, pulmonary, and multidisciplinary care (Snoswell et al., 2021). Telehealth can be equivalent to or more effective than usual care in terms of health outcomes, including blood glucose control, blood pressure management, fewer cardiovascular disease events, fewer chronic obstructive pulmonary disease (COPD) exacerbations, and improved depression (Snoswell et al., 2021).

In psychiatry and psychology, video conferencing is one of the most common forms of telehealth and is used for assessment and treatment. Mental health conditions are well suited to video conferencing because there is less need for a physical examination compared to other chronic conditions. Telepsychiatry dates back to the 1960s and has been shown to be equivalent to face-to-face sessions for counselling and assessment (Drago et al., 2016). Even though symptom reduction is equivalent for video conferencing teletherapy compared to face-to-face delivery, the development of a working alliance can be impeded (Norwood et al., 2018).

Web-based (online) programmes can provide treatments for distress, anxiety, and depression in patients with chronic illness. These programmes mostly use a modular format based on principles of cognitive behavioural treatment (CBT) and are facilitator lead (White et al., 2022). They have been shown to be effective in general, and interventions that included a facilitator were more effective for reducing depression. Interventions that included CBT were more effective at reducing distress and anxiety than those that did not. Evidence to date is stronger for cancer, pain, multiple sclerosis, and diabetes than for other illnesses, for which more studies are needed. Specifically in women with breast cancer, a systematic review of telehealth interventions found reductions in depression, distress, and anxiety, and improved quality of life, sleep, and positive mood (Koç et al., 2022).

An example of a web-based self-management programme is HeLP-Diabetes (Murray et al., 2017). This theory-based intervention included eight sections covering the understanding of diabetes, behaviour change programmes (smoking cessation, obesity, alcohol, diet and exercise, using action planning, goal setting, self-monitoring, reminders, and feedback), explaining the importance of treatments, managing social and work situations, managing feelings (ten CBT based modules), my health record, news, and a moderated forum with videos of patients and additional resources. Health-care professionals registered patients and recommended its use to patients, who could pick and choose which sections to complete. This programme resulted in lower blood glucose in the intervention group compared to the control group, and lower distress in newly diagnosed patients.

Section 3 Connected Devices to Collect and Analyse Data

Telehealth systems can make use of connected devices (also known as the internet of healthy things), which typically comprise sensors that continuously record physiological data, algorithms that analyse the data, and transmitters that share the data with connected smartphones and connect to the cloud for others to access the data. These devices can be implanted into the patient's body (invasive) or be external (non-invasive).

Invasive sensors were developed to be implanted inside the body to continuously measure signals such as blood oxygen. Some invasive sensors can not only monitor signals but also automatically deliver treatment when necessary. A good example is continuous glucose sensing. A small electrochemical sensor is implanted under the skin and is connected to a transmitter that sends signals to a connected device such as a smartphone. Data about interstitial glucose can be sent to a patient or to a health professional who can take action or can be linked to a pump that automatically adjusts insulin levels to maintain an appropriate level. Continuous glucose monitoring significantly improves glycaemic outcomes and patient quality of life (Lin et al., 2021). Another example is implantable cardiac defibrillators, which have been in use since 1980 to prevent sudden cardiac death and treat heart failure (Kuehl et al., 2022). These small battery-powered devices sit in the chest to detect arrhythmias and deliver electric shocks to correct them.

Health wearables are non-invasive devices that collect, process, and share data. They are often placed on the skin (e.g., tattoos and clothing), can be biofluid based (e.g., sweat and tears), or drug delivery systems (e.g., smart bandages, touch-activated, or others (e.g., earphones, contact lenses; Iqbal et al., 2021). Common commercially available wearables are wrist-worn devices (smartwatches) that can continuously measure signals such as heart rate, electrodermal activity, movement, and respiration rate and connect via Bluetooth to a mobile phone, which can upload data to the cloud. These data can be accessible by care teams, and some systems can automatically send alerts when abnormal patterns are detected by algorithms. For example, smartwatches can detect epilepsy seizures from changes in electrodermal activity and send an alert to a carer (Rukasha et al., 2020). A smartwatch with an ECG sensor paired with an app and algorithm has been shown to be accurate compared to an inserted cardiac monitor for detecting atrial fibrillation (Wasserlauf et al., 2019). While further studies are needed, smartwatches may be useful for long-term surveillance and management of patients with chronic illness.

The internet of healthy things can be used in ambient assisted living for older adults (Maskeliūnas et al., 2019). Examples of room-based devices include smart lighting, thermostats, infrared movement detectors in rooms, and pressure sensors in beds. These devices can not only assist with daily living but also be connected to carer networks to allow them to monitor patient safety. However, some patients express concerns over privacy, and interoperability between devices can be an issue.

Smartphones themselves contain many sensors that can measure behaviour: cameras, microphones, location trackers, step trackers, internet history, and keyboard interactions. Data from a person's face, voice, and movements can be analysed for objective patterns of depression and anxiety (Cohn et al., 2019). Decreased smiling and laughing are features of depression that can be assessed through computer models. Slower speech, less pitch variability, and more self-referrals can reflect depression with an accuracy of up to 91% (Koops et al., 2022). Digital phenotyping refers to the use of smartphones to collect data that

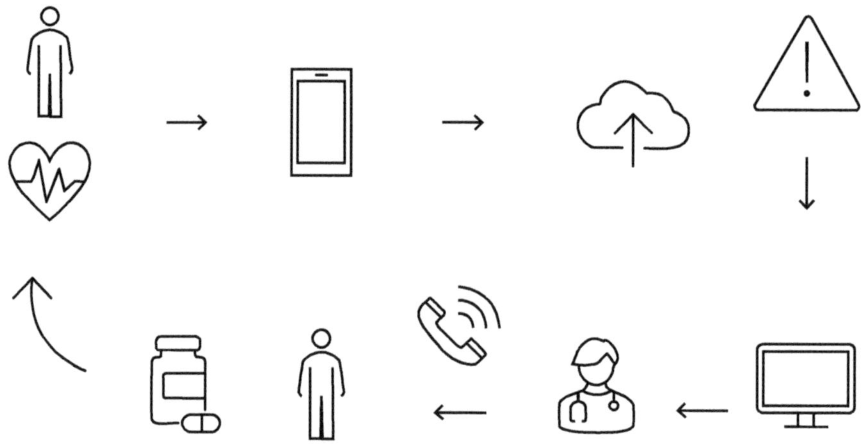

Figure 25.1 Example of a simple telehealth system that includes a health-care provider. A sensing device (e.g., blood pressure monitor) communicates via Bluetooth to a patient's smartphone, which connects to the cloud via the internet. A medical professional checks the results on the cloud through a web portal on their computer, sees changes over time, and contacts the patient to change their medication. The effects of the medication change are detected by the blood pressure monitor in a feedback loop.

can be used to measure behaviour, cognition, and mood for diagnosis, monitoring, and risk prediction (Insel, 2017). In the future, such tools may be able to remotely monitor changes in mood over time and inform patients or providers when treatment is needed.

Figure 25.1 illustrates a telehealth system that includes a connected device and health-care provider, whereas Figure 25.2 illustrates a similar system that provides information to the patient alone.

Devices that monitor a patient's state can inform 'just-in-time' interventions, which adjust the timing, type, and amount of support depending on the patient's state. 'Just-in-time' interventions have been shown to be more effective than control conditions for a number of outcomes, including diabetes management skills, coping with pain, and reduced smoking (Wang & Miller, 2020). However, better theories are needed to describe the temporal dynamics of distress and meaningful levels of change (Nahum-Shani et al., 2018).

Section 4 Technologies for the Delivery of Automated Self-Management Interventions

The previous section described telehealth systems delivered through videoconferencing or web-based portals. It described various implantable, wearable sensors, and external sensors and their uses for monitoring, diagnosis, and treatment delivery tasks within telehealth systems.

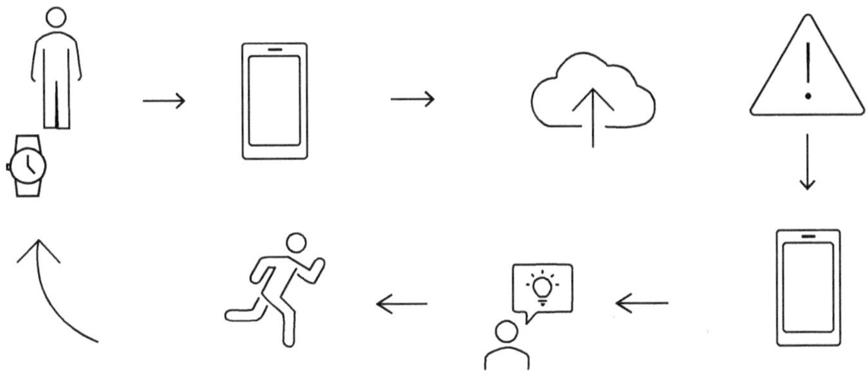

Figure 25.2 A simple example of a telehealth system that does not include a health-care provider. The patient wears a smartwatch that communicates health data (e.g., heart rate and steps) to the patient's phone via Bluetooth, which sends data via the internet to the cloud. An algorithm alerts the patient to inactivity, who decides to increase their exercise behaviour. This behaviour and its subsequent effects on heart rate are detected by the smartwatch in a feedback loop.

The next section focuses on the delivery of automated self-management interventions for chronic illness through mobile phones (mHealth), tablets, computers, smart speakers, and robots. The software used to deliver interventions on these platforms can vary from simple text messages to interactive applications and conversational agents (including chatbots, voice agents, and virtual humans). The section provides some examples of interventions delivered via these modalities and discusses evidence to date for their acceptability and efficacy.

Mhealth: SMS and Smartphone Applications

Many mHealth interventions function autonomously and are administered through text messages. Text or short message service (SMS) interventions are administered through alphanumeric messages of 160 characters or less to a mobile phone (Hall et al., 2015). SMS interventions typically provide health information, reminders, or supportive messages designed by clinicians (Ebuenyi et al., 2021). SMS interventions are simple, low cost, scalable, and highly accessible, with almost three-quarters of the global population estimated to have access to a basic mobile phone (Marcolino et al., 2018). More complex intervention techniques can be used, including message tailoring, personalisation, and repetition (Hall et al., 2015). However, consumers must have cell phone reception to receive an intervention. Moreover, the use of SMS services has decreased in recent years with the uptake of free mobile messaging applications (e.g., WhatsApp), and many SMS interventions are restricted to one-way communication from the health-care provider.

SMS interventions have been shown to be effective in helping people adhere to disease self-management plans, medications, and health-care appointments through regular counselling and reminders (Ebuenyi et al., 2021). Text messages may also be effective for administering lifestyle modification interventions. They have been found to significantly improve diabetes self-care activities and physical activity in people with COPD. Through improving treatment adherence and self-management, SMS interventions have been associated with improvements in disease markers such as HBA_{1C} in diabetes patients and viral load in people with human immunodeficiency virus (HIV; Marcolino et al., 2018). SMS interventions have also been used to provide disease education to people with epilepsy, cardiovascular disease, and asthma and have been associated with improvements in disease knowledge. Moreover, research with SMS interventions in low- and middle-income countries has found promising results (Hall et al., 2014).

A mobile application is software that is designed to run on a smartphone, computer tablet, or smartwatch. There is growing evidence that mobile applications and web-based applications may be suited to delivering interventions for chronic disease management. Like text messaging, intervention content can be delivered to an always-on device. However, a more sophisticated user interface allows for more complex visual approaches to communicating information and delivering interventions.

Research has shown that digitally-delivered visual interventions may be more effective than control conditions at changing health behaviour and illness perceptions in people with chronic disease. A smartphone application that delivered personalised visual imagery based on real-time information about medication and immunoprotection levels in the body was found to improve adherence to antiretroviral therapy and decrease viral load in people living with HIV, compared to a standard application. Tablet applications with visual imagery techniques have also proven effective for improving recovery outcomes in patients with acute coronary syndrome, including symptoms, exercise behaviour, time to return to normal activities, and beliefs about treatment necessity, compared to standard care (Jones et al., 2016). Digital visual interventions have been shown to be acceptable cross-culturally in a diabetes self-management intervention involving patients from New Zealand and Saudi Arabia and their families (Alyami et al., 2022). Visual interventions delivered through mobile applications may more easily communicate complex health information to patients in an accessible and engaging manner than language-based SMS messages.

Evidence of efficacy has been found for mobile applications using other intervention techniques in a range of health areas. These include exercise training programmes for cardiac rehabilitation, disease management for people with asthma, diabetes self-management, and psychological interventions for insomnia and mental health (Marcolino et al., 2018; Weisel et al., 2019). Moreover, mobile applications can collect patient-reported outcome data from home and share insights to care providers (The Clinician, 2022).

Although mobile applications present many advantages over basic SMS interventions, there are some limitations. Mobile applications generally have a higher development cost than SMS interventions, and they may require users to have a smartphone or tablet. This could limit the feasibility of application-based interventions in resource-limited settings. Moreover, many self-directed health applications have been shown to have engagement issues beyond first use and outside of clinical trials, which may be due to the lack of social accountability and engagement that a clinician would typically provide. However, reminders and integration with health-care providers may reduce this issue.

Conversational Agents

Conversational agents (CAs) are computer-based dialogue systems that interact with users (Cassell, 2001). They may present in a text-only (*chatbot*) or voice-only (*voice agent*) form, or they may have a digital embodiment (*embodied conversational agent; ECA*) (see Figure 25.3). Over the past decade, a new form of

(a)

(b)

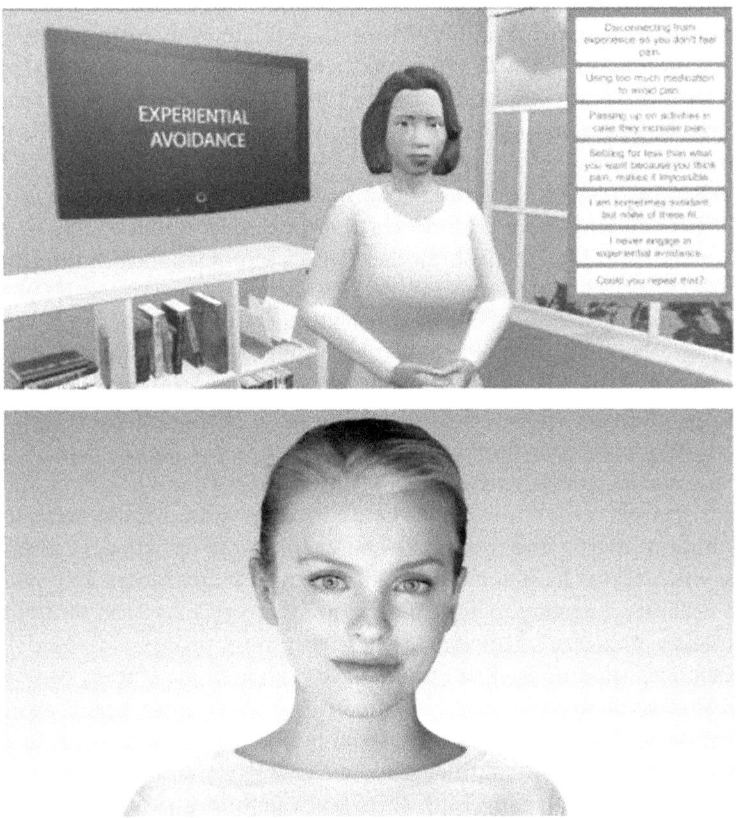

Figure 25.3 (a) ECA ("Relational Agent" by the Relational Agents Group, Northeastern University, USA). From VA Chronic Pain, Relational Agents Group, 2021 https://relationalagents.com/project/vapain/index.html, with permission; (b) VH ("Sam" by Soul Machines Ltd, New Zealand). Photograph taken by Kate Loveys, the University of Auckland, with permission.

ECA called *virtual humans* (VHs) has been tested in health applications. VHs are realistic, autonomous animations in a humanlike form that use artificial intelligence for enhanced social capabilities. They rely on algorithms to make inferences about user states based on their data (e.g., speech, behaviour, physiology), and these inferences inform their social behaviour. VHs can be delivered through websites, as well as other (1) environments (e.g., virtual or augmented reality) for an immersive experience.

An advantage of CAs is that they can provide social and emotional feedback to promote intervention engagement. CAs are capable of building rapport with people through their behaviours, which has been associated with increased engagement (Rizzo & Shilling, 2017). CAs may mimic the sense of social accountability that a human facilitator provides, yet they are as scalable as an SMS intervention.

Some research with CAs has used people's health data to personalise intervention approaches and feedback. One study used a VH integrated with Apple iOS HealthKit data to provide a daily, personalised mental health and exercise intervention to army personnel (Mozgai et al., 2020). Another study integrated a CA with breathing sensors to provide real-time feedback during a meditation intervention (Shamekhi & Bickmore, 2018). The degree of personalisation afforded by sensor integration may boost the acceptability and efficacy of CA interventions.

Systematic reviews of this developing field have found promising results for the efficacy and acceptance of CAs in chronic disease applications. To date, chatbots (text-only agents) have been used to communicate health information and support, collect health data, and provide behavioural interventions to people with chronic disease, and they have been found to improve awareness of disease symptoms, increase treatment adherence, and reduce symptoms of depression and anxiety (Schachner et al., 2020). Chatbots have been acceptable and engaging to people with chronic health conditions in preliminary research, although more randomised controlled trials (RCTs) with larger samples are needed.

Voice agents can also provide behavioural support and health monitoring services to people with chronic illnesses. These services include delivering health information, alerts, and symptom and medication tracking. In these applications, voice agents have achieved high system usability scores with patients, and good usability, interpretability, information delivery, and acceptance scores with health-care providers. However, issues with slow processing speed have been reported in some studies. Few studies have evaluated the efficacy of voice agents, and initial evidence is mixed. Information from a voice agent was shown to change perceptions of the harms of the human papillomavirus (HPV) vaccine (Berube et al., 2021). In another study, an exercise intervention administered by Amazon Alexa and Buddy Link software was found to be safe and feasible in older people, although quality of life and lower extremity function did not change (Jansons et al., 2022).

ECAs and VHs can provide health information and coaching for behavioural interventions. Early studies have shown that ECAs with relational behaviours have received good satisfaction ratings with patients (Bickmore & Gruber, 2010).

ECAs may have benefit in delivering basic psychosocial interventions for mental health and health-related behaviour change (Provoost et al., 2017). Health interventions with VHs have been shown to be more effective than those without agents across an array of outcomes, albeit with a small effect size (Chattopadhyay et al., 2020). This could be due to enhanced engagement in VH interventions; however, additional research is needed. Early trials have found that VHs were acceptable for administering psychological interventions to veterans with mental health conditions (Rizzo & Shilling, 2017) and to younger adults with chronic health conditions and older people (Loveys et al., 2021).

The research to date suggests that CAs show promise for supporting chronic disease management; however, the field is developmental, and more high-quality RCTs are needed in diverse populations. To date, much of the research is based in high-income countries. Moreover, the acceptability of CAs can vary based on their design, the performance of the underlying technology (e.g., animation quality, language model accuracy), and the degree of co-design and tailoring to the target population.

Robots

Social robots are physical machines that are programmed to perceive and act autonomously within the environment and include a social interface (Hegel et al., 2009). They may have robotic, animal, or humanoid forms. Much like CAs, robots are capable of providing companionship (Gasteiger et al., 2021) and building rapport to promote intervention engagement and adherence (Breazeal, 2011). Robots' physical bodies enable additional capabilities, such as touch and physical demonstrations, but have a higher initial cost than web-based interventions.

Social robots can provide a range of services to people with chronic conditions, including psychosocial support, medication management, health data collection, assistance with activities of daily living, and entertainment. Robots used in these applications have included Paro, Pepper, and Care-O-bot, among others (see Figure 25.4).

Robots may be effective and acceptable in several applications for people with chronic diseases. iRobi (Yujin Robot Limited, Korea) was found to improve adherence to long-acting inhalers and rehabilitation exercises in patients with COPD over four months compared to standard care (Broadbent et al., 2018). Several robots have shown benefit in supporting exercise training as part of stroke rehabilitation care (Poli et al., 2013). Robots have also been associated with improvements in distress, quality of life, and loneliness (Robinson et al., 2019). Indeed, Paro has been found to have similar psychosocial benefits to a pet dog in older people. However, most research to date has been in older people or children with autism spectrum disorder, and more studies are needed in broader populations. Moreover, the acceptability of robot interventions may vary depending on the robot's design and factors relating to the user and the implementation.

(a)

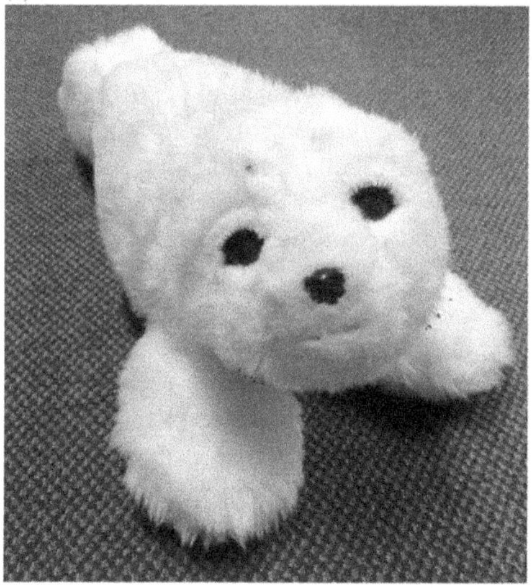

(b)

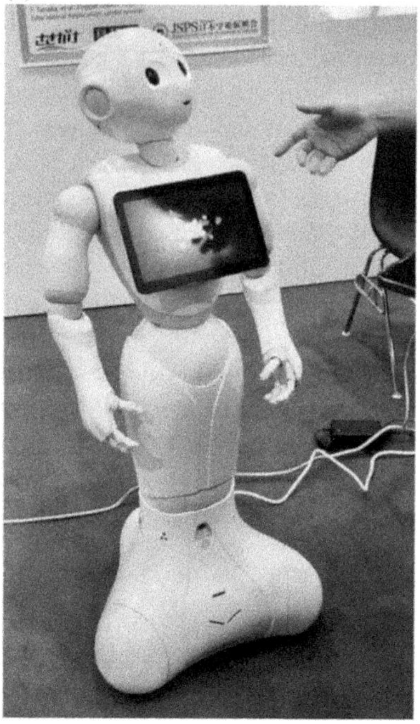

Figure 25.4 Social robots used in support of chronic disease management. Left to right: (A) Paro, a baby seal robot (AIST, Japan). Photograph by Mikaela Law, University of Auckland, with permission. (B) Pepper, a humanoid robot (SoftBank Robotics Group, Japan). Photograph by Elizabeth Broadbent, University of Auckland, with permission.

Section 5 Potential Advantages and Issues of Telehealth

Telehealth technologies present many advantages for chronic disease management. Firstly, they may increase intervention accessibility to people who face barriers to engaging with traditional health services, such as cost, physical distance, stigma, or pandemic-related restrictions (Emerick et al., 2020). Indeed, telehealth services have been associated with lower no-show rates compared to in-person appointments. Telehealth interventions also support people to better monitor their symptoms and disease management from home, enabling a clearer picture of disease progression or improvement for both health-care consumers and providers. Some studies have reported that improved self-monitoring through telehealth provides peace of mind and reassurance for patients and may reduce unnecessary treatment seeking (McFarland et al., 2021). Through the process of engaging in telehealth, consumers may feel more informed, confident, independent, and in control of their condition. This is especially true of older people with chronic diseases, who may be afforded increased independence. Health-care professionals may benefit from the additional information on which to base clinical decisions, reduced workload from improved patient triage, increased scheduling flexibility, and reduced inefficiency (Emerick et al., 2020).

Despite the potential of telehealth interventions, there are several limitations. Some patients may have concerns about reduced face-to-face contact (McFarland et al., 2021), and there may be reduced social accountability when using automated, web-based interventions. An overreliance on telehealth approaches may also introduce bias to patient assessments, as observations of their health, social cues, and home environments will be affected by what the application collects and what is visible over the camera during a telehealth consultation (Emerick et al., 2020). Telehealth approaches may also encounter practical issues such as an unreliable internet connection, creating lag and reducing the fluidity of interactions, sensor batteries running out, and the need for patients to have access to appropriate hardware and internet. Moreover, there may be privacy and confidentiality issues if patients do not have access to a private environment and personal device. Other people present in a patient's environment may provide distraction or biased answers. Physical exams generally cannot be performed through telehealth devices; therefore, they are not suited to consultations with new patients or established patients in need of a physical exam. There may also be upfront costs, and training, and technical support must be given to healthcare providers and consumers.

Many patient-related factors, such as age, education level, digital literacy, cognitive health, and physical disabilities, may affect the acceptability of various telehealth approaches (Marcolino et al., 2018). Thus it is important for developers to adopt co-design processes that involve consumers in the development and implementation process, ensuring the end product meets user needs and preferences. To date, many of the more automated forms of digital health, such as CAs and robots, have not been trained to respond to emergencies (Bickmore et al., 2018). Additionally, some studies have found that users experience separation distress when robots are taken away after extended use (Gasteiger et al., 2021).

Section 6 Conclusions and Future Directions

There have been tremendous advances in telehealth applications for people with chronic conditions. Video communication technology has enabled remote individual consultations, and web-based portals allow the delivery of structured therapies. Sensing devices can be implantable, wearable, or external and enable continuous monitoring of behavioural and physiological data. These data can be stored remotely, where they can be analysed for diagnosis and monitoring purposes by clinicians. Automated personalised treatments can be delivered in a just-in-time manner based on the information collected by these sensors. There are already examples of implantable devices for diabetes and cardiac patients that improve health outcomes.

Psychosocial interventions for patients with chronic illness have been delivered using mobile phones, computers, chatbots, VHs, smart speakers, and robots. Evidence is mounting that these interventions can help improve health outcomes for patients with chronic illnesses. Nevertheless, many technologies are still in the emergent phase and need further development and testing in various patient groups.

The path from research to clinical practice can be a slow one. The adoption of teletherapy consultations by clinicians was accelerated by the recent COVID-19 pandemic. However, the adoption of other forms of telehealth, such as monitoring patient data from remote sensing devices, has been slower. It's important that such technologies are thoughtfully integrated into the workflow of a clinic so that they can be used in a practical and timely fashion. The more we can use technologies to detect problems and intervene early, the better for improving health outcomes with minimal cost and maximum impact.

Further Reading

Luxton, D. D., Nelson, E.-L., & Maheu, M. M. (2024). A practitioner's guide to telemental health: How to conduct legal, ethical, and evidence-based telepractice (2nd ed.). *American Psychological Association*. https://doi.org/10.1037/0000374-000

Linardon, J., Torous, J., Firth, J., Cuijpers, P., Messer, M., & Fuller-Tyszkiewicz, M. (2024). Current evidence on the efficacy of mental health smartphone apps for symptoms of depression and anxiety. A meta-analysis of 176 randomized controlled trials. *World Psychiatry*, *23*(1), 139–149.

Li, H., Zhang, R., Lee, Y. C., Kraut, R. E., & Mohr, D. C. (2023). Systematic review and meta-analysis of AI-based conversational agents for promoting mental health and well-being. *NPJ Digital Medicine*, *6*(1), 236.

References

Alyami, M., Serlachius, A., Law, M., Murphy, R., Almigbal, T. H., Lyndon, M., … Broadbent, E. (2022). Utility and acceptability of a brief type 2 diabetes visual animation: Mixed methods feasibility study. *JMIR Formative Research*, *6*(8), e35079.

Bérubé, C., Schachner, T., Keller, R., Fleisch, E., Wangenheim, F., Barata, F., & Kowatsch, T. (2021). Voice-based conversational agents for the prevention and management of chronic and mental health conditions: systematic literature review. *Journal of Medical Internet Research*, *23*(3), e25933.

Bickmore, T., & Gruber, A. (2010). Relational agents in clinical psychiatry. *Harvard Review of Psychiatry*, *18*(2), 119–130.

Bickmore, T. W., Trinh, H., Olafsson, S., 'Leary, T. K., Asadi, R., Rickles, N. M., & Cruz, R. (2018). Patient and consumer safety risks when using conversational assistants for medical information: an observational study of Siri, Alexa, and Google Assistant. *Journal of Medical Internet Research*, *20*(9), e11510.

Breazeal, C. (2011, August). *Social robots for health applications*. In *2011 Annual international conference of the IEEE engineering in medicine and biology society* (pp. 5368–5371). IEEE.

Broadbent, E., Garrett, J., Jepsen, N., Ogilvie, V. L., Ahn, H. S., Robinson, H., … MacDonald, B. (2018). Using robots at home to support patients with chronic obstructive pulmonary disease: Pilot randomized controlled trial. *Journal of Medical Internet Research*, *20*(2), e8640.

Cameron, J. D., Ramaprasad, A., & Syn, T. (2017). An ontology of and roadmap for mHealth research. *International Journal of Medical Informatics*, *100*, 16–25. https://doi.org/10.1016/j.ijmedinf.2017.01.007

Cassell, J. (2001). Embodied conversational agents: representation and intelligence in user interfaces. *AI Magazine*, *22*(4), 67–67.

Chattopadhyay, D., Ma, T., Sharifi, H., & Martyn-Nemeth, P. (2020). Computer-controlled virtual humans in patient-facing systems: Systematic review and meta-analysis. *Journal of Medical Internet Research*, *22*(7), e18839.

Cohn, J. F., Cummins, N., Epps, J., Goecke, R., Joshi, J., & Scherer, S. (2019). *Multimodal assessment of depression and related disorders based on behavioral signals. In Handbook of multi-modal multi-sensor interfaces: Signal processing, architectures, and detection of emotion and cognition* (Vol. 2, pp. 375–418). Morgan and Claypool. https://doi.org/10.1145/3015783

Drago, A., Winding, T. N., & Antypa, N. (2016). Videoconferencing in psychiatry, a meta-analysis of assessment and treatment. *European Psychiatry*, *36*, 29–37.

Eysenbach, G. (2001). What is e-health? *J Med Internet Res*, *3*(2), e20. https://doi.org/10.2196/jmir.3.2.e20

Ebuenyi, M. C., Schnoor, K., Versluis, A., Meijer, E., & Chavannes, N. H. (2021). Short message services interventions for chronic disease management: A systematic review. *Clinical EHealth*, *4*, 24–29.

Emerick, T., Alter, B., Jarquin, S., Brancolini, S., Bernstein, C., Luong, K., … Wasan, A. (2020). Telemedicine for chronic pain in the COVID-19 era and beyond. *Pain Medicine*, *21*(9), 1743–1748.

Gasteiger, N., Loveys, K., Law, M., & Broadbent, E. (2021). Friends from the future: A scoping review of research into robots and computer agents to combat loneliness in older people. *Clinical Interventions in Aging*, 941–971.

Hall, A. K., Cole-Lewis, H., & Bernhardt, J. M. (2015). Mobile text messaging for health: A systematic review of reviews. *Annual Review of Public Health*, *36*, 393.

Hall, C. S., Fottrell, E., Wilkinson, S., & Byass, P. (2014). Assessing the impact of mHealth interventions in low-and middle-income countries–what has been shown to work? *Global Health Action*, *7*(1), 25606.

Hegel, F., Muhl, C., Wrede, B., Hielscher-Fastabend, M., & Sagerer, G. (2009, February). *Understanding social robots*. In *2009 Second International Conferences on Advances in Computer-Human Interactions* (pp. 169–174). IEEE.

Insel, T. R. (2017). Digital Phenotyping: Technology for a New Science of Behavior. *JAMA*, *318*(13), 1215–1216. https://doi.org/10.1001/jama.2017.11295

Iqbal, S. M. A., Mahgoub, I., Du, E., Leavitt, M. A., & Asghar, W. (2021). Advances in healthcare wearable devices. *npj Flexible Electronics*, *5*(1), 9. https://doi.org/10.1038/s41528-021-00107-x

Jansons, P., Dalla Via, J., Daly, R. M., Fyfe, J. J., Gvozdenko, E., & Scott, D. (2022). Delivery of home-based exercise interventions in older adults facilitated by Amazon Alexa: A 12-week feasibility trial. *The Journal of Nutrition, Health & Aging*, *26*(1), 96–102.

Jones, A. S. K., Ellis, C. J., Nash, M., Stanfield, B., & Broadbent, E. (2016). Using animation to improve recovery from acute coronary syndrome: A randomized trial. *Annals of Behavioral Medicine*, *50*(1), 108–118.

Koç, Z., Kaplan, E., & Tanrıverdi, D. (2022). The effectiveness of telehealth programs on the mental health of women with breast cancer: A systematic review. *Journal of Telemedicine and Telecare*, *0*(0), 1357633X211069663. https://doi.org/10.1177/1357633x211069663

Koops, S., Brederoo, S. G., de Boer, J. N., Nadema, F. G., Voppel, A. E., & Sommer, I. E. (2022). Speech as a Biomarker for Depression. CNS & Neurological Disorders-Drug Targets (Formerly Current Drug Targets-CNS & Neurological Disorders).

Kuehl, M., Tran, P., Osman, F., Panikker, S., Yusuf, S., Dhanjal, T., … Patel, K. (2022). The Evolving Evidence Base of Implantable Cardiac Defibrillators: Past, Present, and Future. INNOVATIONS.
Lin, R., Brown, F., James, S., Jones, J., & Ekinci, E. (2021). Continuous glucose monitoring: A review of the evidence in type 1 and 2 diabetes mellitus. *Diabetic medicine: A Journal of the British Diabetic Association*, *38*(5), e14528. https://doi.org/10.1111/dme.14528
Loveys, K., Sagar, M., Pickering, I., & Broadbent, E. (2021). A digital human for delivering a remote loneliness and stress intervention to at-risk younger and older adults during the COVID-19 pandemic: Randomized pilot trial. *JMIR Mental Health*, *8*(11), e31586.
Marcolino, M. S., Oliveira, J. A. Q., D'Agostino, M., Ribeiro, A. L., Alkmim, M. B. M., & Novillo-Ortiz, D. (2018). The impact of mHealth interventions: Systematic review of systematic reviews. *JMIR mHealth and uHealth*, *6*(1), e8873.
Maskeliūnas, R., Damaševičius, R., & Segal, S. (2019). A review of Internet of Things technologies for ambient assisted living environments. *Future Internet*, *11*(12), 259. http://doi.org/10.3390/fi11120259
McFarland, S., Coufopolous, A., & Lycett, D. (2021). The effect of telehealth versus usual care for home-care patients with long-term conditions: A systematic review, meta-analysis and qualitative synthesis. *Journal of Telemedicine and Telecare*, *27*(2), 69–87.
Mozgai, S., Hartholt, A., & Rizzo, A. S. (2020, March). *An adaptive agent-based interface for personalized health interventions*. In *Proceedings of the 25th International Conference on Intelligent User Interfaces Companion* (pp. 118–119).
Nahum-Shani, I., Smith, S. N., Spring, B. J., Collins, L. M., Witkiewitz, K., Tewari, A., & Murphy, S. A. (2018). Just-in-Time Adaptive Interventions (JITAIs) in mobile health: Key components and design principles for ongoing health behavior support. *Annals of Behavioral Medicine*, *52*(6), 446–462. https://doi.org/10.1007/s12160-016-9830-8
Norwood, C., Moghaddam, N. G., Malins, S., & Sabin-Farrell, R. (2018). Working alliance and outcome effectiveness in videoconferencing psychotherapy: A systematic review and noninferiority meta-analysis. *Clinical Psychology & Psychotherapy*, *25*(6), 797–808.
Perera, A. I., Thomas, M. G., Moore, J. O., Faasse, K., & Petrie, K. J. (2014). Effect of a smartphone application incorporating personalized health-related imagery on adherence to antiretroviral therapy: a randomized clinical trial. *AIDS Patient Care and STDs*, *28*(11), 579–586.
Poli, P., Morone, G., Rosati, G., & Masiero, S. (2013). Robotic technologies and rehabilitation: New tools for stroke patients' therapy. *BioMed Research International*, 2013. https://doi.org/10.1155/2013/153872
Pronovost, A., Peng, P., & Kern, R. (2009). Telemedicine in the management of chronic pain: A cost analysis study. *Canadian Journal of Anesthesia*, *56*(8), 590–596.
Provoost, S., Lau, H. M., Ruwaard, J., & Riper, H. (2017). Embodied conversational agents in clinical psychology: A scoping review. *Journal of Medical Internet Research*, *19*(5), e6553.
Rizzo, A. S., & Shilling, R. (2017). Clinical virtual reality tools to advance the prevention, assessment, and treatment of PTSD. *European Journal of Psychotraumatology*, *8*(sup5), 1414560.
Robinson, N. L., Cottier, T. V., & Kavanagh, D. J. (2019). Psychosocial health interventions by social robots: Systematic review of randomized controlled trials. *Journal of medical Internet research*, *21*(5), e13203.
Rukasha, T. I., Woolley, S., Kyriacou, T., & Collins, T. (2020). Evaluation of wearable electronics for epilepsy: A systematic review. *Electronics*, *9*(6), 968.
Schachner, T., Keller, R., & Von Wangenheim, F. (2020). Artificial intelligence-based conversational agents for chronic conditions: Systematic literature review. *Journal of Medical Internet Research*, *22*(9), e20701.

Scott, R., & Mars, M. (2019). Here we go again-'digital health'. *Journal of the International Society for Telemedicine and eHealth*, *7*, e1–1.
Shamekhi, A., & Bickmore, T. (2018, May). *Breathe deep: A breath-sensitive interactive meditation coach*. In *Proceedings of the 12th EAI International Conference on Pervasive Computing Technologies for Healthcare* (pp. 108–117).
Snoswell, C. L., Chelberg, G., De Guzman, K. R., Haydon, H. H., Thomas, E. E., Caffery, L. J., & Smith, A. C. (2021). The clinical effectiveness of telehealth: A systematic review of meta-analyses from 2010 to 2019. *Journal of Telemedicine and Telecare*, 1357633X211022907.
The Clinician. (2022). *The Clinician completes data colleciton for validating Patient-ReportedExperience-Cancer(PRE-C)measure*.https://theclinician.com/news/the-clinician-completes-data-collection-for-validating-the-patient-reported-experience-cancer-pre-c-measure?fbclid=IwAR1jZ-eIwirnYtaXG-CpFi7YqygdsMLsopVWe6vHr_Ia7zxyHbg513TEANM.
Wang, L., & Miller, L. C. (2020). Just-in-the-Moment Adaptive Interventions (JITAI): A meta-analytical review. *Health Communication*, *35*(12), 1531–1544. https://doi.org/10.1080/10410236.2019.1652388
Wasserlauf, J., You, C., Patel, R., Valys, A., Albert, D., & Passman, R. (2019). Smartwatch performance for the detection and quantification of atrial fibrillation. *Circulation: Arrhythmia and Electrophysiology*, *12*(6), e006834.
Weisel, K. K., Fuhrmann, L. M., Berking, M., Baumeister, H., Cuijpers, P., & Ebert, D. D. (2019). Standalone smartphone apps for mental health—a systematic review and meta-analysis. *NPJ Digital Medicine*, *2*(1), 1–10.
White, V., Linardon, J., Stone, J. E., Holmes-Truscott, E., Olive, L., Mikocka-Walus, A., ... Speight, J. (2022). Online psychological interventions to reduce symptoms of depression, anxiety, and general distress in those with chronic health conditions: A systematic review and meta-analysis of randomized controlled trials. *Psychological Medicine*, *52*(3), 548–573.
WHO (2022) https://www.emro.who.int/health-topics/ehealth/

SECTION 6

Interventions

26
INTRODUCTION
Theoretical Foundations of Health Psychology

Jemma Todd, Amelia J. Scott, and Rachel E. Menzies

Introduction

Most good interventions start with a theory. This section will focus on interventions in health psychology, but first, we need to lay the foundation for these interventions. We provide an overview of some of the key movements in psychology and how they conceptualised behaviour. These waves of psychology and their subsequent interventions have largely focused on mental health, and yet they are also relevant to modifying health behaviour, as well as treatments for chronic health conditions. For key theories specific to health psychology, see Chapter 1.

This chapter will focus on psychological movements, beginning with behaviourism, with its strong emphasis on behaviour and learning principles. Next, we provide an overview of the humanistic movement, the theoretical basis of motivational interviewing, which helped build a client-centred style of care that is still popular today. We then move to current models primarily located within clinical psychology: cognitive behavioural therapy and "third wave" interventions. Finally, we briefly outline some of the advanced applications of these theories to health behaviour.

Freud is generally acknowledged to be the grandfather of psychology, known by many for developing psychodynamics and psychoanalysis. Whilst many of Freud's ideas have shaped psychology even today, we have chosen not to focus on Freudian psychology here for several reasons. Firstly, for Freud, the agent of change was not located in behaviour, and therefore, this was not a primary focus of his theories. Secondly, his theories are widely acknowledged to be unfalsifiable and difficult to quantify. That is, we cannot test whether his claims are true through the scientific method. Finally, and perhaps of most relevance here, his theories have not been applied to health psychology and therefore are of less relevance here. We therefore instead begin our psychology journey with behavioural and learning psychology.

 DOI: 10.4324/9781003318026-32

Behaviourism

Until the late 1800s, psychology was largely focused on introspection. With the coming of behaviourism in the early to mid-1900s, the focus turned squarely towards what could be observed, quantified, and measured. This meant that generally, thoughts and feelings were only considered important so far as they reflected behaviours or behavioural tendencies. Led by figures such as Skinner, Thorndike, Pavlov, and Watson, psychology placed a much greater emphasis on behaviours and their consequences.

Historical Origins

Conditioning is a large part of behaviourism – that is, how events or situations come to be associated with other events, physiological responses, feelings, and behaviours. What is now known as classical or Pavlovian conditioning came about through Pavlov's research with dogs. As is well-known in psychology, Pavlov noticed one day that his dog would salivate (unconditioned response) when presented with food (unconditioned stimulus) before eating, but even simply when he entered the room with food (conditioned stimulus). This led to him repeatedly pairing food with a bell ringing (conditioned stimulus) and the dog eventually salivating on the ringing bell (conditioned response), even if the food did not follow. Pavlov's research was extended by Watson, who focused on the conditioning of emotions. Many will be familiar with his 'little Albert' experiment. In this experiment, a 9-month-old child was presented with a rat. Whilst little Albert did not initially show fear of the rat, the experimenters made a loud noise by hitting a metal rod every time the rat was present, causing little Albert to cry. Following repetition, little Albert showed fear towards the rat, even without the loud noise. Watson also conducted research on 'deconditioning' (known now in its various forms as extinction, systematic desensitisation, and in clinical psychology as exposure therapy). With other children who feared certain animals, he created a positive environment and set about introducing the feared animal in a graded way, where a child could learn that a negative outcome did not follow.

In addition to classical conditioning, behaviourists such as Thorndike (1931) and Skinner (1938) extended this research to instrumental (i.e., operant) conditioning. That is, rather than focusing on the conditioned association between two events or states, Thorndike turned to the association between an event and a behaviour. He found that when a behaviour was followed with a reward, this led to increases in that behaviour (reinforcement), whilst following the same behaviour with something aversive would lead to decreases in the behaviour (punishment). For example, if you pat a dog and it bites you, you may then learn to be afraid of dogs, and this leads you to avoid dogs in the future. In a health context, if someone experienced a pain or twinge in their back when they bent over, they may come to fear certain movements and avoid bending over in that way in the future. Later, these learning principles were extended by Bandura

(1969) to include learning through observation (e.g., watching someone else be bitten by a dog) and instruction (being warned about the perils of patting a dog), both of which can also lead to behaviour (avoiding dogs). It is not hard to imagine how Bandura's learning principles might be relevant to people's health, as we often learn about health information from family, friends, medical professionals, and the media. A friend's negative experience with a vaccine may lead us to be wary of that vaccine, just as a relative's health anxiety concerns may contribute to an increased focus on health and bodily symptoms. The internet is also full of misleading health information that can influence our decisions about health behaviour.

Hence, conditioning remains critical within health psychology, as healthy behaviours can be reinforced by positive outcomes (e.g., feeling energised after exercising) or even by the removal of a negative outcome (e.g., using an asthma inhaler to counteract an asthma attack). Healthy behaviours can also be impacted by negative outcomes (e.g., getting caught in the rain or feeling sore afterwards). Research and theories on conditioning also have important implications for taking active steps to change our health-related behaviours. As an example, we know that repetition is crucial in developing habits, both healthy and not-so-healthy (Lally & Gardner, 2013). Routine can help, as the cues will remind us of the behaviour (e.g., alarm = time to go for a jog).

Later Developments

More recent developments in learning theory focus on factors, such as extinction (how long does it take to learn that dogs are now safe, with repeated exposure to dogs without getting bitten) and renewal (if I go back to where the dog bit me, even after extinction, I might be afraid of dogs). These theories suggest that extinguishing a learned association doesn't 'unlearn' the original behaviour but rather learns another association over the top (Bouton & Swartzentruber, 1991; Vervliet, Craske, & Hermans, 2013). The originally learned association can then sometimes reappear, particularly when back in the original learning environment or if time passes without sufficient reinforcement of the new extinction learning.

These new developments are particularly relevant to health behaviour. For example, imagine a regular smoker who would often smoke with friends. Now, imagine this person is trying to quit smoking. They might manage successfully for a couple of weeks, trying hard not to pick up a cigarette when they normally would. Now, if this person goes back into the environment around friends, it is possible that they may pick up a cigarette without even realising it. Similarly, if someone often snacks in the evening and tries to stop this behaviour but then has a particularly stressful day or they are not at home, they may reach for snacks without even thinking.

Another phenomenon worth considering is the placebo effect. Of relevance to health psychology (Chaput & Herxheimer, 1994), it is often found to be the case that the effectiveness of a medication or procedure is not entirely due to the active ingredient (Wolf, 1950). Sometimes, placebos can have a negative impact, such as physiological side-effects to otherwise inert medications and procedures, often referred to as the nocebo effect. The placebo effect has been attributed to conditioning and expectancy (Stewart-Williams & Podd, 2004). Many medications, including those for health conditions, have a placebo effect, and this has helped to shape best practices for randomised controlled trials by emphasising the importance of having researchers include a placebo-control group in their studies. This area of research has suggested that we need to consider not only active ingredients in medications or procedures but also people's expectations, their experiences, and what is communicated to them.

Behaviour Therapy

Behaviourism had a large influence in clinical psychology, where there was quite a shift away from lengthy psychoanalysis (focused on uncovering unconscious thoughts, feelings, and memories) to a focus almost entirely on behaviour.

Behavioural therapy tends to focus on increasing desirable behaviours through repetition and reward whilst decreasing undesirable behaviours through removing unintended reinforcers, breaking habits, and making the behaviours more aversive. For example, applied behavioural analysis was developed to help people on the autism spectrum or with developmental difficulties reduce problematic behaviours and increase functional activities (Baer, Wol, & Risley, 1968). In addition, exposure therapy incorporates learning principles, where avoidance of a certain situation or object is addressed through graded, repeated exposure to this feared situation until the person no longer fears that situation and does not need to avoid it. Elements of exposure therapy are incorporated into almost all effective anxiety treatments, including those for specific phobias, social anxiety, obsessive-compulsive disorder, post-traumatic stress disorder, and health anxiety.

Many current psychological treatments in health areas rely on principles of behaviour therapy. For example, pacing is a common element of pain management, where the individual will incrementally build up their tolerance to a particular activity, such as sitting or exercising, allowing them to withstand longer and longer periods of these activities whilst their pain remains manageable. As another example, blood-injury phobia may prevent someone from engaging in the proper health treatment that they may need for a particular health condition. Exposure principles can be used to gradually, with repetition, increase that person's ability to be in a medical space and undergo medical procedures.

Humanistic Movements and Motivational Interviewing

Carl Rogers (1902–1987) was a prominent American psychologist, who is best known for establishing person-centred therapy. Rogers was also involved in the early humanistic psychology movement. The person-centred approach, as well as the humanistic movement in general, was intended to be an alternative to the prevailing psychodynamic and behavioural approaches to psychotherapy.

Interestingly, Rogers' theory about human behaviour and change was developed through the process of scientific observation; he and his colleagues were among the first to use recordings of therapy sessions in order to understand what therapist and relationship factors resulted in positive changes during psychotherapy.

Rogers theorised that each person has an innate drive towards growth and fulfilment or a 'self-actualising tendency'. This formed the foundation and central assumption of person-centred therapy. Rogers theorised that people could realise their actualising tendencies so long as they were in the right environment. As such, in the context of therapy, the role of the therapist is to provide an interpersonal climate that facilitates clients' self-actualising tendencies. Rogers proposed three important therapist attitudes that help create the right interpersonal climate:

- Therapists experience and express empathy for their clients.
- Therapists value, respect, and accept their clients, termed 'unconditional positive regard'.
- Therapists demonstrate authenticity and transparency, termed 'congruence'.

Consistent with the theory that clients have their own innate drive toward growth, person-centred therapists avoid directive or prescriptive techniques.

The foundations of humanism and person-centred psychology have significant overlap with the origins of motivational interviewing, which is a very popular intervention in health psychology contexts. Similar to person-centred therapy, the theory behind motivational interviewing was derived from clinical observations and the empirical study of therapy sessions (Moyers, 2004). It was developed by William Miller and Stephen Rollnick, who observed and studied therapy sessions in people with substance use disorders (Miller, Benefield, & Tonigan, 2001; Miller & Rollnick, 2012). They observed that directive and confrontational interventions were associated with worse outcomes, whilst empathic and non-directive interventions were more successful (Miller, Benefield, & Tonigan, 2001).

Similar to person-centred therapy, the assumptions behind motivational interviewing are that clients should be the agents of their own change, and the role of the therapist is to enhance clients' motivation for change without prescribing or directing them towards desired behaviours (Miller & Rollnick, 2012). The assumptions of motivational interviewing overlap with the humanistic belief that people strive for growth and fulfilment in the right conditions. As such, motivational interviewing therapists utilise questioning and reflective listening to focus on clients' ambivalence about change, their ultimate goals, and their perceived discrepancy between their current behaviour and broader goals. These techniques are employed to support clients' innate drive towards improvement (Miller & Rollnick, 2012).

Cognitive Behavioural Therapy

Behaviourism continued to dominate psychology until the 1960s. At this time, American psychiatrist Aaron Beck proposed a divergent conceptualisation of human behaviour. Unlike psychodynamic models, which emphasised unconscious motivations, and learning theory, which focused on observable behavioural responses, the role of cognitions was suddenly brought into the limelight.

The Cognitive Model

Aaron Beck referred to his new conceptualisation as the cognitive model. Whilst this model integrated principles of learning theory, it was the first to emphasise the role of cognition in shaping emotional and behavioural responses. According to the cognitive model, it is a person's interpretation of an event or situation which determines how they feel about it and, consequently, how they will behave.

The cognitive model went on to become the dominant approach to conceptualising human emotion and behaviour and led to the development of cognitive behaviour therapy (CBT). As the name suggests, despite the emphasis on cognitions that differentiated CBT from previous models, CBT interventions do not exclusively address cognition. Instead, they target the interplay between cognitions and behaviour. For example, cognitive strategies may be employed to directly alter the individual's negative beliefs (e.g., "I'm incompetent"), such as by examining the evidence for or against a given thought, evaluating the impact of different styles of thinking, and considering other possible ways of thinking. Subsequent changes in thinking are expected to translate into changes in behaviour (e.g., applying for a promotion at work), which in turn continue to alter the original belief (e.g., by disconfirming their original judgement of their own competence).

In line with this, strategies that directly target behaviours are theorised to subsequently alter cognitions. Behavioural experiments, which involve directly 'testing out' beliefs, are a potent example of this approach (Bennett-Levy et al., 2004). For instance, if an individual believes that worrying about a situation will help reduce the chance of a feared outcome, this can be directly tested out by experimenting with deliberately and excessively worrying about one situation, compared with restricting the degree to which one worries about another situation and evaluating the outcomes. Exposure therapy, which involves systematically facing situations that are usually avoided, can also produce changes in beliefs. Exposure therapy not only challenges a person's estimates of the probability or cost of a feared outcome but also challenges their beliefs regarding their ability to cope with anxiety and discomfort. Behavioural activation for depression (i.e., scheduling and carrying out goal-based activities) is yet another example; increasing one's level of daily activity to build a sense of achievement and enjoyment may disconfirm an individual's beliefs that they are a failure or that their situation is hopeless.

The Role of Avoidance and Thinking Styles

Using a CBT model, it is important to consider the role of maladaptive thinking styles, referred to as 'cognitive distortions' in Beck's early work (1963). These include catastrophising (e.g., jumping to the worst-case scenario), black-and-white thinking (e.g., viewing something as either good or bad), mental filter (e.g., selectively paying attention to certain pieces of evidence, such as one's mistakes), overgeneralising (e.g., assuming that one occurrence will continue to happen over and over again), mind reading (e.g., imagining that we know that others are thinking negatively about us), and fortune telling (e.g., believing that we know how things will turn out; Burns, 1980). Other unhelpful mental behaviours include rumination (i.e., the tendency to repetitively focus on negative thoughts or events).

Although various behaviours are examined in CBT, avoidance is arguably one of the most common, given its relationship to a number of psychosocial outcomes, including anxiety and depression (Jacobson & Newman, 2014), stress, and social support (Li et al., 2018). Whilst learning theory stresses the relationship between avoidance and the extinction of a fear response, CBT models extend this perspective by highlighting the impact of avoidance on cognitions. Specifically, avoidance is problematic not only because it prevents habituation to anxiety, but because it prevents the opportunity to disconfirm original predictions about feared outcomes (that is, to reduce estimates of the probability or cost of a negative event occurring).

Relevance of CBT to Health Psychology

The cognitive behavioural model is of clear value in the context of health psychology. First, it highlights the importance of beliefs that drive health-relevant behaviours. Beliefs about one's own efficacy, and expectations about the difficulty or outcomes of behaviour change, are all argued to contribute to health behaviours (Connor, 2010). Second, negative beliefs about illness or illness symptoms may increase distress about the illness and lead to a range of maladaptive behaviours. For example, in the context of chronic pain, thoughts such as "I can't cope with this pain" may contribute to feelings of anxiety and hopelessness. This may in turn lead to a person withdrawing from their usual activities or isolating from others, consequently worsening the negative emotions, as well as the experience of pain itself.

Several patterns of cognition have been shown to play a key role in a health context. For instance, catastrophic thinking (i.e., the tendency to magnify or feel helpless about symptoms) has been shown to predict symptoms in a range of conditions, including chronic pain (Craner et al., 2017), irritable bowel syndrome (Lackner et al., 2004), insomnia (Harvey & Greenall, 2003), and inflammatory bowel disease (Sweeney et al., 2018). Other key cognitions have been identified in the context of cancer-related distress. Positive beliefs about worry (e.g., beliefs that worry is useful and/or protective), beliefs about the need for certainty and control, and the level to which one's core beliefs about themselves or the world are disrupted by the illness have been shown to impact fear of cancer recurrence, and relevant behaviour (Curran et al., 2020).

The strength of the relationship between cognitions and symptoms should not be underestimated. A patient's beliefs about pain (e.g., the belief that pain signifies damage or disability) have been shown to be one of the strongest predictors of pain and functioning (Jensen et al., 1999) and are more strongly associated with quality of life than is pain intensity itself (Lamé et al., 2005).

Given this body of evidence, it is unsurprising that CBT interventions have been widely implemented in a range of health contexts. Such treatments typically focus on identifying and changing maladaptive cognitions and behaviours (e.g., avoidance) which contribute to the health problem or its impacts on well-being. Numerous meta-analytic findings have demonstrated the efficacy of CBT in patients with medical conditions and chronic illnesses (Bernard et al., 2018; van Straten et al., 2010).

Another important consideration is the interplay between physical and mental well-being. Growing evidence suggests that this relationship is bidirectional; that is, physical health problems can contribute to mental health difficulties, and vice versa (e.g., Vallerand et al., 2019; Schultchen et al., 2019). Numerous studies have also shown that psychological problems impact the efficacy of treatments for physical illnesses (e.g., Zautra et al., 2008). In particular, depression significantly impacts adherence to treatment and, consequently, treatment outcomes (Wing et al., 2002). Specifically, meta-analytic findings reveal that patients with depression are three times more likely to be noncompliant with medical recommendations; no such effect was found for patients with anxiety (DiMatteo et al., 2000). Taken together, addressing psychological comorbidities, particularly low mood, is of key importance in order to produce effective behaviour change.

Mindfulness, Acceptance Commitment Therapy, and Third Wave Psychology

The behaviourism of Pavlov, Skinner and colleagues is often referred to as the 'first wave' of behavioural therapies, and the inclusion of cognition by Aaron Beck is considered the 'second wave'. In more recent decades, a 'third wave' of cognitive behavioural therapies has emerged.

Third wave therapies include a variety of therapy approaches and techniques. The well-documented approaches include acceptance and commitment therapy (ACT), dialectical behaviour therapy, mindfulness-based approaches, and metacognitive therapy. Each therapeutic approach rests on different theories; however, there are some common features across each. In general, these therapeutic approaches emphasise the individual's relationship to their thoughts, emotions, and behaviours (Hayes & Hofmann, 2017). This is in contrast to second wave CBT, which focuses on the *content* of people's thoughts and emotions. For example, the mindfulness-based approaches theorise that the nature of one's awareness and relationship to their thoughts is a key mechanism of suffering. Relational frame theory, which has been central to the development of ACT, suggests that our tendency to identify with our thoughts and beliefs and not see ourselves as separate from them is a key cause of distress and suffering (Hayes, 2004).

To illustrate the difference between second wave CBT and third wave approaches, consider the previous example regarding a client who holds the belief that "I am incompetent". Whilst a CBT therapist would help the client to examine the evidence for and against this belief, an ACT therapist may encourage the client to see these as mere thoughts by reflecting something like "here's that story I tell myself about being incompetent again". Clients would also be encouraged to accept the unpleasant internal experiences that arise from this thought but then continue to engage in valued and meaningful activities. Whilst these approaches look different, they do share some important similarities. For example, both theories agree that thought processes are what bring about one's emotional states. Importantly, both approaches also emphasise the importance of behaviour change in producing improvements to somebody's emotional well-being and day-to-day functioning.

The use of mindfulness-based approaches and ACT have been particularly successful within health psychology contexts (A-Tjak et al., 2015). Because of this, we will elaborate on the premise and applications of each of these in the following sections.

Acceptance and Commitment Therapy (ACT)

As mentioned earlier, a key premise of ACT is that one's suffering results from becoming overly identified with thoughts and feelings. As such, ACT seeks to foster acceptance and mindfulness of these internal experiences without trying to directly change them. The theory follows that this will help people to continue or change their behaviour whilst being aware and accepting of their unpleasant internal experiences. These two ideas (acceptance of unpleasant experiences and engaging in behaviours despite them) in combination are called 'psychological flexibility', which is ultimately intended to help people act in a way that serves their ultimate values and desired directions in life (Hayes, 2004).

ACT was originally devised for people with psychological disorders, such as anxiety and depression. However, many have argued for its utility in other domains, and the evidence for ACT in a variety of contexts (e.g., caregiving, workplace relationships, sporting performance) is growing. In the context of health psychology, ACT shows numerous areas of promise and efficacy. Given its focus on promoting desired behaviours despite unpleasant internal experiences, ACT appears to be an excellent fit in the context of health behaviour interventions (e.g., smoking cessation, increasing physical activity, weight management). For example, somebody who values their health and longevity may have identified a need to increase their physical activity. Working toward this goal inevitably involves unhelpful thoughts (e.g., "I'm too busy and tired") and unpleasant physical sensations (e.g., muscle soreness, discomfort, and fatigue during exercise). This theoretical match is supported by empirical evidence; numerous studies have shown that ACT is efficacious in promoting a range of health behaviours, including physical activity, smoking cessation, and weight management. To illustrate, there is growing interest in the application of ACT to weight loss contexts. It is theorised that the focus on living consistent with one's values and achieving weight loss with these values and goals in mind may be more successful than traditional behavioural weight loss approaches (Forman & Butryn, 2015).

Mindfulness

Mindfulness is a therapeutic technique included in third wave therapies and is also a stand-alone intervention. Mindfulness-based stress reduction (MBSR) and mindfulness-based cognitive therapy (MBCT) have received the most attention as stand-alone interventions and have amassed significant evidence supporting their efficacy for a range of health, interpersonal, and affective outcomes.

There are many theoretical perspectives on the mechanisms and function of mindfulness, and the origins of mindfulness practice date back to Buddhist traditions over 2,500 years ago (Creswell, 2017). Despite this variability, past and current perspectives generally agree on two common mechanisms, or aims, of mindfulness practices:

1 Fostering a greater awareness of the present moment, including internal and external experiences.
2 Adopting an attitude of detachment, acceptance, and openness to these internal and external experiences.

There are also various practices intended to foster these states of awareness and detachment (e.g., paying attention to breath, conducting body scan meditations, mindful walking, and so on). Similar to ACT, the application of mindfulness to health behaviours shows promise given the helpfulness of states such as acceptance and detachment when people are trying to change their behaviour or cope with ill health. For example, numerous studies support the role of mindfulness interventions to help people manage chronic pain conditions, whereby an accepting and non-judgemental attitude may help people to cope and continue to function despite the presence of ongoing pain.

As well as these applications, theories suggest that mindfulness practice may help to improve people's resilience in the face of stress (termed the mindfulness stress-buffering hypothesis; Creswell, 2017). These theories have been supported with empirical evidence too. For example, the body of evidence that examines brain-related changes associated with mindfulness meditation shows that mindfulness practice helps with stress reactivity and overarousal of the nervous system (Tang et al., 2015).

Case Example 1: Pain and Exercise

This case example will elucidate how the different theories described earlier relate to a real-life health psychology context. Take the example of Mark, a person with a history of lower back pain who wishes to engage in daily exercise but is afraid of causing damage to his back. From a behavioural theory perspective, Mark has had past experiences with exercises that have been painful and therefore exercise has been conditioned to be aversive. Consequently, Mark has avoided exercise due to fear of pain. A behavioural theory approach to help Mark work toward his goal of daily exercise would involve graded exposure, or pacing, whereby Mark starts with a short duration of exercise which is gradually increased. With this repeated exposure to the feared situation and with each instance of no pain, the fear reduces, and Mark is more likely to engage in exercise again.

Applying humanistic theory to the case, motivational interviewing would be used to explore the pros and cons of Mark continuing to avoid exercise compared to changing and engaging in daily exercise, such as continuing to avoid exercise is beneficial for avoiding any potential pain but has disadvantages in preventing health benefits of exercise. Motivational interviewing can be further used to highlight discrepancies between current behaviour, e.g., not exercising, and the goals, e.g., exercising, such as "It seems that you have this goal of exercising, but you currently aren't doing any exercise, how do you see yourself achieving your goal?", all whilst emphasising Mark as being the agent of their change.

Within a CBT approach, Mark's cognitions and behaviours would be targeted concurrently. For example, the belief "if I exercise, I will hurt myself" is likely to govern Mark's avoidance of physical activity. A behavioural experiment could be used to test Mark's belief. This would involve Mark engaging in some form of exercise, discussing what happened (i.e., the result of the experiment), and whether the result provides evidence for or against his original belief. In the case where Mark does not hurt themself during exercise, this evidence can be used to weaken the belief, which will encourage Mark to engage in exercise in the future.

From a third wave psychological theory approach, such as ACT, the focus is not necessarily to change Mark's thoughts about exercise and pain but rather to facilitate acceptance of internal experiences (e.g., thoughts and feelings) and encourage desired, value-based action (e.g., exercise). As such, within the ACT approach, Mark's values in life would be explored, using questions like, "What matters to you?", and the answers are then leveraged to encourage value-oriented activity (e.g., exercise as an activity to align with values of freedom and independence). Additionally, Mark's thoughts about hurting themself during exercise would be encouraged to be seen and accepted as merely a thought by reflecting to Mark, "Here's that worry I have about hurting myself", and to accept the fear that may arise from this thought whilst continuing to engage in the valued oriented activity. This case example is further illustrated in Table 26.1.

Conclusion

When we travel, we generally have a good idea of *where* we want to get to, whether it is a particular street, city, or country, but no matter how well we envision our destination, without a map, we may never get there. In the case of psychological interventions and outcomes, theory is our map. Clearly, psychological theory plays an important role in building effective health psychology interventions. Through their underlying assumptions and hypotheses, theories provide a map that guides the clinician toward different interpretations of what an individual's problem is and how it is maintained. Consequently, different

Table 26.1 Theoretical perspectives

Theoretical Perspective	*Explanation of Mark's Difficulties*	*Therapeutic Application*
Behavioural theory	Mark fears exercise because in the past, he has experienced pain in response to increasing his activity levels.	Mark is exposed to the conditioned stimulus (exercise) without the feared response (extreme pain). Eventually, Mark learns that exercise does not result in extreme pain or injury.
Humanistic theory	Whilst Mark has the innate resources and drive to improve his situation, Mark is not currently situated in an interpersonal climate that facilitates these innate drives.	Mark becomes aware of the discrepancy between current lifestyle and intended goals. Mark is empowered to make changes.
Cognitive behavioural therapy	Mark believes that exercise will result in injury, and so thinks, "I will hurt myself if I go for a jog". As a result, Mark avoids exercise.	Mark conducts a behavioural experiment, and engages in some exercise whilst testing the outcome. Mark does not experience an injury and so revises the original belief.
Acceptance and commitment therapy	Mark's pain and fears represent barriers to living in closer alignment with their values and goals.	Mark chooses to engage in physical activity aligned with core goals and values. When fears arise, Mark notices these as only worries and continues to exercise despite these fears.

theoretical perspectives will tend towards different solutions (i.e., interventions) that address these factors. Theoretical movements come and go, and invariably influence each other. The emergence of behaviourist, humanist, and now cognitive behavioural approaches to psychological interventions covers a hundred years of theoretical development, research, and history in psychology. Understanding these different theoretical perspectives and those that will emerge in the future allows us to understand *why* a particular intervention may or may not work. However, more than that, possessing an understanding of different theoretical perspectives and the health psychology interventions that emerge from them allows us to understand how one might integrate interventions in a way that is empirically supported and conceptually sound. As will be discussed in later chapters, in general, interventions that emerge from different theoretical orientations have different degrees of empirical evidence supporting their clinical implementation. However, most good interventions in health psychology start with a good theory.

Further Reading

Bennett-Levy, J., Butler, G., Fennell, M., Hackman, A., Mueller, M., & Westbrook, D. (2004). *Oxford guide to behavioural experiments in cognitive therapy*. Oxford University Press: New York. https://doi.org/10.1093/med:psych/9780198529163.001.0001

Hagger, M.S., Cameron, L.D., Hamilton, K., Hankonen, N., & Lintunen, T. (2020). *The handbook of behavior change*. Cambridge University Press. https://doi.org/10.1017/9781108677318

Michie, S., Campbell, R., Brown, J., & West, R. (2014). *ABC of behaviour change theories*. Silverback Publishing. https://www.behaviourchangetheories.com/

Sallis, J.F., Owen, N., & Fisher, E. (2015). Ecological models of health behavior. In K. Glanz, B.K. Rimer, & K. Viswanath (Eds.), *Health Behavior: Theory, Research, and Practice* (5th ed., 43–64). John Wiley & Sons. https://www.wiley.com/en-au/Health+Behavior:+Theory,+Research,+and+Practice,+5th+Edition-p-9781118628980

References

A-Tjak, J.G., Davis, M.L., Morina, N., Powers, M.B., Smits, J.A., & Emmelkamp, P.M. (2015). A meta-analysis of the efficacy of acceptance and commitment therapy for clinically relevant mental and physical health problems. *Psychotherapy and Psychosomatics*, *84*(1), 30–36.

Baer, D.M., Wolf, M.M., & Risley, T.R. (1968). Some current dimensions of applied behavior analysis. *Journal of Applied Behavior Analysis*, *1*, 91–97.

Bandura, A. (1969). Social-learning theory of identificatory processes. In: Goslin, D., (Ed.), *Handbook of socialization theory and research*. Rand McNally & Co, 213–261.

Beck, A.T. (1963). Thinking and depression: I. Idiosyncratic content and cognitive distortions. *Archives of General Psychiatry*, *9*(4), 324–333.

Bennett-Levy, J., Butler, G., Fennell, M., Hackman, A., Mueller, M., & Westbrook, D. (2004). *Oxford guide to behavioural experiments in cognitive therapy*. New York: Oxford University Press.

Bernard, P., Romain, A.J., Caudroit, J., Chevance, G., Carayol, M., Gourlan, M., Needham Dancause, K., & Moullec, G. (2018). Cognitive behavior therapy combined with exercise for adults with chronic diseases: Systematic review and meta-analysis. *Health Psychology*, *37*(5), 433–450.

Bouton, M.E., & Swartzentruber, D. (1991). Sources of relapse after extinction in Pavlovian and instrumental learning. *Clinical Psychology Review*, *11*, 123–140.

Burns, D.D. (1980). *Feeling good: The new mood therapy*. William Morrow and Company.

Chaput de Saintonge, D.M., Herxheimer, A. (1994). Harnessing placebo effects in health care. *Lancet*, *344*, 995–998.

Connor, M. (2010). Cognitive determinants of health behaviour (pp. 19–30). In A. Steptoe (Ed.) *Handbook of behavioral medicine*. Springer Science and Business Media.

Craner, J.R., Sperry, J.A., Koball, A.M., Morrison, E.J., & Gilliam, W.P. (2017). Unique contributions of acceptance and catastrophizing on chronic pain adaptation. *International Journal of Behavioral Medicine*, *24*, 542–551.

Creswell, J.D. (2017). Mindfulness interventions. *Annual Review of Psychology*, *68*(1), 491–516.

Curran, L., Sharpe, L., MacCann, C., & Butow, P. (2020). Testing a model of fear of cancer recurrence or progression: The central role of intrusions, death anxiety and threat appraisal. *Journal of Behavioral Medicine*, *43*, 225–236.

DiMatteo, M.R., Lepper, H.S., & Croghan, T.W. (2000). Meta-analysis of the effects of anxiety and depression on patient adherence. *Arch Intern Med*, *160*(14), 2101–2107.

Forman, E.M., & Butryn, M.L. (2015). A new look at the science of weight control: How acceptance and commitment strategies can address the challenge of self-regulation. *Appetite*, *84*, 171–180.

Harvey, A.G., & Greenall, E. (2003). Catastrophic worry in primary insomnia. *Journal of Behaviour Therapy and Experimental Psychiatry*, *34*, 11–23.
Hayes, S.C. (2004). Acceptance and commitment therapy, relational frame theory, and the third wave of behavioral and cognitive therapies. *Behavior Therapy*, *35*(4), 639–65.
Hayes, S.C., & Hofmann, S.G. (2017) The third wave of cognitive behavioral therapy and the rise of process-based care. *World Psychiatry*, *16*(3), 245.
Jacobson, N.C., & Newman, M.G. (2014). Avoidance mediates the relationship between anxiety and depression over a decade later. *Journal of Anxiety Disorders*, *28*(5), 437–445.
Jensen, M.P., Romano, J.M., Turner, J.A., Good, A.B., & Wald, L.H. (1999). Patient beliefs predict patient functioning: Further support for a cognitive-behavioural model of chronic pain. *Pain*, *81*, 95–104.
Lackner, J.M., Quigley, B.M., & Blanchard, E.B. (2004). Depression and abdominal pain in IBS patients: The mediating role of catastrophizing. *Psychosomatic Medicine*, *66*, 435–441.
Lally, P., & Gardner, B. (2013). Promoting habit formation. *Health Psychology Review*, *7*, S137–S158.
Lamé, I.E., Peters, M.L., Vlaeyen, J.W.S., Kleef, M.V., & Patijn, J. (2005). Quality of life in chronic pain is more associated with beliefs about pain, than with pain intensity. *European Journal of Pain*, *9*(1), 15–24.
Li, M., Eschenauer, R., & Persaud, V. (2018). Between avoidance and problem solving: Resilience, self-efficacy and social support seeking. *Journal of Counseling & Development*, *96*(2), 132–143.
Moyers, T.B. History and happenstance: How motivational interviewing got its start (2004). *Journal of Cognitive Psychotherapy*, *18*(4), 291–98.
Miller, W.R., Benefield, R.G., & Tonigan, J.S. (2001). Enhancing motivation for change in problem drinking: A controlled comparison of two therapist styles. In C. E. Hill (Ed.), *Helping skills: The empirical foundation* (pp. 243–255). American Psychological Association.
Miller, W.R., & Rollnick S. (2012). *Motivational interviewing: Helping people change*. Guilford Press.
Schultchen, D., Reichenberger, J., Mittl, T., Weh, T.R.M., Smyth, J.M., Blechert, J., & Pollatos, O. (2019). Bidirectional relationship of stress and affect with physical activity and healthy eating. *British Journal of Health Psychology*, *24*(2), 315–333.
Skinner BF (1938). *The behavior of organisms: An experimental analysis*. Oxford, England: Appleton-Century.
Stewart-Williams S, Podd J. (2004). The Placebo effect: Dissolving the expectancy versus conditioning debate. *Psychological Bulletin*, *130*, 324–340.
Sweeney, L., Moss-Morris, R., Czuber-Dochan, W., Meade, L., Chumbley, G., & Norton, C. (2018). Systematic review: Psychosocial factors associated with pain in inflammatory bowel disease. *Alimentary Pharmacology & Therapeutics*, *7*(6), 715–729.
Tang, Y.-Y., Hölzel, B.K., & Posner, M.I. (2015). The neuroscience of mindfulness meditation. *Nature Reviews Neuroscience*, *16*(4), 213–25.
Thorndike, E.L. (1931) *Human learning*. New York; London: The Century Co.
Vallerand, I.A., Patten, S.B., & Barnabe, C. (2019). Depression and the risk of rheumatoid arthritis. *Current Opinion in Rheumatology*, *31*(3), 279–284.
Van Straten, A., Garaedts, A., Verdonck-de Leeuw, I., Andersson, G., & Cuijpers, P. (2010). Psychological treatment of depressive symptoms in patients with medical disorders: A meta-analysis. *Journal of Psychosomatic Research*, *69*, 23–32.
Vervliet, B., Craske, M.G., & Hermans, D. (2013). Fear extinction and relapse: State of the art. *Annual Review of Clinical Psychology*, *9*, 215–248.
Wing, R.R., Phelan, S., & Tate, D. (2002). The role of adherence in mediating the relationship between depression and health outcomes. *Journal of Psychosomatic Research*, *53*(4), 877–881.

Wolf, S. (1950) The effect of suggestion and conditioning on the action of chemical agents in human subjects - The pharmacology of placebos. *Journal of Clinical Investigation, 29*(1), 100–109.
Zautra, A.J., Davis, M.C., Reich, J.W., Nicassario, P., Tennen, H., Finan, P., Kratz, A., Parrish, B., & Irwin, M.R. (2008). Comparison of cognitive behavioral and mindfulness meditation interventions on adaptation to rheumatoid arthritis for patients with and without history of recurrent depression. *Journal of Consulting and Clinical Psychology, 76*(3), 408–421.

27

INTERVENTIONS IN CHRONIC DISEASE

Amelia Williams and Amelia J. Lake

Introduction

Non-communicable diseases, also known as chronic conditions, are a leading cause of morbidity and mortality, a trend projected to continue for decades to come. Forecasts from the Global Burden of Diseases, Injuries, and Risk Factors Study indicate that six of the seven leading causes of death in 2040 will be due to chronic conditions, including respiratory and cardiovascular diseases, chronic kidney disease, Alzheimer's disease, and diabetes (Foreman et al., 2018).

Optimal self-management of existing chronic conditions is crucial if we are to prevent complications and protect health systems worldwide. Living with and managing chronic conditions can be burdensome and significantly impact an individual's physical, emotional, and social well-being.

Diabetes, a chronic condition characterised by impaired glucose regulation, is a typical example. The condition affects 537 million people worldwide and is projected to rise to 783 million by 2045 (International Diabetes Federation, 2021). Diabetes is associated with an increased risk of macro and microvascular complications such as stroke, cardiovascular disease, chronic kidney disease, diabetic retinopathy (i.e., eye condition leading to vision loss and blindness), and peripheral neuropathy (i.e., nerve damage, particularly in the hands and feet).

Self-management of diabetes is central to health outcomes, a primary goal of which is to maintain optimal blood glucose. Diabetes self-management often places an extraordinary level of responsibility on the individual. Daily activities can include self-monitoring blood glucose, regular physical activity, ensuring a healthy diet and carbohydrate calculation (if required), and taking medications as prescribed.

DOI: 10.4324/9781003318026-33

While a multitude of educational, psychological, and behavioural interventions exist to support self-management, there are numerous socioecological factors that can constitute barriers to engagement. This chapter will focus on the factors that influence engagement with self-management interventions and what mediates their outcomes, using diabetes as an example.

Interventions in Chronic Conditions

Interventions to promote health can be conceptualised on three broad levels: policy, system, and individual. Policy-level interventions aim to improve health at the population level. Often population-level initiatives target modifiable risk behaviours to prevent the development of chronic conditions or related complications. Restricting advertisements and increasing taxes on products that are harmful to health, such as alcohol and tobacco, or including risk messaging and plain packaging to reduce consumption are examples of policy-level interventions (World Health Organization, 2017).

Systems-level interventions for chronic conditions aim to improve health-care systems and the quality of care. Health practitioner regulation agencies and professional practice organisations which regulate the quality and implementation of health-care services through clinical guidelines and professional development requirements are examples of systems-level interventions.

Individual-level interventions generally focus on modifiable factors at the personal level. Interventions that focus on increasing a person's knowledge and skills, and addressing psychosocial factors are examples of individual-level interventions. Given the centrality of an individual's behaviour in health psychology and the self-management of chronic conditions, this chapter will focus on individual-level interventions. However, it is important to acknowledge that health outcomes and behaviours are influenced via a complex interplay between individual, interpersonal, system, and population-level factors.

Individual-Level Factors Impacting the Effectiveness of Interventions in Chronic Conditions

Leading factors that can influence the effectiveness of interventions in chronic conditions include modifiable and non-modifiable elements.

Demographic Factors

Social, cultural, and economic factors, such as living and work conditions, cultural background, neighbourhood characteristics, and socio-economic status (SES), are fundamental determinants of health (Cockerham et al., 2017). While individual-level behaviour change interventions cannot directly address some of these non-modifiable factors, they should seek to acknowledge, understand, and accommodate them in health behaviour change interventions.

Often, different populations have varying needs and preferences or face unique barriers to chronic condition self-management. Commonly reported barriers to health-care utilisation among culturally and linguistically diverse (CALD) populations include a lack of cultural safety, lack of culturally sensitive information and services, and language barriers (Zeh et al., 2014). Conceptualisations of health and illness perceptions tend to differ cross-culturally, impacting how individuals engage with self-management. As such, interventions that are not tailored to the priority population are frequently ineffective in the long term (Gwynn et al., 2019). While strategies such as Public and Patient Involvement can be used to optimise the suitability and effectiveness of interventions for specific groups, the extent to which this is exercised in practice is variable (Brett et al., 2014).

The inverse relationship between type 2 diabetes and SES is well established (Connolly et al., 2000). Low SES is associated with poorer health outcomes and reduced access to high-quality diabetes-related health care (Grintsova et al., 2014). Socio-economically disadvantaged populations face unique barriers to health-care utilisation. For example, low health literacy can affect the degree to which an individual understands their condition, their ability to engage in self-management activities, uptake emerging technologies (Box 27.1), and communicate with health-care professionals (Hill-Briggs et al., 2021). Lack of affordability of medications, diabetes products, health-care services, and food insecurity reduces optimal diabetes self-management practices such as healthy eating and exercise habits. Low availability and accessibility of health-care services in underserved or remote communities and lack of transport further reduce opportunities to access care. Such factors influence the extent to which some interventions to improve diabetes self-management are feasible or acceptable.

Box 27.1 Are Diabetes Technologies Widening Health Inequalities?

Technology is playing an increasing role in the management of chronic conditions, including diabetes (see Chapter 25 in this volume for more information). Scientific advancements offer a range of diabetes-specific technologies that have been rapidly integrated as a standard of care. Such technologies, such as continuous glucose monitoring and insulin pumps, show widespread benefits for self-management, clinical outcomes, and patient self-efficacy. However, disparities in usage based on SES and ethnicity have been well documented (Agarwal et al., 2022). Prominent factors that impact an individual's ability to utilise diabetes technologies include accessibility, affordability, mismatch between consumer preferences and care models, lack of user education and wrap-around support to initiate and sustain use, language and numeracy-related barriers.

Psychological and Behavioural Factors

Optimal chronic condition self-management requires significant skills and motivation to successfully execute the complex and varied daily self-care activities (see Chapter 23). Educational and practical support are crucial for equipping individuals with the appropriate knowledge and skills. Beyond knowledge, psychological and behavioural characteristics and attributes play a significant role in shaping health-related behaviours. Research has consistently demonstrated the important role of personal-level characteristics, such as motivation, attitudes, self-efficacy, illness beliefs, emotions, and risk perception in self-management of chronic conditions, and their implications for intervention effectiveness (Schulman-Green et al., 2016).

Psychological distress, adjustment to the initial diagnosis, and ongoing emotional responses to living with a chronic condition are important and often overlooked aspects of self-management (see Chapter 24). Individuals with a chronic physical condition are more likely to be diagnosed with comorbid psychological disorders such as anxiety or depression (Clarke & Currie, 2009). In the longer term, the pervasive and relentless nature of managing a chronic condition may lead to condition-specific distress with implications for quality of life, emotional health, and physical health outcomes. For example, diabetes-related distress and mental health comorbidities are equally associated with reduced engagement in self-care behaviours, poorer quality of life, and suboptimal diabetes outcomes (Skinner et al., 2020).

Behavioural theory provides a basis for exploring the influence of psychological and behavioural factors on self-management which can be incorporated to optimise interventions in chronic conditions (more detail on theories and methodology in Chapters 1 and 4). For example, theory-based structured Diabetes Self-Management Education (DSME) programmes are widely considered a critical element of care (Zare et al., 2020). DSMEs are increasingly incorporating behavioural and psychological techniques into intervention elements (Winkley et al., 2020). Such interventions are often characteristically complex, given the multiple components and intervention targets, ranging modes of delivery, and variability of provider characteristics and training. This poses a challenge for design and evaluation, particularly with respect to selecting and specifying elements theorised to address psychological and behavioural factors and lead to change. Pragmatic approaches to integrating theory may offer a viable solution. The case study on p. 476 provides an example of such an approach, illustrating a systematic process of identifying determinants of sustained type 1 diabetes management, many of which were social and emotionally driven, leading to the inclusion of additional intervention components.

Interpersonal Factors

Self-management of chronic conditions exists in often complex and dynamic social contexts involving family, friends, peers, workplaces, communities, and health-care professionals. Interpersonal factors and social relationships play an important role in the effectiveness of interventions for chronic conditions (see Section 4 for more information on interpersonal relationships and health). For example, social support or influence from health professionals, family members, and peers is associated with improved diabetes self-management, psychological health, and clinical outcomes (Song et al., 2017). Social influences may also serve to impede self-management. For example, unsupportive or unempathetic interactions with health professionals, non-supportive behaviour or 'misguided helping' from family members, and negative judgement are known barriers to self-management (Litterbach et al., 2020; Miller & DiMatteo, 2013; Puhl et al., 2020).

Interventions to improve health outcomes for people with chronic conditions need to consider the social world of the individual. Ways through which this can be achieved are through mobilisation of social support and seeking to reach people or systems that influence self-management behaviour. For example, there is strong support for integrating peer support into diabetes self-management interventions which offers social support through a non-hierarchical, reciprocal relationship where illness-specific experiences and challenges can be shared (Azmiardi et al., 2021).

It is important to note that the emotional impacts of a chronic condition can extend beyond the individual. Increased burden, emotional distress, and lower quality of life are also common among family members of those living with a chronic condition (Kovacs Burns et al., 2013). For example, diabetes can have an all-encompassing effect on daily life for the entire family, particularly when the family member with diabetes is a child (Bluebond-Langner, 1996). Therefore, balancing the needs of the whole family when developing interventions for chronic disease is an important area of consideration.

The following case study describes a trial of a theory-based psychosocial intervention involving people living with type 2 diabetes and their partners.

Case study 1 "Two for one"? A couples-based behaviour change intervention to optimise outcomes for people with type 2 diabetes (Trief et al., 2019)

Background: Health risks associated with diabetes may provoke worry and anxiety among family members. Studies show that increased burden, emotional distress, and lower quality of life are common. Conversely, spouses or partners can influence self-management among people with diabetes. Interventions in chronic conditions that promote partner involvement and optimise communication may improve psychosocial and physical health outcomes. A three-armed, randomised controlled trial was conducted to explore the efficacy of a couples-based, telephone-delivered lifestyle behaviour change intervention for people with type 2 diabetes.

Intervention overview: A theory-based approach was used to develop the intervention, based on Social Learning Theory and Interdependence Theory. Participants in the intervention arm received couple's calls (CC), which included lifestyle behaviour education and relationship-focused content focusing on communication, collaboration, and interdependence. The remaining two groups received the behavioural intervention via independent calls (IC) or diabetes education alone (DE).

Results: There were significant improvements in HbA1c (average blood glucose levels over the past two to three months) and improved psychosocial outcomes among the participants with diabetes in the CC arm. Improvements in partner distress and relationship satisfaction were also observed among the CC group. However, no 'ripple effects' in lifestyle behaviour were observed. The acceptability of telephone delivery was supported by the participants, with a proportion indicating that they would not have participated had the intervention been face-to-face.

Key Points

- Including partners in a behaviour change intervention can improve physical health and psychosocial outcomes for people with type 2 diabetes.
- Partners may derive beneficial effects for psychosocial outcomes from the intervention but may need to be directly targeted to improve behavioural outcomes.
- Telephone delivery is feasible and may reduce attendance-related barriers.

Best Practice Recommendations for Design, Implementation, and Reporting of Interventions in Chronic Conditions

Interventions that improve population health and the outcomes for individuals living with a chronic condition need to be well designed, implemented, evaluated, and subsequently reported if they are to be effective. Many high-quality guidance and frameworks are available to support researchers in this process. Two of the most comprehensive are an updated (2021) framework for developing and evaluating complex interventions commissioned by the UK Medical Research Council and National Institute for Health Research (Skivington et al., 2021) and an intervention development approach called Intervention Mapping (Bartholomew Eldredge et al., 2016). Other notable examples include the very accessible Behaviour Change Wheel (BCW), an intervention development framework underpinned by a synthesis of 19 frameworks of behaviour change (Michie et al., 2014b) and guidance published by leaders in the field (Abraham & Denford, 2020; O'Cathain et al., 2019).

Common intervention planning processes and actions are summarised in Box 27.2. This section provides a brief overview of each theme. Importantly, intervention development processes are not strictly sequential. Rather, experts suggest that health behaviour change interventions be conducted iteratively, moving between activities until development is complete (O'Cathain et al., 2019).

Understand the Problem and Context

"The determinants of health must be diagnosed before the intervention is designed; if they are not, the intervention will be based on guesswork and will run a greater risk of being misdirected and ineffective."

(Green & Kreuter, 1999)

Box 27.2 Common Intervention Planning Processes and Actions

- Understand the problem and context.
- Involve stakeholders from inception and at every stage.
- Utilise behaviour change theories and frameworks.
- Plan for implementation and evaluation from the beginning.
- Register, report, and disseminate.

Developing a comprehensive understanding of the health problem of interest involves defining precisely what the health problem is, what the impacts are, and for whom, and in what context. The first steps can clarify if the problem is amenable to change via an intervention, and if so, what needs to change, who it should target, and at what level (e.g., individual, practice, policy).

An appropriate first step is a needs assessment, a systematic process of collecting evidence to understand the determinants of the health problem and the mechanisms that would lead to change. Needs assessment studies can comprise a variety of methods including primary (e.g., qualitative interviews, quantitative surveys) or secondary methodologies (e.g., reviews of the literature). A mixed-methods approach is often preferred. For example, a qualitative study may identify the personal-level factors impacting a behaviour for a specific population, while a review of the literature may identify existing interventions that could be implemented or adapted to the priority population/context.

Once data has been collected, appropriate intervention targets and expected behavioural outcomes can be identified. These, and the hypothesised causal pathway from the intervention to the programme outcomes and anticipated health and quality of life benefits, can be illustrated via logic modelling. Importantly, this work is not done in isolation. Conceptualisation of the problem can be enriched via the involvement of a multidisciplinary project team and other key stakeholders.

Involve Stakeholders from Inception and at Every Stage

Stakeholders are defined as persons with an interest or concern in something. In the context of interventions for the management of chronic conditions, the term applies to members of the priority population who are experts in their own care and who have a right to be involved in decisions that affect them. Meaningful involvement of members of the priority population from the outset is vital. The approach is known as Patient and Public Involvement and aims to promote research and interventions that are more likely to appropriately meet the needs of those it is designed for.

Culturally appropriate diabetes self-management interventions are associated with improved glycaemic outcomes compared with conventional care (Creamer et al., 2016). The following case study describes the co-design of a culturally sensitive intervention that identified unique barriers to self-management and the adoption of existing guidelines among the priority population.

Case study 2 Design of a culturally sensitive self-management intervention for African and Caribbean communities in the United Kingdom (Moore et al., 2019)

Background: African and Caribbean (AfC) communities in the United Kingdom (UK) are disproportionately impacted by type 2 diabetes. Barriers to optimal diabetes self-management include low health literacy, knowledge gaps, unmet social needs, distrust, and lack of culturally appropriate advice.

Intervention overview: The Healthy Eating and Active Lifestyles for Diabetes (HEAL-D) programme involved the development of a culturally sensitive self-management and support programme for AfC communities in the UK using a co-design approach.

Focus groups with 41 members of the AfC population explored perceptions of diet and lifestyle and barriers and enablers to the adoption of evidence-based type 2 diabetes management guidelines. Themes were validated through stakeholder consultation, which included community advocates and members of the priority population.

Utilising a co-design approach, 27 members of the AfC population took part in two co-design workshops to review intervention content and strategies to ensure the cultural acceptability of the intervention. These included the following:

- Reduced focus on weight loss as an outcome measure and preference for waist measurements over BMI-based targets (the latter considered culturally inappropriate).
- Verbal demonstration of practical intervention elements (e.g., culturally relevant cooking and health guidance, exercise classes, practical educational games).
- Inclusion of group discussion to meet social support and social comparison needs.

The involvement of other key stakeholders can also provide valuable insight. Family members are important stakeholders, and a lack of clarity about family involvement is commonly reported (Thirsk & Schick-Makaroff, 2021). Defining how the intervention is expected to improve health outcomes requires consideration of existing mechanisms and dynamics in the family unit. For example, interventions that focus on increasing knowledge alone are likely ineffective in promoting supportive behaviour (Thirsk & Schick-Makaroff, 2021), while parent-focused interventions for adolescents with type 1 diabetes may limit benefits to the child (Rey Velasco et al., 2020). Some other stakeholder groups to be considered in programme planning include those who are likely to implement an intervention, such as health-care professionals, those with specific expertise in the health condition, policymakers, and funding bodies.

Once the intervention has been designed, a key activity involves piloting (or pretesting) with key stakeholders, including members of the priority population. This important step can provide the preliminary measurement of the feasibility, acceptability, and efficacy of the intervention, allowing for iterative refinement.

Utilise Behaviour Change Theories and Frameworks

Theories of behaviour change describe the influences and mechanisms that govern a specified behaviour. They provide a scaffolding or framework to support programme developers to systematically identify and target behavioural determinants and inform intervention content (see Chapter 2). Moreover, behaviour change theories inform the understanding of the causal mechanisms involved in a particular health behaviour. Leading guidance recommends the explicit use of theory in developing and evaluating interventions (Abraham & Denford, 2020; Bartholomew Eldredge et al., 2016; Michie et al., 2014b; O'Cathain et al., 2019; Skivington et al., 2021).

While the relative effectiveness of theory-based interventions is a point of debate (Dalgetty et al., 2019), it is argued that this can be attributed to the ineffective use of theory which fails to link theorised determinants with intervention techniques (Hagger & Weed, 2019; Winkley et al., 2020). While the use of a single theory may not account for all change processes, taking an 'eclectic' approach by linking the relevant determinants of a health behaviour to 'useful' theories is recommended (Bartholomew Eldredge et al., 2016). Importantly, interventions with an explicit underlying theoretical rationale can assist evaluation by enabling the use of a common language for intervention elements and identification of the underlying mechanisms of change via mediation analyses.

Models and frameworks that synthesise behaviour change theories can support this process. For example, the BCW is a multi-layered intervention development framework that supports the programme developer from the identification of behavioural determinants to the selection of intervention components and implementation settings (Michie et al., 2014b). Further detail about the BCW components and their utility for intervention development is provided in Figure 27.1. The following case study illustrates the use of Capability, Opportunity, Motivation – Behaviour (COM-B) to sustain diabetes self-management (see Chapter 29 for more details on COM-B).

Plan for Implementation and Evaluation from the Beginning

Implementation is concerned with the translation and movement of evidence-based interventions to routine, widespread usage (see Chapter 30 for more details). Interventions that focus on efficacy alone may not be adopted or sustained because they do not meet the needs of the users, are inappropriate for the context they are implemented in, or are not cost-effective.

Implementation activities are varied. They can address and guide implementation processes, identify determinants of implementation, and guide process

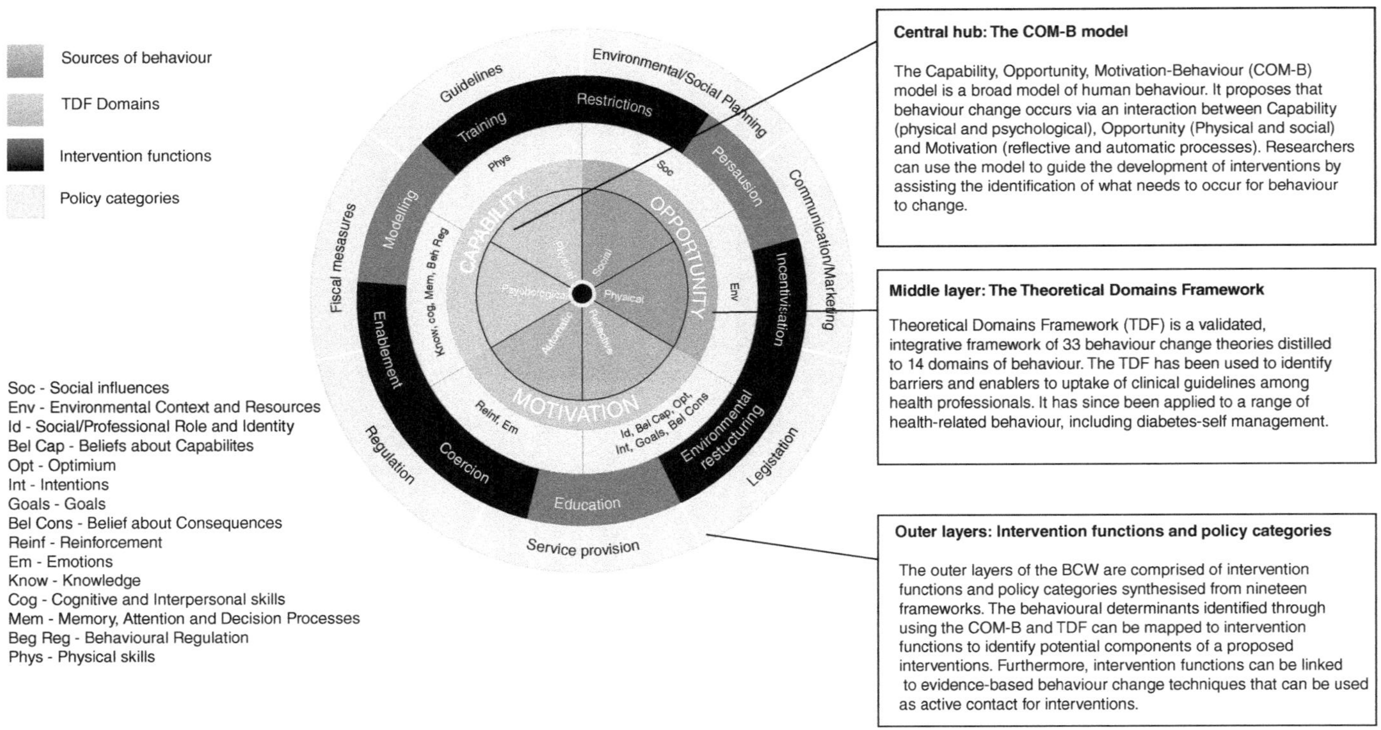

Figure 27.1 The BCW. *Figure based on Michie S, Atkins L, West R. (2014) The Behaviour Change Wheel: A Guide to Designing Interventions. London: Silverback Publishing*. www.behaviourchangewheel.com.

Case study 3 Use of a behaviour change framework to identify psychological influences on sustained self-management in type 1 diabetes (Stanton-Fay et al., 2021)

Background: Diabetes self-management interventions are often effective in the short term, but positive outcomes are challenging to sustain. The Dose Adjustment for Normal Eating (DAFNE) *Plus* study aimed to optimise an existing DSME intervention to promote sustained self-management.

Summary: Key behaviours required for optimal type 1 diabetes self-management were identified by key stakeholders. Barriers and enablers of sustained self-management were identified through a systematic review and health-care provider and participant-generated responses. Using the COM-B Model, a framework analysis was conducted to identify key determinants. The determinants were mapped to behaviour change techniques (BCTs), the irreducible components of an intervention (see Chapter 29). Existing content was evaluated to determine which BCTs were already included. The intervention was then refined to include additional BCTs to address key determinants.

Results: One hundred fifty distinct behaviours involved in managing type 1 diabetes were identified. Findings suggest that long-term management is driven primarily by cognitive and emotional influences. Common barriers included low self-efficacy related to implementing skills independently, beliefs about diabetes and self-management, difficulty with routines, and balancing self-management and life challenges. Emotional factors included anxiety about hypoglycaemia and complications, low diabetes acceptance, feeling burdened by self-management, and a sense of hopelessness when glycaemic targets were not met. Specific components were added to address psychological determinants and develop skills to integrate self-management into daily life.

Key Points

- Psychological influences play a major role in sustained diabetes self-management.
- Use of theory and frameworks enables clear specification of intervention components expected to lead to behaviour change.

and outcome evaluations (Luszczynska et al., 2020). Key questions to be answered when planning the implementation of an intervention for chronic conditions relate to the feasibility, acceptability, and effectiveness (see Chapter 30). These elements are critical if one is to increase the likelihood that the intervention will be used in the 'real world' and lead to intended outcomes.

It is important to gain perspectives from both the recipient of the intervention, and those who will deliver it and consider the goodness of fit of the intervention within the context it is intended to be implemented. For example, diabetes self-management interventions are commonly delivered by health professionals in primary or tertiary care settings. In primary care settings, time and resources are often strained, and available staff may lack the appropriate skills or expertise to deliver an intervention with fidelity (Rushforth et al., 2016). Training may be required, as will planning to ensure that workloads are not exceeded and roles are clearly agreed upon. Identifying and addressing such factors during the development phases can facilitate strategies that may help to overcome potential barriers.

Finally, without a well-planned, appropriately powered, and conducted evaluation, we do not know whether an intervention is effective. We will also not know how well it worked, how it worked, or for whom. Ensuring that intervention aims, outcomes, and hypothesised underlying mechanisms of behaviour change are clearly specified is a crucial task of effective evaluation planning (see Chapter 10). This is because if we are unsure about the specific changes that are expected to arise from an intervention, or the process that this occurs through, then the likelihood of conducting a meaningful evaluation is limited.

The task of selecting appropriate measures to quantify change is also important. HbA1c is a common outcome measure to assess the effectiveness of interventions designed to improve diabetes self-management. However, it is also recommended that other measures be used to verify whether an effect was gained through the proposed mechanisms. For example, a hypothetical intervention based on the Health Belief Model may propose that change is occurring via increasing the perceived threat of diabetes-related complications, perceived benefit of self-care behaviour, and self-efficacy. Biomedical and self-care measures would likely be included to determine if the intervention resulted in improvements in these constructs. Thus, in this instance, measures of specified components of the Health Belief Model proposed to promote change should be included both pre- and post-intervention to determine whether the intervention is exerting its effect in the way it was designed and hypothesised to.

A process evaluation seeks to determine whether outcomes were impacted by the way they were delivered and the context they were delivered in, with consideration to the fidelity and quality of implementation. Interventions in chronic conditions are inherently complex, often including numerous components and variations in delivery methods and provider characteristics. It is therefore necessary to understand the aspects of interventions or delivery that impact effectiveness to enhance wider implementation. This requires explicit measurement of fidelity, a clear description of intervention components, the context of delivery, and provider/participant factors. This can assist in elucidating why it may have been ineffective, what the barriers to implementation were, and how it can be optimised to better fit the context or population.

Evaluations of interventions in chronic conditions should also explore variation in outcomes and whether the intervention is reaching the target population. If an intervention is ineffective among certain subgroups, this is a potential indicator that the adaptation, tailoring, or design of a new intervention is inadequate or unsuitable. If the demographic characteristics of participants and adopters are not representative of the priority population, it is unlikely that it will result in meaningful outcomes for the groups for whom it was intended.

Register, Report, and Disseminate

Outcomes of intervention trials in chronic conditions should be reported irrespective of the outcome if knowledge is to be extended and research waste prevented. Guidance from the International Committee of Medical Journal Editors recommends the registration of clinical trials in a public trials registry (e.g., ClinicalTrials.gov) *at or before* the time of first participant enrolment. Once completed, programme developers have an obligation to disseminate their findings for the benefit of others and in recognition of the contribution of study participants. The Enhancing the QUAlity and Transparency Of health Research (EQUATOR) network, an international initiative provides reporting guidance for all main study types (EQUATOR network, 2022).

Conclusion

Chronic conditions have a major impact on people's lives. Interventions in chronic conditions typically seek to improve the health and quality of life outcomes of the person living with the condition while minimising the risk of developing future health complications. Those targeting the individual are grounded in health psychology and are known as health behaviour change interventions. Such interventions are inherently 'complex' due to the multi-factorial components of the intervention, range of behaviours and underlying psychosocial mechanisms that can be targeted, and the knowledge, skills, and capabilities required to implement them.

The first part of this chapter sought to demonstrate the scope and range of individual-level factors that can impact the adoption, sustainment, and effectiveness of health psychology and behaviour change interventions in chronic conditions. The second part synthesised the key themes of leading guidance and frameworks to assist the aspiring intervention developer with planning, design, development, and execution of health behaviour change interventions.

Further Reading

Hagger M.S., Cameron L.D., Hamilton K., Hankonen N., & Lintunen T. (2020) Changing behavior: A theory- and evidence-based approach. In: M.S. Hagger, L.D. Cameron, K. Hamilton, N. Hankonen, & T. Lintunen (Eds). The Handbook of Behavior Change. Cambridge Handbooks in Psychology. Cambridge: Cambridge University Press. http://doi.org/10.1017/9781108677318.001

Michie, S., Campbell, R., Brown, J., & West, R. (2014). *ABC of Behaviour Change Theories*. Silverback Publishing. https://silverbackpublishing.org/products/abc-of-behaviour-change-theories

Sallis, J. F., Owen, N., & Fisher, E. (2015). Ecological models of health behavior. In K. Glanz, B. K. Rimer, & K. Viswanath (Eds.), *Health behavior: Theory, research, and practice* (5th ed., 43–64). John Wiley & Sons. https://www.wiley.com/en-au/Health+Behavior%3A+Theory%2C+Research%2C+and+Practice%2C+5th+Edition-p-9781118629000

References

Abraham, C., & Denford, S. (2020). Design, Implementation, and Evaluation of Behavior Change Interventions: A Ten-Task Guide. In M. S. Hagger, L. D. Cameron, K. Hamilton, N. Hankonen, & T. Lintunen (Eds.), *The handbook of behavior change* (pp. 269–284). Cambridge University Press.

Agarwal, S., Simmonds, I., & Myers, A. K. (2022). The use of diabetes technology to address inequity in health outcomes: Limitations and opportunities. *Current Diabetes Reports*, *22*(7), 275–281. https://doi.org/10.1007/s11892-022-01470-3

Azmiardi, A., Murti, B., Febrinasari, R. P., & Tamtomo, D. G. (2021). The effect of peer support in diabetes self-management education on glycemic control in patients with type 2 diabetes: a systematic review and meta-analysis. *Epidemiology and Health*, *43*, e2021090. https://doi.org/10.4178/epih.e2021090

Bartholomew Eldredge, L. K., Markham, C. M., Ruiter, R. A. C., Fernandez, M. E., Kok, G., & Parcel, G. S. (2016). *Planning health promotion programs: An intervention mapping approach* (4th ed.). Jossey-Bass.

Bluebond-Langner, M. (1996). *In the shadow of illness: parents and siblings of the Chronically Ill Child.* Princeton University Press.

Brett, J., Staniszewska, S., Mockford, C., Herron-Marx, S., Hughes, J., Tysall, C., & Suleman, R. (2014). Mapping the impact of patient and public involvement on health and social care research: a systematic review. *Health Expectations*, *17*(5), 637–650. https://doi.org/10.1111/j.1369-7625.2012.00795.x

Clarke, D. M., & Currie, K. C. (2009). Depression, anxiety and their relationship with chronic diseases: a review of the epidemiology, risk and treatment evidence. *Medical Journal of Australia*, *190*(S7). https://doi.org/10.5694/j.1326-5377.2009.tb02471.x

Cockerham, W. C., Hamby, B. W., & Oates, G. R. (2017). The social determinants of chronic disease. *American Journal of Preventive Medicine*, *52*(1), S5–S12. https://doi.org/10.1016/j.amepre.2016.09.010

Connolly, V., Unwin, N., Sherriff, P., Bilous, R., & Kelly, W. (2000). Diabetes prevalence and socioeconomic status: a population based study showing increased prevalence of type 2 diabetes mellitus in deprived areas. *Journal of Epidemiology & Community Health*, *54*(3), 173–177. https://doi.org/10.1136/jech.54.3.173

Creamer, J., Attridge, M., Ramsden, M., Cannings-John, R., & Hawthorne, K. (2016). Culturally appropriate health education for Type 2 diabetes in ethnic minority groups: an updated Cochrane Review of randomized controlled trials. *Diabetic Medicine*, *33*(2), 169–183. https://doi.org/10.1111/dme.12865

Dalgetty, R., Miller, C. B., & Dombrowski, S. U. (2019). Examining the theory-effectiveness hypothesis: A systematic review of systematic reviews. *British Journal of Health Psychology*, *24*(2), 334–356. https://doi.org/10.1111/bjhp.12356

EQUATOR Network. (n.d.). EQUATOR Network: Enhancing the QUAlity and Transparency Of Health Research. Retrieved October 18, 2022, from https://www.equator-network.org/

Foreman, K. J., Marquez, N., Dolgert, A., Fukutaki, K., Fullman, N., McGaughey, M., Pletcher, M. A., Smith, A. E., Tang, K., Yuan, C.-W., Brown, J. C., Friedman, J., He, J., Heuton, K. R., Holmberg, M., Patel, D. J., Reidy, P., Carter, A., Cercy, K., … Murray, C. J. L. (2018). Forecasting life expectancy, years of life lost, and all-cause and cause-specific mortality for 250 causes of death: reference and alternative scenarios for 2016–40 for 195 countries and territories. *The Lancet*, *392*(10159), 2052–2090. https://doi.org/10.1016/S0140-6736(18)31694-5

Green, L. W., & Kreuter, M. W. (1999). *Health promotion planning: An educational and ecological approach.* Mayfield Publishing Company.

Grintsova, O., Maier, W., & Mielck, A. (2014). Inequalities in health care among patients with type 2 diabetes by individual socio-economic status (SES) and regional deprivation: a systematic literature review. *International Journal for Equity in Health*, *13*(1), 43. https://doi.org/10.1186/1475-9276-13-43

Gwynn, J., Sim, K., Searle, T., Senior, A., Lee, A., & Brimblecombe, J. (2019). Effect of nutrition interventions on diet-related and health outcomes of Aboriginal and Torres Strait Islander Australians: a systematic review. *BMJ Open*, *9*(4), e025291. https://doi.org/10.1136/bmjopen-2018-025291

Hagger, M. S., & Weed, M. (2019). DEBATE: Do interventions based on behavioral theory work in the real world? *International Journal of Behavioral Nutrition and Physical Activity*, *16*(1), 36. https://doi.org/10.1186/s12966-019-0795-4

Hill-Briggs, F., Adler, N. E., Berkowitz, S. A., Chin, M. H., Gary-Webb, T. L., Navas-Acien, A., Thornton, P. L., & Haire-Joshu, D. (2021). Social determinants of health and diabetes: A scientific review. *Diabetes Care*, *44*(1), 258–279. https://doi.org/10.2337/dci20-0053

International Diabetes Federation. (2021). *IDF Diabetes Atlas* (10th ed.). http://www.diabetesatlas.org/

Kovacs Burns, K., Nicolucci, A., Holt, R. I. G., Willaing, I., Hermanns, N., Kalra, S., Wens, J., Pouwer, F., Skovlund, S. E., & Peyrot, M. (2013). Diabetes Attitudes, Wishes and Needs second study (DAWN2™): Cross-national benchmarking indicators for family members living with people with diabetes. *Diabetic Medicine*, *30*(7), 778–788. https://doi.org/10.1111/dme.12239

Litterbach, E., Holmes-Truscott, E., Pouwer, F., Speight, J., & Hendrieckx, C. (2020). "I wish my health professionals understood that it's not just all about your HbA_{1c}!". Qualitative responses from the second Diabetes MILES – Australia (MILES-2) study. *Diabetic Medicine*, *37*(6), 971–981. https://doi.org/10.1111/dme.14199

Luszczynska, A., Lobczowska, K., & Horodyska, K. (2020). Implementation Science and Translation in Behavior Change. In M. S. Hagger, L. D. Cameron, K. Hamilton, N. Hankonen, & T. Lintunen (Eds.), *The handbook of behavior change* (pp. 333–348). Cambridge University Press.

Michie, S., Atkins, L., & West, R. (2014b). *The behaviour change wheel: A guide to designing interventions*. Silverback Publishing.

Miller, T., & DiMatteo, R. (2013). Importance of family/social support and impact on adherence to diabetic therapy. *Diabetes, Metabolic Syndrome and Obesity: Targets and Therapy*, *421*. https://doi.org/10.2147/DMSO.S36368

Moore, A. P., Rivas, C. A., Stanton-Fay, S., Harding, S., & Goff, L. M. (2019). Designing the Healthy Eating and Active Lifestyles for Diabetes (HEAL-D) self-management and support programme for UK African and Caribbean communities: a culturally tailored, complex intervention under-pinned by behaviour change theory. *BMC Public Health*, *19*(1), 1146. https://doi.org/10.1186/s12889-019-7411-z

O'Cathain, A., Croot, L., Duncan, E., Rousseau, N., Sworn, K., Turner, K. M., Yardley, L., & Hoddinott, P. (2019). Guidance on how to develop complex interventions to improve health and healthcare. *BMJ Open*, *9*(8), e029954. https://doi.org/10.1136/bmjopen-2019-029954

Puhl, R. M., Himmelstein, M. S., Hateley-Browne, J. L., & Speight, J. (2020). Weight stigma and diabetes stigma in U.S. adults with type 2 diabetes: Associations with diabetes self-care behaviors and perceptions of health care. *Diabetes Research and Clinical Practice*, *168*, 108387. https://doi.org/10.1016/j.diabres.2020.108387

Rey Velasco, E., Pals, R. A. S., Skinner, T. C., & Grabowski, D. (2020). Pre-empting the challenges faced in adolescence: A systematic literature review of effects of psychosocial interventions for preteens with type 1 diabetes. *Endocrinology, Diabetes & Metabolism*, *3*(2). https://doi.org/10.1002/edm2.120

Rushforth, B., McCrorie, C., Glidewell, L., Midgley, E., & Foy, R. (2016). Barriers to effective management of type 2 diabetes in primary care: qualitative systematic review. *British Journal of General Practice*, *66*(643), e114–e127. https://doi.org/10.3399/bjgp16X683509

Schulman-Green, D., Jaser, S. S., Park, C., & Whittemore, R. (2016). A metasynthesis of factors affecting self-management of chronic illness. *Journal of Advanced Nursing*, *72*(7), 1469–1489. https://doi.org/10.1111/jan.12902

Skinner, T. C., Joensen, L., & Parkin, T. (2020). Twenty-five years of diabetes distress research. *Diabetic Medicine*, *37*(3), 393–400. https://doi.org/10.1111/dme.14157
Skivington, K., Matthews, L., Simpson, S. A., Craig, P., Baird, J., Blazeby, J. M., Boyd, K. A., Craig, N., French, D. P., McIntosh, E., Petticrew, M., Rycroft-Malone, J., White, M., & Moore, L. (2021). A new framework for developing and evaluating complex interventions: update of Medical Research Council guidance. *BMJ*, n2061. https://doi.org/10.1136/bmj.n2061
Song, Y., Nam, S., Park, S., Shin, I., & Ku, B. J. (2017). The impact of social support on self-care of patients with diabetes: What is the effect of diabetes type? Systematic review and meta-analysis. *The Diabetes Educator*, *43*(4), 396–412. https://doi.org/10.1177/0145721717712457
Stanton-Fay, S. H., Hamilton, K., Chadwick, P. M., Lorencatto, F., Gianfrancesco, C., de Zoysa, N., Coates, E., Cooke, D., McBain, H., Heller, S. R., & Michie, S. (2021). The DAFNEplus programme for sustained type 1 diabetes self management: Intervention development using the Behaviour Change Wheel. *Diabetic Medicine*, *38*(5). https://doi.org/10.1111/dme.14548
Thirsk, L. M., & Schick-Makaroff, K. (2021). Family interventions for adults living with type 2 diabetes mellitus: A qualitative meta-synthesis. *Patient Education and Counseling*, *104*(12), 2890–2899. https://doi.org/10.1016/j.pec.2021.04.037
Trief, P. M., Fisher, L., Sandberg, J., Hessler, D. M., Cibula, D. A., & Weinstock, R. S. (2019). Two for one? Effects of a couples intervention on partners of persons with Type 2 diabetes: a randomized controlled trial. *Diabetic Medicine*, *36*(4), 473–481. https://doi.org/10.1111/dme.13871
Winkley, K., Upsher, R., Stahl, D., Pollard, D., Kasera, A., Brennan, A., Heller, S., & Ismail, K. (2020). Psychological interventions to improve self-management of type 1 and type 2 diabetes: a systematic review. *Health Technology Assessment*, *24*(28), 1–232. https://doi.org/10.3310/hta24280
World Health Organization. (2017). *Tackling NCDs: "best buys" and other recommended interventions for the prevention and control of noncommunicable diseases*. https://www.who.int/publications/i/item/WHO-NMH-NVI-17.9
Zare, S., Ostovarfar, J., Kaveh, M. H., & Vali, M. (2020). Effectiveness of theory-based diabetes self-care training interventions; a systematic review. *Diabetes & Metabolic Syndrome: Clinical Research & Reviews*, *14*(4), 423–433. https://doi.org/10.1016/j.dsx.2020.04.008
Zeh, P., Sandhu, H. K., Cannaby, A. M., & Sturt, J. A. (2014). Cultural barriers impeding ethnic minority groups from accessing effective diabetes care services: a systematic review of observational studies. *Diversity & Equality in Health and Care*, *11*(1). https://doi.org/10.21767/2049-5471.100001

28

COMMUNITY-BASED INTERVENTIONS

Hamsini Sivaramakrishnan, Matthew McDonald, and Eleanor Quested

Introduction

Health behaviours that form part of everyday life, such as physical activity, have been known to contribute significantly to the risk of non-communicable diseases (NCDs), as well as quality and longevity of life (World Health Organisation [WHO], 2022). Although there may be small variations in national recommendations, overall, there is a consensus that increasing physical activity is a health behaviour that should be encouraged for primary and secondary prevention of NCDs such as diabetes, heart disease, and several cancers (WHO, 2022). However, most adults do not meet these guidelines, and the number of adults living with, or at risk of, NCDs is high and growing exponentially (WHO, 2022). As a result, considerable research effort has been invested into designing, evaluating, and implementing interventions to support people to be sufficiently active.

Oftentimes, health behaviour change programmes targeting physical activity for people with or at risk of NCDs are delivered in exercise facilities under the supervision of a health professional (see Chapter 27 in this volume for more information). For example, patients with cardiovascular disease may participate in physical activity in a hospital gym or community sports hall supervised by a physiotherapist. However, using exercise facilities and expert facilitators tends to be expensive, resource intensive, and has limited potential for sustainability or expansion outside of resource-rich metropolitan areas (Servio et al., 2019). Other solutions to promote health behaviours include exercise-on-prescription type interventions, whereby a health practitioner such as a general practitioner attempts to promote self-managed behaviour modification during very brief interactions as part of routine practice. However, research has shown that these types of programmes face a number of challenges, including limited adoption and feasibility in 'real-world' settings, and there is limited evidence of short- and long-term efficacy (e.g., Pavey et al., 2013). Other options for health behaviour

DOI: 10.4324/9781003318026-34

change may include commercial programmes, workplace programmes, and online programmes. Although there is support for the potential of these formats (e.g., Grimani et al., 2019), there remain numerous barriers to participation for large proportions of the population, and in many cases, those are also the populations most at risk. For example, people from low socio-economic circumstances, culturally and linguistically diverse people, and those residing in rural and regional areas tend to be disproportionally underrepresented in health behaviour change programmes, yet over-represented in the statistics of those 'at risk' (Lorenc et al., 2013). Such individuals and groups are sometimes described as 'hard to reach', while in actuality, it may be that the opportunities to develop and sustain healthy behaviours are hard to reach for those individuals. As we discuss later in this chapter, the social and environmental determinants of whether one does or does not (or can, or cannot) engage in or adhere to health behaviours are substantially more nuanced than simply 'lifestyle' choices that one does or does not make.

Community-based health behaviour change interventions provide an alternative approach to promoting healthy behaviours that circumnavigates some (but not all) of the limitations of the aforementioned facility-based or individually driven approaches. For clarity, in this chapter, we define 'community-based approaches' to be those health programmes that can capitalise on existing infrastructures in the community – for example, by being delivered in community facilities or settings by local, non-clinically trained facilitators. Programmes that utilise settings such as workplaces, schools, Universities, or clinical locations or staff would not be considered within this category. In their design, context, and content, community-based programmes can align with the cultural values, needs, and preferences of particular communities. As such, community-based interventions have the potential to be accessible, appropriate, and appealing when designed and implemented appropriately. Research supports this assertion; for example, cultural considerations in the design and delivery of a community intervention for African American adults living with diabetes in Detroit supported compliance and adherence (Two Feathers et al., 2005). In addition, community-based programmes have reduced reliance on specialist facilities, expertise, and resources, which is likely to increase cost-effectiveness which in turn may accelerate translation (Phillips et al., 2014).

Aims of the Chapter

The overarching aim of this chapter is to explore the role that community-based interventions can play in supporting the health behaviours of adults with or at risk of NCDs. Drawing from contemporary literature, and with a specific focus on interventions using sport as a vehicle to promote health behaviours, we will describe some of the key considerations when designing interventions for delivery in community settings. Next, we will provide an overview of the research that has capitalised on the appeal of sport as a means to engage people in physical activity and other positive health behaviours. Before offering our reflections on the challenges of this work, and recommendations, we will reflect more specifically on some of the equity issues often observed in research and practice related to community-based interventions. Overall, we hope this chapter will provide a broad summary of the state of play with regard to health behaviour change interventions delivered in the community. We also hope to provide stimulus to encourage the development of equitable, scalable, and sustainable community-based interventions in the future.

Considerations for the Design of Sustainable Community-Based Interventions

Community-based interventions can be designed for particular subsets of a community, distinguished by particular cultural or social characteristics. Or, they can be designed as community-wide interventions that target an entire population with a focus on one or more risk factors (e.g., physical activity, diet) or self-management behaviours (see Chapter 27). These may include person-focused programmes, including behaviour change interventions (see Chapter 29), delivered to groups in community facilities with the goal of fostering individual change. Mass media campaigns and environmental change programmes are also examples of community-based interventions. In this chapter, we focus predominantly on person-focused interventions.

Principles of best practice for the design of interventions for delivery in community settings mirror recommendations for designing interventions for delivery in other contexts or for specific populations. For example, there is merit in using models or frameworks such as the Medical Research Council guidelines, Intervention Mapping approaches (see Chapter 29), and the Behaviour Change Wheel (see Chapter 27) to guide intervention development and evaluation. The PRACTIS guide (Koorts et al., 2018b) is a model that draws on existing frameworks and has been illustrated as relevant to the design and scale-up of physical activity interventions in community settings such as the Football Fans in Training (FFIT) programme (Hunt et al., 2020), discussed both later in this chapter and in Chapter 30. The initial step of the PRACTIS framework focuses on characterising the parameters of the intervention setting using the 'five Ps' (people, place, process, provisions, principles) and, as such, is particularly useful for designing community-based interventions. From the outset, the five Ps highlights consideration of who will be involved and necessary for effective implementation, which settings and organisations will be needed to contribute, the process required for intervention delivery, the resources needed for success, and the principles (such as behaviour change theories) underlying the intervention and implementation process.

An important second step in the PRACTIS guide is stakeholder engagement. Stakeholders play a critical role in delivering and supporting the intervention, and may be responsible for the intervention or staff, equipment, or venue needed to deliver the intervention. They also have an important role to play in the development of strategies to help optimise the potential for successful implementation of effective interventions (see Chapter 30). Reliance on community stakeholders is therefore a central feature of successful community interventions, but equally, it can be a source of vulnerability. In many cases, the role of a stakeholder in delivering or advocating for an intervention may be left-of-centre to their primary responsibilities. Sustaining stakeholders' motivation and engagement, and establishing interventions that meet their expectations, is therefore particularly important. Hence, involving stakeholders and agencies and considering their priorities from the outset may be especially important for community-based interventions that are delivered outside of healthcare systems. Regardless of the setting, establishing and scaling up successful interventions is a complex process, and the potential for success is in part influenced by the level of congruence in the goals and expectations of stakeholders at the outset (Koorts et al., 2022). Consideration of how an intervention can embed within or complement existing initiatives may also be a strategy that can be adopted to improve the pace of community engagement, as existing structures and relationships can be utilised (Koorts et al., 2022). Other steps within the PRACTIS guide include identifying and overcoming barriers to implementation. Koorts et al. (2022) use a social-ecological model to illustrate the potential barriers to implementation and the importance of working with stakeholders to overcome those and design sustainable community-based interventions. We outline some examples of these social-ecological barriers later in this chapter.

Sport-Themed Community-Based Interventions

Providing appropriate community-based opportunities for sport participation may not only increase long-term engagement in physical activity but may also cultivate a sense of well-being (Walsh et al., 2018). Furthermore, the appeal of and connection with sport among large segments of the population creates opportunities for it to be used to package community-based health behaviour change interventions in a way that may be more appealing to or congruent with individuals' self-identity. This section of the chapter describes novel community-based sport or sport-themed interventions that have capitalised on this appeal and are geared towards tackling barriers to engaging individuals in physical activity and other positive health behaviours.

Football Fans in Training (FFIT)

Given the widespread appeal of sport, situating behaviour change interventions in community settings is one means to help engage men (and more recently, women) that may otherwise be reluctant to participate in interventions that have diet or weight management components. One such programme, which draws on the attraction of professional football (soccer), is FFIT. FFIT was designed to use the attraction of professional soccer clubs and settings to engage male supporters in a structured behavioural weight management programme (Hunt et al., 2020). By delivering the programme at football clubs, FFIT enhanced physical and symbolic proximity to professional football clubs and fostered a sense of team spirit among participants. FFIT included 12 weekly sessions of coach-led education and football-themed physical activity. This programme was effective at supporting men to lose weight, with a large proportion of participants losing a clinically meaningful amount of weight and keeping it off even after 3.5 years (Hunt et al., 2020).

Dads and Daughters Exercising and Empowered (DADEE)

Sport can also be used as a hook to engage parents and their children in physical activity. Girls are consistently less likely than boys to be physically active and participate in sports. Fathers have a vital role in influencing their children's physical activity behaviours and typically spend more time supporting and co-participating in physical activity with male children (Zahra et al., 2015). The Dads and Daughters Exercising and Empowered (DADEE) programme is a novel community health programme that uses sport to engage fathers and their daughters in a health behaviour change intervention that tackles gender stereotypes around physical activity (Morgan et al., 2022). DADEE demonstrated effectiveness in increasing fathers' and daughters' physical activity and improving daughters' social-emotional well-being. By incorporating behaviour change techniques (e.g., self-monitoring, goal setting) and psychological theory (e.g., Self-Determination Theory) in their delivery (see Chapter 293 for more information on behaviour change techniques), the FFIT and DADEE programmes provide examples of how gender can be considered in the design of community health interventions.

Walking Sports

Walking sports offer an innovative approach to promoting physical activity among older adults. Walking sport initiatives have used popular sporting rules and modified them to cater to older adults' physical activity needs. Adaptation of such sports that typically attract younger participants can help extend the reach of opportunities to individuals who would otherwise be unable or unlikely to participate (see Chapter 30). Walking sports are specifically adapted to lessen the cardiovascular demands of playing traditional sports such as soccer and netball (McEwan et al., 2019). By replacing running with walking, walking sports are low-impact, non-contact alternatives that may be particularly attractive to a less mobile, older demographic who may wish to be physically active and participate in sports but are unable to meet the physical demands of traditional sports. Walking versions of soccer, netball, hockey, and basketball are offered at local sports clubs across the globe, with walking soccer being the most widespread (Corepal et al., 2020). Pilot walking soccer programmes demonstrated high participant retention rates, were feasible and acceptable to males aged over 50 years, and were sustainable to conduct in a community-based setting (McEwan et al., 2019). Similarly, a large-scale evaluation found walking netball programmes to be acceptable, feasible, and effective in increasing physical activity in middle-aged and older women (Kinnafick et al., 2021).

Walking sport participation (much like traditional sport participation, see Sivaramakrishnan et al., 2021) is linked with a wide range of physical, psychological, and social benefits (Corepal et al., 2020). These benefits include reduced body fat mass and percentage, improved cardiovascular and metabolic fitness, and enhanced quality of life and psychosocial well-being (Arnold et al., 2015; Kinnafick et al., 2021). For middle-aged men experiencing mental health concerns, the inclusive environment cultivated within walking soccer programmes enabled participants to experience improvements in their mental health and well-being (Taylor & Pringle, 2022). For people living with dementia, walking soccer participation provided a feeling of pride associated with achievement and improved their mood, while the physical exertion involved improved their quality of sleep (MacRae et al., 2022). Walking sport programmes provide an example of how age and physical ability can be considered in the implementation and delivery of community health interventions. Yet, a range of other characteristics can play an influencing role in who interventions reach. The following section highlights equity-related considerations in community-based health interventions and research.

Equity Issues in Community-Based Health Interventions and Research

When implementing and evaluating community-based health interventions, it is important to assess equity issues that may impact access and/or emerge as a result. Health inequalities can be defined as the systematic, avoidable, and unfair differences in health outcomes between populations and different social groups within the same population or as a gradient across a population ranked by social position (McCartney et al., 2019). An 'inverse prevention law' describes how those most in need may be amongst the least likely to receive and benefit from appropriate preventative health interventions (Lorenc et al., 2013). Interventions designed to support individuals to make health behaviour changes without structural change typically require high levels of personal resources, education, and agency from participants to maximise the potential participation benefits (Adams et al., 2016). The degree of 'agency' individuals exert over their health behaviours is socio-economically patterned, with lower socio-economic groups more likely to have lower levels of health literacy and less likely to have the resources necessary to enact positive health behaviour changes based on their participation in community-based interventions.

Inequalities can occur at any stage of an intervention or research study. That is, interventions could be more accessible or attractive to, more easily adhered to, and/or more effective for individuals from more 'advantaged' groups, such as those with higher education levels (Birch et al., 2022). Individuals from 'disadvantaged' population groups, such as those from lower socio-economic areas or with lower levels of education, often face a disproportionately high burden of disease. If effective health behaviour interventions are not accessed by these groups, or if they reach across social groups but are more effective in more 'advantaged' groups, they may serve to augment health inequalities. Any such widening of health outcomes between population sub-groups is termed 'intervention-generated inequalities' (Lorenc et al., 2013).

Intervention-generated inequalities can occur across a range of demographic characteristics. The PROGRESS-Plus framework summarises these factors: place of residence, race/ethnicity/culture/language, occupation, gender/sex, religion, education, socio-economic status, social capital, and other additional factors ('Plus') (O'Neill et al., 2014b). In the context of behavioural weight management, a recent systematic review found no inequalities as per PROGRESS-Plus criteria; however, there was some evidence that groups classified as 'more advantaged' may be more likely to be recruited, adhere to interventions, and be retained (Birch et al., 2022). Indeed, some intervention types may be more prone to intervention-generated inequalities; for example, digital interventions for increasing physical activity were ineffective in low socio-economic groups but were effective in high socio-economic groups receiving the same interventions (Western et al., 2021). There may be a 'digital divide' due to differing levels of e-health literacy across social groups. Community-based interventions create opportunities to close such divides if additional efforts are taken to co-design appropriate interventions, adapt intervention content, or adopt more suitable research methodologies to engage specific sub-groups.

Unrepresentative research can sometimes be used to underpin health policy, potentially contributing to systemic health inequalities. For example, women, older adults, and racial minorities were underrepresented in randomised trials that informed cardiovascular care guidelines in the United States (Sardar et al., 2014). Participant characteristics relevant to health equity, such as indices of socio-economic status, can be inadequately reported or considered in the design of trials and interventions (McDonald et al., 2022). Recent UK guidelines to optimise the recruitment and retention of participants from ethnic minority groups to randomised trials highlight four key recommendations: (i) ensure recruitment methods and eligibility criteria do not unintentionally limit participation, (ii) develop trial materials with inclusion in mind, (iii) ensure cultural competence of staff, and (iv) build trusted partnerships with community organisations that represent ethnic minority groups (Dawson et al., 2022). These recommendations are designed to promote diversity without specific inclusion criteria related to ethnicity.

To engage some population groups, it may be more appropriate for community-based health programmes to have inclusion criteria that restrict participation to the specific target group/s. For example, supporting Indigenous people's participation in randomised controlled trials requires actively involving Indigenous research partners and respectfully drawing on Indigenous knowledge and values (Glover et al., 2015). In the Australian context, adherence to biomedical understandings of health and research methodologies (e.g., randomised controlled trials) may be divisive amongst some Aboriginal and Torres Strait Islander communities (Lin et al., 2016). For these types of interventions to play a role in addressing health inequalities for Aboriginal and Torres Strait Islander people, interventions should be co-developed with the community, integrate culturally safe person-centred approaches (e.g., clinical yarning, which combines cultural communication preferences with biomedical understandings of health), and utilise Indigenous worldviews and research frameworks and practices (e.g., decolonisation methodologies) (Gidgup et al., 2021; Lin et al., 2016). While some of these considerations are unique to Indigenous populations, the need for researchers to consider how community-based programmes may or may not be acceptable to or engaging for specific sub-population groups is evident.

Public health policy typically emphasises the need for community-based interventions to support improved health outcomes in priority population groups, and at a minimum, they should not contribute to the widening of health inequalities between groups. In some circumstances, community-based health interventions can be differentially attractive, engaging, and/or effective across different sections of the population. The reasons for these differences are complex but include factors related to health literacy, personal resources or agency, gender norms, cultural safety, and a lack of community consultation/involvement. The following section highlights further challenges to implementing community-based health interventions.

Challenges and Recommendations for Practice

As signalled at the start of this chapter, engaging and/or adhering to health behaviour recommendations is complex and substantially more nuanced than simply 'lifestyle' choices that one does or does not make. Several variables are known to influence whether an individual 'chooses' to engage (or is capable of engaging) in health behaviours. These include social, environmental, and political factors. A key challenge to delivering engaging and effective community-based interventions lies in shifting focus away from solely attributing health behaviours to 'lifestyle' choices and, instead, addressing the multitude of social and environmental barriers that may preclude engagement of the target population. In this section, in keeping with our focus on sport-themed interventions, we illustrate some challenges, limitations, and recommendations for implementing and delivering community-based interventions and specifically discuss some key considerations for implementing sport interventions targeted towards older adults.

Another challenge lies in tailoring interventions to the needs of the target population. Boulton et al. (2018) suggested that ageing adults who saw themselves as capable of participating in an activity, led fairly active lifestyles, and perceived physical and mental health benefits from participation were more likely to engage in physical activity. Although enhanced physical health was identified as a key outcome of sport participation, such activities may also increase the risk of injury, a risk that may be further exacerbated by age, thereby limiting the capacity of ageing adults to participate in sports (Jenkin et al.,

2018). Walking sports, as discussed previously, are modified to a slower pace and limit the risk of injury, illustrating how community-based interventions can be appropriately adapted to successfully overcome such limitations to suit the target population.

Some of the most important influences on individual health behaviours are social determinants of health (e.g., housing, income, cultural norms). However, one limitation of community-based interventions is that they are typically unable to tackle such social determinants. Among ethnic minority populations who may hold differing cultural and social norms surrounding physical activity and sport participation, inadequate social support and prevailing social norms may discourage involvement (Fleury & Lee, 2006). Sport tends to be viewed as being aimed at younger age groups and in some cultures for males rather than females; therefore, ageing adults and females may perceive their involvement in such activities to be inappropriate (Jenkin et al., 2018). As indicated previously, to overcome barriers for specific sub-populations, community-based interventions would benefit from co-design and adaptation of intervention content to fit their needs.

Aspects of the physical environment, such as walkability, traffic, and safety, were found to determine participation in community-based interventions (Bauman et al., 2012). Also, the affordability of the activity, whether in terms of equipment or membership fees, was an important participation determinant (Boulton et al., 2018; Jenkin et al., 2018). Notably, these aspects of the perceived and neighbourhood environment were linked with adults' physical activity behaviours even after controlling for demographic and psychosocial factors (Saelens et al., 2012). Therefore, to support individuals to make health behaviour changes, stakeholders responsible for community-based interventions would need to prioritise and facilitate structural change.

Barriers to participation present challenges to the effective rollout of community interventions. For example, older adults reported that a key barrier to participation was a lack of appropriate playing opportunities, particularly those in close proximity with appropriate facilities that catered for senior ages (Jenkin et al., 2018). Furthermore, organisational challenges have meant that these interventions are limited in their capacity to cater to varied demographic groups (e.g., gender, age, physical activity level). At a policy level, sustainability of the physical activity/sport offering was a key determinant – in Australia, stakeholders (i.e., sport organisations) reported a tendency to adopt a strategic focus on (younger and elite athlete) demographics that may be more engaged in sports (Jenkin et al., 2016). In terms of funding, to survive a precarious funding landscape, a strong evidence base generated from randomised control trials is required to establish intervention efficacy. Stakeholder support must also be strong and sustainable. Koorts et al. (2022) note however that the weight of the evidence base or community support could be diminished if the political environment was unfavourable and support was insufficient. With increasing neoliberal narratives and policies surrounding sport participation in ageing adults, there is a shift in responsibility, placing an undue burden on individuals to make healthy 'lifestyle' choices. Yet, stakeholders and the prevailing political landscape ultimately regulate the availability and sustainability of community-based interventions.

Little is known of behaviour change maintenance following participation in community-based interventions; some evidence indicates that integrating psychological mechanisms such as motivation, self-regulation, habit formation, and providing physical and psychological resources (e.g., behaviour change techniques) can support long-term behavioural maintenance (Kwasnicka et al., 2016). This growing body of research illustrates that in order to facilitate effective interventions to promote physical activity (and other health behaviours), it is imperative to consider not just the individual (and individual determinants of health behaviours) but equally the broader social and environmental factors that may influence the engagement of the target population. The social-ecological model (see Chapter 26) provides a framework to understand the complexities of individuals' behaviour within the context of their unique environment (Sallis et al., 2006). This model considers the interrelations between various nested social-ecological (i.e., personal, psychosocial, environment, organisational, and policy) levels with regard to specific health behaviours. To design sustainable community-based interventions, it is important to work with stakeholders to identify and overcome barriers at each level of the social-ecological framework. In theory, with appropriate stakeholder support and political will, effective community-based health interventions that align with public health policy should be well-placed for implementation on a wider population level (see Chapter 30). Yet, public health policy requires a specific focus to address matters related to health inequalities.

Conclusion

The literature is rich with an array of health behaviour change interventions delivered via different formats and settings, such as existing clinical services or online. Community-based interventions fill a gap for those who are not currently engaging in health services, and who find the possibility of taking part in a group-based intervention to be appealing. These types of interventions can capitalise on existing spaces and facilities, perhaps sometimes used for another purpose, making conduct feasible and sustainable. Integration with a setting or activity that may be of personal interest de-clinicalises such interventions and thereby may enhance the potential appeal to many. Community-based interventions may also benefit from further integration of key principles from health psychology research and theory to optimise behaviour change in these settings. Growth in collaboration between community organisations, community members, and academics would strengthen the possibilities to link research with practice. Yet, health inequalities need to be considered in intervention design to support improved health outcomes and minimise the risk of intervention-generated inequalities. The efficacy and sustainability of community interventions rely on the concordance between the target population, stakeholders, and public health policy.

Further Reading

Koorts, H., Eakin, E., Estabrooks, P., Timperio, A., Salmon, J., & Bauman, A. (2018). Implementation and scale up of population physical activity interventions for clinical and community settings: the PRACTIS guide. *International Journal of Behavioral Nutrition and Physical Activity*, *15*(1), 1–11.

O'Neill, J., Tabish, H., Welch, V., Petticrew, M., Pottie, K., Clarke, M., ... & Tugwell, P. (2014). Applying an equity lens to interventions: using PROGRESS ensures consideration of socially stratifying factors to illuminate inequities in health. *Journal of Clinical Epidemiology*, *67*(1), 56–64.

References

Adams, J., Mytton, O., White, M., & Monsivais, P. (2016). Why are some population interventions for diet and obesity more equitable and effective than others? The role of individual agency. *PLoS Medicine*, *13*(4), e1001990.

Arnold, J. T., Bruce-Low, S., & Sammut, L. (2015). The impact of 12 weeks walking football on health and fitness in males over 50 years of age. *BMJ Open Sport & Exercise Medicine*, *1*, e000048.

Bauman, A. E., Reis, R. S., Sallis, J. F., Wells, J. C., Loos, R. J., Martin, B. W., & Lancet Physical Activity Series Working Group. (2012). Correlates of physical activity: Why are some people physically active and others not?. *The Lancet*, *380*(9838), 258–271.

Birch, J. M., Jones, R. A., Mueller, J., McDonald, M. D., Richards, R., Kelly, M. P., Griffin, S. J., & Ahern, A. L. (2022). A systematic review of inequalities in the uptake of, adherence to, and effectiveness of behavioral weight management interventions in adults. *Obesity Reviews*, 23(6), e13438.

Boulton, E. R., Horne, M., & Todd, C. (2018). Multiple influences on participating in physical activity in older age: Developing a social ecological approach. *Health Expectations*, *21*(1), 239–248.

Corepal, R., Zhang, J. Y., Grover, S., Hubball, H., & Ashe, M. C. (2020). Walking soccer: A systematic review of a modified sport. *Scandinavian Journal of Medicine & Science in Sports*, *30*(12), 2282–2290.

Dawson, S., Banister, K., Biggs, K., Cotton, S., Devane, D., Gardner, H., Gillies, K., Gopalakrishnan, G., Isaacs, T., & Khunti, K. (2022). Trial Forge Guidance 3: randomised trials and how to recruit and retain individuals from ethnic minority groups—practical guidance to support better practice. *Trials*, *23*(1), 1–12.

Fleury, J., & Lee, S. M. (2006). The social ecological model and physical activity in African American women. *American Journal of Community Psychology*, *37*(1), 129–140.

Gidgup, M. J., Kickett, M., Weselman, T., Hill, K., Coombes, J., Ivers, R., ... Hill, A. M. (2021). Barriers and enablers to older indigenous people engaging in physical activity—A qualitative systematic review. *Journal of Aging and Physical Activity*, *30*(2), 340–352.

Glover, M., Kira, A., Johnston, V., Walker, N., Thomas, D., Chang, A. B., Bullen, C., Segan, C., & Brown, N. (2015). A systematic review of barriers and facilitators to participation in randomized controlled trials by Indigenous people from New Zealand, Australia, Canada and the United States. *Global Health Promotion*, *22*(1), 21–31.

Grimani, A., Aboagye, E., & Kwak, L. (2019). The effectiveness of workplace nutrition and physical activity interventions in improving productivity, work performance and workability: A systematic review. *BMC Public Health*, *19*(1), 1–12.

Hunt, K., Wyke, S., Bunn, C., Donnachie, C., Reid, N., & Gray, C. M. (2020). Scale-up and scale-out of a gender-sensitized weight management and healthy living program delivered to overweight men via professional sports clubs: The wider implementation of Football Fans in Training (FFIT). *International Journal of Environmental Research and Public Health*, *17*(2), 584.

Jenkin, C. R., Eime, R. M., Westerbeek, H., & van Uffelen, J. G. (2018). Sport for adults aged 50+ years: Participation benefits and barriers. *Journal of Aging and Physical Activity*, *26*(3), 363–371.

Jenkin, C., Eime, R., Westerbeek, H., & van Uffelen, J. (2016). Why don't older adults participate in sport. *Reported prepared for the Australian Sports Commission.*

Kinnafick, F.E., Brinkley, A.J., Bailey, S.J., & Adams, E. J. (2021). Is walking netball an effective, acceptable and feasible method to increase physical activity and improve health in middle- to older age women?: A RE-AIM evaluation. *International Journal of Behavioural Nutrition and Physical Activity*, *18*, 136.

Koorts, H., Eakin, E., Estabrooks, P., Timperio, A., Salmon, J., & Bauman, A. (2018b). Implementation and scale up of population physical activity interventions for clinical and community settings: The PRACTIS guide. *International Journal of Behavioral Nutrition and Physical Activity*, *15*(1), 1–11.

Koorts, H., Maple, J. L., Eakin, E., Lawrence, M., & Salmon, J. (2022). Complexities and context of scaling up: A qualitative study of stakeholder perspectives of scaling physical activity and nutrition interventions in Australia. *Frontiers in Public Health*, *662*.

Kwasnicka, D., Dombrowski, S. U., White, M., & Sniehotta, F. (2016). Theoretical explanations for maintenance of behaviour change: A systematic review of behaviour theories. *Health Psychology Review*, *10*(3), 277–296.

Lin, I., Green, C., & Bessarab, D. (2016). 'Yarn with me': Applying clinical yarning to improve clinician–patient communication in Aboriginal health care. *Australian Journal of Primary Health*, *22*(5), 377–382.

Lorenc, T., Petticrew, M., Welch, V., & Tugwell, P. (2013). What types of interventions generate inequalities? Evidence from systematic reviews. *Journal of Epidemiology and Community Health*, *67*(2), 190–193.

MacRae, R., Macrae, E., & Carlin, L. (2022). Modifying walking football for people living with dementia: Lessons for best practice. *Sport in Society*, *25*(8), 1405–1418.

McCartney, G., Popham, F., McMaster, R., & Cumbers, A. (2019). Defining health and health inequalities. *Public Health*, *172*, 22–30.

McDonald, M. D., Hunt, K., Sivaramakrishnan, H., Moullin, J., Avenell, A., Kerr, D. A., Birch, J. M., Ntoumanis, N., & Quested, E. (2022). A systematic review examining socioeconomic factors in trials of interventions for men that report weight as an outcome. *Obesity Reviews*, *23*(7), e13436.

McEwan, G., Buchan, D., Cowan, D., Arthur, R., Sanderson, M., & Macrae, E. (2019). Recruiting older men to walking football: A pilot feasibility study. *Explore*, *15*(3), 206–214.

Morgan, P. J., Rayward, A. T., Young, M. D., Pollock, E. R., Eather, N., Barnes, A. T., ... Lubans, D. R. (2022). Establishing effectiveness of a community-based, physical activity program for fathers and daughters: A randomized controlled trial. *Annals of Behavioral Medicine*, *56*(7), 698–711.

O'Neill, J., Tabish, H., Welch, V., Petticrew, M., Pottie, K., Clarke, M., Evans, T., Pardo, J. P., Waters, E., & White, H. (2014b). Applying an equity lens to interventions: Using PROGRESS ensures consideration of socially stratifying factors to illuminate inequities in health. *Journal of Clinical Epidemiology*, *67*(1), 56–64.

Pavey, T. G., Campbell, J. L., Fox, K. R., Green, C., Moxham, T., Taylor, R. S., ... Searle, J. (2013). Effect of exercise referral schemes in primary care on physical activity and improving health outcomes: Systematic review and meta-analysis. *British Journal of Sports Medicine*, *47*(8), 526.

Phillips, S. M., Alfano, C. M., Perna, F. M., & Glasgow, R. E. (2014). Accelerating translation of physical activity and cancer survivorship research into practice: Recommendations for a more integrated and collaborative approach. *Cancer Epidemiology, Biomarkers & Prevention*, *23*(5), 687–699.

Saelens, B. E., Sallis, J. F., Frank, L. D., Cain, K. L., Conway, T. L., Chapman, J. E., ... Kerr, J. (2012). Neighborhood environment and psychosocial correlates of adults' physical activity. *Medicine and Science in Sports and Exercise*, *44*(4), 637–646.
Sallis, J. F., Cervero, R. B., Ascher, W., Henderson, K. A., Kraft, M. K., & Kerr, J. (2006). An ecological approach to creating active living communities. *Annual Review of Public Health*, *27*, 297–322.
Sardar, M. R., Badri, M., Prince, C. T., Seltzer, J., & Kowey, P. R. (2014). Underrepresentation of women, elderly patients, and racial minorities in the randomized trials used for cardiovascular guidelines. *JAMA Internal Medicine*, *174*(11), 1868–1870.
Sérvio, T. C., Britto, R. R., de Melo Ghisi, G. L., da Silva, L. P., Silva, L. D. N., Lima, M. M. O., ... Grace, S. L. (2019). Barriers to cardiac rehabilitation delivery in a low-resource setting from the perspective of healthcare administrators, rehabilitation providers, and cardiac patients. *BMC Health Services Research*, *19*(1), 1–10.
Sivaramakrishnan, H., Gucciardi, D., McDonald, M., Quested, E., Cheval, B., & Ntoumanis, N. (2021). Psychosocial outcomes of sport participation for middle-aged and older adults: A systematic review and meta-analysis. *International Review of Sport and Exercise Psychology*, *17*(1), 398–419.
Taylor, D., & Pringle, A. (2022). Investigating the effect of walking football on the mental and social wellbeing of Men. *Soccer & Society*, *23*(7), 805–820.
Two Feathers, J., Kieffer, E. C., Palmisano, G., Anderson, M., Sinco, B., Janz, N., et al. (2005). Racial and ethnic approaches to community health (REACH) detroit partnership: Improving diabetes-related outcomes among African American and Latino adults. *American Journal of Public Health*, *95*, 1552–1560.
Walsh, B., Whittaker, E. M., Cronin, C., & Whitehead, A. E. (2018). 'Net Mums': A narrative account of participants' experiences within a netball intervention. *Qualitative Research in Sport, Exercise and Health*, *10*(5), 604–619.
Western, M. J., Armstrong, M. E., Islam, I., Morgan, K., Jones, U. F., & Kelson, M. J. (2021). The effectiveness of digital interventions for increasing physical activity in individuals of low socioeconomic status: A systematic review and meta-analysis. *International Journal of Behavioral Nutrition and Physical Activity*, *18*(1), 1–21.
World Health Organisation. (2022). *Global status report on physical activity 2022*. https://www.who.int/publications/i/item/9789240059153
Zahra, J., Sebire, S. J., & Jago, R. (2015). "He's probably more Mr. sport than me"–a qualitative exploration of mothers' perceptions of fathers' role in their children's physical activity. *BMC Pediatrics*, *15*(1), 1–9.

29

HEALTH BEHAVIOUR CHANGE INTERVENTIONS

Barbara A. Mullan, Caitlin Liddelow, Hayley Breare, and Chloe Maxwell-Smith

Introduction

Many of the leading causes of death in the world are preventable (WHO, 2022). Non-communicable diseases (NCDs) such as heart disease, cancer, and diabetes and communicable diseases such as influenza and COVID-19 are easily preventable through lifestyle changes, as has been highlighted in Chapter 27 and Chapter 28. Behaviours such as smoking, alcohol consumption, sedentary behaviour, poor diet, and inadequate hygiene practices are all preventable risk factors for the increased risk of developing an NCD or infection from communicable diseases (AIHW, 2021). Despite many people knowing the risks of engaging in such behaviours as binge drinking, many people still struggle to make positive changes to their behaviour. Changing health behaviours is hard (Kelly & Barker, 2016) for many reasons, and this is where interventions are crucial. Behaviour change interventions can be defined as "a coordinated set of activities designed to change specified behaviour patterns" (Michie, Van Stralen, et al., 2011). Often, the components that make up a behaviour change intervention are termed 'behaviour change techniques' (BCTs; Michie et al., 2013).

Over the last 30 years, there has been abundant research on the development, implementation, and evaluation of behaviour change interventions. During the height of the COVID-19 pandemic, the importance of behaviour change interventions for public health became a talking point in science and government (Bavel et al., 2020; Sibony, 2020). However, despite decades of research and implementation, most attempts to change behaviour have had zero to small success (Kelly & Barker, 2016). It is therefore important that to ensure successful behaviour change interventions, researchers and policymakers have an in-depth understanding of (1) the behaviours that precede non-communicable and communicable diseases and infections, (2) why people engage in behaviours knowing their risk, (3) what psychological theories and frameworks can be applied to

DOI: 10.4324/9781003318026-35

better understand human health behaviours, (4) how different behaviours can be changed via different psychosocial constructs and techniques, (5) how to select and implement BCTs, and (6) how to conduct a successful behaviour change intervention.

The aim of this section is to answer the previous questions to improve understanding of interventions in health psychology. Firstly, we will introduce to you, in greater depth, why behaviour change interventions are needed, with a particular focus on the need to prevent both communicable and non-communicable diseases. Second, we will highlight and discuss what makes a successful behaviour change intervention with some worked examples from key global behavioural health and science researchers. We will then provide an overview of the use of psychosocial theories and frameworks that can assist in developing, implementing, and evaluating behaviour change interventions. Chapter 29 will provide an in-depth discussion of the advancements in behaviour change, particularly focusing on BCTs and the strengths and limitations of their use. Finally, in Chapter 30, we will discuss how to maintain behaviour change in the long term through interventions, with examples of specific interventions that have successfully maintained behaviour.

Why Do We Need Behaviour Change Interventions?

Behaviour change interventions are a significant focus of health psychology research. Health psychology models often adopt a biopsychosocial framework and seek to explain the psychological underpinnings of behaviour from a contextualised understanding of health (Schwartz, 1982). Behaviour change interventions have a volitional focus. That is, the measurable change in an action, such as smoking behaviour or alcohol consumption, are key outcomes in behaviour change interventions, despite underlying psychological and individual factors impacting these outcomes. Indeed, the biopsychosocial model acknowledges psychological predictors of behaviour, such as intention to engage in the behaviour, attitudes towards the behaviour, and perceived control over behaviour, yet a hurdle lies in translating psychological change to the volitional stage (Schwarzer & Hamilton, 2020) or in bridging the intention-behaviour gap (Sniehotta et al., 2005). Consequently, interventions that target behaviour change as a primary outcome hinge on the assumptions that (1) the behaviour is modifiable, and (2) the change in behaviour will have implications for survival, longevity, or quality of life following a health threat (Conner & Norman, 1996). The potential for behaviour change interventions to improve survival, longevity, and quality of life outcomes spans modifiable risk factors for non-communicable and communicable diseases.

Behaviour Change Interventions for Non-communicable Disease

As rates of chronic disease rise (WHO, 2022), initiatives seeking to reduce health risk behaviours and promote protective health behaviours have become imperative. NCDs are those that cannot be transmitted from one person to another, such as cardiovascular disease, cancer, and metabolic diseases. NCDs are the leading cause of death globally, with an estimated 74% of global deaths attributed to NCDs (WHO, 2022). Many risk factors linked with disease morbidity are behavioural in nature, with Smoking, Nutrition, Alcohol, and Physical (SNAP) activity factors accounting for a significant proportion of the behavioural burden of disease (AIHW, 2021). Some characteristics, such as being part of a lower socioeconomic group, having poorer access to health services, and being culturally and linguistically diverse, put individuals at greater risk of NCDs and are therefore greater priorities for behaviour change. Advances in scientific knowledge, technology, and therapeutic approaches mean that people are living longer, many with NCDs (Cao et al., 2018). While NCD prevention efforts are important, controlling risk factors and management of comorbidity while living with NCDs have become necessary ventures. As such, a shift has occurred whereby reducing disease morbidity and improving quality of life while living with chronic disease have become primary concerns in research and public health.

Behaviour Change Interventions for Communicable Disease

Recent years have seen an upsurgence of behaviour change interventions to reduce the burden of communicable diseases. Communicable diseases include those that can be transmitted from one person to another. These diseases include COVID-19, influenza, and sexually transmitted infections. Some health risk behaviours, such as illicit drug use and unsafe sex, and protective health behaviours, such as medication adherence and health screening behaviours, have substantive roles in modifiable communicable disease burden. Behavioural determinants of such diseases have brought about interventions to promote protective behaviours against communicable diseases, including vaccination uptake (Ling et al., 2019), safe sex (De Vasconcelos et al., 2018), and food hygiene (Charlesworth et al., 2021).

The burden of disease permeates individual, societal, and political domains, warranting effective interventions for primary behavioural determinants (Michie, 2008). From a political perspective, effective health behaviour change interventions are financially advantageous, reduce the prevalence of morbidity and disability in the population, and reduce the burden on health sectors. On a societal level, behaviour change interventions can promote prosocial behaviours, harness community infrastructure to foster change, and increase health literacy. Finally, individuals have significant benefits to glean from effective behaviour change interventions. Impacts on an individual can encompass change associated with disease awareness and prevention through improved quality of life and disease management. Notwithstanding the promise of behaviour change interventions, the process of designing and delivering an effective behaviour change intervention requires a tailored and targeted approach.

What Makes a Successful Behaviour Change Intervention?

Deeming an intervention 'successful' may be based on the efficacy of the primary outcome of the intervention, like changes in behaviour or achieving the desired health-related outcome (e.g., weight loss, knowledge). Alternatively, success might be thought of as the utility and the potential implementation of the intervention into real-world practices. It is important that we consider both the effectiveness and translation of behaviour change interventions when designing and delivering interventions, with the intention of achieving community benefits and improved health outcomes. There are many options to consider when designing an intervention that may affect its success. While it is important to include evidence-based content, supported and informed by BCTs, there are practical decisions that influence the intervention's success. This is important when success is conceptualised in terms of real-world delivery and impact.

Delivery and E-interventions

Recent innovations in technology have seen an influx in the ways that interventions can be delivered. While face-to-face delivery was once considered the 'gold standard' for intervention delivery, variations in the procedure and delivery of interventions are now common and, indeed, may better suit diverse and priority populations. A prime example is the use of mass media campaigns. These include the delivery of public health messaging via television, radio, community exposure, and social media. Despite the strengths of mass media campaigns as wide-reaching vehicles for increasing awareness about health risks, the capacity for mass media campaigns to elicit behaviour change beyond awareness and education is an area for discussion (Charlesworth et al., 2021). The Australian Cancer Council's LiveLighter campaign has been effective at increasing awareness and eliciting subsequent healthy dietary behaviours (Morley et al., 2018). However, evaluation of other mass media campaigns by the Cancer Council, such as Find Cancer Early, suggests intensive and action-oriented initiatives are important, beyond increasing awareness, to prompt subsequent behaviour change (Croager et al., 2018).

Digital means for provoking behaviour change had previously been limited to mass media campaigns, telephone-delivered counselling, or non-interactive digital tools (i.e., videos, pedometers). However, the last decade has seen an exponential rise in varieties of digital interventions focused on behaviour change. Recent advances in technology, particularly smartphones, have facilitated opportunities for effective and targeted 'e-interventions'. One significant development has been the prevalence of smartphones in the general population and the utility of smartphones for hosting applications (apps). Apps provide an interactive and accessible vehicle for data collection and the delivery of intervention materials, such as BCTs. For example, apps can incorporate educational material, feedback, social networks, and behavioural prompts while capturing logs of health behaviours, such as nutritional intake and physical activity. Indeed, apps, when coupled with smart wearable devices, such as physical activity trackers, can be seen as powerful and scale intervention packages (McKay et al., 2019). Moreover, this resource-effective delivery may reduce the demand on research staff and health professionals and has the potential to bridge some disparities in intervention delivery (Hardcastle et al., 2019). However, they also highlight differences in technological literacy and access across target populations. Hybrid intervention models, incorporating face-to-face and remotely delivered components, mitigate these disparities (Maxwell-Smith et al., 2019). Other programmes that have included remotely delivered and digital components show promise for continued use of digital interventions, despite this being relatively new (Shoneye et al., 2020).

Length and Intensity

Interventions can differ in terms of their length and intensity, which both have strengths and limitations. Brief interventions are shorter (e.g., from five minutes to a couple of months), require fewer resources, can be less demanding overall for participants, and can result in meaningful changes in health behaviours (Aveyard et al., 2016), whereas long-term interventions (i.e., from six months onwards) require more resources, time and financial support. Importantly, interventions, whether short or long term, need to include longer-term follow-ups of behaviour change to judge the maintenance of behaviour change as it is common for many studies not to evaluate intervention effects beyond 12 months, making it difficult to understand if behavioural maintenance occurs after the intensive intervention period (Curioni & Lourenco, 2005).

To move towards future implementation of interventions, one strategy may involve slowly phasing out intervention components over time rather than having a sudden ending to the intervention. This may allow participants to maintain the target behaviour beyond the boundaries of the study. For example, for colorectal and endometrial cancer survivors at cardiovascular risk, the use of wearable technology supported by BCTs resulted in significant change in physical activity over 12 weeks, and improvements in physical activity remained at 24 weeks, even when intervention materials other than wearing a tracker tapered off (Maxwell-Smith et al., 2019). This strategy of tapering off interventions may help us to bridge the gap into translation, giving a real-world indication of whether an intervention has been successful.

Directions for Future Interventions

While there are no strict guidelines for creating a successful intervention, there are key considerations to be made when designing and delivering behaviour change interventions. Formative research that is accompanied by consumer representative and stakeholder involvement can support decision-making on intervention content, mode of delivery, and intervention structure. This co-design approach provides an opportunity to understand populations' preferences and support needs and the anticipation of barriers that may hinder behaviour change.

While 'no one size fits all', we can tailor interventions for populations with diverse preferences and needs, such as those with NCD, risk factors for disease, remote or marginalised populations, and culturally and linguistically diverse groups. Therefore, to be able to deliver successful behaviour change interventions, we need to design behaviour change interventions for and with the population of interest and embed these interventions with tailored, evidence-based BCTs.

What Theories and Frameworks Are Useful?

Theories and frameworks are useful tools that guide the development of effective behaviour change interventions. Interventions informed by theory and BCTs, for example, in dietetic practice and physical activity, demonstrate greater potential to improve health-related outcomes compared to interventions without theoretical underpinning (Rigby et al., 2020).

The Health Action Process Approach (HAPA)

The gap between intention and behaviour is one of the most highly studied areas within behavioural science. While intention is important, it does not always lead to behaviour change (Sniehotta et al., 2005). The Health Action Process Approach (HAPA) addresses this, as it encompasses both motivational and volitional phases (Schwarzer & Luszczynska, 2008). This social-cognitive model encompasses both motivational and volitional phases. The motivational stage includes risk awareness, self-efficacy, and outcome expectancies, leading to intention. Once intention towards a behaviour exists, planning occurs in the volitional phase. This motivational stage outlines that risk awareness, self-efficacy, and outcome expectancies are vital components that form intention to engage in a target behaviour. Once intention towards a behaviour exists, a process of planning must occur in the volitional phase. This phase involves developing action and coping planning, strategies for maintenance, and self-regulation.

HAPA acknowledges the roles of situational barriers and resources. For example, if there is a lack of social support, difficulties to continue to quit smoking are theorised to persist. Further, if there is a time barrier to engaging in physical activity, sedentary behaviours may continue, despite an intention to be physically active. Therefore, it is essential to consider and identify challenges where there may be constraints on opportunities and capabilities that play into the engagement of health behaviours.

Capability, Opportunity, Motivation – Behaviour (COM-B) Model

The COM-B Model can be a starting point to understand the determinants of a target behaviour and guide intervention design (Michie et al., 2011). The COM-B Model involves three components: capability, opportunity, and motivation, which are essential for behaviour.

'Capability' involves the physical and/or psychological ability to engage in the target behaviour. For example, when looking at handwashing behaviours, capability involves having the physical skills to wash your hands and further having the psychological skills to use the correct handwashing technique.
'Opportunity' refers to the combination of physical and social resources that are required for the target behaviour. This might include having social support from family and friends when quitting smoking and having access to a space to engage in physical activity.
'Motivation' is separated into reflective and automatic motivation that drives an individual's intentions to engage or not engage in the target behaviour. Both capability and opportunity can interact with and increase motivation when addressed during an intervention. West and Michie (2020) describe reflective motivation as the conscious motivation that requires intentional planning and evaluation towards the behaviour. Automatic motivation, rather, involves motivation from personal desires, habits, and routines that exist without conscious thought.

Taken together, these components are critical to understanding influences on behaviour. By breaking down the constructs needed to achieve the target behaviour, COM-B can provide direction towards tailored intervention designs and support decisions surrounding the use of BCTs. Across health contexts, the COM-B Model has been useful for guiding behaviour change interventions such as in digital weight management (Shoneye et al., 2020) and training health professionals (Mullan et al., 2022). An example case study of how the COM-B Model could be applied in diabetes self-management can be found in Chapter 27.

Intervention Mapping Frameworks

Intervention mapping frameworks provide a guide for designing interventions to address feasibility, intervention structure and content, stakeholder engagement, and implementation (Bartholomew et al., 1998). The Theoretical Domains Framework (TDF; Cane et al., 2012) is broadly used and outlines 14 key domains that help to identify and specify influences of the target behaviour. The TDF uses a behaviour change theoretical lens to address both behavioural problems and implementation challenges (Atkins et al., 2017). The refined and validated framework by Cane et al. (2012) outlines 14 key domains that help to identify and specify influences of the target behaviour. Examples include social influences, knowledge, goals, environmental context, and resources. Many studies have used the TDF to identify barriers and enablers of the target behaviour to support the intervention design (Alexander et al., 2014).

In summary, the intervention design process is important not only for determining feasibility but also for making practical decisions based on the influences on behaviour, barriers and enablers to behaviour, and strategies for implementation. We must distil the 'active ingredients' of interventions, taxonomised as BCTs, to draw conclusions and build knowledge of the particular units that comprise behaviour change interventions.

Behaviour Change Techniques

As highlighted and discussed in other parts of this chapter, changing behaviour is not easy. To overcome inconsistencies in behavioural interventions, and to improve the replicability and quality assessment of interventions, BCTs were developed (Michie et al., 2011). BCTs are the "irreducible, observable, and replicable components" of a behaviour change intervention (Michie et al., 2011). They are often termed the 'active ingredients' of interventions and target the psychological, social, physical, and environmental variables that influence behaviour. Michie et al. (2013) hierarchically clustered 93 individual BCTs, which were then further classified into 16 groups based on their mechanism of action or targeted theoretical construct.

Strengths and Limitations of Behaviour Change Techniques

While there are many positives to using BCTs in interventions targeted at changing health or social behaviours, the use of BCTs is not void of criticisms and limitations.

Strengths of BCTs:

- The BCT taxonomy (Michie et al., 2013) is the *only* current comprehensive and validated classification of active intervention components. It is a reliable method for selecting, specifying, and implementing techniques to change behaviour.
- BCTs and the taxonomy can be easily used and applied. Examples of researchers using BCTs in interventions can be seen in Chapter 29. In the London Borough of Havering, the local council employed the COM-B framework (see Chapter 29) and BCTs to develop several initiatives to improve vaccine hesitancy and uptake during the pandemic (Local Government Association UK, 2021).
- Many BCT clusters and individual BCTs are flexible in their use with different target populations (e.g., age, gender, ethnicity, religion), through different modes of delivery (e.g., online vs. in-person), and in different doses (Michie et al., 2013). Evidence suggests BCTs are effective both in-person and through digital technologies (e.g., phone applications, online) (Mullan et al., 2022; Engels et al., 2022).
- There is variation and choice in the number and combination of BCTs used in an intervention. The use of three BCTs has been suggested to be the best for increasing physical activity (Schroé et al., 2020), while the specific combination of the BCTs 'problem-solving' and 'providing rewards' in online interventions showed the smallest change across a range of healthy behaviours, compared to other combinations (van Genugten et al., 2016).

Limitations of BCTs:

- The current taxonomy does not provide explicit linkings with behaviour change theories (see Chapter 29), such that the taxonomy does not provide clear links between the BCTs and the theoretical constructs they are said to modify (Hailey et al., 2022), despite being clustered in this way. This means that sometimes incorrect BCTs are chosen when developing interventions, thus potentially being a waste of finite time and resources.

- Researchers, practitioners, and policymakers developing interventions or applying BCTs must have an in-depth understanding of the processes that underly and generate behaviours. Without this understanding, incorrect BCTs may be chosen that do not accurately target the underlying behavioural processes. In short, the use of BCTs requires a strong understanding of the target behaviour and how and why it works (Kelly & Barker, 2016).
- While some BCTs may be effective and successful for a specific behaviour or target group, this does not necessarily mean the same BCTs will be effective for other behaviours and groups (Michie, van Stralen, et al., 2011) despite some evidence to suggest this. The underlying determinants of a particular behaviour, as well as influences external to the behaviour (for that target group), need to be considered prior to selecting BCTs to form an intervention. The consideration of formative research and change theory are important first steps before using BCTs.
- The developers of the taxonomy acknowledge that all BCTs may not be as flexible as others. For example, BCTs related to environmental change or incentives which are often used in large-scale public health interventions are said to actually be more effective in smaller, personally delivered interventions (Michie et al., 2013)
- Recent research has suggested the taxonomy is limited, with other types of BCTs such as relational BCTs (e.g., sharing experiential knowledge) not included. Many of these 'missing' BCTs have been identified through qualitative research and case studies (Marks et al., 2022).
- The effectiveness of individual BCTs and select combinations of BCTs need to be critically considered. Researchers and policymakers need to consider if it is an individual BCT driving the change in behaviour (or lack thereof), a combination of selected BCTs, or other external factors (e.g., individual differences) (Hailey et al., 2022). Often, when an intervention is deemed to be effective, not all of the individual BCTs contributed to eliciting behaviour change.

Maintaining Behaviour Change in Interventions

The effects of interventions to change behaviour are still relatively small and not maintained in the long term (Kwasnicka et al., 2016). It may be that the increased use of BCTs will allow transparency into the mechanisms by which behaviour change can be maintained over time. Kwasnicka et al. (2016) make theoretical suggestions to improve behaviour change maintenance. These include motivation, self-regulation, habits, resources, and the environment. Thus interventions, including BCTs that target these constructs, are needed. Early research into the maintenance of physical activity found that planning, maintenance self-efficacy, and action control were all important in maintaining behaviour change over time

(Sniehotta et al., 2005). While the authors did not specifically mention BCTs, there are a number of BCTs that are designed specifically to target these constructs, e.g., 'focusing on past success' targets self-efficacy and 'goal planning (behaviour)' targets planning.

A recent study exploring the long-term effects of an intervention to change behaviour found that habit was important to maintaining changes in behaviour over time (Charlesworth et al., 2023). Further recent research has proposed some unanswered questions in developing habit-based interventions, and specifically looked at behaviour maintenance and real-world interventions. BCTs that are commonly used to change habits include restructuring the environment and habit formation (Mullan et al., 2022) and can be used to develop interventions to maintain behaviour change. More research is needed to look at any consistencies in BCTs, across populations and particularly across behaviours, as most maintenance research seems to be focused on maintaining weight loss or maintaining increased physical activity.

Conclusion

While there are no strict guidelines for creating a successful intervention, there are key considerations to be made when designing and delivering behaviour change interventions. Selecting an appropriate evidence-based theoretical background is an essential first step when designing an intervention in health psychology. Formative research that is accompanied by consumer representative and stakeholder involvement, can support decision-making on intervention content, mode of delivery, and intervention structure. This co-design approach provides an opportunity to understand populations' preferences and support needs and the anticipation of barriers that may hinder behaviour change. While 'no one size fits all', we can tailor interventions for populations with diverse preferences and needs, such as those with an NCD, risk factors for disease, remote or marginalised populations, and culturally and linguistically diverse groups. It can also be said that as long as the BCTs you choose to incorporate in an intervention are appropriate for the target behaviour and population, and are effective, there is no need to include several of them. Therefore, to be able to deliver successful behaviour change interventions, we need to design behaviour change interventions for and with the population of interest and embed these interventions with tailored evidence-based BCTs. It is also imperative that moving forward, researchers and intervention developers aim to longitudinally assess the outcomes of the intervention to greater our understanding of long-term behaviour change and maintenance.

Further Reading

Michie, S., Atkins, L., & West, R. (2014). The behaviour change wheel. *A guide to designing interventions. 1st ed. Great Britain: Silverback Publishing*, 1003–1010.

Schwarzer, R., & Hamilton, K. (2020). Changing behavior using the health action process approach. In M. Hagger, L. Cameron, K. Hamilton, N. Hankonen, & T. Lintunen (Eds.), *The handbook of behavior change* (pp. 89–103). Cambridge University Press.

References

AIHW. (2021). *Australian Burden of Disease Study 2018 – Key findings*. AIHW. https://www.aihw.gov.au/reports/burden-of-disease/burden-of-disease-study-2018-key-findings

Alexander, K. E., Brijnath, B., & Mazza, D. (2014). Barriers and enablers to delivery of the Healthy Kids Check: An analysis informed by the Theoretical Domains Framework and COM-B model. *Implementation Science*, *9*(1), 60. https://doi.org/10.1186/1748-5908-9-60

Atkins, L., Francis, J., Islam, R., O'Connor, D., Patey, A., Ivers, N., Foy, R., Duncan, E. M., Colquhoun, H., Grimshaw, J. M., Lawton, R., & Michie, S. (2017). A guide to using the Theoretical Domains Framework of behaviour change to investigate implementation problems. *Implementation Science*, *12*(1). https://doi.org/10.1186/s13012-017-0605-9

Aveyard, P., Lewis, A., Tearne, S., Hood, K., Christian-Brown, A., Adab, P., Begh, R., Jolly, K., Daley, A., Farley, A., Lycett, D., Nickless, A., Yu, L.-M., Retat, L., Webber, L., Pimpin, L., & Jebb, S. A. (2016). Screening and brief intervention for obesity in primary care: A parallel, two-arm, randomised trial. *The Lancet*, *388*(10059), 2492–2500. https://doi.org/10.1016/s0140-6736(16)31893-1

Bartholomew, L. K., Parcel, G. S., & Kok, G. (1998). Intervention mapping: A process for developing theory and evidence-based health education programs. *Health Education & Behavior*, *25*(5), 545–563. https://doi.org/10.1177/109019819802500502

Bavel, J. J. van, Baicker, K., Boggio, P. S., Capraro, V., Cichocka, A., Cikara, M., Crockett, M. J., Crum, A. J., Douglas, K. M., Druckman, J. N., Drury, J., Dube, O., Ellemers, N., Finkel, E. J., Fowler, J. H., Gelfand, M., Han, S., Haslam, S. A., Jetten, J., … Willer, R. (2020). Using social and behavioural science to support COVID-19 pandemic response. *Nature Human Behaviour*, *4*(5), 460–471. https://doi.org/10.1038/s41562-020-0884-z

Cane, J., O'Connor, D., & Michie, S. (2012). Validation of the theoretical domains framework for use in behaviour change and implementation research. *Implementation Science*, *7*(1), 37. https://doi.org/10.1186/1748-5908-7-37

Cao, B., Bray, F., Ilbawi, A., & Soerjomataram, I. (2018). Effect on longevity of one-third reduction in premature mortality from non-communicable diseases by 2030: a global analysis of the Sustainable Development Goal health target. *The Lancet Global Health*, *6*(12), e1288–e1296. https://doi.org/10.1016/S2214-109X(18)30411-X

Charlesworth, J., Liddelow, C., Mullan, B., Tan, H., & Abbott, B. (2023). Examining the long-term effects of a safe food-handling media campaign. *Food Control*, *149*, 109690 https://doi.org/10.1016/j.foodcont.2023.109690

Charlesworth, J., Mullan, B., Howell, J., Tan, H., Abbott, B., & Potter, A. (2021). Evaluating the impact of a pilot safe food-handling media campaign among consumers in Western Australia: Implications for public health messaging. *Food Control*, *126*, 108070. https://doi.org/10.1016/j.foodcont.2021.108070

Conner, M., & Norman, P. (1996). *Predicting health behaviour: Research and practice with social cognition models*. Open University Press.

Croager, E. J., Gray, V., Pratt, I. S., Slevin, T., Pettigrew, S., Holman, C. D., & Bulsara, M., & Emery, J. (2018). Find cancer early: Evaluation of a community education campaign to increase awareness of cancer signs and symptoms in people in Regional Western Australians [Evaluation]. *Frontiers in Public Health*, *6*. https://doi.org/10.3389/fpubh.2018.00022

Curioni, C., & Lourenco, P. (2005). Long-term weight loss after diet and exercise: A systematic review. *International Journal of Obesity*, *29*(10), 1168–1174. https://doi.org/10.1038/sj.ijo.0803015

De Vasconcelos, S., Igor, T., Cooper, B., Chollier, M., Stephenson, R., Blondeel, K., Troussier, T., & Kiarief, J. (2018). Behaviour change techniques in brief interventions to prevent HIV, STI and unintended pregnancies: A systematic review. *PLoS One*, *13*(9). https://doi.org/10.1371/journal.pone.0204088

Engels, L., Monns, C., Mergelsberg, E., Kothe, E., Hamilton, K., Gardner, B., ten Hoor, G., & Mullan, B. (2022). How to imrpove the diet of toddlers? The feasibility of an online, habit-based intervention targeting parental feeding behaviour. *Health Psychology and Behavioral Medicine*, *10*(1) 1020–1037. https://doi.org/10.1080/21642850.2022.2134869

Hailey, V., Rojas-Garcia, A., & Kassianos, A. P. (2022). A systematic review of behaviour change techniques used in interventions to increase physical activity among breast cancer survivors. *Breast Cancer*, *29*(2), 193–208. https://doi.org/10.1007/s12282-021-01323-z

Hardcastle, S. J., Hince, D., Jiménez-Castuera, R., Boyle, T., Cavalheri, V., Makin, G., Tan, P., Salfinger, S., Tan, J., Ganendra Raj, M., Levitt, M., Cohen, P. A., Saunders, C., & Platell, C. (2019). Promoting physical activity in regional and remote cancer survivors (PPARCS) using wearables and health coaching: Randomised controlled trial protocol. *BMJ Open*, *9*(5). https://doi.org/10.1136/bmjopen-2018-028369

Kelly, M. P., & Barker, M. (2016). Why is changing health-related behaviour so difficult? *Public Health*, *136*, 109–116. https://doi.org/10.1016/j.puhe.2016.03.030

Kwasnicka, D., Dombrowski, S. U., White, M., & Sniehotta, F. (2016). Theoretical explanations for maintenance of behaviour change: A systematic review of behaviour theories. *Health Psychology Review*, *10*(3), 277–296. https://doi.org/10.1080/17437199.2016.1151372

Ling, M., Kothe, E. J., & Mullan, B. A. (2019). Predicting intention to receive a seasonal influenza vaccination using Protection Motivation Theory. *Social Science & Medicine*, *233*, 87–92. https://doi.org/10.1016/j.socscimed.2019.06.002

Local Government Association UK. (2021). *The London Borough of Havering: Using the COM-B framework to develop a vaccine take up strategy.*

Marks, J., Sriskandarajah, N., Aurelio, M. M., Gillard, S., Rinaldi, M., Foster, R., & Ussher, M. (2022). Experiences of peer workers and mental health service users with a peer support intervention: applying and critiquing a behaviour change techniques taxonomy. *Advances in Mental Health*, *20*(2), 91–101. https://doi.org/10.1080/18387357.2021.2012088

Maxwell-Smith, C., Hince, D., Cohen, P. A., Bulsara, M. K., Boyle, T., Platell, C., Tan, P., Levitt, M., Salama, P., Tan, J., Salfinger, S., Makin, G., Mohan, G. R. K. A., Jiménez-Castuera, R., & Hardcastle, S. J. (2019). A randomized controlled trial of WATAAP to promote physical activity in colorectal and endometrial cancer survivors. *Psycho-Oncology*, *28*(7), 1420–1429. https://doi.org/10.1002/pon.5090

McKay, F. H., Slykerman, S., & Dunn, M. (2019). The App behavior change scale: Creation of a scale to assess the potential of apps to promote behavior change. *JMIR mHealth and uHealth*, *7*(1), e11130. https://doi.org/10.2196/11130

Michie, S.(2008). Designing and implementing behaviour change interventions to improve population health. *Journal of Health Services Research & Policy*, *13*(3), 64–69. https://doi.org/10.1258/jhsrp.2008.008014

Michie, S., Ashford, S., Sniehotta, F. F., Dombrowski, S. U., Bishop, A., & French, D. P. (2011). A refined taxonomy of behaviour change techniques to help people change their physical activity and healthy eating behaviours: The CALO-RE taxonomy. *Psychology & Health*, *26*(11), 1479–1498. https://doi.org/10.1080/08870446.2010.540664

Michie, S., Van Stralen, M. M., & West, R. (2011). The behaviour change wheel: A new method for characterising and designing behaviour change interventions. *Implementation Science*, *6*(1), 1–12. https://doi.org/10.1186/1748-5908-6-42

Michie, S., Wood, C., Johnston, M., Abraham, C., Francis, J., Hardeman, W., Eccles, M., Richardson, M., & Cane, J. (2013). The Behaviour Change Technique Taxonomy (BCTTv1) of 93 hierarchically-clustered techniques: Testing reliability of the taxonomy in specifying the content of behaviour change interventions. *Annals of Behavioral Medicine*, *46*(1), 81–95. https://doi.org/10.1007/s12160-013-9486-6

Morley, B. C., Niven, P. H., Dixon, H. G., Swanson, M. G., McAleese, A. B., & Wakefield, M. A. (2018). Controlled cohort evaluation of the LiveLighter mass media campaign's impact on adults' reported consumption of sugar-sweetened beverages. *BMJ Open*, *8*(4). https://doi.org/10.1136/bmjopen-2017-019574

Mullan, B., Liddelow, C., Haywood, D., & Breare, H. (2022). Behavior change training for health professionals: Evaluation of a 2-hour workshop. *JMIR Formative Research*, *6*(11), e42010. https://doi.org/10.2196/42010

Rigby, R. R., Mitchell, L. J., Hamilton, K., & Williams, L. T. (2020). The use of behavior change theories in dietetics practice in primary health care: A systematic review of randomized controlled trials. *Journal of the Academy of Nutrition and Dietetics*, *120*(7), 1172–1197. https://doi.org/10.1016/j.jand.2020.03.019

Schroé, H., van Dyck, D., de Paepe, A., Poppe, L., Loh, W. W., Verloigne, M., Loeys, T., de Bourdeaudhuij, I., & Crombez, G. (2020). Which behaviour change techniques are effective to promote physical activity and reduce sedentary behaviour in adults: a factorial randomized trial of an e- and m-health intervention. *International Journal of Behavioral Nutrition and Physical Activity*, *17*(1), 127. https://doi.org/10.1186/s12966-020-01001-x

Schwartz, G. E. (1982). Testing the biopsychosocial model: The ultimate challenge facing behavioral medicine? *Journal of Consulting and Clinical Psychology*, *50*, 1040–1053. https://doi.org/10.1037/0022-006X.50.6.1040

Schwarzer, R., & Hamilton, K. (2020). Changing behavior using the health action process approach. In M. Hagger, L. Cameron, K. Hamilton, N. Hankonen, & T. Lintunen (Eds.), *The handbook of behavior change* (pp. 89–103). Cambridge University Press.

Schwarzer, R., & Luszczynska, A. (2008). How to Overcome Health-Compromising Behaviors. *European Psychologist*, *13*(2), 141–151. https://doi.org/10.1027/1016-9040.13.2.141

Shoneye, C. L., Mullan, B., Begley, A., Pollard, C. M., Jancey, J., & Kerr, D. A. (2020). Design and Development of a Digital Weight Management Intervention (ToDAy): Qualitative Study. *JMIR mHealth and uHealth*, *8*(9), e17919. https://doi.org/10.2196/17919

Sibony, A.-L. (2020). The UK COVID-19 Response: A Behavioural Irony? *European Journal of Risk Regulation*, *11*(2), 350–357. https://doi.org/10.1017/err.2020.22

Sniehotta, F. F., Scholz, U., & Schwarzer, R. (2005). Bridging the intention–behaviour gap: Planning, self-efficacy, and action control in the adoption and maintenance of physical exercise. *Psychology & Health*, *20*(2), 143–160. https://doi.org/10.1080/08870440512331317670

van Genugten, L., Dusseldorp, E., Webb, T. L., & van Empelen, P. (2016). Which Combinations of Techniques and Modes of Delivery in Internet-Based Interventions Effectively Change Health Behavior? A Meta-Analysis. *Journal of Medical Internet Research*, *18*(6), e155. https://doi.org/10.2196/jmir.4218

West, R., & Michie, S. (2020). A brief introduction to the COM-B Model of behaviour and the PRIME Theory of motivation. *Qeios*. https://doi.org/10.32388/ww04e6.2

WHO. (2022). *Global health estimates: Leading causes of death*. Retrieved 14/11/2022, from https://www.who.int/data/gho/data/themes/mortality-and-global-health-estimates/ghe-leading-causes-of-death

30

IMPLEMENTATION STRATEGIES

From Lab to Field

Matthew McDonald, Matthew McLaughlin, and Joanna C. Moullin

Introduction

Implementation science aims to improve the efficiency and effectiveness by which evidence moves from 'lab to field'. Its goal is for evidence-based interventions to be implemented equitably, sustainably, and at scale. Implementation science is the "study of methods to promote the introduction and integration of research findings and evidence into healthcare policy and practice" (NIH Fogarty International Centre, n.d.). Once positioned at the end of a linear research pipeline, implementation science now positions itself across the spectrum of research, whereby interventions and implementation strategies should be developed with the end goal of sustainment at scale in mind (A. Milat et al., 2020; Moullin et al., 2020).

The core components of implementation are having an evidence-based *intervention*, to be implemented into a multi-level *context*, over a multi-phasic implementation *process*, which is influenced by a range of *implementation factors* (barriers and facilitators) and *implementation strategies* to achieve positive *implementation outcomes* (Moullin, Sabater-Hernández, Fernandez-Llimos, & Benrimoj, 2015).

The central feature and first core component of implementation research and practice is an evidence-based *intervention*, innovation, practice, technique, programme or tool. The intervention's characteristics influence the ease and likelihood of successful implementation across all stages of the implementation process. As such, it is important intervention developers and researchers consider implementation and design 'implementable' interventions from the start (Klaic et al., 2022). To assist with this, we encourage stakeholder identification, engagement, and collaboration during intervention development. Another consideration is the balance of delivering the intervention as it was designed and

DOI: 10.4324/9781003318026-36

intended – that is, with fidelity versus adapting the intervention to fit the context. This is discussed further later.

The second core component of implementation is the *context* where the intervention is to be implemented. Ecological multi-level models of context are useful to remember and embrace the complexity of the system. Generally, one should consider the readiness and agency of all stakeholders involved with the implementation process, the conditions, and characteristics of the setting(s) in which the intervention is to operate, the circumstances immediately surrounding the organisation(s), including the community, patients (for whom the intervention is targeting) and their social networks, and finally the system's economic, political, and professional milieu. In addition, the complexity of the interrelationships between the levels should be considered. These have been termed bridging factors (Lengnick-Hall et al., 2021).

The crux of implementation is the *process*, an often long and complex series of phases or stages to introduce and integrate an intervention into practice. Initially, stakeholders need to explore the programme, gap, or need and determine whether an intervention(s) will address the problem, concluding with a decision to either adopt or reject the intervention (exploration phase). If the decision is to adopt, planning for implementation occurs, whereby all levels of the context, including the intervention itself (e.g., adapted to improved intervention fit), should be prepared (preparation phase). Next, once an intervention starts to be delivered in practice, implementation is truly beginning (implementation phase). Finally, sustainability occurs once an intervention is delivered without additional implementation support, indicating sufficient capacity, and intervention benefits are maintained (sustainment phase). This includes continuous monitoring, evaluation, quality improvement, and ongoing adaptation.

More recently, two other implementation concepts have gained deserving attention. These are equity and scalability, both scale-up and scale-out. Equity is a goal of implementation; in particular, focus on implementation strategies is required for this to be achieved (e.g., adaptation). Scalability typically focuses on increasing adoption to extend the reach of effective interventions to a greater proportion of the target population under real-world conditions whilst retaining effectiveness (Milat et al., 2013). Scale-up is whereby the implementation of an intervention is expanded to similar settings under which it was tested (Aarons et al., 2017). Scale-out is the concept of implementation occurring in circumstances that are similar to, but distinct from, the contexts and populations by which intervention and/or implementation has been tested (Aarons et al., 2017).

Implementation *factors* are a widely explored component of implementation science. Often called investigation of barriers and facilitators or enablers, implementation factors are the variables that may affect the implementation process either positively or negatively. These exist across the implementation process, but different factors may be more prominent at different stages of the process.

Implementation *strategies* are the activities and techniques that are directed towards improving the adoption, implementation, and integration of an intervention, including building the context's capability and capacity (individuals', organisations', and systems') (Powell et al., 2015; Proctor et al., 2013). Implementation strategies can use identified facilitators and overcome the barriers during the steps and stages of the implementation process. They may be directed towards the intervention, or any level of the context, at any stage of the implementation process. As such, any change theory may be appropriate, e.g., systems change, organisational change, behavioural change, and service adaptation.

Improving implementation *outcomes* is the final core component of implementation science. Implementation outcomes precede clinical outcomes and include outcomes such as reach/penetration: how many patients receive an intervention; adoption: how many providers (clinicians or organisations) deliver an intervention; implementation cost: costs associated with implementation. Other more proximal outcomes or antecedents include intervention feasibility, acceptability, and appropriateness. Measures of other implementation factors could also be included (Reilly et al., 2020).

Implementation theories, models, and frameworks provide a shared language, guidance, and tools for planning, conducting, and evaluating implementation studies and projects. They can be broadly aligned to one of the core components of implementation and thus classified as a process, determinant, evaluation, implementation, and/or classic theory (Nilsen, 2020). Ten of the more commonly used implementation theories, models, and frameworks are presented in Table 30.1. Theories, models, and frameworks should be dynamic, evolving through revisions and enhancements. As such, it is possible to contextualise and adapt frameworks for individual situations, such as dividing contextual domains into further levels depending on the desired analysis and research question or adding in influencing factors that don't appear in a given framework. Moullin et al. (2020) have provided recommendations for using implementation frameworks in research and practice.

Table 30.1 Ten highly cited implementation frameworks, models, and theories

Title	*Acronym*	*Brief Summary*
Consolidated Framework for Implementation Research (Damschroder et al., 2009)	CFIR	A pragmatic structure that can guide evaluations and help build implementation evidence in different settings. CFIR includes five domains (intervention characteristics, outer setting, inner setting, characteristics of individuals and process) and various constructs that could influence implementation.

(*Continued*)

Table 30.1 (Continued)

Title	*Acronym*	*Brief Summary*
Exploration, Preparation, Implementation, and Sustainment (Aarons et al., 2011)	EPIS	The EPIS framework is a comprehensive multi-phasic, multi-level implementation framework to guide implementation research and practice. EPIS consists of the implementation process (divided into four phases) and implementation factors (i.e., outer/ inner innovation and bridging factors).
Reach, Effectiveness, Adoption, Implementation, Maintenance (Glasgow et al., 1999)	RE-AIM	RE-AIM supports the evaluation of public health interventions via five dimensions: reach, effectiveness, adoption, implementation, and maintenance.
Theoretical Domains Framework (Cane et al., 2012)	TDF	This framework provides a comprehensive theoretical assessment of implementation problems and consists of 12 theoretical domains with exemplar questions for each to use in interviews.
Capability, Opportunity, Motivation – Behaviour Model of the Behaviour Change Wheel (Michie et al., 2014)	COM-B and BCW	A comprehensive theory-based guidance for developing interventions. The BCW connects behavioural influences identified by COM-B with intervention functions, policy categories, and behaviour change techniques.
Practical, Robust Implementation and Sustainability Model (Feldstein & Glasgow, 2008)	PRISM	PRISM is a tool for implementing and evaluating health interventions, which focuses on the characteristics and perspectives of organisational workers and the need to plan for an implementation and sustainability infrastructure from the outset.
Integrated-Promoting Action on Research Implementation in Health Services (Harvey & Kitson, 2015)	i-PARIHS	i-PARIHS adopts a flexible approach to implementation and positions facilitation as the active ingredient in the process. This tool recognises that implementation in practice is complex, unpredictable, and non-linear.

(*Continued*)

Table 30.1 (Continued)

Title	*Acronym*	*Brief Summary*
Interactive Systems Framework (Wandersman et al., 2008)	ISF	ISF supports stakeholders to understand the needs of other stakeholders and systems, including needs, barriers, and resources. It also provides a structure for summarising existing literature and highlighting priority areas.
Knowledge to Action (Wilson et al., 2011)	KTA	The KTA framework recognises decision points, interactions, and support structures within three phases (research, translation, and institutionalisation) to help support moving knowledge into sustainable action.
Normalisation Process Theory (Murray et al., 2010)	NPT	NPT provides trialists with a consistent framework for describing, assessing, and enhancing implementation potential.

Implementation Strategies and Stakeholder Involvement

Implementation science is multidisciplinary in nature, and a core tenet of the field is meaningful engagement with a range of stakeholders who may be involved in designing, delivering, and/or receiving an evidence-based intervention. The term 'stakeholder' can refer to a broad range of partners, including those involved in delivering the intervention (i.e., individuals and organisations), expert researchers in the intervention field, implementation scientists, organisational leaders', policymakers, and other key decision-makers, and members of the target audience for the evidence-based intervention. The push towards more inclusive trials, tackling health inequalities, and participatory research methods that involve consumers and the community in interventions and research studies (see Chapter 28) is highly relevant across the research pathway. Given that stakeholders often include individuals involved in adopting, implementing, maintaining, and/or advocating for the evidence-based intervention, they can play a key role in helping to ensure a good fit to context and that consumer or organisation priorities are met. Thus, stakeholders have an important role to play in deciding which implementation strategies should be selected for implementing evidence-based interventions.

Implementation strategies can be discrete individual components (e.g., sharing an educational flyer) but are usually multi-faceted, multi-level, and encompass a package of different components. Taxonomies of implementation strategies, such as the Expert Recommendations for Implementing Change ('ERIC'; which comprises 73 strategies), provide a useful resource for researchers and implementors (Powell et al., 2015). However, there is limited understanding of which specific strategies, or combination of strategies, may work best in which contexts or circumstances. Implementation strategies are often poorly or inconsistently described or a part of a package of different components that make them difficult to understand. As would be done in the evaluation of intervention effectiveness, it is essential to report implementation strategies. Proctor and colleagues outline the importance of implementation strategies being named, defined, and specified based on seven components (actor, action, action targets, temporality, dose, outcomes, and theory/justification) to allow for their measurement and potential replication (Proctor et al., 2013). Reporting implementation strategies in this manner allows for their comparison and synthesis for evaluation across different studies, interventions, and contexts.

Selecting appropriate implementation strategies for evidence-based intervention can be a complex task. The design of implementation strategies should be reported explicitly, undertaken with purpose, and informed by theory. The BCW provides comprehensive theory-based guidance for developing interventions (Michie et al., 2014). At the BCW's core is the Capability Opportunity Motivation – Behaviour (COM-B) Model, which is designed to help identify influences on behaviour. The BCW connects these influences on behaviour with intervention functions, policy categories, and behaviour change techniques (Michie et al., 2014). Michie and colleagues integrate BCW-COM-B with the Theoretical Domains Framework (TDF), which comprises 14 theoretical domains (Cane et al., 2012). This ultimately provides a framework for a more elaborate analysis that can help identify implementation factors and inform the process of selecting or tailoring implementation strategies (Michie et al., 2014).

Another systematic approach to help plan for and select implementation strategies is implementation mapping (Fernandez et al., 2019). Implementation mapping (which is based on intervention mapping) follows a five-step process. The first step of implementation mapping is to undertake an initial implementation needs assessment. This is an essential step mirrored across different approaches to developing implementation strategies and is often referred to as identifying implementation barriers and facilitators (implementation factors). A variety of methods can be used in this step, such as consensus approaches (discussed next), qualitative research, and participatory research. The implementation strategies (both in implementation mapping and other approaches) are then selected or designed based on overcoming the implementation barriers identified and capitalising on facilitators. The four implementation mapping steps that follow the initial needs assessment are (1) stating implementation outcomes/performance objectives, identifying determinants, and creating matrices of change objectives; (2) choosing mechanisms of change and selecting or designing implementation strategies; (3) producing implementation protocols and materials; and (4) evaluating implementation outcomes (Fernandez et al., 2019). Throughout the implementation mapping process, principles of participatory research and stakeholder involvement are emphasised. With potential adopters and implementers involved from the beginning of the implementation planning process, a realistic understanding of the resources and requirements for evidence-based practice implementation can be ascertained.

One strategy to help identify implementation factors and decide on or tailor implementation strategies is involving stakeholders in consensus approaches (e.g., nominal group technique and concept mapping). The aim of consensus methods is to overcome issues with group decision-making, such as influential individuals or groups with vested interests in a particular outcome (Jones & Hunter, 1995). Thus, stakeholder views are considered and incorporated in an equitable manner. One such structured consensus method is concept mapping, which is a mixed-methods approach that engages stakeholders in brainstorming, sorting, and rating activities (Kane & Trochim, 2007). The initial brainstorming task can be used to prompt stakeholders to generate implementation strategy suggestions (e.g., *"A strategy to implement this evidence-based programme in our organisation is…"*); then the statements are compiled, reduced, and organised into concepts before finally being rated on dimensions, such as 'importance' and 'feasibility' (Kane & Trochim, 2007). In this way, consensus can be generated on implementation strategies or types of strategies that may be most likely to be feasible, efficient, and effective for overcoming implementation barriers.

Implementation strategies can be considered an intervention that can be studied using a variety of research methods and study designs comparable to research undertaken to examine the effectiveness of evidence-based interventions aiming to improve health outcomes or behaviours. The next chapter summarises some of the different types of study designs and evaluation methods used in implementation science.

Implementation of Research Study Designs and Evaluation

Traditional study design approaches in implementation science have sought to gradually scale-up interventions found to be effective in order to achieve population-wide health improvement (Indig et al., 2018). This linear research 'pipeline' of study designs starts with piloting and feasibility research, then efficacy, effectiveness, implementation, and, finally, dissemination research (Indig et al., 2018). For each of the different stages of the pipeline, there is a shift in focus of implementation outcomes. Pilot and feasibility designs tend to focus on reach, acceptability, feasibility, and appropriateness. Efficacy trials focus on establishing the impact of the intervention under ideal and controlled circumstances. Effectiveness trials evaluate impact under more 'real-world' conditions. These efficacy and effectiveness trials are conducted prior to trials to assess models of intervention delivery for scale, dissemination, and large-scale implementation.

The traditional pipeline approach has been met with a number of challenges. The main challenge has been moving research along this pipeline at sufficient speed to address public health risks (Contopoulos-Ioannidis et al., 2008) whilst retaining effect sizes by avoiding the scale-up penalty (Lane et al., 2021). To date, more than 98% of research published in public health journals has used study designs at the early stages of this study design pipeline (Wolfenden et al., 2016).

More novel approaches to implementation science research study designs have emerged, aiming to more efficiently bridge the gap between implementation science research and public health policy and practice. Type I, II, and III effectiveness-implementation hybrid evaluation designs are a novel means of accelerating the research translation process in public health (Curran et al., 2012). The aim of these designs is to provide key information to inform policy and practice, in a timely manner. Unlike the traditional pipeline approach to implementation science research translation, hybrid designs seek to accelerate the translation process through the collection of effectiveness and implementation information simultaneously. Hybrid designs collect health outcomes (effectiveness), as well as the effects of an implementation strategy in improving intervention implementation (implementation). Hybrid designs are favourable for policymakers and practitioners, as they concurrently provide information regarding intervention effects and implementation approaches in a timely manner.

Type I hybrid designs primarily aim to test the effectiveness of interventions in improving health outcomes, whilst simultaneously collecting information about their implementation (Curran et al., 2012). Type I trials are best suited to demonstrating the effect of an intervention on a small scale, but they provide only preliminary data about the potential suitability of implementation strategies if implemented under real-world ecological conditions. See *Case Example 1* for an example of a type I hybrid design.

Type II hybrid designs concurrently examine, with similar or equal emphasis, the effectiveness of an intervention and an implementation strategy (Curran et al., 2012). Type II designs assess both the effects of the intervention in improving public health behaviour and of an implementation strategy in improving the implementation of the intervention components. Implementation outcomes for type II trials typically involve assessing the cost, acceptability, and feasibility of both the intervention and the implementation strategy. Type II hybrid designs may be particularly useful when efficacy has been established, but a new implementation approach needs to be evaluated to see if it preserves the intervention effects.

Type III hybrid designs primarily focus on examining the impact of an implementation strategy in achieving the implementation of a specific evidence-based policy recommendation or practice. Such designs are particularly suited to scale-up studies, where they are powered to detect meaningful changes in the implementation of an evidence-based intervention. Type III designs also collect information about the impact of the intervention on health outcomes. Given this is a secondary emphasis of these designs, the evaluations of health outcomes may be less rigorous and conducted only in a nested sample of sites. Such trials are particularly appropriate where there is existing evidence of an intervention's health effects but where adapted or alternate implementation strategies are being tested. An example of a type III implementation trial is provided in *Case Example 1*.

Increasingly important is the selection of implementation outcomes suitable to assess scalability of public health interventions. Effectiveness and implementation data from hybrid effectiveness-implementation trials is important, but not sufficient, for decision-making regarding the scalability of interventions (Milat et al., 2020). Assessing implementation outcomes specific to scalability helps to avoid lengthy research processes (Contopoulos-Ioannidis et al., 2008) and superfluous expenditure of evaluation resources – for example, by conducting multiple large trials. Implementation outcomes for scalability, derived from the Implementation Scalability Assessment Tool (ISAT) (Milat et al., 2020), include examining the strategic and political context, evidence of effectiveness, costs and benefits, fidelity, adaptation, reach, acceptability, delivery setting, infrastructure and workforce, and sustainability (Milat et al., 2020). The ISAT tool has ten domains of scalability and can be used to develop scalable interventions from the outset, as well as to assess the suitability of public health interventions for scale-up. The ISAT can also be used as an evaluation framework for scale-up studies. In the next section (after the case example), a focus is given to adaptation, context and fidelity – as important outcomes for assessing the implementation and scalability of interventions.

Case Example 1: **Scaling-up Physical Activity 4 Everyone (PA4E1): A Multi-component School-Based Physical Activity Programme for Adolescents**

Physical Activity 4 Everyone (PA4E1) is a physical activity programme designed to address inactivity in secondary schools in New South Wales, Australia. PA4E1 was designed for delivery by a government health service, Hunter New England Local Health District. PA4E1 consists of both school physical activity practices (i.e., the intervention) and implementation strategies to support schools in the uptake of these practices (Sutherland et al., 2019). The seven physical activity practices were designed using socio-ecological theory and were informed by existing evidence – to increase schools' physical activity opportunities and environments.

The first trial of PA4E1 (from 2012 to 2014) used a randomised controlled trial type I hybrid effectiveness-implementation study design, evaluating primarily the effectiveness of the intervention to increase students' physical activity (primary outcome). The results were significant, with a 49-minute-a-week difference between intervention and control groups in moderate to vigorous physical activity (primary outcome; Sutherland et al., 2021). Implementation of the intervention, as well as cost, were also measured with positive results. Therefore, based on a number of scalability domains (Milat et al., 2020), including effectiveness, cost, implementation, and an identified delivery model for scale-up, the intervention was deemed suitable for scale-up.

In 2016, PA4E1 was adapted for scale-up (for fivefold the number of schools) and scale-out (for delivery by four Local Health Districts). The adaptation process focused on adapting the implementation strategies for scale-up using a four-step iterative, theory and stakeholder-involved process (Sutherland et al., 2019). In total, 20 pre-planned adaptations were made (Mclaughlin et al., 2021), and systematically detailed and coded using the Framework for Reporting Adaptations and Modifications FRAME (Stirman et al., 2019). The primary pre-planned adaptations involved the introduction of digital delivery mode (a website) for implementation support, as well as a shift in the delivery agent from an external champion employed by the research team to an internal school champion (an existing PE teacher from the school).

The scale-up trial (from 2017 to 2019) utilised a type III hybrid implementation-effectiveness design in 49 schools, as evidence of the intervention's health effects was established in the first trial, but the adapted implementation strategy needed to be tested. As such, the primary aim was focused on implementation, specifically to evaluate the implementation uptake of the seven evidence-based PA4E1 intervention practices by schools. Secondary evaluation aims included student physical activity (health outcome), cost-effectiveness, and a comprehensive process evaluation, including a detailed evaluation of the new digital delivery mode, fidelity, reach, adaptations, and modifications. Findings from the scale-up trial indicated that, at 24-month follow-up, school uptake of four or more of seven practices (primary outcome) was significantly higher in the programme group (16/23, 69%) than the control group (0/25, 0%) ($p < 0.001$) (Sutherland et al., 2021). The cost to deliver the intervention was considerably reduced from the first trial. Modifications made during intervention delivery were adjudged to be 'fidelity-consistent' (i.e., the core intervention elements were retained) (Mclaughlin et al., 2021).

Adaptation, Context, and Fidelity

Adapting effective interventions and the strategies to support their implementation can play an important role in the scaling of interventions to different contexts. Adaptation may be particularly important to help address health inequalities where the unmodified intervention may be unappealing, ineffective, or otherwise inappropriate for sub-group populations that may have a higher risk of ill health than the general population (see Chapter 28). Adaptation can be defined as the thoughtful and deliberate alteration of intervention design or delivery, to improve intervention fit or effectiveness within a given context (Miller et al., 2021). To this end, adaptations can be conceptualised as implementation strategies themselves, whereby the adaptation of an intervention is designed to support a better intervention fit to context. Guidelines for adapting interventions for different contexts emphasise the importance of involving a diverse range of stakeholders throughout the process (Moore et al., 2021). Modification can be defined as encompassing any alteration, either proactive and deliberate (adaptation) or unplanned and ad-hoc in response to implementation challenges (Miller et al., 2021). Modifications to effective interventions have typically been viewed as undesirable and likely to negatively impact intervention effects, particularly in medical interventions. However, modifications can have a positive impact, and they are most likely to when made systematically and are proactively aimed at improving intervention fit (e.g., to align with target population values), have a stated goal or reason, and retain the integrity of core intervention elements or functions (Moore et al., 2013).

Core elements of interventions (e.g., behaviour change techniques, theoretical underpinnings, and mechanisms of action), that are adjudged crucial for effectiveness, are typically considered unavailable for adaptation. Recently, these core intervention elements have been conceptualised as 'core functions' that should be preserved but can vary in form (Wahlen et al., 2022). That is, a different form of delivering the same component could be used without retracting from the core functions, such as delivering a goal-setting activity through encouraging discussion with other participants rather than individually via handouts. As far as possible, evidence-based interventions should be delivered with fidelity (as intended) to the core intervention elements or functions. However, behavioural community-based interventions are inevitably adapted to some extent upon implementation. For example, in a study examining adaptations to an evidence-based chronic disease prevention programme implemented by community-based organisations, adaptations were noted for a variety of reasons, including to enhance engagement, reach specific groups, increase programme fit, and reinforce programme messages (Carvalho et al., 2013).

Interventions are typically trialled under research conditions that utilise infrastructure, resources, and expertise that may not be readily available in 'real-world' settings. After the more controlled research phase of intervention testing, a reduction in intervention effectiveness is often observed (known as a 'scale-up penalty' or 'voltage drop'). For example, in a systematic review of 'scaled-up' physical activity, intervention effects were markedly lower than in pre-scale trials (Lane et al., 2021). Intervention adaptations that are incongruent with core elements or functions during scale-up, may be particularly susceptible to reduced intervention effects. Thus, it may be appropriate to monitor the fidelity of delivery to core intervention elements or functions upon implementation beyond the more controlled research phase. Inconsistent and inadequate reporting of adaptations has resulted in a lack of understanding of what types of adaptations may or may not work in new contexts (Moore et al., 2021). Thus, guidelines for reporting modifications to interventions and implementation strategies have been developed (Miller et al., 2021; Moore et al., 2021). The PA4E1 case study previously discussed provides a case example of how the extent, type, and rationale for adaptations and modifications made before and during scale-up can be systematically reported (Mclaughlin et al., 2021).

Assessment of the similarities and differences between new and old contexts is an important initial step before adaptation (Moore et al., 2021). If differences between contexts are adjudged to be significant or in the absence of sufficient evidence, the adapted intervention may require feasibility or pilot testing in the new context. Whereas in cases where effective evidenced-based interventions are being implemented in or scaled out to a "*moderately different setting or with a different population*", it may be considered appropriate to '*borrow strength*' from prior research without undertaking another another randomised controlled trial to assess intervention effects (RCT; Aarons et al., 2017).

Case Example 2: Adaptation, Scale-Up, and Scale-Out of Football Fans in Training

Football Fans in Training (FFIT) is a rigorously tested health behaviour change intervention that uses the appeal of professional sports clubs and settings to engage male supporters (see Chapter 28). FFIT is effective at supporting participants in losing weight and improving a variety of secondary health outcomes (Hunt et al., 2014). The programme has been scaled up in Scotland with ongoing routine programme deliveries managed by a voluntary sector organisation (Scottish Professional League-Trust), which work closely with the University of Glasgow programme developers (Hunt et al., 2020). The geographical distribution of football clubs in the Scottish professional league set-up and investment of stakeholders (i.e., delivery partners, football clubs, funders, policymakers) has helped support the roll-out of FFIT and sustained deliveries in association with clubs spanning the country (Hunt et al., 2020). Data from routine 'scaled-up' FFIT deliveries in Scotland and England ($n > 3000$) suggests little or no 'voltage drop' in intervention effects when compared to the effectiveness RCT weight outcomes (Hunt et al., 2020; Hunt et al., 2014).

FFIT has also been adapted (or 'scaled out') to different countries, sports, and populations (Hunt et al., 2020). In several of these scaled-out programmes, based on the differences between new and old contexts, it was deemed necessary to undertake pilot RCTs to assess the feasibility of the adapted intervention and trial procedures to inform full-scale effectiveness trials in the new context. For example, the Aussie-Fans in Training Programme, which was adapted for and piloted in professional Australian Football contexts, successfully engaged men in Australia to inform parameters for a full-scale trial. In Scotland, the FFIT programme was minimally adapted for and tested in a non-randomised feasibility trial for women, with the programme delivery systems and sporting contexts remaining consistent. In Germany, due to minimal intervention adaptations and similarities in the targeted population (i.e., men 35–65 years with BMI > 28) and sporting context (i.e., football) to those utilised in the original effectiveness RCT, further effectiveness data was considered unnecessary. In the latter two examples, the similarities between the delivery contexts allowed for the minimally adapted interventions to be implemented based on '*borrowed strength*' from the prior RCT outcomes. The example of FFIT provides a case study of how interventions can be scaled up, scaled out, and adapted for new contexts and under which circumstances different types of evaluation may be warranted.

Conclusion

Effective evidence-based interventions that support improved health behaviours or health outcomes should be widely available and reach those most in need of support. To do this, studies that are either focused solely on implementation or that have a combined focus on intervention effects and implementation outcomes are required.

A range of implementation frameworks, models, and research methods exist to guide the process. In some cases, adapting interventions that have an evidence base may be a more efficient process than developing new interventions. Whichever methods or guiding frameworks are utilised, effective stakeholder engagement and multi-disciplinarity are central to the success of implementation efforts.

Further Reading

Bauer, M. S., & Kirchner, J. (2020). Implementation science: What is it and why should I care? *Psychiatry Research*, *283*, 112376.

Brown, C. H., Curran, G., Palinkas, L. A., Aarons, G. A., Wells, K. B., Jones, L., … Wallace, A. (2017). An overview of research and evaluation designs for dissemination and implementation. *Annual Review of Public Health*, *38*, 1–22.

Brownson, R. C., Colditz, G. A., & Proctor, E. K. (2017). *Dissemination and implementation research in health: translating science to practice*: Oxford University Press.

References

Aarons, G. A., Hurlburt, M., & Horwitz, S. M. (2011). Advancing a conceptual model of evidence-based practice implementation in public service sectors. *Administration and Policy in Mental Health and Mental Health Services Research*, *38*(1), 4–23.

Aarons, G. A., Sklar, M., Mustanski, B., Benbow, N., & Brown, C. H. (2017). "Scaling-out" evidence-based interventions to new populations or new health care delivery systems. *Implementation Science*, *12*(1), 111.

Cane, J., O'Connor, D., & Michie, S. (2012). Validation of the theoretical domains framework for use in behaviour change and implementation research. *Implementation Science*, *7*(1), 1–17.

Carvalho, M. L., Honeycutt, S., Escoffery, C., Glanz, K., Sabbs, D., & Kegler, M. C. (2013). Balancing fidelity and adaptation. *Journal of Public Health Management and Practice*, *19*(4), 348–356.

Contopoulos-Ioannidis, D. G., Alexiou, G. A., Gouvias, T. C., & Ioannidis, J. P. (2008). *Life cycle of translational research for medical interventions*. In (Vol. 321, pp. 1298–1299): American Association for the Advancement of Science.

Curran, G. M., Bauer, M., Mittman, B., Pyne, J. M., & Stetler, C. (2012). Effectiveness-implementation hybrid designs: Combining elements of clinical effectiveness and implementation research to enhance public health impact. *Medical Care*, *50*(3), 217.

Damschroder, L. J., Aron, D. C., Keith, R. E., Kirsh, S. R., Alexander, J. A., & Lowery, J. C. (2009). Fostering implementation of health services research findings into practice: A consolidated framework for advancing implementation science. *Implementation Science*, *4*(1), 1–15.

Feldstein, A. C., & Glasgow, R. E. (2008). A practical, robust implementation and sustainability model (PRISM) for integrating research findings into practice. *The Joint Commission Journal on Quality and Patient Safety*, *34*(4), 228–243.

Fernandez, M. E., Ten Hoor, G. A., Van Lieshout, S., Rodriguez, S. A., Beidas, R. S., Parcel, G., … Kok, G. (2019). Implementation mapping: using intervention mapping to develop implementation strategies. *Frontiers in Public Health*, *7*, 158.

Glasgow, R. E., Vogt, T. M., & Boles, S. M. (1999). Evaluating the public health impact of health promotion interventions: the RE-AIM framework. *American Journal of Public Health*, *89*(9), 1322–1327.

Harvey, G., & Kitson, A. (2015). PARIHS revisited: from heuristic to integrated framework for the successful implementation of knowledge into practice. *Implementation Science*, *11*(1), 1–13.

Hunt, K., Wyke, S., Bunn, C., Donnachie, C., Reid, N., & Gray, C. M. (2020). Scale-Up and Scale-Out of a Gender-Sensitized Weight Management and Healthy Living Program Delivered to Overweight Men via Professional Sports Clubs: The Wider Implementation of Football Fans in Training (FFIT). *International Journal of Environmental Research And Public Health, 17*(2), 584. Retrieved from https://www.mdpi.com/1660-4601/17/2/584

Hunt, K., Wyke, S., Gray, C. M., Anderson, A. S., Brady, A., Bunn, C., ... Leishman, J. (2014). A gender-sensitised weight loss and healthy living programme for overweight and obese men delivered by Scottish Premier League football clubs (FFIT): a pragmatic randomised controlled trial. *The Lancet, 383*(9924), 1211–1221.

Indig, D., Lee, K., Grunseit, A., Milat, A., & Bauman, A. (2018). Pathways for scaling up public health interventions. *BMC Public Health, 18*(1), 1–11.

Jones, J., & Hunter, D. (1995). Consensus methods for medical and health services research. *BMJ: British Medical Journal, 311*(7001), 376.

Kane, M., & Trochim, W. M. (2007). *Concept mapping for planning and evaluation*. Sage Publications, Inc.

Klaic, M., Kapp, S., Hudson, P., Chapman, W., Denehy, L., Story, D., & Francis, J. J. (2022). Implementability of healthcare interventions: an overview of reviews and development of a conceptual framework. *Implementation Science, 17*(1), 1–20.

Lane, C., McCrabb, S., Nathan, N., Naylor, P.-J., Bauman, A., Milat, A., ... Wolfenden, L. (2021). How effective are physical activity interventions when they are scaled-up: A systematic review. *International Journal of Behavioral Nutrition and Physical Activity, 18*(1), 1–11.

Lengnick-Hall, R., Stadnick, N. A., Dickson, K. S., Moullin, J. C., & Aarons, G. A. (2021). Forms and functions of bridging factors: Specifying the dynamic links between outer and inner contexts during implementation and sustainment. *Implementation Science, 16*(1), 1–13.

Mclaughlin, M., Campbell, E., Sutherland, R., McKenzie, T., Davies, L., Wiggers, J., & Wolfenden, L. (2021). Extent, Type and Reasons for Adaptation and Modification When Scaling-Up an Effective Physical Activity Program: Physical Activity 4 Everyone (PA4E1).

Michie, S., Atkins, L., & West, R. (2014). The behaviour change wheel. *A guide to designing interventions. 1st ed. Great Britain: Silverback Publishing*, 1003–1010.

Milat, A., Lee, K., Conte, K., Grunseit, A., Wolfenden, L., Van Nassau, F., ... Bauman, A. (2020). Intervention Scalability Assessment Tool: A decision support tool for health policy makers and implementers. *Health Research Policy and Systems, 18*(1), 1–17.

Milat, A. J., King, L., Bauman, A. E., & Redman, S. (2013). The concept of scalability: increasing the scale and potential adoption of health promotion interventions into policy and practice. *Health Promotion International, 28*(3), 285–298.

Miller, C. J., Barnett, M. L., Baumann, A. A., Gutner, C. A., & Wiltsey-Stirman, S. (2021). The FRAME-IS: A framework for documenting modifications to implementation strategies in healthcare. *Implementation Science, 16*(1), 1–12.

Moore, G., Campbell, M., Copeland, L., Craig, P., Movsisyan, A., Hoddinott, P., ... Rehfuess, E. (2021). Adapting interventions to new contexts—the ADAPT guidance. *BMJ, 374*, n1679.

Moore, J. E., Bumbarger, B. K., & Cooper, B. R. (2013). Examining adaptations of evidence-based programs in natural contexts. *The Journal of Primary Prevention, 34*(3), 147–161.

Moullin, J. C., Dickson, K. S., Stadnick, N. A., Albers, B., Nilsen, P., Broder-Fingert, S., ... Aarons, G. A. (2020). Ten recommendations for using implementation frameworks in research and practice. *Implementation Science Communications, 1*(1), 1–12.

Moullin, J. C., Sabater-Hernández, D., Fernandez-Llimos, F., & Benrimoj, S. I. (2015). A systematic review of implementation frameworks of innovations in healthcare and resulting generic implementation framework. *Health Research Policy and Systems, 13*(1), 1–11.

Murray, E., Treweek, S., Pope, C., MacFarlane, A., Ballini, L., Dowrick, C., ... 'Donnell, C. (2010). Normalisation process theory: A framework for developing, evaluating and implementing complex interventions. *BMC Medicine*, *8*(1), 1–11.

Nilsen, P. (2020). Making sense of implementation theories, models, and frameworks. In *Implementation Science 3.0* (pp. 53–79): Springer.

NIH Fogarty International Center (n.d.). Toolkit Part 1: Implementation Science Methodologies and Frameworks. https://www.fic.nih.gov/About/center-global-health-studies/neuroscience-implementation-toolkit/Pages/methodologies-frameworks.aspx

Powell, B. J., Waltz, T. J., Chinman, M. J., Damschroder, L. J., Smith, J. L., Matthieu, M. M., ... Kirchner, J. E. (2015). A refined compilation of implementation strategies: Results from the Expert Recommendations for Implementing Change (ERIC) project. *Implementation Science*, *10*(1), 1–14.

Proctor, E. K., Powell, B. J., & McMillen, J. C. (2013). Implementation strategies: Recommendations for specifying and reporting. *Implementation Science*, *8*(1), 1–11.

Reilly, K. L., Kennedy, S., Porter, G., & Estabrooks, P. (2020). Comparing, contrasting, and integrating dissemination and implementation outcomes included in the RE-AIM and implementation outcomes frameworks. *Frontiers in Public Health*, *8*, 430.

Stirman, S. W., Baumann, A. A., & Miller, C. J. (2019). The FRAME: An expanded framework for reporting adaptations and modifications to evidence-based interventions. *Implementation Science*, *14*(1), 58.

Sutherland, R., Campbell, E., McLaughlin, M., Nathan, N., Wolfenden, L., Lubans, D. R., ... Searles, A. (2021). Scale-up of the Physical Activity 4 Everyone (PA4E1) intervention in secondary schools: 24-month implementation and cost outcomes from a cluster randomised controlled trial. *International Journal of Behavioral Nutrition and Physical Activity*, *18*(1), 1–18.

Sutherland, R., Campbell, E., Nathan, N., Wolfenden, L., Lubans, D. R., Morgan, P. J., ... Reeves, P. (2019). A cluster randomised trial of an intervention to increase the implementation of physical activity practices in secondary schools: Study protocol for scaling up the Physical Activity 4 Everyone (PA4E1) program. *BMC Public Health*, *19*(1), 1–14.

Wahlen, M. M., Schroeder, M. C., Johnson, E. C., Lizarraga, I. M., Engelbart, J. M., Tatman, D. J., ... Birken, S. A. (2022). Identifying Core Functions of an Evidence-Based Intervention to Improve Cancer Care Quality in Rural Hospitals. *Frontiers in Health Services*, *2*.

Wandersman, A., Duffy, J., Flaspohler, P., Noonan, R., Lubell, K., Stillman, L., ... Saul, J. (2008). Bridging the gap between prevention research and practice: the interactive systems framework for dissemination and implementation. *American Journal of Community Psychology*, *41*(3), 171–181.

Wilson, K. M., Brady, T. J., Lesesne, C., & Translation, N. W. G. (2011). Peer reviewed: an organizing framework for translation in public health: the knowledge to action framework. *Preventing Chronic Disease*, *8*(2).

Wolfenden, L., Milat, A. J., Lecathelinais, C., Skelton, E., Clinton-McHarg, T., Williams, C., ... Yoong, S. L. (2016). A bibliographic review of public health dissemination and implementation research output and citation rates. *Preventive Medicine Reports*, *4*, 441–443.

SECTION 7

Global Health Psychology

31
AN INTRODUCTION TO 'GLOBAL HEALTH PSYCHOLOGY'

Bronwynè Coetzee, Rizwana Roomaney, and Lucie Byrne-Davis

Understanding the 'Global' in Global Health Psychology

The fact that there is a section on 'global health psychology' in this handbook is both good and bad. It is good because there is an increasing desire for our science and practice to reach across international borders and, indeed, an increasing acknowledgement that our science is incomplete without considering the health psychology of the majority of the Earth's population. It is bad, however, because it reflects that much of health psychology is firmly centred on the global minority: those people living in high-income countries. Indeed, the field of psychology, generally, has been of concern in this regard since a landmark publication detailed how much of what we think we know of human psychology is based on research conducted with and by people in Western, Education, Industrialised, Rich, and Democratic (so-called WEIRD) populations (Henrich, Heine & Norenzayan, 2010). In this section, we will outline some of the key issues emerging from these needs, desires, and attempts to globalise the science and practice of health psychology, although we are aware that, as authors who span three continents and six countries, there will be much happening in health psychology around the world of which we are unaware. We hope that in presenting our collective views of global health psychology, we will pique the curiosity of readers and identify what we do not know, as well as what we do know. Our content is intended to stimulate thought and debate, as these topics are not amenable to fixing or finalising.

Global health psychology may be considered a relatively new sub-discipline of health psychology. Indeed, in 2019, the inaugural summit on Psychology and Global Health: A Leader in Climate Action took place in Lisbon, Portugal, led by the American Psychological Association (APA). At this meeting, psychologists around the world met to consider the application of psychological science and behaviour change principles to address the ever-growing climate crises/

 DOI: 10.4324/9781003318026-38

climate breakdown. Indeed, global crises, such as climate change/breakdown and the COVID-19 pandemic, have been key occurrences in driving forward a 'global' health psychology agenda. In response to the outbreak of COVID-19 at the end of 2019 and beginning of 2020, governments around the world put together expert advisory committees consisting of experts across various fields and disciplines, including global health experts and health psychologists, as well as psychologists with extensive experience in behaviour change techniques. Perhaps for many health psychologists, the appointment to these committees provided some affirmation of the key role that health psychologists (who are behaviour change experts) can play in global health. In global health, there has been a recent acknowledgement of the crucial role that behavioural research can play. The World Health Organisation (WHO) made the first global resolution on behavioural sciences for health on 29 May 2023 (Habersaat & Altieri, 2023). This resolution is a crucial signal that member states are recognising the powerful impact that the study and practice of behavioural, and other social/cultural, science can have on health. Although not all health psychology is behavioural science and not all behavioural science is health psychology, a large element of the research and practice of health psychology includes an understanding of behaviour.

The fields of 'global health', 'global public health', and 'health psychology' have traditionally been distinct and separate. However, these fields share the collective focus of promoting health and well-being for all. Health, of course, can have different meanings in different contexts but broadly encompasses a focus on the physical, biological, mental, emotional, social, and even spiritual dimensions of well-being (WHO, 2022). Global health is a field and discipline dedicated to promoting and improving the health and well-being of the global community. Koplan et al. (2009) define global health as

> an area for study, research, and practice that places a priority on improving health and achieving equity in health for all people worldwide. Global health emphasises transnational health issues, determinants, and solutions; involves many disciplines within and beyond the health sciences and promotes interdisciplinary collaboration; and is a synthesis of population-based prevention with individual-level clinical care.
>
> *(Koplan et al., 2009, p. 1995)*

As such, the field is largely concerned with health promotion and disease prevention. The field thus broadly involves multidisciplinary teams with specialties in epidemiology, behavioural medicine, medicine, psychology, and so on.

Health psychology, on the other hand, is a specific sub-discipline of psychology, and the field is primarily concerned with both the role that psychologists play in promoting health and well-being and improving quality of life and the interactions between cognition, emotion, and behaviour in health. Specifically, the sub-discipline focuses on understanding and addressing the biological, social, psychological, and structural determinants of health (Coetzee et al., 2022b). While the focus of global health is on the broader population and larger scale disease prevention and health promotion, the focus of health psychology and the role of health psychologists has largely entailed supporting the individual regarding the various psychosocial factors that impact health and well-being but also, crucially, contextualising this within specific contexts and settings. The important field of critical health psychology, which focuses on critical rather than positivist approaches, has perhaps the greatest synergy with global health since it focuses on "health and illness as socially, culturally, politically and historically situated" (Lyons & Chamberlain, 2017, p. 533). Often seen as 'critical' of health psychology, Maclachlan stressed how critical health psychology is critical for disciplines i.e., that thinking critically can and does improve the conduct of research (MaClachlan, 2006).

Taken together, 'global health psychology' might then be considered as the overlap between health psychology and global health. Although there is no accepted definition of the term, 'global health psychology' may be defined as seeking "to address health problems that transcend national boundaries, that may be influenced by circumstances and experiences in other countries, and that require co-operative actions and solutions" (Maclachlan, 2006, p. 363). This definition promotes the idea that global health problems require global health solutions, and that these solutions should be informed by all in order to be relevant and equally accessible to all. Reference to 'all' is important here, as global health psychology also then means a coming together of researchers in the Global North and Global South with knowledge and expertise in health psychology to work collaboratively towards promoting health and well-being. However, this coming together and working collaboratively is not as easy as it seems, and the North-South divide still feels quite prominent for many in the field.

In 2017, well before the COVID-19 pandemic, health psychologists affiliated with the European Society for Health Psychology (EHPS) wrote about global health psychology and their experiences of research, volunteering, and consultancy in the global context (Byrne-Davis et al., 2017). This article, featured in the *European Health Psychologist* (a key journal of the EHPS), provides an account of the challenges experienced by health psychologists working across the world and finding opportunities and ways in which to lend their expertise to address important health issues. In this article, the authors share their surprise and concern about the struggles of contributing solutions to global health issues, given a call for the help of psychologists (Shelton, 2013) to use their "knowledge and skills in behaviour change" to address global health priorities (p. 321) by a public health specialist in 2013. The authors go on to reflect on their own experiences of working in global health partnerships.

The challenges highlighted by health psychologists attempting to work in global health might reflect the relatively problematic notion of health psychology as a 'privileged speciality'. Health psychology is far more established in the Global North than it is in the Global South. Indeed, in the United States, United Kingdom, and Australia, registration with professional bodies as a health psychologist is possible and provides those trained as health psychologists in these countries with an opportunity to work in a variety of health settings to address health behaviours. Further, the professionalisation of health psychology in these settings means that health psychologists might have access to funding, opportunities, and other resources that may be harder to come by for those in the Global South, where health psychology is not yet firmly established. Indeed, in South Africa, the route to establishing health psychology as a recognised and professional registration category remains challenging (Coetzee et al., 2022b). However, great strides have been made by psychologists working broadly within the field since the 1980s (Kagee, 2006). At present, there exists a health psychology division within the Psychological Society of South Africa (PSySSA).

The Importance of Engaging in Global Health Psychology

Health psychology is about much more than behaviour, but behavioural science has received a large increased focus since the COVID-19 pandemic and its curtailment relying on prosocial behaviours (mask-wearing, distancing, handwashing) and health protective behaviours (vaccination). Of course, the impact of communicable diseases has remained high in low- and middle-income countries (LMICs), long after this became a less important issue in high-income countries (HICs). Indeed, the fact that interest in communicable disease prevention through behaviour change has increased recently is itself evidence of the bias towards problems experienced in HICs in health psychology and health behavioural science.

It is not only communicable disease prevention that has been identified as important in global health behavioural science. In 2013, the US Agency for International Development (USAID) launched an open-access journal funded by USAID and therefore without an author processing charge. This journal led, in its first issue, with an editorial about how crucial it is to develop behavioural science in global health. The editorial identified six 'domains' of behavioural change for global health, calling them the "missing health system building block": freestanding, personal, or lifestyle behaviours; care-seeking behaviours or demand; client adherence and collaboration; provider behaviour; prosocial and antisocial behaviour; and policy and priority-setting behaviours. In fact, behaviours can be directly associated with a substantial part of the global burden of disease (Kivimäki, Vineis & Brunner, 2015). Beyond these 'behavioural risk factors', which are typically lifestyle health behaviours, such as smoking, high fat and sugar diets, and poor child nutrition, behaviour is also an upstream influence on environmental risk factors, such as air pollution and some of the most important risks to health, including antimicrobial resistance and climate change. It is clear, then, that the behavioural aspects of health psychology are crucial to human health across the globe. The question we need to ask ourselves is, How ready is our science to be applied to these real-world health problems?

There are two issues that have called into question the readiness of psychological science generally for application to important real-world health problems. Over the last decade or so, psychology experienced what is known as a 'replication crisis'. In 2015, the Open Science Collaboration replicated 100 experimental or correlational studies in psychology (including cognitive and social psychology, both of which provide some underpinnings of health psychology). They found that approximately two-thirds of studies did not replicate (Aarts et al., 2015). A further issue, particularly salient in global health, is the issue of the populations from which samples are taken for many of our psychology studies. In 2010, a study made two important findings: (1) that the majority of behavioural studies are based on samples taken from so-called WEIRD populations, but that these populations make up only 12% of the global population, and (2) that researchers imply or state that their findings could be generalised to this global majority (Henrich, Heine & Norenzayan, 2010b). These two issues, coupled with the importance of psychology to global health, must then surely push for a health psychology that has an increasing global focus.

Hopefully, we have made a good case for health psychologists engaging across borders, both to improve the science we produce and to make it more meaningful and useful in tackling real-world health issues. A final reason for engaging globally is one of social accountability and justice. The Inverse Care Law, the perverse findings that people most in need of care are the people least likely to receive it (Hart, 1971), is as relevant now as it was when it was coined 50 years ago, particularly in LMICs. In HICs, the issue is that the health disadvantages experienced by people of lower incomes are not adequately met even by a greater proportion of care being directed at them. In LMICs, people with more social and financial advantages are more likely to receive good health care than those who are poorer (Cookson, Doran, Asaria, et al., 2021b). In an increasingly global world, it is surely important for health researchers to be focusing on health issues affecting the global majority and this requires a shift in our focus from problems and populations who make up only a minority of the world. How to engage in a way that is meaningful, useful, and ethical is an important consideration.

Working across Low- Middle- and High-Income Countries

When we were first asked to edit a section on global health psychology for this important handbook, we felt excited to do so. We were grateful to the editors of the handbook for acknowledging that this section was needed and would add value to this handbook. We also felt privileged and honoured that we were asked to contribute to this section by editing it. As researchers who work in the field but are also located outside the health psychology hubs of Europe and North America, we often experience ourselves as being on the outside looking in, especially when we engage with colleagues from the Global North. We thought that we knew what global health psychology was (we are less certain now) and wasted no time reaching out to colleagues who work in health psychology in countries where the field was not well-established or who collaborated with researchers from these countries. We hoped to share with readers the experiences of others working in health psychology who were located on the periphery. We invited researchers in these locations to contribute to this section in the hope that it would give the reader some insights into what working in health psychology is like for those who do not work in settings where the field is well-established.

We cannot overlook the fact that health psychology has been firmly established both as a profession and research field in several countries. In many countries, the profession of health psychology does not exist, and there are no postgraduate courses in health psychology. The establishment of health psychology in some countries has only been possible because of the interest from psychologists and the availability of resources to support and expand the field. One of the reasons that health psychology is not established in other countries is that there is fierce competition for resources, and health psychology can be considered a luxury and is therefore not prioritised. This has not stopped many from engaging in the field either by conducting research or teaching health psychology to university students. Often, this means transplanting health psychology knowledge and theory developed in well-resourced settings to lesser-resourced settings. This transplanting of knowledge and theory helps to encourage health psychology as a universal field. It works because health psychology, similar to psychology in general, is very much aimed at creating positive changes in individuals to improve health.

However, within resource-constrained settings, more attention may need to be paid to structural social elements and the role that they play in health. For example, studies on healthy eating habits often place an emphasis on the importance of family meal practices, which are based on the nuclear family. However, in many under-resourced countries, this nuclear family is replaced by extended families, single-parent households, and even child-headed households. In addition, families may struggle with food insecurity, and parents may work long, irregular hours and be unable to eat with their children. Our point is that even though we know that contexts differ, we continue to transplant knowledge between vastly different contexts. Furthermore, the research methods used may not be appropriate or culturally sensitive in different settings.

One way through which health psychology research has been expanded in the Global South is through North-South research collaborations. This section of the handbook is co-authored by psychologists and researchers who have experience with these types of collaborations. While there are many positive experiences, these chapters also highlight several challenges pertaining to North-South research collaboration. These include a mismatch in motivation for collaboration, knowledge, and power dynamics that play out during the course of data collection and publication, and tokenism. As researchers, we have also experienced many of these challenges.

We considered what drives these collaborations. For those of us from the Global South, we are driven by a need to expand the field of health psychology and improve the health of people in our home countries. We are often eager to collaborate and learn from more experienced researchers. Sometimes we enter into collaborations without considering power dynamics, which may emerge later on. For example, in some cases, funding is made available from collaborators or funders from the more resourced settings, and this may set up certain power dynamics. Collaborators from the North may see themselves as leading the projects as they bring the funding. This may lead to collaborations where researchers from the local contexts where the research is conducted are seen as little more than data collectors. Their indigenous knowledge and expertise may be overlooked in favour of the knowledge held by those from contexts where health psychology is more established. In this way, we should caution against research colonialism and encourage collaborators to embrace principles that allow for deeper critical engagement and the development of new knowledge. For those of us in the Global North, we are sometimes driven by interesting new research questions, a desire to travel and see more of the world, and, hopefully, to play our part in redressing the imbalanced focus of health psychology on the problems of the global minority. What undoubtedly occurs, as has been found with a wide range of health professionals (Tyler, Chatwin, Byrne, et al., 2018), is that working in contexts that are profoundly different from our own provides us with a push to reflect and a widening of our minds. This two-way gain from working across the Global North and South is often overlooked, with a narrative of 'aid' or 'volunteering' being espoused. It is crucial that we do not accept this narrative but instead seek to create ethical and fair collaborations.

Indeed, the collaboration space is an exciting one, and we have much to gain from global health psychology. There is potential for the development of new methods, theories, and interventions, and in a world that is becoming increasingly globalised, this may yield tremendous contributions that can be used in the Global North and South. While this section highlights many experiences, pitfalls, and challenges associated with global health psychology, it also provides some of our thoughts and some guidelines that can lead to better collaborations for researchers endeavouring to work together in the future.

In the remainder of this section, we cover a range of topics that we considered were the most current and crucial to highlight. Chapter 32 presents the authors' perceptions of the state of health psychology in the Global South. They outline what is available on the internet that describes health psychology across a variety of countries. In Chapter 33, the authors highlight and discuss the challenges researchers, embedded within the field of health psychology, face in terms of finding funding opportunities to promote health psychology research in the Global South. The authors also discuss the challenges that arise when applying health psychology theories developed in the Global North to health and behavioural issues in the Global South. Finally, the authors reflect on the challenges related to disseminating research in the Global South to a global audience. Chapter 34 highlights an area of health psychology which is highly advanced in the Global South: action research and community participatory research. These authors define the approach and provide a range of examples related to health psychology where this research approach has been implemented successfully in LMICs. Finally, in Chapter 35, the authors bring together some of the key issues in ethics and collaboration. The authors highlight the importance of health partnerships and the challenges in achieving equal and fair health partnerships in global health research. Ending with a hopeful outlook, the authors propose ways in which key role players can form health partnerships both locally and internationally. As we said at the start of this chapter, global health psychology is not a fixed thing, something that we can wholly cover in a book section. We have undoubtedly highlighted the topics of most concern to us and will have unfortunately not touched on areas that others will consider to be important. Above all, we hope that this section sparks interest and thoughts about the place of health psychology in an increasingly globalised world.

Further Reading

Coetzee, B. J., Vogel, L., Sander, S., Field, C., Kagee, A., & Roomaney, R. (2022). Revisiting the relevance and importance of Health Psychology in South Africa. *South African Journal of Psychology*, *53*(1), 57–67. https://doi.org/10.1177/00812463221094728

Cookson, R., Doran, T., Asaria, M., Gupta, I., & Mujica, F. P. (2021). The inverse care law re-examined: A global perspective. *The Lancet*, *397*(10276), 828–838. https://doi.org/10.1016/s0140-6736(21)00243-9

Crisp, N. (2010). *Turning the World Upside Down: The search for global health in the 21st Century*. http://www.gtc.ox.ac.uk/images/ems/F.%20Turning%20the%20World%20Upside%20Down%20-%20Oxford%204%20December%202009.pdf

Henrich, J., Heine, S., & Norenzayan, A. (2010). The weirdest people in the world? *Social Science Research Network*. https://doi.org/10.2139/ssrn.1601785

References

Aarts, A. A., Anderson, J. E., Anderson, C. J., Attridge, P. R., Attwood, A., Axt, J., Babel, M., Bahník, Š., Baranski, E., Barnett-Cowan, M., Bartmess, E., Beer, J. S., Bell, R., Bentley, H., Beyan, L., Binion, G., Borsboom, D., Bosch, A., Bosco, F. A., … Graham, J. (2015). Estimating the reproducibility of psychological science. *Science*, *349*(6251). https://doi.org/10.1126/science.aac4716

Byrne-Davis, L., Bull, E., Burton, A., Dharni, N., Gillison, F., Maltinsky, W., Mason, C., Sharma, N., & Hart, J. (2017). Global health psychology: Research, volunteering consultancy. *The European Health Psychologist*, *19*(2), 321–325.

Coetzee, B. J., Vogel, L., Sander, S., Field, C., Kagee, A., & Roomaney, R. (2022b). Revisiting the relevance and importance of Health Psychology in South Africa. *South African Journal of Psychology*, *53*(1), 57–67. https://doi.org/10.1177/00812463221094728

Cookson, R., Doran, T., Asaria, M., Gupta, I., & Mujica, F. P. (2021b). The inverse care law re-examined: A global perspective. *The Lancet*, *397*(10276), 828–838. https://doi.org/10.1016/s0140-6736(21)00243-9

Habersaat, K. B., & Altieri, E. (2023). Behavioural Sciences for Better Health: WHO resolution and Action framework. *European Journal of Public Health*, *33*(Supplement_2). https://doi.org/10.1093/eurpub/ckad160.463

Hart, J. T. (1971). The inverse care law. *The Lancet* (London, England), *1* 297(7696), 405–412. https://doi.org/10.1016/s0140-6736(71)92410-x

Henrich, J., Heine, S., & Norenzayan, A. (2010b). The weirdest people in the world? *Social Science Research Network*. https://doi.org/10.2139/ssrn.1601785

Kagee, A. (2006). A milestone for South African psychology. *South African Journal of Psychology*, *36*(4), 661–665. https://doi.org/10.1177/008124630603600401

Kivimäki, M., Vineis, P., & Brunner, E. J. (2015). How can we reduce the global burden of disease? *The Lancet*, *386*(10010), 2235–2237. https://doi.org/10.1016/s0140-6736(15)00129-4

Koplan, J. P., Bond, T. C., Merson, M. H., Reddy, K. S., RodrńGuez, M. H., Sewankambo, N., & Wasserheit, J. N. (2009). Towards a common definition of global health. *The Lancet*, *373*(9679), 1993–1995. https://doi.org/10.1016/s0140-6736(09)60332-9

Lyons, A. C., & Chamberlain, K. (2017). *Critical Health Psychology*. In Palgrave Macmillan UK eBooks (pp. 533–555). https://doi.org/10.1057/978-1-137-51018-1_26

MacLachlan, M. (2006). Towards a global health contribution for critical health psychology. *Journal of Health Psychology*, *11*(3), 361–365. https://doi.org/10.1177/1359105306063304
Shelton, J. D. (2013). The 6 domains of behavior change: the missing health system building block. *Global Health, Science and Practice*, *1*(2), 137–140. https://doi.org/10.9745/ghsp-d-13-00083
Tyler, N., Chatwin, J., Byrne, G., Hart, J., & Byrne-Davis, L. (2018). The benefits of international volunteering in a low-resource setting: Development of a core outcome set. *Human Resources for Health*, *16*(1). https://doi.org/10.1186/s12960-018-0333-5
World Health Organization (WHO) (2022). *Achieving well-being: A global framework for integrating well-being into public health utilizing a health promotion approach*. https://cdn.who.int/media/docs/default-source/health-promotion/framework4wellbeing_16dec22.pdf?sfvrsn=32a0e228_5&download=true Last accessed 30th October 2023.

32

WHAT IS THE STATE OF HEALTH PSYCHOLOGY IN THE GLOBAL SOUTH?

Enoch Teye-Kwadjo, Darlina Hani Fadil Azim, Asma Bibi, and Jo Hart

Introduction

Concerned with "the promotion and maintenance of health, the prevention and treatment of illness" (Matarazzo, 1982, p. 4) across different social contexts, health psychology emerged in the Global North in the 1970s (APA Task Force on Health Research, 1976). Since then, as the role of psychologists in health care gains momentum in the 21st century, increasing numbers of psychologists are identifying themselves with health psychology (https://www.apa.org/about/division/div38), with clinical health psychology (Bogucki et al., 2022; https://www.apa.org/ed/graduate/specialize/health), or with other related disciplines such as behavioural medicine (Davidson et al., 2021; Smith, 2020) and medical psychology (King, 2013). There is also evidence that most psychologists who trained as clinical psychologists, social psychologists, and public health professionals have been undertaking health promotion and maintenance work that could be described as health psychology work (Kobau et al., 2011; Taylor, 2011).

Recent articles by Plass et al. (2017) and McSharry and colleagues (2017) explored health psychology presence and training in countries represented by the European Health Psychology Society (EHPS), which included some Global South countries. Yet, comprehensive information about the state of health psychology in the Global South is limited. There is a need for health psychologists to be interested in where and how health psychology is taught, practiced, and regulated as a professional division in the Global South. This information could elucidate our understanding of how health psychology is practiced as a science and a profession in a variety of settings across the Global South and support its development.

In this chapter, we first assess the state of health psychology as a professional division in the Global South, defined as "the regions of Latin America, Asia,

DOI: 10.4324/9781003318026-39

Africa, and Oceania" (Dados & Connell, 2012, p. 12). In order to explore the presence and structures around health psychology in the Global South, an extensive search was carried out using the number of countries ($N = 137$) in the Global South categorised by region (see OWSD, n.d.). Next, we describe the presence of health psychology interest groups or bodies in the Global South. We adopt the APA's definition of 'division of psychology' as a professional home organised by interest groups (APA, 2023). Thus, throughout this chapter, we use professional division/category of psychology to represent a subdiscipline of psychology and 'professional group/body' to represent the members identifying with or belonging to this professional interest group, who, through their teaching, research, practice, and advocacy, are promoting the goals of this professional division or subdiscipline of psychology. Then, for each Global South country where health psychology is present, we provide an indication of the health psychology research being conducted in that country. Finally, we provide a summary of the state of health psychology in the Global South.

Search Strategy

The search for information was conducted in two phases. In Phase One, we searched for information on the presence of health psychology as a professional division and healthy psychology groups/bodies on the World Wide Web and on Google for specific countries in the Global South. We also searched on the websites of universities for the listing of health psychology and on the websites of psychological associations/societies as listed on the website of the International Union of Psychological Science (https://www.iupsys.net/) and the Memoranda of Understanding Partners section of the American Psychological Association's website (https://www.apa.org/international/programs/memorandum-understanding/partners). We also searched the grey literature and social media platforms for information on health psychology and health psychology groups/bodies in the Global South. The search strategy was guided by a research question: "What is the state of health psychology in the Global South?" To make the search manageable, we broke the research question into major concepts and themes. We listed important synonyms or alternative terms (e.g., health psychology or health psychologist (s) or clinical health psychology). We developed a search planner and entered all of the concepts and thematic areas into it. Following the classification of Global South Countries by the OWSD, we categorised the Global South nations into four regions: (a) Africa, (b) Asia and the Pacific, (c) Latin America and the Caribbean, and (d) the Arab Region. Within each region, we searched for a number of countries. The search terms/concepts were 'health psychology', 'health psychologist(s)', 'clinical health psychology', 'health psychology body', 'health psychology division', and 'health psychology group'. The terms for the countries were the names of the Global South countries (e.g., Ghana, South Africa, Nigeria). We used the appropriate Boolean operator "OR" to link our search terms and combined them with the "AND" operator. For example, ("health psychology" 'OR' "health psychologist" 'OR' "clinical health psychology", 'OR' "health psychology association", 'OR' "health psychology division", 'OR' "healthy psychology group") 'AND' ("Ghana"). The main language for the search was English language but websites of psychological associations/societies that were not in the English language were also searched and translated using Google Translate. Where available, the electronic information gathered is supplemented by information from authors' own countries and contacts, as well as contacting organisations directly. Figure 32.1 is a flow diagram to summarise the search in Phase One.

In Phase Two, we searched on Google Scholar and Scopus for health psychology research in the Global South countries where we found evidence of the presence of health psychology as a professional division. The search terms used

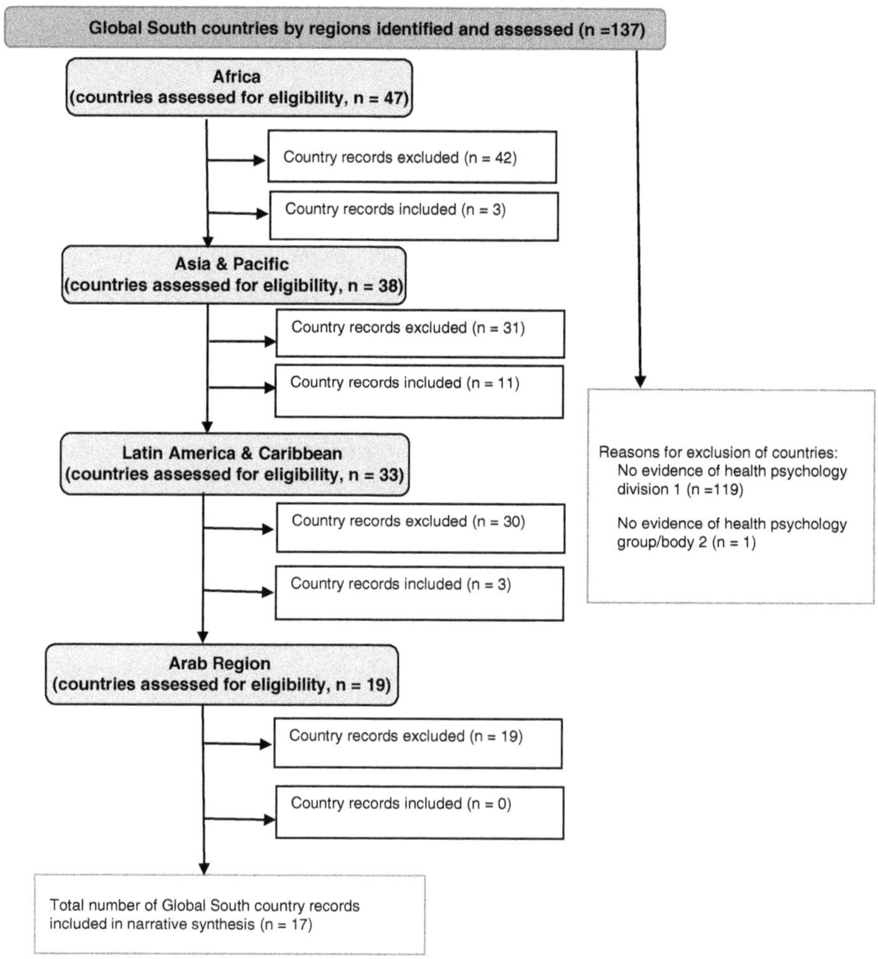

Figure 32.1 Flow diagram showing the number of global south countries assessed and selected.

reflected popular topics in health psychology as well as theories of health behaviour. The health psychology research topic-related terms used were 'dietary behaviour', 'smoking cessation', 'health screening uptake', 'medication adherence', 'treatment adherence', 'sexual risk behaviour', 'chronic disease self-care behaviour', 'sedentary behaviour', 'physical activity', 'health beliefs', and 'health behaviour'. The health behaviour theory-based search terms included 'health belief model', 'theory of planned behaviour', 'protection motivation theory', and 'socio-cognitive theory'. These search terms were combined with the 'AND' Boolean operator and linked with the "OR" Boolean operator. Full articles, titles, and abstracts were searched.

Data Extraction

The data were extracted using data extraction and assessment matrix we developed in Microsoft Word. For each country, the data extracted included whether or not health psychology is present in that country, the name of the health psychology association or group, list of members, website of the association, and names of universities where health psychology is taught as a course. A thematic narrative review was used to synthesise the health psychology information obtained in the countries. Regarding the indicator of health psychology research in a Global South country, the main information that was extracted was the country of the research participants, the health-enhancing behaviour or health-compromising behaviour studied, and findings of the study, as well as the references.

Inclusion Criteria

Being a Global South country where health psychology is recognised as a professional division, with the presence of a health psychology interest group/body, having this information on the World Wide Web or on social media, or having this information on the website of a higher education institution, or on the website of a national psychological association/society, or on a specific website meant for the health psychology interest group. Global South countries were also included if they have health psychology as an academic course on a university's website. Health psychology information on Global South countries was also included if the information was in the English language or in other languages translatable by the use of Google Translate. Regarding the indicator of health psychology research undertaken in the countries where health psychology is present as a professional division, the research was included if the title of the study reflects a health psychology research topic/theme (i.e., health-enhancing behaviour change or health-compromising behaviour), uses health behaviour theory to guide this research or intervention, and the sample used in the study is from the Global South country in question. We included these studies irrespective of whether or not the author(s) self-identifies or self-identify as health psychologists (via their departmental affiliations).

Exclusion Criteria

Being a Global South country where health psychology is not recognised as a professional division, with no presence of health psychology interest group/body, not having this information on the World Wide Web or on social media, or not having this information on the website of a higher education institution, or on the website of a national psychological association/society, or on a specific website meant for the health psychology interest group. Global South countries were also excluded if they did not have health psychology as an academic course on a university's website. Health psychology information on Global South countries was also excluded if the information was in a language other than the English language and was not translatable by the use of Google Translate. Regarding the indicator of health psychology research undertaken in the countries where health psychology is present as a professional division, the research was excluded if the title of the study does not reflect a health psychology research topic/theme (i.e., health-enhancing behaviour change or health-compromising behaviour), does not use health behaviour theory to guide this research or intervention, and the sample used in the study is not from the Global South country in question. We excluded these studies irrespective of whether or not the author(s) self-identifies or self-identify as health psychologists (via their departmental affiliations).

Health Psychology as a Professional Division and the Presence of Health Psychology Groups or Bodies in Africa

Ghana

Established by an Act of Parliament (Act 857), the Ghana Psychology Council (GPC) makes it mandatory for psychologists to identify themselves with a specialty or subfield of psychology when applying for licensure and certification. One of the specialties named in the licensure application form is health psychology (see https://ghanapsychologycouncil.gov.gh/downloads/). The Ghana Psychological Association (GPA) also recognises health psychology as a professional category. In addition, health psychology and clinical health psychology are taught as undergraduate and graduate courses at two Ghanaian universities, the University of Ghana (2023) and the University of Cape Coast (2023), respectively. This information indicates that there is a group of health psychologists and clinical health psychologists in Ghana. This group, according to the GPA, conducts its activities mostly on WhatsApp and is yet to migrate its activities to its website. There is evidence that some psychologists who self-identified as health psychologists are teaching and practising in Ghana (see de-Graft Aikins, 2018). The first author of this chapter is a health psychologist who is teaching and conducting health psychology research in Ghana.

There is substantial evidence to suggest that health psychology research is being conducted in Ghana. For example, the theory of planned behaviour was found to be useful in understanding safe sexual behaviour among school-going adolescents (Teye-Kwadjo et al., 2017) and seatbelt-wearing behaviour among drivers in Ghana (Teye-Kwadjo et al., 2020). In addition, in a sample of 200 Ghanaian women, Ampofo et al. (2020) found that the health belief model's constructs of perceived benefits, perceived threat, perceived barriers, and cues for action were important determinants of cervical cancer screening uptake. Further, health behaviours such as diabetes self-care and self-management were examined among Ghanaian patients (Hushie, 2019; Obirikorang et al., 2022). Other health psychology research in Ghana investigated illness perceptions and antiretroviral medication adherence among people living with HIV (Anakwa et al., 2021; Fosu et al., 2022) and illness perceptions and health-related quality of life in Ghanaian breast cancer survivors (Dadzie et al., 2023; Ofei et al., 2023).

Nigeria

There is evidence that the Nigerian Psychological Association (NPA) recognises health psychology and clinical health psychology as professional categories, as can be seen in the specialties of the members on the NPA's website (see https://npass.org.ng/). This information suggests that the NPA requires psychologists in Nigeria to self-identify with a subfield during registration for membership. While there is little evidence to suggest that there is a professional group or body of health psychologists in Nigeria, the presence of psychologists identifying themselves with this professional category indicates that there are scores of health psychologists working as individuals in Nigeria.

We found some evidence of health psychology research in Nigeria. For example, Sripad et al. (2019) examined health beliefs, attitudes, and health-care-seeking behaviour among Nigerian women who experienced pre-eclampsia and eclampsia during pregnancy, applying the health beliefs model. They found that perceived threat and perceived susceptibility to health complications predicted care-seeking behaviours in this sample. Using the theory of planned behaviour, Ojedokun et al. (2022) examined littering preventive behaviour in a sample of 300 Nigerians. Results showed that perceived behaviour control was positively associated with littering prevention intentions, and littering prevention intentions, in turn, predicted littering prevention behaviour. Moreover, consistent condom use behaviour of young Nigerians was assessed by researchers (Adebiyi & Asuzu, 2009; Ajayi et al., 2019; Sunmola et al., 2007).

South Africa

The Psychological Society of South Africa (PsySSA) created a professional interest group for health psychology (Psychological Society of South Africa, 2021). It is important to note that the creation of this professional division follows many years of professional consciousness-raising for such a specialised subfield by South African scholars (see. e.g., Yen, 2016; Yen & Vaccarino, 2018). Recent research in South Africa has reported that a growing number of psychologists are self-identifying with health psychology (see Coetzee et al., 2023). Thus, a professional health psychology group is present in South Africa. South Africa also has a national delegate in the EHPS (https://ehps.net/national-delegates/south-africa/).

Health psychology research is present in South Africa despite health psychology as a professional category being new in South Africa. The theory of planned behaviour has been applied to various health-enhancing behaviours, including consistent condom use among South African adolescents (Jemmott et al., 2007) and adherence to antiretroviral therapy among HIV patients (Saal & Kagee, 2012). Blood pressure (BP) control behaviour in patients with hypertension, as well as treatment adherence, was undertaken by Onwukwe and Ngene (2022). They found that poor treatment adherence was a strong predictor of high BP and called for effective behaviour change interventions to address hypertension. Other South African work also examined key health behaviours, such as smoking cessation (Morar & Robertson, 2022) and quality of life in women living with endometriosis (Roomaney & Kagee, 2018).

Health Psychology as a Professional Division and the Presence of Health Psychology Groups or Bodies in Asia and the Pacific

China

The Chinese Psychological Society recognises health psychology as a professional category and has created divisions for Emotional and Health Psychology and Behavior and Health Psychology (https://www.cpsbeijing.org/about/leaders/index.htm). In addition, health psychology is taught as an academic discipline at the Department of Psychology, Beijing Normal University (https://psych.bnu.edu.cn/rcpy/bkspy/kcjsa/b537a0f63f7344b1b53679cf011b65f6.htm). Further, sponsored by the China Mental Health Association, the China Association for Science and Technology publishes an academic journal entitled *Chinese Journal of Health Psychology* (see the journal's website at https://www.zazhi.com.cn/zgjkxlx/). All these pieces of information point to the fact that there is a professional group of health psychologists present in China.

Health psychology research abounds in China. Wang et al. (2022) examined the healthy eating intentions and behaviour of 1,281 Chinese residents across 21 provinces, 3 autonomous regions, and 4 municipalities using the health belief model (HBM). They found that the HBM provided a good explanatory framework for understanding healthy eating behaviour. Other results demonstrated that perceived severity, perceived benefits, self-efficacy, and perceived susceptibility were associated with residents' healthy eating intentions. In addition, Shi et al. (2021) applied the theory of planned behaviour (TPB) to understand the intention to improve oral health behaviours among Chinese students. The researchers found that the TPB accounted for 28.30% of the variance in intentions to improve their oral health. Attitudes, subjective norms, and perceived behavioural control were found to be significantly associated with the intentions to improve oral health behaviours. Moreover, Hu et al. (2022) examined the factors influencing self-care behaviours of 1,140 Chinese patients with type 2 diabetes using the HBM. The results showed that perceived severity, perceived benefits, and perceived barriers were associated with diabetes self-care behaviours in this sample. Other health behaviours such as medication adherence (Ge et al., 2022), dementia preventive health-promoting lifestyle behaviour (Li et al., 2022), diabetic complication screening uptake (Jiang et al., 2021), and adherence to COVID-19 preventive behaviour were investigated in Chinese samples.

Hong Kong

There is a social and health psychology course at the University of Hong Kong (https://psychology.hku.hk/social-and-health-psychology/). The course operates a social and health psychology lab (https://www.psychology.hku.hk/sopsylab/). In addition, there is a health psychology course for undergraduate students at the Hong Kong Shue Yan University (https://counpsy.hksyu.edu/UndergraduateProgrammes/UGCourseoutline/PSY/PSY303%20Health%20Psychology). The Hong Kong University of Science and Technology also runs a health psychology programme (https://hkust.edu.hk/). Further, there is a clinical health psychology Centre at the Hong Kong Sanatorium and Hospital. However, the Hong Kong Psychological Society Ltd does not have health psychology as one of the professional divisions of psychology available in Hong Kong (https://www.hkps.org.hk/en/). Nonetheless, the available information on health psychology in Hong Kong thus far suggests that there are individuals or interest groups teaching and/or practising health psychology in Hong Kong.

We found evidence of health psychology research in Hong Kong. Cheung et al. (2021) assessed the knowledge of and behaviour towards a reduction in salt intake among 426 adults in Hong Kong. Results showed that most participants were not aware that excessive salt intake could bring about coronary heart disease. They observed a low salt reduction behaviour among the participants because the participants were not interested in checking the salt content listed on their food labels. Similarly, Siu et al. (2019) investigated unhealthy eating behaviours of adolescents from low-income families in Hong Kong. The results showed that most participants skipped meals and practiced irregular meal patterns because of poverty. Siu et al. (2019) also found that some of the participants perceived healthy eating to be expensive and was thus unappealing. Moreover, health psychology topics such as vaccination uptake behaviour (Mo & Lau, 2015), smoking cessation (Ho et al., 2021; Li et al., 2020), and physical activity behaviour (Ha et al., 2010; Huang et al., 2014; Zhang et al., 2022) have been undertaken by participants in Hong Kong.

India

India's National Academy of Psychology (NAOP) recognises clinical health psychology as a professional category (NAOP, 2022). This professional category has several psychologists identifying themselves with it (https://naopindia.org/divisions). There is also evidence that health psychology is recognised as crucial in the Indian health-care system (see Hariharan et al., 2022).

Hariharan et al. (2022) underscore the need for health psychologists and medical professionals to work together to promote health and prevent illness, given the shift from biomedical to the biopsychosocial model of health care. As an example, there is a specific Centre devoted to the study of health psychology at the University of Hyderabad (https://medicalsciences.uohyd.ac.in/healthpsychology/). There is also the India Academy of Health Psychology, which is a professional organisation of psychologists who identify themselves with this specialty (Indian Academy of Health Psychology, 2023). From the foregoing, it seems clear that there is a professional health psychology group or body present in India.

There is evidence of health psychology research in India. For example, Mishra et al. (2021) investigated adherence to antidiabetic medication and quality of life among 227 patients with T2 diabetes mellitus in Uttarakhand, India. They found that, compared with patients who were non-adherent, patients who were adherent to their antidiabetic medication reported higher quality of life. Further, Sahoo and Pradhan (2021) examined reproductive health-care beliefs and behaviours among displaced tribal communities in Odisha and Chhattisgarh, India, using the HBM. The study found that the HBM's constructs provided a useful framework for understanding participants' perceived susceptibility to disease and the severity of disease relative to their traditional health-care beliefs and behaviours. Tarkar (2023) assessed the utility of the TPB and HBM in predicting COVID-19 vaccine uptake in India. Results showed the integrated model explained 71% of the variance in vaccine uptake intentions, while attitudes, subjective norms, and perceived behavioural control from the TPB were positively associated with vaccine uptake intentions. Other results showed that perceived benefits and perceived susceptibility from the HBM had indirect effects on vaccine uptake intentions through attitudinal beliefs.

Indonesia

We found evidence indicating that the Himpunan Psikologi Indonesia (HIMPSI) (Indonesian Psychological Association) has created health psychology as a professional division known as the Indonesian Health Psychology Association (https://himpsi.or.id/asosiasi). The Indonesian Health Psychology Association has a leadership and secretariat, which can be found on HIMPSI's website. This information confirms that health psychology as a professional group or body is present in Indonesia.

There is evidence of health psychology research in Indonesia. Dewi et al. (2019) examined breast self-examination (BSE) as health behaviour among women living in Surabaya, Indonesia, employing the HBM. Results showed that perceived benefits, perceived self-efficacy, perceived barriers, and cues to action were associated with BSE and that the HBM was useful in explaining BSE practice. Similarly, Sumarmi et al. (2021) assessed the factors associated with pap smear uptake intentions in the rural areas of Indonesia using the HBM. They found that the HBM accounted for 31% of the variance in intentions to undergo pap smear testing among Indonesian women. Other health psychology topics investigated in Indonesia include, but are not limited to, physical activity and sedentary behaviour (Andriyani et al., 2021) and COVID-19 vaccine uptake (Adiyoso et al., 2023).

Iran

The Iranian Psychological Association (https://iranpa.org/Default-EN.aspx) has a professional category for health psychology, as can be seen in the creation of the Iranian Health Psychology Association on its website. The list of members of the Iranian Health Psychology Association can be found at this link (https://civilica.com/l/434/). This information suggests that there is a professional body of health psychologist teaching, researching, and/or practising in Iran. In addition, there are two health psychology journals in Iran. They are *Health Psychology* (https://hpj.journals.pnu.ac.ir/article_1393.html?lang=en) published by the Payame Noor University and the Iranian Health Psychology Association, and the *Iranian Journal of Health Psychology* (https://ijohp.journals.pnu.ac.ir/). Other research also described the state of medical psychology in Iran (see Ghobari & Bolhari, 2001). The goals of medical psychology are similar to those of health psychology.

Health psychology research is growing in Iran. Shahsavari et al. (2022) applied the HBM to understand genital warts preventive behaviour among Iranian women. They found that perceived susceptibility, perceived severity, and self-efficacy were positively associated with genital warts preventive behaviour among the women. Hosseini et al. (2021) examined retinopathy preventive behaviour among patients with type 2 diabetes using the TPB. They reported that the TPB provided a useful framework for understanding health-related behaviour and should be used to design effective blood sugar control programmes among patients with diabetes in Iran. Further, Dadipoor et al. (2023) assessed waterpipe smoking cessation among Iranian women, applying the TPB. They reported that an increase in the attitude score, perceived behavioural control score, and subjectives norms score led to the odds of smoking cessation increasing by 31%, 0.02%, and 16%, respectively, whereas an increase in the intention score triggered a 26% increase in smoking cessation. Other researchers have investigated hypertension preventive behaviours among Iranian University workers (Azadi et al., 2021) and self-care behaviours of 100 patients with hypertension living in Toyserkan, Iran.

Japan

Health psychology is recognised as a professional category in Japan because there is the Japanese Association of Health Psychology (https://kenkoshinri.jp/english/message.html). Early research in Japan provided information on the motivations for the development of health psychology in Japan (Kyoto, 1989). Japan, therefore, has a professional group of health psychologists working in the country.

We found evidence of health psychology research in Japan. Research in Japan examined smoking cessation behaviour and found that smoking cessation behaviour varied by levels of nicotine dependency (Goto et al., 2007). Kajiwara and Morimoto (2023) examined illness representations and differences in self-care behaviour among 212 patients with chronic kidney disease (CKD) in western Japan. They found that self-care behaviour scores differed by three clusters of illness representational patterns. They concluded that the self-care behaviour of CKD patients in Japan was contingent on illness representations. Other health psychology work looked at healthy dietary behaviour patterns of Japanese adults and found that various factors such as food selection, cooking frequency, and food disposal practices predicted healthy dietary behaviours. Matsuda et al. (2023) investigated dietary behaviours of Japanese lactating women. Using the protection motivation theory, Okuhara et al. (2020) found that perceived severity and self-efficacy predicted greater levels of staying at home as a COVID-19 preventive behaviour, whereas response efficacy and perceived vulnerability did not predict staying at home.

Malaysia

The Malaysian Psychological Association/Persatuan Psikologi Malaysia (https://www.psima.org.my/) has professional divisions of psychology, such as positive psychology (https://www.isqols.org/news/11142981) and clinical psychology (https://www.mscp.my/about-us) but not health psychology. However, there is a health psychology clinic at the Universiti Kebangsaan Malaysia that provides health psychology services to clients (https://www.ukm.my/fsk/health-psychology-clinic/). A look at the clinic's website suggests that most of the psychologists offering this service received training in clinical psychology. This information also suggests that there are scores of psychologists in Malaysia with a background in clinical psychology who are offering a hybrid service in clinical health psychology. Thus, it is possible that there is a health psychology interest group in Malaysia, but this group's activities are not available online. This information corroborates that of a personal communication by the second author of this chapter (from Malaysia), who revealed that most psychologists providing health psychology services in Malaysia received training in clinical psychology. The second author is a clinical psychologist who is teaching and practising health psychology in Malaysia.

There is considerable evidence that health psychology research is being conducted in Malaysia. Lim et al. (2019) examined the factors associated with smoking cessation in Malaysia and found that older age, being married, and having tertiary education were associated with smoking cessation behaviour. Other results showed smokers with low nicotine addiction were likely to quit smoking. Similarly, Chean et al. (2019) explored the barriers to smoking cessation among

57 smokers in Malaysia using individual interviews. The themes that emerged that participants considered to be important barriers to smoking cessation were personal and lifestyle behaviours (i.e., failure to resist smoking temptation), nicotine addiction, social cultural norms, and misconceptions. Relatedly, Zamzuri et al. (2021) assessed the factors associated with successful smoking cessation among 285 smokers in Malaysia and found the predictors of cessation to be nicotine replacement therapy, attending frequent medical appointments, and having diabetes comorbidity. Further, physical activity behaviours were examined among women by Hanlon et al. (2019). They found that availability of social support to women, location of the physical activity, and women-specific physical activity programmes encouraged greater participation by women. Other researchers reported a positive association between social support and physical activity behaviour among rural-dwelling women in Malaysia (Marthammuthu et al., 2021). Moreover, Dahlui et al. (2013) investigated breast screening uptake and health issues among rural women in Malaysia and found that having knowledge of breast cancer and being married were important predictors of BSE and clinical breast examination. Similar breast cancer screening uptake work was undertaken among Malaysian women by Schliemann et al. (2020).

Pakistan

Health psychology is recognised by the Pakistan Psychological Association as a professional category (http://www.psychologypak.org/divisions.php). This information suggests that there are scores of psychologists who identify themselves with this subfield of psychology in Pakistan. For example, the third author of this chapter is a health psychologist who is practising health psychology in Pakistan. The Pakistan Psychological Association also aims to train and develop professionals in many specialties of psychology (Rahman, 2004). Information gathered from direct sources suggests that while some psychologists are practising health psychology in Pakistan, they are yet to come together as a professional interest group to promote the ideals of health psychology.

Scholars in Pakistan have conducted health psychology research. For example, Ajani et al. (2021) assessed the self-care behaviour of 402 patients living with hypertension in Pakistan. They found that self-care behaviour was related to abstinence from alcohol, smoking cessation, and medication adherence. Age, male gender, and level of education were also found to be associated with self-care behaviour in this sample. Similarly, other researchers examined self-care practices of Pakistani patients living with type 2 diabetes mellitus (Bukhsh et al., 2019). In addition, Tariq et al. (2022) investigated the role of physical activity in patients living with type 2 diabetes in Pakistan and reported that most women viewed walking as the only acceptable form of physical activity for patients with diabetes. Hussain et al. (2020) studied the influence of health literacy on medication adherence in 524 female patients with type 2 diabetes in Pakistan and observed that patients high in health literacy were more likely to engage in optimal medication adherence. Other researchers looked at the sexual risk-taking behaviour of Pakistani homeless youth (Noor et al., 2021) and hepatitis B and C protective health behaviours among Pakistani ever-married women (Maqsood et al., 2021).

Singapore

The Singapore Psychological Society (https://singaporepsychologicalsociety.org/about-us/about-sps/) has six special interest groups aimed at promoting psychological services in Singapore. These special interest groups include coaching psychology, clinical psychology, group psychotherapy, and counselling psychology (https://singaporepsychologicalsociety.org/join-sps/). Available information shows that all members of the Singapore Psychological Society must register with the association by identifying themselves with a subfield of psychology, including health psychology (Singapore Psychological Society, 2023). There is a Clinical and Health Psychology Centre (CHPC) at the National University of Singapore (https://fass.nus.edu.sg/psy/clinical-and-health-psychology-centre/). According to information on the CHPC's website, it provides psychological services that include assessment and intervention. In addition, there is a modular undergraduate course in health psychology at the Singapore University of Social Sciences (https://www.suss.edu.sg/courses/detail/psy265). Further, there is a department devoted to the provision of Psychological Medicine at the National University Hospital (National University Health System, 2023). Psychological medicine is considered by psychologists to be similar to health psychology in many respects. While the Singapore Psychological Society does not have health psychology as a special interest group yet, evidence available on university websites in Singapore suggests that there are scores of Singaporean psychologists who identify themselves with health psychology and are providing health psychological services, including teaching health psychology. It is possible that the activities of these psychologists who identify themselves with health psychology (e.g., as lecturers in health psychology) have yet to be migrated to the World Wide Web.

There is evidence health psychology research is being conducted in Singapore. For example, Hoong et al. (2023) examined chronic disease self-management among 461 patients in Singapore and found that, compared with pre-intervention participants, post-intervention participants reported greater improvement in self-rated health, self-management behaviour, self-efficacy, and medication adherence. Lim et al. (2020) examined healthy eating behaviours (dietary behaviour) of 358 Singaporean mothers of young children and found that children's eating behaviours correlated positively with mothers' perceived behaviour control and self-efficacy. Other work found that the HBM is consistent in predicting colorectal cancer screening uptake and preventive health behaviours (Lau et al., 2020), and advocated for the health preventive interventions to be based on health behaviour theory. Moreover, Wong et al. (2010) examined smoking cessation and cancer risk in the Singaporean population and reported that, compared with current smokers, those who quit smoking were 28 times less likely to get lung cancer. Similarly, in a study among physicians and patient smokers in Singapore, Joshi et al. (2010) found that the motivators for smoking cessation included concern with smoker's own health and that of their families and friends as well as the cost of cigarettes. Other results showed that the barriers to smoking cessation in this sample were cravings and concern with withdrawal symptoms. Further, health psychology topics such as healthy lifestyle intentions (Banerjee & Ho, 2020), medication adherence (Yoon et al., 2023), and physical activity (Tay et al., 2023; Teh et al., 2023) were examined among Singaporeans.

South Korea

The Korean Psychological Association (KPA) has a division for health psychology as a professional category, named the Korean Health Psychological Association (https://www.koreanpsychology.or.kr/eng/eng01_5.asp). The Korean Health Psychological Association has the mandate to certify its members as health psychology experts, as can be seen on its website (https://www.healthpsy.or.kr:6028/). This information demonstrates that there is a professional health psychology group in Korea.

Health psychology research in Korea has examined safe sexual behaviour among young adults using the TPB (Moon et al., 2023). This research found that sexual attitudes and sexual communication influenced safe sexual behaviours and that the TPB model explained a total of 49% of the variance in safe sexual behaviours. Other work examined unhealthy weight control behaviour and substance use among young Koreans (Lee & Lee, 2019). Lee and Lee (2019) found that increased energy drink intake, cigarette smoking, and electronic cigarette use influenced unhealthy weight control behaviours of adolescent Koreans. Moreover, Je et al. (2020) assessed the factors that affect the reproductive health promotion behaviour of Korean young women from 13 Korean universities using the TPB. The results showed that sexual autonomy predicted reproductive health-promoting behaviour in this sample, whereas attitudes, subjective norms, and perceived behavioural control were positively associated with reproductive health-promoting intentions. Further, Kang et al. (2018) studied the influence of physical activity, perceived social support, and loneliness on quality of life among older adults in South Korea. They observed that physical activity and perceived social support had a significant positive effect on quality of life.

Sri Lanka

Health psychology is taught at the Institute of Mental Health in Sri Lanka (https://www.imhlk.com/diploma-course-in-health-psychology/), suggesting the presence of health psychologists in Sri Lanka, perhaps not as a group but as individuals. We, however, did not find any information on health psychology as a professional category on the Sri Lanka Psychological Association's social media handles.

We found suggestions that some health psychology research is being done in Sri Lanka. For example, Amraei et al. (2020) applied the HBM to understand the cardiovascular disease preventive behaviours of nurses. Applying the HBM, Mahindarathne (2021) examined COVID-19 preventive behaviour and found that perceived benefits, self-efficacy, and health motivation influenced cues to action, which, in turn, influenced COVID-19 preventive behaviour. Other research investigated sedentary behaviour and physical activity levels among Sri Lankans (De Silva Weliange et al., 2016; Godakanda et al., 2018) and healthy eating behaviour (Sirasa et al., 2021).

Health Psychology as a Professional Division and the Presence of Health Psychology Groups or Bodies in Latin America and the Caribbean

Brazil

The Brazilian Society of Psychology (Sociedade Brasileira de Psicologia – SBP; https://www.iupsys.net/about/members/national-members/brazil/) recognises health psychology as a professional division. Health psychology is present in Brazil as a professional category, with universities offering courses in health psychology at the undergraduate and graduate levels. There is a national, professional health psychology body named Associação Brasileira de Psicologia da Saúde (ABPSA; https://abpsa.org.br/). Brazil also has a national delegate with the EHPS (2023). Other literature has provided important information about health psychology in Brazil (Spink, 2018; Spink et al., 2016). Thus, there is substantial evidence to suggest that health psychology work in Brazil is promoted and regulated by a national, professional health psychology body. *Trends in Psychology*, an important psychology journal published by the Brazilian Society of Psychology, accepts a broad range of manuscripts, including those that investigate health psychology research topics (https://www.springer.com/journal/43076).

There is burgeoning health psychology research in Brazil. This research has examined various health psychology research topics, including diabetes self-care behaviour (Binhardi et al., 2021; Macedo et al., 2022), medication adherence (Albuquerque et al., 2022), cervical cancer screening uptake (da Silva et al., 2017), tobacco smoking cessation (Daldegan-Bueno et al., 2022), breast cancer screening uptake (Hudson et al., 2016), sedentary behaviour (Werneck et al., 2021), eating behaviours and dietary intake (de Castro et al., 2019), and poor dietary habits and physical inactivity (Christofaro et al., 2016). Other health psychology research assessed the healthy walking behaviour of 3,296 Brazilian residents in the Distrito Federal, Florianópolis, and Porto Alegre, using the TPB and found that perceived behavioural control and intention were the strongest predictors of walking behaviour (Neto et al., 2020). Moreover, Deshpande et al. (2009) assessed the factors that determine healthy eating habits among Brazilian college students, applying the HBM. They found that the constructs of the HBM provided a useful framework for understanding students' healthy eating habits.

Costa Rica

The Costa Rican Psychologists' Professional Association/Colegio de Profesionales en Psicología de Costa Rica (CPPCR) (https://www.iupsys.net/about/members/national-members/costa-rica/). The CPPCR (http://www.psicologiacr.com/) is a creature of law and regulates the activities of professional psychologists in Costa Rica. There is evidence that the CPPCR recognises health psychology as a professional division (https://ehps.net/national-delegates/costa-rica/). Health psychology practice in Costa Rica is also closely linked to that of clinical health psychology or medicinal psychology. In addition, Costa Rica has a national representation at the EHPS. There are undergraduate and graduate courses in health psychology/clinical health psychology in Costa Rica. This information suggests that there is a professional health psychology group/body present in Costa Rica (https://ehps.net/national-delegates/costa-rica/).

There is health psychology research in Costa Rica. This research has examined nonadherence to antiretroviral therapy in an HIV-positive patient population in Costa Rica and found that transportation difficulties, taking drugs on an empty stomach, and lack of pill management skills were determinants of non-adherence (Stout et al., 2004). Feldman et al. (2020) examined smoking cessation among workers in Costa Rica and found that, compared with non-quitters who lived with a smoker, quitters did not live with a smoker, and quitters were less likely to have a friend. Correspondingly, Feldman et al. (2020) have engaged in promoting smoking cessation in Costa Rica. Moreover, other health psychology research topics such as healthy eating habits (Monge-Rojas et al., 2015), diabetes and hypertension self-management (Fort et al., 2013), and casual sexual behaviour (Romero-Daza & Freidus, 2008) have been investigated among Costa Ricans.

Jamaica

There is evidence that the Jamaican Psychological Society (JamPsych) recognises health psychology as a professional category and requires psychologists to indicate their specialties during registration (https://www.jampsych.com/copy-of-membership). Health psychology is also taught at the undergraduate level at the University of the West Indies (Marks et al., 2022). We did not find express information on JamPsych's website indicating that health psychology groups or bodies are present in Jamaica. However, the recognition of health psychology as a professional category and the fact that it is being taught as an academic discipline suggests that there are scores of individuals teaching, researching, and practising health psychology in Jamaica. Recent research on the state of health psychology in Jamaica corroborates this information (Marks et al., 2022).

There is an indication of health psychology research in Jamaica. Singh et al. (2023) investigated health-related quality of life (HRQoL) among Jamaican adolescents with chronic illness and found that, compared with healthy adolescents, those with chronic illness reported poor HRQoL. Patterson (2022) examined health beliefs about male condom use and condom negotiation among Jamaican women living in Islington, Saint Mary, and observed that women reported both enablers of and barriers to condom use communication and negotiation. Other work also examined the lifestyles of Jamaicans living with hypertension and found that lifestyles such as exercise, alcohol restriction, smoking cessation, medication adherence, and healthy dietary behaviours were engaged in by the participants to control their hypertension. Moreover, various studies have examined cervical cancer screening uptake (Bessler et al., 2007; Ncube et al., 2015) and health beliefs about pap smear screening (Linton, 2021) among Jamaican women.

Limitations

We acknowledge the following limitations of this chapter. First, we relied heavily on electronic information on the World Wide Web, university websites, and grey literature for the presence of health psychology in the Global South. It is possible that health psychology is present in some countries in the Global South but that this presence is not available online (i.e., via the World Wide Web, websites, or social media platforms). We focused exclusively on health psychology information available via verifiable means to enhance validity evidence. We note that we could have included personal communication or interviews with psychologists in Global South countries that did not have an online presence. However, this was beyond what was possible in researching this chapter and would require a funded study to do so. Relying on individual accounts as to whether or not health psychology is present in a Global South country could also give rise to biases and inaccurate information. Second, we searched for information on health psychology in the Global South using websites, the World Wide Web, and social media platforms that were mostly in the English language as well as in other languages that could be translated by Google Translate. It is possible that our reliance on English language databases limited information on health psychology available in other languages that we could not access. Readers should take these limitations into consideration when interpreting information in this chapter.

Conclusion

In this chapter, we found ample evidence suggesting that health psychology is recognised as a professional division in some countries in the Global South. There is also evidence that professional health psychology interest groups or bodies are present in some of the countries surveyed. However, there is little information on the activities of the professional health psychology groups or bodies in some of the countries surveyed, suggesting that more work remains to be done in this regard. As discussed at the start, there might well be health psychologists and health psychology research which has not been discovered as part of the research for this chapter. Encouraging academics and practitioners to label their work as health psychology can support the development of the profession internationally and provide communities of practice.

Despite health psychology being a relatively young subfield of psychology, it seems to be a fast-growing subfield of psychology not only in the Global North but also in the Global South, corroborating the work of Benjamin (2014), who stated that health psychology was one of the fastest growing psychology specialties. By understanding health psychology globally, the health psychology international community can provide advocacy and support to enable countries to develop embedded health psychology as a training and career route. Internationally, we can provide examples of best practices and develop persuasive arguments for governments – for example, how health psychology can be a powerful tool in tackling health inequalities, enhancing health-care systems, and improving health outcomes.

Further Reading

Harris, M. (2024) *Decolonising healthcare innovation low-cost solutions from low-income countries*. Routledge.

Yen, J. (2016). Psychology and health after apartheid: Or, Why there is no health psychology in South Africa. *History of Psychology*, *19*(2), 77–92. https://doi.org/10.1037/hop0000025

Yen, J., & Vaccarino, O. (2018). 'Health psychology'or 'psychology for health'? A history of psychologists' engagement with health in South Africa. *Journal of Health Psychology*, *23*(3), 408–424. https://doi.org/10.1177/1359105317708201

References

Adebiyi, A. O., & Asuzu, M. C. (2009). Condom use amongst out of school youths in a local government area in Nigeria. *African Health Sciences*, *9*(2), 92–97.

Adiyoso, W., Wilopo, W., Nurbaiti, B., & Suprapto, F. A. (2023). The use of Health Belief Model (HBM) to explain factors underlying people to take the COVID-19 vaccine in Indonesia. *Vaccine: X*, *14*, 100297. https://doi.org/10.1016/j.jvacx.2023.100297

Ajani, K., Gowani, A., Gul, R., & Petrucka, P. (2021). Levels and predictors of self-care among patients with hypertension in Pakistan. *International Journal of General Medicine*, 1023–1032. https://doi.org/10.2147/IJGM.S297770

Ajayi, A. I., Ismail, K. O., & Akpan, W. (2019). Factors associated with consistent condom use: A cross-sectional survey of two Nigerian universities. *BMC Public Health*, *19*, 1–11. https://doi.org/10.1186/s12889-019-7543-1

Albuquerque, E. S., Pinto, L. D., Neto, V. L., & Fragoso, T. S. (2022). Medication adherence in systemic lupus erythematosus during Brazilian COVID-19 pandemic. *Lupus*, *31*(2), 221–227. https://doi.org/10.1177/09612033221074177

Ampofo, A. G., Adumatta, A. D., Owusu, E., & Awuviry-Newton, K. (2020). A cross-sectional study of barriers to cervical cancer screening uptake in Ghana: An application of the health belief model. *PloS One*, *15*(4), e0231459. https://doi.org/10.1371/journal.pone.0231459

Amraei, S. G., Malekshahi, F., Goudarzi, F., & Ebrahimzadeh, F. (2020). Using an educational program based on health belief model to improve the preventive behaviors of nurses against cardiovascular diseases. *Journal of Education and Health Promotion*, *9*, 100.

Anakwa, N. O., Teye-Kwadjo, E., Kretchy, I. A. (2021). Illness perceptions, social support and antiretroviral medication adherence in people living with HIV in the greater Accra region, Ghana. *Nursing Open*, *8*, 2595–2604. https://doi.org/10.1002/nop2.797

Andriyani, F. D., Biddle, S. J., & De Cocker, K. (2021). Adolescents' physical activity and sedentary behaviour in Indonesia during the COVID-19 pandemic: A qualitative study of mothers' perspectives. *BMC Public Health*, *21*(1), 1–14. https://doi.org/10.1186/s12889-021-11931-1

APA Task Force on Health Research. (1976). Contributions of psychology to health research: Patterns, problems, and potentials. *American Psychologist*, *31*(4), 263–274. https://doi.org/10.1037/0003-066X.31.4.263

APA. (2023). *APA divisions: Professional homes organized by members of APA*. Available at https://www.apa.org/about/division, accessed September 12, 2023.

Azadi, N. A., Ziapour, A., Lebni, J. Y., Irandoost, S. F., Abbas, J., & Chaboksavar, F. (2021). The effect of education based on health belief model on promoting preventive behaviors of hypertensive disease in staff of the Iran University of Medical Sciences. *Archives of Public Health*, *79*(1), 69. https://doi.org/10.1186/s13690-021-00594-4

Banerjee, S., & Ho, S. S. (2020). Applying the theory of planned behavior: Examining how communication, attitudes, social norms, and perceived behavioral control relate to healthy lifestyle intention in Singapore. *International Journal of Healthcare Management*, *13*(supl), 496–503.

Benjamin, L. T. (2014) *A brief history of modern psychology* (2nd ed.). John Wiley & Sons.

Bessler, P., Aung, M., & Jolly, P. (2007). Factors affecting uptake of cervical cancer screening among clinic attendees in Trelawny, Jamaica. *Cancer Control*, *14*(4), 396–404. https://doi.org/10.1177/107327480701400410

Binhardi, B. A., de Souza Teixeira, C. R., de Almeida-Pititto, B., Barbosa-Junior, F., Franco, L. J., de Melo, K. F. S., … de Oliveira, R. E. M. (2021). Diabetes self-care practices and resilience in the Brazilian COVID-19 pandemic: Results of a web survey: DIABETESvid. *Diabetology & Metabolic Syndrome*, *13*, 1–11. https://doi.org/10.1186/s13098-021-00706-8

Bogucki, O. E., Kacel, E. L., Schumann, M. E., Puspitasari, A. J., Pankey, T. L., Seime, R. J., … Morrison, E. J. (2022). Clinical health psychology in healthcare: Psychology's contributions to the medical team. *Journal of Interprofessional Education & Practice*, 100554. https://doi.org/10.1016/j.xjep.2022.100554

Bukhsh, A., Khan, T. M., Sarfraz Nawaz, M., Sajjad Ahmed, H., Chan, K. G., & Goh, B. H. (2019). Association of diabetes knowledge with glycemic control and self-care practices among Pakistani people with type 2 diabetes mellitus. *Diabetes, Metabolic Syndrome and Obesity: Targets and Therapy*, 1409–1417. https://doi.org/10.2147/DMSO.S209711

Chean, K., Goh, L. G., Liew, K., Tan, C., Choi, X., & Tan, K. (2019). Barriers to smoking cessation: A qualitative study from the perspective of primary care in Malaysia. *BMJ Open*, *9*, e025491. http://doi.org/10.1136/bmjopen-2018-025491

Cheung, J., Neyle, D., & Chow, P. P. K. (2021). Current knowledge and behavior towards salt reduction among Hong Kong citizens: A cross–sectional survey. *International Journal of Environmental Research and Public Health*, *18*(18), 9572. https://doi.org/10.3390/ijerph18189572

Christofaro, D. G. D., De Andrade, S. M., Mesas, A. E., Fernandes, R. A., & Farias Junior, J. C. (2016). Higher screen time is associated with overweight, poor dietary habits and physical inactivity in Brazilian adolescents, mainly among girls. *European Journal of Sport Science*, *16*(4), 498–506. https://doi.org/10.1080/17461391.2015.1068868

Coetzee, B. J., Vogel, L., Sander, S., Field, C., Kagee, A., & Roomaney, R. (2023). Revisiting the relevance and importance of health psychology in South Africa. *South African Journal of Psychology*, *53*(1), 57–67. https://doi.org/10.1177/00812463221094728

Dadipoor, S., Heydari, G., Abu-Rmeileh, N. M., Mohseni, S., Kakhaki, H. E. S., Aghamolaei, T., & Shahabi, N. (2023). A predictive model of waterpipe smoking cessation among women in southern Iran: application of the theory of planned behavior. *BMC Public Health*, *23*(1), 1151. https://doi.org/10.1186/s12889-023-16053-4

Dados, N., & Connell, R. (2012). The global south. *Contexts*, *11*(1), 12–13.

Dadzie, H. A. N., Teye-Kwadjo, E., Oppong Asante, K., Amankwah-Poku, M., Gyasi-Gyamerah, A. A., Akotia, C. S., Osafo, J., Amankwaa-Frempong, E., Roomaney, R., & Kagee, A. (2023). Psychological factors associated with mental adjustment to breast cancer: A hospital-based observational study. *Illness, Crisis & Loss*. https://doi.org/10.1177/10541373231117601. Advanced online publication.

Dahlui, M., Gan, D. E. H., Taib, N. A., & Lim, J. N. W. (2013). Breast screening and health issues among rural females in Malaysia: How much do they know and practice?. *Preventive Medicine*, *57*, S18–S20. https://doi.org/10.1016/j.ypmed.2012.12.010

Daldegan-Bueno, D., Maia, L. O., Massarentti, C. M., & Tófoli, L. F. (2022). Ayahuasca and tobacco smoking cessation: Results from an online survey in Brazil. *Psychopharmacology*, *239*(6), 1767–1782. https://doi.org/10.1007/s00213-022-06063-2

da Silva, E. R. P., de Souza, A. S., de Souza, T. G. B., Tsuha, D. H., & Barbieri, A. R. (2017). Screening for cervical cancer in imprisoned women in Brazil. *Plos One*, *12*(12), e0187873. https://doi.org/10.1371/journal.pone.0187873

Davidson, K. W., Bacon, S. L., Bennett, G. G., Brondolo, E., Czajkowski, S. M., Diefenbach, M. A., Epel, E. S., Matthews, K., Revenson, T. A., Ruis, J. M., Segerstrom, S. C., & Behavioural Medicine Research Council. (2021). Accomplishing breakthroughs in behavioural medicine research. *Nature Human Behaviour*, *5*(7), 813–815. https://doi.org/10.1038/s41562-021-01134-4

de Castro, M. A., Garcez, M. R., Pereira, J. L., & Fisberg, R. M. (2019). Eating behaviours and dietary intake associations with self-reported sleep duration of free-living Brazilian adults. *Appetite*, *137*, 207–217. https://doi.org/10.1016/j.appet.2019.02.020

De Silva Weliange, S., Fernando, D., & Gunatilake, J. (2016). Pattern of physical activity among Sri Lankan adults in the District of Colombo: A cross-sectional study. *Asia Pacific Journal of Public Health*, *28*(8), 725–736. https://doi.org/10.1177/1010539516660191

de-Graft Aikins, A. (2018). Health psychology in Ghana: A review of the multidisciplinary origins of a young sub-field and its future prospects. *Journal of Health Psychology*, *23*(3), 425–441. https://doi.org/10.1177/1359105317752805

Deshpande, S., Basil, M. D., & Basil, D. Z. (2009). Factors influencing healthy eating habits among college students: An application of the health belief model. *Health Marketing Quarterly*, *26*(2), 145–164. https://doi.org/10.1080/07359680802619834

Dewi, T. K., Massar, K., Ruiter, R. A., & Leonardi, T. (2019). Determinants of breast self-examination practice among women in Surabaya, Indonesia: An application of the health belief model. *BMC Public Health*, *19*(1), 1–8. https://doi.org/10.1186/s12889-019-7951-2

EHPS. (2023). *Brazil*. Available at https://ehps.net/national-delegates/brazil/#:~:text=Health%20psychology%20research%20groups%20have,psychology%20services%20and%20mental%20health

Feldman, R. H., Villalobos, A., & Rodriguez, R. (2020). Promoting smoking cessation in Costa Rica: A focus group study of smokers and ex-smokers. *International Quarterly of Community Health Education*, *40*(4), 331–336. https://doi.org/10.1177/0272684X19896722

Feldman, R. H., Villalobos-Pérez, A., & Rodríguez, R. G. (2020). Workplace smoking cessation in Costa Rica: Pilot study findings. *Workplace Health & Safety*, *68*(11), 508–512. https://doi.org/10.1177/2165079920907933

Fort, M. P., Alvarado-Molina, N., Peña, L., Mendoza Montano, C., Murrillo, S., & Martínez, H. (2013). Barriers and facilitating factors for disease self-management: A qualitative analysis of perceptions of patients receiving care for type 2 diabetes and/or hypertension in San José, Costa Rica and Tuxtla Gutiérrez, Mexico. *BMC Family Practice*, *14*, 1–9. https://doi.org/10.1186/1471-2296-14-131

Fosu, M., Teye-Kwadjo, E., & Salifu Yendork, J. (2022). Patient-reported experiences of medication adherence at a community-based HIV clinic, Ghana. *Journal of Patient Experience*, *9*, 23743735221107263. https://doi.org/10.1177/23743735221107263

Ge, P., Liu, S. T., Xu, S. X., Zhang, J. Z., Lai, Y. J., Fu, R. C., … Wu, Y. B. (2022). The influence of parents on medication adherence of their children in China: A cross-sectional online investigation based on health belief model. *Frontiers in Public Health*, *10*, 845032. https://doi.org/10.3389/fpubh.2022.845032

Ghobari, B., & Bolhari, J. (2001). The current state of medical psychology in Iran. *Journal of Clinical Psychology in Medical Settings*, *8*, 39–43. https://doi.org/10.1023/A:1011323822372

Godakanda, I., Abeysena, C., & Lokubalasooriya, A. (2018). Sedentary behavior during leisure time, physical activity and dietary habits as risk factors of overweight among school children aged 14–15 years: Case control study. *BMC Research Notes*, *11*(1), 1–6. https://doi.org/10.1186/s13104-018-3292-y

Goto, R., Nishimura, S., & Ida, T. (2007). Discrete choice experiment of smoking cessation behaviour in Japan. *Tobacco Control*, *16*(5), 336–343. http://doi.org/10.1136/tc.2006.019281

Ha, A. S., Macdonald, D., & Pang, B. O. (2010). Physical activity in the lives of Hong Kong Chinese children. *Sport, Education and Society*, *15*(3), 331–346. https://doi.org/10.1080/13573322.2010.493313

Hanlon, C., Khoo, S., Morris, T., & Eime, R. (2019). Factors influencing women in physical activity programs in Malaysia. *Health Promotion International*, *34*(3), 389–399. https://doi.org/10.1093/heapro/dax093

Hariharan, M., Padhy, M., & Chivukula, U. (Eds.). (2022). *Health Psychology: Contributions to the Indian Health System*. Taylor & Francis. https://doi.org/10.1037/0033-295X.98.2.224

Ho, R., Fok, P. W. Y., & Chan, H. C. H. (2021). Pattern and determinants of alcohol and tobacco co-use and its relationship with smoking cessation in Hong Kong. *Tobacco Prevention and Cessation*, *7*(March), 1–9. https://doi.org/10.18332/tpc/132288

Hoong, J. M., Koh, H. A., Wong, K., & Lee, H. H. (2023). Effects of a community-based chronic disease self-management programme on chronic disease patients in Singapore. *Chronic Illness*, *19*(2), 434–443. https://doi.org/10.1177/17423953221089

Hosseini, S. S., Shamsi, M., Khorsandi, M., & Moradzadeh, R. (2021). The effect of educational program based on theory of planned behavior on promoting retinopathy preventive behaviors in patients with type 2 diabetes: RCT. *BMC Endocrine Disorders*, *21*, 1–7. https://doi.org/10.1186/s12902-021-00680-2

Hu, Y., Liu, H., Wu, J., & Fang, G. (2022). Factors influencing self-care behaviours of patients with type 2 diabetes in China based on the health belief model: A cross-sectional study. *BMJ Open*, *12*(8), e044369. http://doi.org/10.1136/bmjopen-2020-044369

Huang, R., Ho, S. Y., Lo, W. S., & Lam, T. H. (2014). Physical activity and constipation in Hong Kong adolescents. *Plos One*, *9*(2), e90193. https://doi.org/10.1371/journal.pone.0090193

Hudson, S., Brazil, D., Teh, W., Duffy, S. W., & Myles, J. P. (2016). Effectiveness of timed and non-timed second appointments in improving uptake in breast cancer screening. *Journal of Medical Screening*, *23*(3), 160–163. https://doi.org/10.1177/0969141315624937

Hushie, M. (2019). Exploring the barriers and facilitators of dietary self-care for type 2 diabetes: A qualitative study in Ghana. *Health Promotion Perspectives*, *9*(3), 223.

Hussain, N., Said, A. S., & Khan, Z. (2020). Influence of health literacy on medication adherence among elderly females with type 2 diabetes in Pakistan. *International Quarterly of Community Health Education*, *41*(1), 35–44. https://doi.org/10.1177/0272684X19896724

Indian Academy of Health Psychology. (2023, November 30-December 2). The 8th International Conference of the Indian Academy of Health Psychology (ICIAHP 2023). Peninsula Beach Resort, Goa, India. Available at https://rsamadhan.com/wp-content/uploads/2023/08/ICIAHP-23-brochure_compressed.pdf, accessed March 5, 2024

Je, M., Ju, H. O., & Lee, J. (2020). Factors affecting reproductive health promotion behavior among late-adolescent girls in South Korea: A cross-sectional descriptive study. *Children and Youth Services Review*, *118*, 105347. https://doi.org/10.1016/j.childyouth.2020.105347

Jemmott, J. B. III, Heeren, G. A., Ngwane, Z., Hewitt, N., Jemmott, L. S., Shell, R., & O'Leary, A. (2007). Theory of planned behavior predictors of intention to use condoms among Xhosa adolescents in South Africa. *AIDS Care*, *19*(5), 677–684. https://doi.org/10.1080/09540120601084308

Jiang, L., Liu, S., Li, H., Xie, L., & Jiang, Y. (2021). The role of health beliefs in affecting patients' chronic diabetic complication screening: A path analysis based on the health belief model. *Journal of Clinical Nursing*, *30*(19–20), 2948–2959. https://doi.org/10.1111/jocn.15802

Joshi, V., Suchin, V., & Lim, J. (2010). Smoking cessation: Barriers, motivators and the role of physicians—a survey of physicians and patients. *Proceedings of Singapore Healthcare*, *19*(2), 145–153. https://doi.org/10.1177/201010581001900209

Kajiwara, Y., & Morimoto, M. (2023). Identification of illness representational patterns and examining differences of self-care behavior in the patterns in chronic kidney disease. *Plos One*, *18*(3), e0283701. https://doi.org/10.1371/journal.pone.0283701

Kang, H. W., Park, M., & Wallace, J. P. (2018). The impact of perceived social support, loneliness, and physical activity on quality of life in South Korean older adults. *Journal of Sport and Health Science*, *7*(2), 237–244. https://doi.org/10.1016/j.jshs.2016.05.003

King, P.S. (2013). Medical psychology. In: Gellman, M.D., Turner, J. R. (eds.), *Encyclopedia of Behavioral Medicine*. Springer, New York, NY. https://doi.org/10.1007/978-1-4419-1005-9_970

Kobau, R., Seligman, M. E., Peterson, C., Diener, E., Zack, M. M., Chapman, D., & Thompson, W. (2011). Mental health promotion in public health: Perspectives and strategies from positive psychology. *American Journal of Public Health*, *101*(8), e1–e9. https://doi.org/10.2105/AJPH.2010.300083

Kyoto, T. K. (1989). Health psychology in Japan. *Applied Psychology*, *38*(4), 379–395. https://doi.org/10.1111/j.1464-0597.1989.tb01215.x

Lau, J., Lim, T. Z., Wong, G. J., & Tan, K. K. (2020). The health belief model and colorectal cancer screening in the general population: A systematic review. *Preventive Medicine Reports*, *20*, 101223. https://doi.org/10.1016/j.pmedr.2020.101223

Lee, Y., & Lee, K. S. (2019). Relationship between unhealthy weight control behaviors and substance use patterns among Korean adolescents: Results from the 2017 national youth risk behavior survey. *Public Health*, *174*, 56–64. https://doi.org/10.1016/j.puhe.2019.06.005

Li, H., Zhang, J., Wang, L., Yang, T., & Yang, Y. (2022). A health promoting-lifestyle prediction model for dementia prevention among Chinese adults: Based on the health belief model. *BMC Public Health*, *22*(1), 2450. https://doi.org/10.1186/s12889-022-14828-9

Li, W. H. C., Ho, K. Y., Wang, M. P., Cheung, D. Y. T., Lam, K. K. W., Xia, W., … Lam, T. H. (2020). Effectiveness of a brief self-determination theory–based smoking cessation intervention for smokers at emergency departments in Hong Kong: A randomized clinical trial. *JAMA Internal Medicine*, *180*(2), 206–214. doi:10.1001/jamainternmed.2019.5176

Lim, K. H., Heng, P. P., Nik Mohamed, M. H., Teh, C. H., Mohd Yusoff, M. F., Ling, J. M. Y., … Ab Rahman, J. (2019). Prevalence and factors associated with attempts to quit and smoking cessation in Malaysia. *Asia Pacific Journal of Public Health*, *31*(7_suppl), 22S–31S. https://doi.org/10.1177/1010539519874944

Lim, S. L., Teoh, C., Zhao, X., Umareddy, I., Grillo, V., Singh, S. S., & Khouw, I. (2020). Attitudes & beliefs that influence healthy eating behaviours among mothers of young children in Singapore: A cross-sectional study. *Appetite*, *148*, 104555. https://doi.org/10.1016/j.appet.2019.104555

Linton, D. (2021). Beliefs related to Pap smear intention among Jamaicans: A qualitative research study. *The Nurse Practitioner*, *46*(3), 51–55. https://doi.org/10.1097/01.NPR.0000733696.44874.ec

Macedo, J. C. L., Soares, D. A., de Carvalho, V. C. H. D. S., Cortes, T. B. A., Mistro, S., Kochergin, C. N., … Oliveira, M. G. (2022). Self-Care in Patients with Non-Optimal Diabetes Management in Brazilian Rural Areas: A Mixed-Methods Study. *Patient Preference and Adherence*, 1831–1842. https://doi.org/10.2147/PPA.S373302

Mahindarathne, P. P. (2021). Assessing COVID-19 preventive behaviours using the health belief model: A Sri Lankan study. *Journal of Taibah University Medical Sciences*, *16*(6), 914–919. https://doi.org/10.1016/j.jtumed.2021.07.006

Maqsood, S., Iqbal, S., Zakar, R., Zakar, M. Z., & Fischer, F. (2021). Determinants of overall knowledge and health behaviours in relation to hepatitis B and C among ever-married women in Pakistan: Evidence based on Demographic and Health Survey 2017–18. *BMC Public Health*, *21*(1), 2328. https://doi.org/10.1186/s12889-021-12406-z

Marks, L. R., Stenersen, M., Coleman, M., Sanders, S., & Wilkins-Yel, K. (2022). Health psychology in Jamaica: A qualitative analysis. *Counselling Psychology Quarterly*, *35*(1), 155–172. https://doi.org/10.1080/09515070.2021.1927670

Marthammuthu, T., Hairi, F. M., Choo, W. Y., Salleh, N. A. M., & Hairi, N. N. (2021). A qualitative investigation on the roles of social support on physical activity behaviour among the rural-Dwelling older women in Malaysia. *International Journal of Environmental Research and Public Health*, *18*(18), 9609. https://doi.org/10.3390/ijerph18189609

Matarazzo, J. D. (1982). Behavioral health's challenge to academic, scientific, and professional psychology. *American Psychologist*, *37*(1), 1–14. https://doi.org/10.1037/0003-066X.37.1.1

Matsuda, K., Shiraishi, M., Hori, N., Horiguchi, H., & Matsuzaki, M. (2023). Psychosocial experiences related to dietary behavior of Japanese Lactating Women: A qualitative study. *Nutrients*, *15*(3), 789. https://doi.org/10.3390/nu15030789

McSharry, J., Chater, A. M., Lučanin, J. D., Höfer, S., Paschali, A., & Warner, L. (2017). Health psychology education and training in countries represented in the EHPS. *European Health Psychologist*, *19*(6), 375–381.

Mishra, R., Sharma, S. K., Verma, R., Kangra, P., Dahiya, P., Kumari, P., Sahu, P. K., Bhakar, P., Kumawat, R., Kaur, R., & Kant, R. (2021). Medication adherence and quality of life among type-2 diabetes mellitus patients in India. *World Journal of Diabetes*, *12*(10), 1740–1749. https://doi.org/10.4239/wjd.v12.i10.1740

Mo, P. K. H., & Lau, J. T. F. (2015). Influenza vaccination uptake and associated factors among elderly population in Hong Kong: The application of the Health Belief Model. *Health Education Research*, *30*(5), 706–718. https://doi.org/10.1093/her/cyv038

Monge-Rojas, R., Fuster-Baraona, T., Garita, C., Sánchez, M., Smith-Castro, V., Valverde-Cerros, O., & Colon-Ramos, U. (2015). The influence of gender stereotypes on eating habits among Costa Rican adolescents. *American Journal of Health Promotion*, *29*(5), 303–310. https://doi.org/10.4278/ajhp.130904-QUAL-462

Moon, N., Kang, H., Heo, S. J., & Kim, J. H. (2023). Factors affecting the safe sexual behaviors of Korean young adults by gender: A structural equation model. *Korean Journal of Women Health Nursing*, *29*(2), 115–127. https://doi.org/10.4069/kjwhn.2023.06.16

Morar, T., & Robertson, L. (2022). Smoking cessation among people with mental illness: A South African perspective. *South African Family Practice*, *64*(1). a5489. https://doi.org/10.4102/safp.v64i1.5489

NAOP. (2022). *NAOP Divisions*. Available at https://naopindia.org/divisions, accessed August 22, 2023.

National University Health System. (2023). *Psychological medicine*. Available at https://www.nuh.com.sg/our-services/Specialties/Psychological-Medicine/Pages/default.aspx, accessed August 6, 2023.

Ncube, B., Bey, A., Knight, J., Bessler, P., & Jolly, P. E. (2015). Factors associated with the uptake of cervical cancer screening among women in Portland, Jamaica. *North American Journal of Medical Sciences*, *7*(3), 104. https://doi.org/10.4103/1947-2714.153922

Neto, I. L., Matsunaga, L. H., Machado, C. C., Günther, H., Hillesheim, D., Pimentel, C. E., … d'Orsi, E. (2020). Psychological determinants of walking in a Brazilian sample: An application of the Theory of Planned Behavior. *Transportation Research Fart F: Traffic Psychology and Behaviour*, *73*, 391–398. https://doi.org/10.1016/j.trf.2020.07.002

Noor, M. N., Holt, M., Qureshi, A., de Wit, J., & Bryant, J. (2021). Sexual risk-taking among homeless young people in Pakistan. *Health & Social Care in the Community*, *29*(5), 1550–1558. https://doi.org/10.1111/hsc.13220

Obirikorang, Y., Acheampong, E., Anto, E. O., Afrifa-Yamoah, E., Adua, E., Taylor, J., … Obirikorang, C. (2022). Nexus between constructs of social cognitive theory model and diabetes self-management among Ghanaian diabetic patients: A mediation modelling approach. *PLOS Global Public Health*, *2*(7), e0000736. https://doi.org/10.1371/journal.pgph.0000736

Ofei, S. D., Teye-Kwadjo, E., Amankwah-Poku, M., Gyasi-Gyamerah, A. A., Akotia, C. S., Osafo, J., Roomaney, R., & Kagee, A. (2023). Determinants of post-traumatic growth and quality of life in Ghanaian breast cancer survivors. *Cancer Investigation*, *41*(4), 379–393. https://doi.org/10.1080/07357907.2023.2181636

Ojedokun, O., Henschel, N., Arant, R., & Boehnke, K. (2022). Applying the theory of planned behaviour to littering prevention behaviour in a developing country (Nigeria). *Waste Management*, *142*, 19–28. https://doi.org/10.1016/j.wasman.2022.02.006

Okuhara, T., Okada, H., & Kiuchi, T. (2020). Predictors of staying at home during the covid-19 pandemic and social lockdown based on protection motivation theory: A cross-sectional study in Japan. *Healthcare*, *8*(4), 475. https://doi.org/10.3390/healthcare8040475

Onwukwe, S. C., & Ngene, N. C. (2022). Blood pressure control in hypertensive patients attending a rural community health centre in Gauteng Province, South Africa: A cross-sectional study. *South African Family Practice*, *64*(1), a5403. https://doi.org/10.4102/safp. v64i1.5403

OWSD (n.d.). [*Countries in the Global South (by region)*]. Available at https://owsd.net/sites/default/files/OWSD%20138%20Countries%20-%20Global%20South.pdf, accessed August 3, 2023.

Patterson, Y. (2022). An exploratory study of Jamaican women's health beliefs around male condom use and negotiation in Jamaica. *Social Work in Public Health*, *37*(6), 510–522. https://doi.org/10.1080/19371918.2022.2039829

Plass, A. M., Gruszczynska, E., Andersson, S. I., & Kassianos, A. P. (2017). Health psychology practice in Europe and other countries represented in EHPS: A first step to moving forward together. *European Health Psychologist*, *19*(6), 399–400.

Psychological Society of South Africa. (2021, July 20). *Health psychology: Special interest group*. Available at https://www.psyssa.com/category/health-psychology/, accessed July 4, 2023.

Rahman, N. K. (2004). Psychology in Pakistan. In M. J. Stevens & D. Wedding (Eds.), *Handbook of International Psychology* (pp. 243–260). Brunner-Routledge.

Romero-Daza, N., & Freidus, A. (2008). Female tourists, casual sex, and HIV risk in Costa Rica. *Qualitative Sociology*, *31*, 169–187.

Roomaney, R., & Kagee, A. (2018). Salient aspects of quality of life among women diagnosed with endometriosis: A qualitative study. *Journal of Health Psychology*, *23*(7), 905–916. https://doi.org/10.1177/1359105316643069

Saal, W., & Kagee, A. (2012). The applicability of the Theory of Planned Behaviour in predicting adherence to ART among a South African sample. *Journal of Health Psychology*, *17*(3), 362–370. https://doi.org/10.1177/1359105311416875

Sahoo, M., & Pradhan, J. (2021). Reproductive healthcare beliefs and behaviours among displaced tribal communities in Odisha and Chhattisgarh: An analysis using health belief model. *Journal of the Anthropological Survey of India*, *70*(1), 87–102. https://doi.org/10.1177/2277436X211005922

Schliemann, D., Htay, M. N. N., Dahlui, M., Paramasivam, D., Cardwell, C. R., Tamin, N. S. B. I., … Donnelly, M. (2020). Impact of a mass media campaign on breast cancer symptoms awareness and screening uptake in Malaysia: Findings from a quasi-experimental study. *BMJ Open*, *10*(8), e036503. http://doi.org/10.1136/bmjopen-2019-036503

Shahsavari, S., Alavi, A., Razmjoue, P., Mohseni, S., Ranae, V., Hosseini, Z., & Dadipoor, S. (2022). A predictive model of genital warts preventive behaviors among women in the south of Iran: Application of health belief model. *BMC Women's Health, 22*(1), 63. https://doi.org/10.1186/s12905-022-01649-6

Shi, H., Wang, J., Huang, R., Zhao, J., Zhang, Y., Jiang, N., … Xu, X. (2021). Application of the extended theory of planned behavior to understand Chinese students' intention to improve their oral health behaviors: A cross-sectional study. *BMC Public Health, 21*, 1–9. https://doi.org/10.1186/s12889-021-12329-9

Singapore Psychological Society. (2023). *Directory of SPS members*. Available at https://singaporepsychologicalsociety.org/members-directory/, accessed August 14, 2023.

Singh, I., Asnani, M. R., & Harrison, A. (2023). Health-related quality of life in adolescents with chronic illness in Jamaica: Adolescent and parent reports. *Journal of Adolescent Health, 72*(1), 12–20. https://doi.org/10.1016/j.jadohealth.2022.07.013

Sirasa, F., Mitchell, L., Azhar, A., Chandrasekara, A., & Harris, N. (2021). A 6-week healthy eating intervention with family engagement improves food knowledge and preferences but not dietary diversity among urban preschool children in Sri Lanka. *Public Health Nutrition, 24*(13), 4328–4338. https://doi.org/10.1017/S1368980021001877

Siu, J. Y. M., Chan, K., & Lee, A. (2019). Adolescents from low-income families in Hong Kong and unhealthy eating behaviours: Implications for health and social care practitioners. *Health & Social Care in the Community, 27*(2), 366–374. https://doi.org/10.1111/hsc.12654

Smith, T. W. (2020). Health psychology and behavioral medicine: Methodological issues in the study of psychosocial influences on disease. In A. G. C. Wright & M. N. Hallquist (Eds.), *The Cambridge handbook of research methods in clinical psychology* (pp. 287–298). Cambridge University Press. https://doi.org/10.1017/9781316995808.027

Spink, M. J. P. (2018). Interlaced strands: Health psychology in Brazil from an autobiographic perspective. *Journal of Health Psychology, 23*(3), 397–407. https://doi.org/10.1177/1359105317738259

Spink, M. J. P., Brigagão, J. M., Menegon, V. M., & Vicentin, M. C. G. (2016). SIB health psychology in Brazil: The challenges for working in public health settings. *Journal of Health Psychology, 21*(3), 273–280. https://doi.org/10.1177/1359105316628759

Sripad, P., Kirk, K., Adoyi, G., Dempsey, A., Ishaku, S., & Warren, C. E. (2019). Exploring survivor perceptions of pre-eclampsia and eclampsia in Nigeria through the health belief model. *BMC Pregnancy and Childbirth, 19*, 1–11. https://doi.org/10.1186/s12884-019-2582-2

Stout, B. D., Leon, M. P., & Niccolai, L. M. (2004). Nonadherence to antiretroviral therapy in HIV-positive patients in Costa Rica. *AIDS Patient Care and STDs, 18*(5), 297–304. https://doi.org/10.1089/108729104323076034

Sumarmi, S., Hsu, Y. Y., Cheng, Y. M., & Lee, S. H. (2021). Factors associated with the intention to undergo Pap smear testing in the rural areas of Indonesia: A health belief model. *Reproductive Health, 18*(1), 1–10. https://doi.org/10.1186/s12978-021-01188-7

Sunmola, A. M., Olley, B. O., & Oso, G. E. (2007). Predictors of condom use among sexually active persons involved in compulsory national service in Ibadan, Nigeria. *Health Education Research, 22*(4), 459–472. https://doi.org/10.1093/her/cyl100

Tariq, O., Rosten, C., & Huber, J. (2022). Experiences of living with type 2 diabetes in Pakistan: the role of culture and family in physical activity. *International Journal for Equity in Health, 21*(1), 1–11. https://doi.org/10.1186/s12939-022-01706-4

Tarkar, P. (2023). Predicting intentions to get the COVID-19 vaccine in India: An integration of theory of planned behaviour and health belief model. *The International Journal of Health Planning and Management, 38*(1), 214–238. https://doi.org/10.1002/hpm.3582

Tay, Z., Chen, B., Kui, K. Y., Padmapriya, N., Chong, M. F. F., Müller, A. M., … Müller-Riemenschneider, F. (2023). Results from the Singapore 2022 report card on physical activity for children and adolescents. *Journal of Exercise Science & Fitness, 21*(1), 20–25. https://doi.org/10.1016/j.jesf.2022.10.005

Taylor, S. (2011). The future of social-health psychology: Prospects and predictions. *Social and Personality Psychology Compass*, *5*(5), 275–284. https://doi.org/10.1111/j.1751-9004.2011.00360.x

Teh, W. L., Abdin, E., Siva Kumar, F. D., Roystonn, K., Wang, P., … Subramaniam, M. (2023). Measuring social desirability bias in a multi-ethnic cohort sample: its relationship with self-reported physical activity, dietary habits, and factor structure. *BMC Public Health*, *23*(1), 1–10. https://doi.org/10.1186/s12889-023-15309-3

Teye-Kwadjo, E., Kagee, A., & Swart, H. (2017). Determinants of condom use among heterosexual young men and women in southeastern Ghana: A mediation analysis. *Psychology & Sexuality*, *8*(4), 291–305. https://doi.org/10.1080/19419899.2017.1391870

Teye-Kwadjo, E., Salia, S., Mensah, G. O., & Ofori, R. (2020). Exploring Ghanaian commercial drivers' intentions to wear a seat belt. *Case Studies on Transport Policy*, *8*, 453–459. https://doi.org/10.1016/j.cstp.2019.10.009

University of Cape Coast. (2023). *Clinical health psychology*. Available at https://ucc.edu.gh/programmes/master-philosophy-clinical-health-psychology, accessed July 20, 2023.

University of Ghana. (2023). *PSYC463: Health psychology*. Available at https://www.ug.edu.gh/psychology/courses/psyc-463-health-psychology, accessed July 20, 2023

Wang, Y., Wen, X., Zhu, Y., Xiong, Y., & Liu, X. (2022). Chinese Residents' Healthy Eating Intentions and Behaviors: Based on an Extended Health Belief Model. *International Journal of Environmental Research and Public Health*, *19*(15), 9037. https://doi.org/10.3390/ijerph19159037

Werneck, A. O., Silva, D. R., Malta, D. C., Gomes, C. S., Souza-Júnior, P. R., Azevedo, L. O., … Szwarcwald, C. L. (2021). Associations of sedentary behaviours and incidence of unhealthy diet during the COVID-19 quarantine in Brazil. *Public Health Nutrition*, *24*(3), 422–426. https://doi.org/10.1017/S1368980020004188

Wong, K. Y., Seow, A., Koh, W. P., Shankar, A., Lee, H. P., & Yu, M. C. (2010). Smoking cessation and lung cancer risk in an Asian population: Findings from the Singapore Chinese Health Study. *British Journal of Cancer*, *103*(7), 1093–1096. https://doi.org/10.1038/sj.bjc.6605782

Yen, J. (2016). Psychology and health after apartheid: Or, Why there is no health psychology in South Africa. *History of Psychology*, *19*(2), 77–92. https://doi.org/10.1037/hop0000025

Yen, J., & Vaccarino, O. (2018). 'Health psychology'or 'psychology for health'? A history of psychologists' engagement with health in South Africa. *Journal of Health Psychology*, *23*(3), 408–424. https://doi.org/10.1177/1359105317708201

Yoon, S., Kwan, Y. H., Yap, W. L., Lim, Z. Y., Phang, J. K., Loo, Y. X., … Low, L. L. (2023). Factors influencing medication adherence in multi-ethnic Asian patients with chronic diseases in Singapore: A qualitative study. *Frontiers in Pharmacology*, *14*, 1124297. https://doi.org/10.3389/fphar.2023.1124297

Zamzuri, M. A. I. A., Kamarudin, S. A. A., Ariffin, A. H., Ibrahim, A. A., Othman, M. H., Johari, A., … Pang, N. T. P. (2021). Rate of smoking cessation and factors associated with successful quit smoking in Seremban District of Malaysia. *Clinical Epidemiology and Global Health*, *12*, 100862. https://doi.org/10.1016/j.cegh.2021.100862

Zhang, T., Huang, B., Wong, H., Wong, S. Y. S., & Chung, R. Y. N. (2022). Built environment and physical activity among adults in Hong Kong: Role of public leisure facilities and street centrality. *Land*, *11*(2), 243. https://doi.org/10.3390/land11020243

33
CHALLENGES CURRENTLY FELT IN THE GLOBAL SOUTH

Vica Tomberge, Asma Bibi, Enoch Teye-Kwadjo, and Benjamin Ambuehl

Introduction

There are particular challenges arising in the conduct and dissemination of health psychology research and practice in the many countries where 'health psychology' is not a distinct and well-established field. These challenges are certainly at least partly the result of inequalities in knowledge production and research resources. These are themselves a result of the history of colonisation and imbalances in structural power and intellectual labour force between the Global South and Global North (Connell, 2014; Flint et al., 2022). Research funding schemes, for example, and with them resources to conduct and disseminate research and drive research interests, are more easily accessible for researchers affiliated with institutions in the Global North than the Global South (Connell, 2014; Flint et al., 2022). The imbalances in the field of health psychology are, for example, that health psychology theories and methodological approaches most often applied, cited, and taught originate from research institutions in the Global North (e.g., Ajzen, 1991; Bandura, 1998; Rosenstock, 1974; Schwarzer, 1992), leading to a representation bias of researchers, research participants, and the topics being explored in international journals and conferences (Barrett, 2020). Researchers from the Global North predominantly decide the research being funded, conducted, and published, contributing to a vicious cycle of inequalities in knowledge production (Posada & Chen, 2018). Figure 33.1 visualises the cycle of knowledge production and the fields of challenges it can pose for health psychology research in the Global South.

This chapter reflects on where researchers and practitioners may face challenges when conducting health psychology research in the Global South. First, we will reflect on challenges that arise from the funding of research and its interrelatedness with power-balanced collaborations in Global North-South research partnerships, leading to potential challenges if not properly established. Second, we will discuss challenges that may arise when applying established health

DOI: 10.4324/9781003318026-40

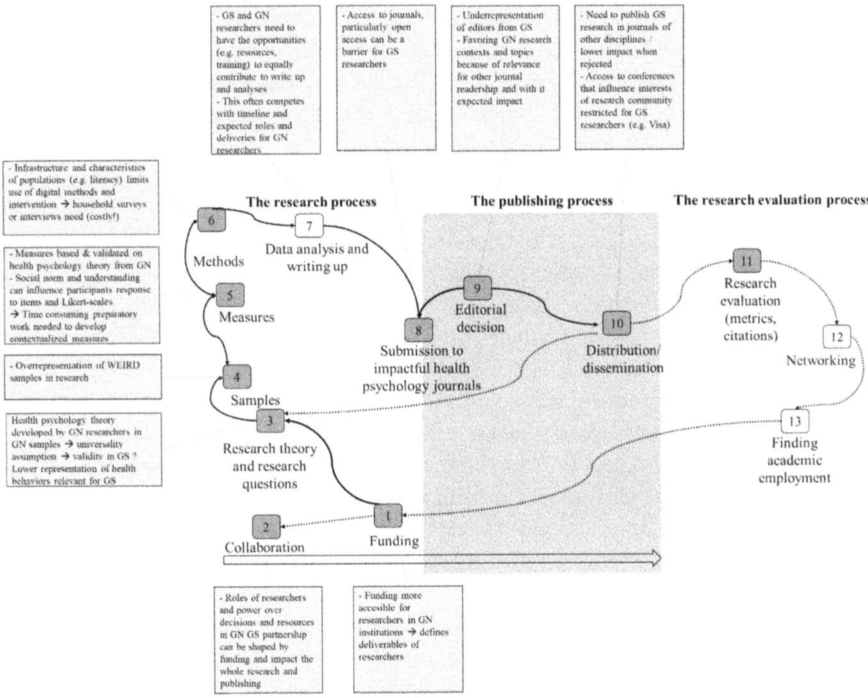

Note: GN = Global North, GS = Global South, Note that this figure simplifies challenges and only covers a small range of nuances of inequalities in knowledge production between GN and GS. The challenges greyed out are discussed in this chapter. Figure based on Posada, A., & Chen, G. (2018). Inequality in knowledge production: The integration of academic infrastructure by big publishers. *ELPUB 2018*. 10.4000/proceedings.elpub.2018.30. hal-01816707

Figure 33.1 Challenges for health psychology research in the Global South in the cycle of knowledge production.

psychology theory in research in the Global South, using an example of the applicability of the theory of planned behaviour (TPB: Ajzen, 1991) and the health belief model (HBM: Janz & Becker, 1984). Third, we will outline challenges that may arise when conducting research using common health psychology methods and measures. Finally, challenges in disseminating research to the international research community will be discussed. Although it is difficult to generate universal recommendations to overcome these challenges, the subsections will include reflections and avenues of further research to advance the consideration of different health psychology research fields and perspectives.

Challenges in Funding and North-South Collaborations

In times of widespread discussions about identity, origin, and cultural appropriation, researchers around the globe also reflect on their roles, work ethics, and partnership principles when conducting research across societies (Zingerli, 2010). For example, in collaborations of health-related research in the Global South, researchers from the North and South often work on joint projects. However, due to colonisation and/or structural power imbalances, ideas, rules, and decisions are often asymmetric. For example, when defining the aims of research projects (Flint et al., 2022) and establishing research partnerships, it is necessary to follow the rules of the funders, who are mostly from Global North countries (Erondu et al., 2021b). Furthermore, journals for the dissemination of research are dominated and edited by scientists from the Global North (Carbonnier & Kontinen, 2015), and so researchers must follow the rules and decisions of the Global North. It is worth stating here that there have been strong and decisive moves to right this wrong, with journals making statements about the authorship they expect to see of papers where the research is conducted in the Global South (*Nature*, 2022). This imbalance has practical implications: in a scoping review, Voller et al. (2022) summarise that many research partnerships still do not apply principles, guidelines, and models for equal partnerships, even though these have been developed and are readily available. Topics featuring most prominently in the guidelines were partner roles, responsibilities, and ways of working; capacity strengthening; motivation and goals; resource contributions; agenda setting and study design; governance structures and institutional agreements; dissemination; respect for affected populations; funding and long-term commitments; data handling and ownership.

Especially in health research, as it concerns the physical and mental health of humans globally and, indeed, the planet itself, the burden and benefits of doing research should be shared equally by the North and South partners (Edejer, 1999). This is not always the case. Sometimes researchers from the Global North delegate all field work to researchers of the Global South. There seems to be a rationale for that because the researchers in the Global South have the cultural proximity and understanding of the field and the capabilities to conduct this fieldwork. However, this results in researchers involved in fieldwork having an increased workload and exposing themselves to potential health threats, whilst researchers of the Global North benefit more from the data and research findings. There is a lack of indigenous researchers in the more senior and management roles (Kalinga, 2019) and a lack of including researchers from the Global South when setting the research agendas (Bradley, 2017b) and when writing guidelines (Voller et al., 2022).

Successful research partnerships are inclusive partnerships. Much has been written about the foundations or principles of partnership. Larkan and colleagues introduced the 'seven pillars': common focus and vision among partners, shared values, equitable and inclusive relationships, mutually beneficial and exchanging knowledge, transparent and honest communication, balanced responsibilities, shared management and mutual accountability, and conflict resolution (Larkan et al., 2016). The Tropical Health and Education Trust, a UK non-governmental organisation that managed the UK government Health Partnership Scheme, outlines the nine principles of partnership: strategic, harmonised and aligned, effective and sustainable, respectful and reciprocal, organised and accountable, responsible, flexible, resourceful and innovative, committed to joint learning and embed equity and inclusion (THET, n.d.). The intercultural practice of reflective relationships

(Fisher et al., 2016) is represented by the theory of psychological ownership (Pierce et al., 2001), where several participatory mechanisms (e.g., involvement in decision-making; contributions of labour, ideas, and time; detailed knowledge about the characteristics and processes in the project) and characteristics of the environment (e.g., trust, power distance, institutional climate) make people start feeling like they own their job, project, or organisation and thus elicits positive work outcomes (job performance, organisational performance, citizenship behaviour). By promoting psychological ownership, a more collaborative, equitable, and effective research partnership is possible. To prevent the negative consequences of psychological ownership (i.e., territoriality and knowledge protection) and reinforce equitable partnerships, every team member contributes to routes to ownership and subsequently beneficial consequences amongst the collective (Batool et al., 2023). It seems that those of us who are researchers and practitioners in psychology should be even more attuned to these psychological issues arising from our work. Furthermore, ownership serves as a determinant for sustainable partnerships, especially with mutual accountability, respectful communication, and flexible support from the project management that foster jointly built trust, expertise, and commitment of everyone and successfully co-create knowledge (Andriessen et al., 2023; OECD, 2011). Participatory activities and how they relate to psychological ownership are discussed in more detail in Chapter 34 of this volume. Much has been written to guide researchers, and we suggest following journal requirements and author guidelines (e.g., from *Nature* https://www.nature.com/nature-portfolio/editorial-policies/ethics-and-biosecurity) when planning collaborations. Further, general codes of conduct (e.g., TRUST global code of conduct https://www.globalcodeofconduct.org/) and ethical considerations for research participants and staff (e.g., declaration of Helsinki) apply for research collaborations in health psychology in low- and middle-income countries (LMICs) in the same way as for any other partnerships. We specifically recommend strengthening partnerships based on the seven pillars, fostering collective ownership, respect, and reflection within and about the collaboration to negotiate tasks, responsibilities, and power and social relations in international research partnerships to help develop more respectful and reflexive conduct of research projects starting from the very beginning when applying for funding. Further, advocating that funding bodies should distribute the funding and responsibilities equally across both institutions directly may be a way for us to affect changes in inequalities in collaboration at a structural level. This might require funding bodies to learn more about financial management and policies in countries that might differ from those in the Global North.

Challenges Associated with Using Health Behaviour Theories in the Global South

Behaviour is central to health maintenance and illness prevention across social contexts and populations (see, e.g., Fisher et al., 2011; Kwasnicka et al., 2016; Leventhal et al., 2008). Defined as "overt behavioral patterns, actions and habits that relate to health maintenance, to health restoration and to health improvement" (Gochman,

1997, p. 3), health behaviours, such as binge drinking, eating a healthy diet, physical activity, condom use, smoking, risky driving, medication adherence, health screening uptake, vaccination uptake, and sexual risk behaviour, can be difficult to change (Conner & Norman, 2017; Gardner et al., 2021; Kelly & Barker, 2016). Consequently, health psychology researchers have developed various health behaviour theories/models to explain, predict, and modify health-compromising behaviour and health-enhancing behaviour (Glanz & Bishop, 2010; Prestwich et al., 2015). They include the theory of reasoned action/theory of planned behaviour (TRA/TPB: Ajzen, 1991), health belief model (HBM: Janz & Becker, 1984), social cognitive theory (SCT: Bandura, 1998), protection motivation theory (PMT: Maddux & Rogers, 1983), transtheoretical model of change (TTM: Prochaska & DiClemente, 1983), health action process approach (HAPA: Schwarzer, 2016), and others. Our experience is that popular theoretical models which are commonly applied in the Global South are the TPB and HBM (Ajzen, 2011; Dsouza et al., 2021).

Health psychologists have long recognised that an individual's health or illness is determined by the interaction of biological, psychological, and socio-cultural factors (i.e., biopsychosocial model (Engel, 1977)). Yet, most of the theories and models developed to guide the conduct of evidence-based health psychology research have been developed with social and behavioural data in the Global North, which could potentially limit their utility and applicability to settings and populations in the Global South. However, research has shown that the way individuals think about health and well-being can differ significantly across cultures, even when there are similar concepts across cultures (Diener et al., 2010). In addition, Kline et al. (2018) argued that whilst culture remains a human universal, it should be viewed as a fundamental source of variation in human behaviour. They warned psychologists against engaging in what the authors described as the (i) *deficit assumption*: "that population-level differences in developmental timing or outcomes are necessarily due to something lacking among non-Western populations" (p. 1), (ii) *Western centrality assumption*: "that Western populations represent a normal and/or healthy standard against which development in all societies can be compared" (p. 1), and (iii) *equivalency assumption*: "that using identical research methods will necessarily produce equivalent and externally valid data, across disparate cultural contexts" (p. 1).

Using Global North theories can, without proper contextualisation, lead to challenges on several levels. On the one hand, theoretical constructs in themselves, for example, social support or relationship quality, may be understood and expressed differently by populations across cultures. Psychological models are typically built by a range of constructs, such as health behaviour models, including self-efficacy, motivation, or social support. We need to question whether psychological models and theories developed in the Global North contain constructs that are the same in the Global South. For example, in psychological ownership, a theory that stems from the organisational context in the Global North, authors found that the core of the feeling is different in the Global South. In the original context, psychological ownership is conceptualised with core feelings of possessiveness only, but when the authors investigated the understanding of psychological ownership in India, they found a core trinity: besides possessiveness, the authors also found controlling and social perception (Ambuehl & Inauen, 2022). Similarly, a psychometric assessment of the popular Big Five personality inventory in the South African population found evidence of a 6-dimensional factor structure, including four of the original five dimensions and two new dimensions, which the authors named "Positive Social-Relational" and "Negative Social-Relational" factors (see Fetvadjiev et al., 2015).

In recent years, the social-cognition models of health behaviours that were in widespread use in the Global North – namely, the TPB and the HBM – have been criticised (Sniehotta et al., 2014). The criticism stems from a lack of evidence that the constructs predict behaviour and the lack of unconscious influences on behaviour. Nonetheless, the constructs within these models are still of interest when studying the multiple influences on health behaviours. In the following section, we present illustrative evidence of the challenges associated with using the constructs of popular health behaviour models in the Global South, specifically the TPB and the HBM.

Utility of the Model Constructs of the TPB and HBM in the Global South

There is considerable evidence of the successful application of the TPB and HBM to predict and change health behaviour in the Global South. Yet, there is evidence that some model constructs of the TPB and HBM are often found not to be salient in some settings and populations in the Global South. As can be seen in Table 33.1, across various settings and populations in the Global South, health behaviour researchers have found evidence suggesting that some model constructs of the TPB and HBM did not work as conceptualised by the theory developers. These findings suggest that such constructs are not considered to be important modifiable determinants of health behaviour in those social contexts and by extension should not be included in health behaviour interventions.

Whilst a full evaluation of why some TPB/HBM-based theoretical constructs are not considered salient in some settings and populations in the Global South is beyond the scope of this chapter, the reasons may not be far-fetched. For example, classified as socio-cognitive theories, health behaviour theories/models generally assess health-compromising or health-enhancing behaviour at the level of the individual. Thus, whilst these theoretical concepts may demonstrate sufficient predictive validity in social contexts that emphasise personal achievement and independence, such as in countries of the Global North, their predictive validity in social contexts that emphasise interdependence, embeddedness, and group norms, such as in countries of the Global South, would be limited. The bidirectional interaction between the individual and their social context (Markus & Kitayama, 2010) suggests that efforts aimed at understanding health and illness beliefs ought to take social context into consideration, particularly in collectivist cultures. McBride and Morgan (2022) and Nilsen and Bernhardsson (2019) highlighted the role of context in the implementation of science and health, which warrants the attention of health psychologists. Further, Schwarzer (2011) argued that health should be viewed as a psychosocial question because

Table 33.1 Illustrative example of the theoretical challenges of applying health behaviour theories/models in the Global South

Authors, year of publication	*Health behaviour theory used, model constructs examined*	*Health behaviour studied*	*Study population, sample size (N), country*	*Study results*	*Model constructs found to be problematic in the research setting*	*Authors' notes on problematic theoretical constructs*
1 Teye-Kwadjo et al. (2017)	TPB: Attitudes Subjective norms Perceived control Intention Behaviour	Condom use	High school adolescents (N = 684), Ghana	Attitudes and perceived control were positively associated with condom use intention; intention was associated with condom use behaviour.	Subjective norms were not associated with condom use intentions.	Subjective norms are not salient for condom use in the study setting.
2 Teye-Kwadjo et al. (2020)	TPB: Attitudes Subjective norms Perceived control Intention	Seat belt use	Drivers of passenger-carrying vehicles (N = 303), Ghana	Attitudes were associated with intentions to use seat belts.	Subjective norms and perceived control were not associated with intentions to use seat belts.	Seat belt use norms are non-existent in the study setting, and thus drivers lack control over their use.

3 Sumarmi et al. (2021)	HBM: Perceived susceptibility Perceived severity Perceived benefits Perceived barriers	Cervical cancer and pap smear testing uptake	Rural married women (*N* = 687), Indonesia	Perceived severity, perceived benefits, and perceived barriers were associated with pap smear testing.	Perceived susceptibility was not associated with pap smear testing.	Perceived susceptibility was not considered salient for pap smear testing in the study setting.
4 Aboelmaged (2021)	TPB: Attitudes Subjective norms Perceived control Intention	E-waste recycling intentions	University students (*N* = 379), United Arab Emirates	Attitudes were positively associated with e-waste recycling intention.	Subjective norms and perceived control were not associated with e-waste recycling intentions.	Subjective norms and perceived control were not considered salient for e-waste recycling intentions in the study setting.

(*Continued*)

Table 33.1 (Continued)

Authors, year of publication	*Health behaviour theory used, model constructs examined*	*Health behaviour studied*	*Study population, sample size (N), country*	*Study results*	*Model constructs found to be problematic in the research setting*	*Authors' notes on problematic theoretical constructs*
5 Lin et al. (2021)	TPB: Attitudes Subjective norms Perceived control Intention	Safe sex intentions	College students (*N* = 460), China	Subjective norms and perceived control were positively associated with safe sex intentions.	Attitudes towards safe sex were not associated with safe sex intentions.	Attitudes were not considered salient for safe sex intentions in the study setting.
6 Ojedokun et al. (2022)	TPB: Attitudes Subjective norms Perceived control Intention Behaviour	Littering-preventive intentions and behaviour	Community residents in Akure (*N* = 300), Nigeria	Subjective norms and perceived control were positively associated littering-preventive intentions. Littering-preventive intentions were associated with littering-preventive behaviour.	Attitudes were not associated with littering-preventive intentions in the sample.	Attitudes were not considered salient for littering-preventive intentions in the study setting.

7 Saal and Kagee (2012)	TPB: Attitudes Subjective norms Perceived control Intention Behaviour	Adherence to ART treatment intentions	Patients receiving anti-retroviral treatment (*N* = 101), South Africa	Perceived control was positively associated with ART treatment intentions.	Attitudes and subjective norms were not associated with ART treatment intentions in the sample.	Attitudes and subjective norms were not considered salient for ART treatment intentions in the study setting.
8 Jemmott et al. (2007)	TPB: Attitudes Subjective norms Perceived control Intention	Condom use intentions	School-going adolescents (*N* = 390), South Africa	Attitudes and perceived control were positively associated with condom use intentions.	Subjective norms were not associated with condom use intentions in the sample.	Attitudes were not considered salient for condom use intentions in the study setting.

(*Continued*)

Table 33.1 (Continued)

Authors, year of publication	*Health behaviour theory used, model constructs examined*	*Health behaviour studied*	*Study population, sample size (N), country*	*Study results*	*Model constructs found to be problematic in the research setting*	*Authors' notes on problematic theoretical constructs*
9 Hu et al. (2022)	HBM: Perceived susceptibility Perceived severity Perceived benefits Perceived barriers	Diabetes self-care behaviour	Patients with type 2 diabetes (*N* = 1140), China	Perceived severity, perceived barriers, and perceived benefits were positively associated with self-care behaviours.	Perceived susceptibility was not associated with diabetes self-care in the sample.	Perceived susceptibility was not considered salient for diabetes self-care in the study setting.
10 Khan et al. (2022)	HBM: Perceived susceptibility Perceived severity Perceived benefits Perceived barriers Self-efficacy Cues to action	COVID-19 vaccine uptake	Young adult men and women (*N* = 560), Pakistan	Perceived severity, perceived susceptibility, perceived barriers, self-efficacy, and cues to action were associated with COVID-19 vaccine uptake.	Perceived benefits were not associated with COVID-19 vaccine uptake in the sample.	Perceived benefits were not considered salient for COVID-19 vaccine uptake in the study setting.

Note: TBP = Theory of planned behaviour, HBM = Health belief model the individual's interactions with the social-ecological systems can influence their cognitive, emotional, and behavioural processes. It should be noted, however, that modern theories and frameworks, notably the Capability Opportunity Motivation – Behaviour (COM-B) framework (Michie, Van Stralen & West, 2011), explicitly situate a person within their context.

Another challenge in the use of models and theories is that model constructs often have psychological assessments associated with them, which were developed and normed using behavioural data in the Global North. This practice obviously limits their generalisability and perhaps their applicability to health behaviour in Global South settings and populations (see, e.g., Einarsdottir et al., 2010, 2020). For example, Morgan et al. (2019) argued that the socio-cultural context of the individual can influence how they perceive, interpret, and endorse test items. Health psychologists working in the Global South should make efforts to validate health behaviour measures before applying them to research settings and populations in the Global South (Clark & Watson, 2019; Morgan et al., 2021) or, indeed, develop novel, culturally appropriate, valid measures. Other researchers have demonstrated that there is much to be gained from using a mixed method research approach, specifically qualitative methods (see, e.g., Ambuehl et al., 2021; Tomberge et al., 2022), to investigate health behaviour research questions and adapt theoretical constructs and models in the Global South. Besides all these attempts to contextualise established health psychology theory to overcome challenges towards its validity in the Global South, asserting alternative knowledge systems might be even more crucial to target the roots of their limited validity (Connell, 2014).

Finally, there is a need for health psychologists to undertake cultural competency training (Kaihlanen et al., 2019; Marja & Suvi, 2021) to increase their knowledge of the social contexts, particularly those in the Global South in which they may be applying health behaviour theory cross-culturally to predict and modify behaviour. Training is important because biological, psychological, and socio-cultural factors contribute to the aetiology of illness, suggesting that social factors have important effects on health and well-being across settings and populations (Kumsta, 2019; Osazuwa & Moodley, 2023).

Challenges in the Applicability of Health Psychology Methods

Besides theory construction and theory testing, another challenge is the application of health psychology methods in the Global South. We have discussed the assumptions around the universality of theories, and it is a similar issue that impacts conducting health psychology research and practice, i.e., we make assumptions about the generalisability of our methods. There are challenges in application concerning researchers, participants, measurement methods, and context.

Research Participants and Researchers

In Chapter 31, we introduced the acronym "WEIRD" (Western, Educated, Industrialised, Rich, and Democratic) to describe participants who make up the majority of the samples used in psychological research. By definition, many research participants in the Global South will differ in their characteristics from these WEIRD samples used in research in the Global North. It is an obvious and serious threat to evidence-based psychological research and practice that samples are taken only from specific populations that do not reflect the global majority. Using digital health as an example, despite the potential benefits afforded by emerging technologies, many individuals will remain without access (Naslund et al. 2017). Those without access might include individuals in the most impoverished settings, women who have less access to mobile devices than men, individuals in rural areas without electricity or reliable network coverage, and those living in regions without access to mobile phones or the internet because of governmental policies and strict regulation of telecommunications sectors (Naslund et al. 2017). Having researchers predominantly from WEIRD populations might also pose an issue, as the research questions they choose to address or the way they interpret findings will also be influenced by who they are.

Measurement Methods

Much health psychology research is mixed methods, and questionnaires are often used to assess or measure psychological constructs (Miles & Gilbert, 2005). There are several potential sources of bias in measurement, including the meaning of constructs and the equivalence of language in questions and in answer scales. Even the choices health psychologists make about what constructs to measure can be heavily influenced by their own contexts, experiences, and previous research, all of which have a strong bias towards WEIRD populations.

Language Bias

Language is used to create and share categories, identities, attitudes, and values, influencing our perception (Harzing et al., 2009). If studies use self-reported questionnaires, they are based on formulated questions and response options. Since formulations might be understood differently and wordings have different nuances or several synonyms in different languages, simply translating questionnaires across contexts can be problematic (Harzing et al., 2009). For example, negatively keyed scale items (inverse formulated items) can be difficult to understand because this way of formulating sentences might not be regularly used in some languages (Ambuehl & Inauen, 2022; Teye-Kwadjo, 2021).

Also, semantic nuances of item wordings are a challenge when translating questionnaires. The methodological foundation of minimising error variance in psychological scales requires that multiple explicit (manifest) items ask for the same implicit (latent, underlying) psychological construct in slightly different ways, providing variance for statistical analysis. In order to translate these nuances, back-translation approaches are used, and special care is needed when translating sensory and emotional terms (Ares, 2018). However, challenges in translation go beyond linguistic translations (Ambuehl & Inauen, 2022), as the concepts themselves have to be equivalent, not just the language. Beyond the questions that have been posed, there might also be implicit and biased assumptions in how people are expected to answer the questions.

Response Bias

Response styles are a tendency to systematically respond to questionnaire items regardless of item content and can differ across countries (Harzing et al., 2009). Thus, responses to health psychological questionnaires also require pragmatic adaptation. In our experience, conceptually, answer options formats such as Likert scales particularly offer difficulties in validity and reliability. Extreme responses from both ends of the scale offer a simplified response pattern corresponding to "Yes"/"No" dichotomic answer options. The systematic choice of extreme answer options is linked to understanding and acceptability (Harzing, 2006). This can be due to several reasons, such as difficulties to understand for a population not used to and neither familiar with research questions (Harzing et al., 2009) and also because of low literacy rates in the study sample (Kemmelmeier, 2016b). Using visually supported scales, e.g., the five dots scale (Harter et al., 2020), facial expressions, or representing the degree of agreement/emotion by different amounts of everyday objects, e.g., wood or manioc, and ranking scales instead can help to mitigate these challenges. De Jong et al. (2016), for example, have assessed the degree of complaint through a visualisation of different amounts of wood carried on a person's back in humanitarian settings, and Sharma et al. (2017) have developed culture-specific visualisation of emotional faces to rate pain in Nepal. The World Health Organisation Quality of Life Group worked to create the equivalence of Likert scales across multiple countries by creating a large pool of potential descriptors in each country and language and asking participants to place the descriptors along a visual analogue scale. They selected the descriptors that clustered around the points on the scale where there would be a statement, i.e., the interquartiles (for example, see Skevington & Tucker, 1999).

Social desirability can also influence how people respond to measurements, and this might be culturally and contextually dependent. Social desirability describes a situation when respondents answer questions in a way that is perceived to be accepted by the social environment (Graeff, 2005). It has been proposed that social desirability can be minimised by asking questions with neutral formulations (so that the participant is less sure of the socially desirable answer) and in a setting of privacy and confidentiality (Chung & Monroe, 2003). These countermeasures might not always be appropriate or practical in some cultures and settings and so countermeasures themselves need to be adapted carefully to the respective context (Chillag et al., 2019).

Health psychologists can tackle the challenges set out earlier through careful translation of research materials. The new model of translation (TRAPD model) comprises translation, review, adjudication, pretesting and documentation. Through this, key contextual issues are explicitly incorporated into the translation process, and health psychologists are not relying on a more traditional forward and backward translation of the language approach. It is clear that adaptation and validation of research instruments according to established guidelines and tutorials is a minimum (e.g., Ambuehl & Inauen, 2022).

Contextual Challenges Relating to Data Collection

Data collection in the Global South may be impacted by several factors. Low levels of literacy and digital literacy might make online data collection challenging, and in some circumstances impossible, and researchers may need to rely on interviewer-administered questionnaires. The mode of data collection can influence participants' responses as these may differ in the presence of a data collector. Lack of infrastructure (e.g., internet connection, power supply) can make the use of modern and efficient data collection methods such as computer-assisted personal interviews (CAPI; Böhme & Stör, 2014) expensive or even impossible. Some more advanced data collection and analysis methods (e.g., biosamples and water quality measurement; biomarkers with high technology measurement tools) are impossible to use or depend on previous construction of facilities (e.g., local laboratories to analyse water quality in Nepal; Schertenleib et al., 2019).

We suggest that when engaging in research in contexts which are new (for researcher and /or participants) and in which methods have not been developed, funding needs to be available for extensive training for researchers and for the time required to do this preparatory work. Training should include theoretical explanations and discussions on translations and understandings of questionnaires, challenges, and resources. This will help to ensure the highest standards of proficiency, ethics, and transparency in data collection and processing (Burger et al., 2022). We recommend following good scientific practice by conducting pilot research work and preliminary qualitative studies prior to data collection, as well as checking the equivalent understanding of the terms and questions in the target population. Conducting research in the Global South can require extensive preparatory work if all scales and constructs are adapted, piloted, and validated before using them. And during data collection, we recommend using visually supported scales when asking questions in the rating scale format, e.g., five dots scale, facial expressions, or representing degree of agreement/emotion by different amounts of everyday objects, e.g., wood or manioc.

Challenges in Disseminating Health Psychology Research

Disseminating health psychology research from the Global South can be a challenge. It is to be noted that most of the research cited in the following section stems from disciplines other than health psychology, e.g., public health (Sumathipala et al., 2004), social sciences, and general psychology (Barrett, 2020; Kline et al., 2018). Due to the lack of literature that analyses the representations in health psychology research, some of the points are based on the experience of the authors. Systematic analyses and qualitative research assessing experiences in the dissemination of health psychology research from the perspective of Global South researchers are yet to be conducted. These challenges manifest, on the one hand, as a representation bias of topics (i.e., funders and editors deciding that research topics are perceived as specific for the Global South and are not of general relevance to the readership and thus reject to offer a publication).

Representation Bias in Research Topics Concerning the Global South

Assuming the universality of theory derived from the Global North implies that psychological research conducted in the Global North is often perceived as more generalisable than psychological research conducted in the Global South (Kline et al., 2018). In contrast, it is often assumed that 'non-WEIRD' populations in psychological research show traits and health behaviours that would be less applicable to other contexts and therefore less relevant to building and testing health psychology theory (Barrett, 2020; Kline et al., 2018). In our transnational and interdisciplinary psychological research, we encountered that high-ranking journals may show less interest in health behaviours that are specific for the Global South, such as health behaviours related to safe sanitation or water access, arguing that these behaviours were too niche: "*[T]here were concerns regarding the overall fit of the manuscript with the journal, as this manuscript assesses a highly specific behavior of water-carrying and may therefore be better suited for a more specialized outlet*" (editor of international journal). At this very moment, no international journals exist that target the dissemination of health psychology research from the Global South, and journals that have their origin in the Global South have lower impact factors, thus limiting the recognition when publishing research like this. This results in a lack of representation of research conducted in the Global South in high-ranking journals, international scientific conferences, and university classrooms. And if they appear, they are often specifically classified as research from the Global South or case studies of a certain country, whilst research from the Global North rarely makes a reference to their geographical location (Baber, 2003). Additionally, the publication costs and the financial support to write publications pose a barrier to dissemination of research. Only a few journals have waivers if the corresponding author is from a country on the development assistance committee (DAC) list. As a consequence, researchers may publish in less prestigious journals or journals of the Global South that may be considered reputable, which contributes to the common finding that researchers from the Global South are less often cited among scientific disciplines (Confraria et al., 2017). On the other hand, challenges manifest as limited publications authored by researchers from the Global South.

Representation Bias of Researchers from the Global South

As a cause, consequence, or manifestation of the representation bias in research topics and populations, one may also find a representation bias in authors, editors, and researchers in leadership positions from the Global South (Dada et al.,

2022; Keiser et al., 2004; Palser et al., 2021), particularly at the intersection of female gender (Baobeid et al., 2022). This likely accounts for health psychology in the same way as in many other disciplines. Analyses in several research fields show that editors from the Global North are overrepresented in editorial boards (Dada et al., 2022; Keiser et al., 2004; Palser et al., 2021), which affects the selection of research topics and manuscripts that get accepted for publication (Sumathipala et al., 2004). For example, in the field of global health research, only 33% of editors are based in LMICs (Nafade et al., 2019).

Also, most of the authors in high-impact journals are researchers from the Global North (Keiser et al., 2004). This may be explained by a lower density of research institutions and a lower number of researchers in the Global South than in the Global North (World Bank, 2022) or by barriers to Global South researchers to disseminate their work in high-ranking journals and international scientific conferences. A systematic review in the field of global health showed that only 4% of global health conferences were held in the Global South, and only 39% of attendees were from the Global South (Velin et al., 2021). Obstacles identified for Global South researchers were visa restrictions, high travel cost coverage, and lesser acceptance of research presentations at conferences.

Further, in publications that include authors from Global North and South, researchers from the Global South are underrepresented in recognised authorship positions, i.e., first and last authors in publications (Langer et al., 2004; Merriman et al., 2021; Sumathipala et al., 2004). This issue is closely related to other challenges, such as who is leading research projects and who receives funding, because most journals have demanding criteria for authorship positions: Researchers from the Global North have higher opportunities for funds to conduct studies in the Global South, which often specify a certain scientific output within a specific timeline. The Global North researchers would then take care of deciding who is writing the manuscript, as they are often the principal investigators. If partnerships are not planned equally (see Chapter 34), researchers and health experts from the Global South would then manage the study, deliver interventions, and collect data due to their local expertise (Karlsson et al., 2007). Those who write or substantially revise the drafted paper most often will take the role of first author, whilst the lead/PI will take the role of last author. Thus those who primarily contribute to data collection or field administration (Smith et al., 2014) are excluded from these roles. This is clearly a structural imbalance that needs to be addressed for parity. This is further exacerbated by the insistence on 'academic English' (Ransing et al., 2023). Authorship in published papers is important for further funding and career opportunities, and thus this representation bias contributes to a vicious cycle of inequalities. It is always within the control of the collaborators to decide who takes authorship positions. It is clear that partnerships should carefully consider and make agreements about who the authors are and the positions that they take.

On another note, one also needs to consider that South-North collaborations are often transdisciplinary, particularly in areas where health psychology is not an established field. Public health researchers, health practitioners, or non-governmental organisation workers may have other ambitions for the project agenda and would focus on their field of expertise and ways of dissemination (e.g., stakeholder informing), obviously not prioritising a publication in a health psychology journal. This difference in ambition should also contribute to decisions about responsibilities and authorship.

One way to address the dissemination bias in North-South collaborations is to reflect potential biases at the beginning of a research project and actively address them as a team, following the seven pillars of equal partnership (Larkan et al., 2016). Researchers could reserve more time for information and manuscript exchange and make sure they are aware of the barriers that may occur along the way of authorship determination and dissemination of research. Reflection of ways to distribute authorship more equally needs to be made a priori, e.g., through shared first authorship, customised rules in terms of task distribution and merit of authorship.

Smith et al. (2014) suggest deliberately putting researchers from the Global South as first authors to actively compensate for inequality. Even though we agree that this would definitely bring more inequality in terms of recognition given for working hours invested, simply changing the orders of authorships and then still having another person take over the first authorship role would not contribute to a diversified perspective in health psychology research. To structurally enable Global South researchers to lead authorship tasks, possible barriers need to be identified already when planning a research project. Support staff such as research assistants can support the researcher's teaching responsibilities whilst writing; a scientific writing course, if they do not have access to one or even a person to support caretaking tasks, may need to be discussed and budgeted in research agendas. Particularly in times of crisis like the COVID-19 pandemic, persons with caring responsibilities worldwide and even more in the Global South find themselves thrown back into traditional family roles (Raj, 2022).

One more general way to promote research by researchers from the Global South and start breaking the cycle of representation bias is being committed to citing a diversity of literature in terms of selected journals, authors (including representation of gender), examined populations, and health behaviours in our work. If we cannot find any, or only a little, corresponding research representing the Global South, there is a need to mention that potentially limited universality for certain health psychology theories and methods exists. Persons who lecture students in health psychology may integrate this reflection in their lectures and motivate students to invest time in a diversified search of the literature in terms of authors and examined populations in their work. They can raise awareness amongst colleagues and students that what is considered as standard is not inherently universal. If health psychologists encourage others to critically scrutinise the status quo of research and help broaden the knowledge of diverse health behaviours, researchers, and study populations, they can push equality in the dissemination of research and ultimately develop a deeper understanding of human health behaviour.

Conclusions

Overall, structural imbalances and unequal distribution of power in the intellectual knowledge production between North and South do manifest on the level of conducting health psychology research. This can lead to challenges and inequalities in assessing funding, power in research collaborations, application of established health psychology theory, psychological research methods and measures, and dissemination of research. All these challenges are interrelated and may exacerbate one another. Research teams may overcome or even avoid some of these challenges by establishing sustainable and equal partnerships, testing and adapting established theories, valuing alternative knowledge systems and sources, and developing context-specific research methods and measures. Some of these challenges can be targeted by researchers and research teams directly, such as the distribution of labour and fairness in authorship. Challenges such as the centrality of Global North–based research for funding schemes and journal guidelines or a limited base of research measures validated in the Global South may, however, be more complex.

Overall, reflecting on the historical and ongoing division of power between the Global North and South production, dissemination, and use of knowledge in the field of health psychology are essential to identify and address challenges at the level of collaboration and the use of theory and methods. We do not claim that the points being raised are exhaustive and consider the discussion of challenges in health psychology research in the Global South an ongoing process of reflection and collaborative exchange.

Further Reading

Bradley, M. (2017a). *Chapter 2: Whose agenda? Power, policies, and priorities in North–South research partnerships*. In Putting Knowledge to work: Collaborating, influencing and learning for international development. 37–70. https://doi.org/10.3362/9781780449586.002

Connell, R. (2013). Using southern theory: Decolonizing social thought in theory, research and application. *Planning Theory*, *13*(2), 210–223. https://doi.org/10.1177/1473095213499216

Erondu, N., Aniebo, I., Kyobutungi, C., Midega, J., Okiro, E. A., & Okumu, F. O. (2021a). Open letter to international funders of science and development in Africa. *Nature Medicine*, *27*(5), 742–744. https://doi.org/10.1038/s41591-021-01307-8

Kemmelmeier, M. (2016a). Cultural differences in survey responding: Issues and insights in the study of response biases. *International Journal of Psychology*, *51*(6), 439–444. https://doi.org/10.1002/ijop.12386

Nature addresses helicopter research and ethics dumping. (2022). *Nature*, *606*(7912), 7. https://doi.org/10.1038/d41586-022-01423-6

References

Aboelmaged, M. (2021). E-waste recycling behaviour: An integration of recycling habits into the theory of planned behaviour. *Journal of Cleaner Production*, *278*, 124182. https://doi.org/10.1016/j.jclepro.2020.124182

Ajzen, I., (1991) The theory of planned behavior. *Organizational Behavior and Human Decision Processes*, 50(2): 179–211

Ajzen, I. (2011) The theory of planned behaviour: Reactions and reflections, *Psychology & Health*, 26(9): 1113–1127, DOI: 10.1080/08870446.2011.613995

Ambuehl, B. & Inauen, J. (2022) Contextualized Measurement Scale Adaption: A 4-Step Tutorial for Health Psychology Research. *International Journal of Environmental Research and Public Health*, 19(19): 12775.

Ambuehl, B., Tomberge, V.M.J., Kunwar, B.M., Schertenleib, A., Marks, S.J. & Inauen, J. (2021) The Role of Psychological Owndership in Safe Water Management: A Mixed-Methods Study in Nepal. *Water*, 13(5): 589. https://doi.org/10.3390/w13050589

Andriessen, N., Appiah-Effah, E., Browne, S. J. I., al Jahjah, R., Kabika, J., Kinobe, J. R., … Strande, L. (2023). Quantities and qualities of fecal sludge: Experiences from field implementation with a Volaser in 7 countries during a pandemic. *Frontiers in Water*, 5, 1130081.

Ares, G. (2018) Methodological issues in cross-cultural sensory and consumer research. *Food Quality and Preference*, 64: 253–63. https://doi.org/10.1016/j.foodqual.2016.10.007

Baber, Z. (2003). Provincial Universalism: The Landscape of Knowledge Production in an Era of Globalization. *Current Sociology*, *51*(6), 615–623. https://doi.org/10.1177/00113921030516004

Bandura, A. (1998) Health promotion from the perspective of social cognitive theory. *Psychology and Health*, 13(4): 623–49. https://doi.org/10.1080/08870449808407422

Baobeid, A., Faghani-Hamadani, T., Sauer, S., Boum, Y., Hedt-Gauthier, B. L., Neufeld, N., Odhiambo, J., Volmink, J., Shuchman, M., Ruggiero, E. D., & Condo, J. U. (2022). Gender equity in health research publishing in Africa. *BMJ Global Health*, *7*(7), e008821. https://doi.org/10.1136/bmjgh-2022-008821

Barrett, H. C. (2020). Towards a Cognitive Science of the Human: Cross-Cultural Approaches and Their Urgency. *Trends in Cognitive Sciences*, 24(8), 620–638. https://doi.org/10.1016/j.tics.2020.05.007

Batool, U., Raziq, M.M., Obaid, A. et al. Psychological ownership and knowledge behaviors during a pandemic: role of approach motivation. *Current Psychology*, 42, 25089–25099 (2023). https://doi.org/10.1007/s12144-022-03450-y

Böhme, M. & Stör, T. (2014) Household Interview Duration Analysis in CAPI Survey Management. *Field Methods*, 26(4): 390–405. https://doi.org/10.1177/1525822X14528450

Bradley, M. (2017b). Whose agenda? Power, policies, and priorities in North–South research partnerships. Putting Knowledge to Work: Collaborating, influencing and learning for international development, 37–69.

Burger, O., Chen, L., Erut, A., Fong, F.T.K. Rawlings, B., Legare, C.H. (2022) Developing cross-cultural data infrastructures (CCDIs) for research in cognitive and behavioral sciences. *Review of Philosophy and Psychology*, 14: 565–85. https://doi.org/10.1007/s13164-022-00635-z

Carbonnier, G. & Kontinen, T. (2015), Institutional Learning in North-South Research Partnerships. *Revue Tiers Monde*, 221: 149–62. https://doi.org/10.3917/rtm.221.0149

Chillag, K., Guest, G., Bunce, A., Johnson, L., Kilmarx, P.H. & Clark, L.A. & Watson, D. (2019) Constructing validity: New developments in creating objective measuring instruments. *Psychological Assessment*, 31(2): 1412–27. https://psycnet.apa.org/doi/10.1037/pas0000626

Chung, J. & Monroe, G. S. (2003). Exploring social desirability bias. *Journal of Business Ethics*, *44*, 291–302.

Clark, L. A., & Watson, D. (2019). Constructing validity: New developments in creating objective measuring instruments. *Psychological assessment*, *31*(12), 1412.

Confraria, H., Mira Godinho, M., & Wang, L. (2017). Determinants of citation impact: A comparative analysis of the Global South versus the Global North. *Research Policy*, *46*(1), 265–279. https://doi.org/10.1016/j.respol.2016.11.004

Connell, R. (2014) Using southern theory: Decolonizing social thought in theory, research and application. *Planning Theory*, 13(2), 210–223. https://doi.org/10.1177/1473095213499216

Conner, M., & Norman, P. (2017). Health behaviour: Current issues and challenges. *Psychology & health*, 32(8), 895–906.

Dada, S., van Daalen, K. R., Barrios-Ruiz, A., Wu, K.-T., Desjardins, A., Bryce-Alberti, M., Castro-Varela, A., Khorsand, P., Zamorano, A. S., Jung, L., Malolos, G., Li, J., Vervoort, D., Hamilton, N. C., Patil, P., Omrani, O. E., Wangari, M.-C., Sibanda, T., Buggy, C., & Mogo, E. R. I. (2022). Challenging the "old boys club" in academia: Gender and geographic representation in editorial boards of journals publishing in environmental sciences and public health. *PLOS Global Public Health*, *2*(6), e0000541. https://doi.org/10.1371/journal.pgph.0000541

de Jong, K., Ariti, C., van der Kam, S., Mooren, T., Shanks, L., Pintaldi, G., & Kleber, R. (2016). Monitoring and evaluating psychosocial intervention outcomes in humanitarian aid. *PLOS ONE*, 11(6), e0157474. https://doi.org/10.1371/journal.pone.0157474

Diener, E., Kahneman, D., & Helliwell, J. (2010). *International differences in well-being*. Oxford University Press.

Dsouza, J.P., Van den Brouke, S., Pattanshetty, S. & Dhoore, W. (2021) The application of health behavior theories to promote cervical cancer screening uptake. *Public Health Nursing*, 38(6): 1039–79.

Edejer, T. T. North-South research partnerships: the ethics of carrying out research in developing countries BMJ 1999; 319:438, doi:10.1136/bmj.319.7207.438

Einarsdottir, S., Bjornsdottir, M. D., & Lerkkanen, J. (2020). Cross-cultural validation of assessment instruments used in career counselling and guidance in the Nordic countries. In E. H. Haug, T. Hooley, J. Kettunen & R. Thomsen (Eds.), *Career and career guidance in the Nordic countries* (pp. 177–189). Brill Sense. https://doi.org/10.1163/9789004428096.

Einarsdottir, S., Rounds, J., & Su, R. (2010). Holland in Iceland revisited: An emic approach to evaluating U.S. vocational interest models. *Journal of Counseling Psychology*, 57, 361–367. https://doi.org/10.1037/a0019685.

Engel, G. L. (1977). The need for a new medical model: a challenge for biomedicine. *Science*, 196(4286), 129–136.

Erondu, N. A., Aniebo, I., Kyobutungi, C., Midega, J., Okiro, E., & Okumu, F. (2021b). Open letter to international funders of science and development in Africa. *Nature Medicine*, 27(5), 742–744.

Fetvadjiev, V. H., Meiring, D., van de Vijver, F. J. R., Nel, J. A., & Hill, C. (2015). The South African Personality Inventory (SAPI): A culture-informed instrument for the country's main ethnocultural groups. Psychological Assessment, 27(3), 827–837. https://doi.org/10.1037/pas0000078

Fisher, E.B., Fitzgibbon, M.L., Glasgow, R.E., Haire-Joshu, D., Hayman, L.L., Kaplan, R.M., Nanney, M.S. & Ockene, J.K., (2011) Behavior Matters. *American Journal of Preventive Medicine*, 40(5), E15–30.

Fisher, K. R., Shang, X., & Xie, J. (2016). Global South–North partnerships: Intercultural methodologies in disability research. Disability in the Global South: The Critical Handbook, 567–582.

Flint, A., Howard, G., Baidya, M., Wondim, T., Poudel, M., Nijhawan, A., Mulugeta, Y., & Sharma, S. (2022). Equity in Global North–South research partnerships: interrogating UK funding models. *Global Social Challenges Journal*, 1(1), 76–93. https://doi.org/10.1332/VQIL8302

Gardner, B., Arden, M. A., Brown, D., Eves, F. F., Green, J., Hamilton, K., Hankonen, N., Inauen, J., Keller, J., Kwasnicka, D., Labudek, S., Marien, H., Masaryk, R., McCleary, N., Mullan, B. A., Neter, E., Orbell, S., Potthoff, S., & Lally, P. (2021): Developing habit-based health behaviour change interventions: Twenty-one questions to guide future research, *Psychology & Health*. https://doi.org/10.1080/08870446.2021.2003362. Advanced online publication.

Glanz, K. & Bishop, D.B. (2010) The Role of Behavioral Science Theory in Development and Implementation of Public Health Interventions. *Annual Review of Public Health* 31(1), 399–418.

Gochman, D. S. (Ed.). (1997). *Handbook of health behavior research* (vol. 1–4). Plenum.

Graeff, T.R. (2005) Response Bias. Encyclopedia of Social Measurement (pp. 411–8), Elsevier ISBN 978-0-12-369398-3

Harter, M., Inauen, J. & Mosler, H.J. (2020) How does community-led total sanitation (CLTS) promote latrine construction, and can it be improved? A cluster-randomized controlled trial in Ghana. *Social Science & Medicine*, 245(112705). https://doi.org/10.1016/j.socscimed.2019.112705

Harzing, A.W., Baldueza, J., Barner-Rasmussen, W., Barzanty, C., Canabal, A., Davila, A., Esperjo, A., Ferreira, R., Giroud, A., Koester, K., Liang, Y.K., Moockaitis, A., Morley, M.J., Myloni, B., Odusanya, J.O.T., O'Sullivan, S.L., Palaniappan, A.K., Prochno, P., Choudhury, S.R., Saka-Helmhout, A., Siengthai, S., Viswat, L., Soydas, A.U., Zander, L. (2009) Rating versus ranking: What is the best way to reduce response and language bias in cross-national research? *International Business Review*, 18(4): 417–32. https://doi.org/10.1016/j.ibusrev.2009.03.001

Harzing, A.W. (2006) Response styles in cross-national survey research: A 26-country Study. *International Journal of Cross Cultural Management*, 6(2). https://doi.org/10.1177/1470595806066332

Hu, Y., Liu, H., Wu, J., & Fang, G. (2022). Factors influencing self-care behaviours of patients with type 2 diabetes in China based on the health belief model: A cross-sectional study. *BMJ open*, *12*(8), e044369. https://doi.org/10.1136/bmjopen-2020-044369

Janz, N.K. & Becker, M.H. (1984) The health belief model: A decade later. *Health Eduation & Behavior*, 11(1), 1–47. https://doi.org/10.1177/109019818401100101

Jemmott III, J. B., Heeren, G. A., Ngwane, Z., Hewitt, N., Jemmott, L. S., Shell, R., & O'Leary, A. (2007). Theory of planned behaviour predictors of intention to use condoms among Xhosa adolescents in South Africa. *AIDS Care*, *19*(5), 677–684. https://doi.org/10.1080/09540120601084308

Kaihlanen, A.M., Hietapakka, L. & Heponiemi, T. (2019) Increasing cultural awareness: qualitative study of nurses' perceptions about cultural competence training. *BMC Nursing*, *18*(38). https://doi.org/10.1186/s12912-019-0363-x

Kalinga, C. (2019) Caught between a rock and a hard place: Navigating global research partnerships in the global South as an indigenous researcher, *Journal of African Cultural Studies*, *31*(3), 270–272, DOI: 10.1080/13696815.2019.1630261

Karlsson, S., Srebotnjak, T., & Gonzales, P. (2007). Understanding the North–South knowledge divide and its implications for policy: a quantitative analysis of the generation of scientific knowledge in the environmental sciences. *Environmental Science & Policy*, *10*(7-8), 668–684.

Keiser, J., Utzinger, J., Tanner, M., & Singer, B. H. (2004). Representation of authors and editors from countries with different human development indexes in the leading literature on tropical medicine: Survey of current evidence. *BMJ (Clinical Research Ed.)*, *328*(7450), 1229–1232. https://doi.org/10.1136/bmj.38069.518137.F6

Kelly, M.P. & Barker, M. (2016) Why is changing health-related behaviour so difficult? *Public Health*, *136*, 109–116. https://doi.org/10.1016/j.puhe.2016.03.030

Kemmelmeier, M. (2016b). Cultural differences in survey responding: Issues and insights in the study of response biases. *International Journal of Psychology*, *51*(6), 439–444.

Khan, B., Khan, A., & Khan, R. (2022). Measuring the intention in favour and against getting vaccinated from COVID-19 using the health belief model: Cross-sectional study of Pakistan. *Illness, Crisis & Loss*, 10541373221118149. https://doi.org/10.1177/10541373221118149

Kline, M.A., Shamsudheen, R. & Broesch, T. (2018) Variation is the universal: making cultural evolution work in developmental psychology. *Philosophical Transactions of the Royal Society B*, *373*(1743). https://doi.org/10.1098/rstb.2017.0059

Kumsta, R. (2019) The role of epigenetics for understanding mental health difficulties and its implications for psychotherapy research. *Psychology and Psychotherapy: Theory, Research and Practice*, *92*(2): 190–207. https://doi.org/10.1111/papt.12227

Kwasnicka, D., Dombrowski, S.U., White, M. & Sniehotta, F.F. (2016) Theoretical explanations for maintenance of behaviour change: a systematic review of behaviour theories, *Health Psychology Review*, *10*(3), 277–296, DOI: 10.1080/17437199.2016.1151372

Langer, A., Díaz-Olavarrieta, C., Berdichevsky, K., & Villar, J. (2004). Why is research from developing countries underrepresented in international health literature, and what can be done about it? *Bulletin of the World Health Organization*, *82*(10), 802–803.

Larkan, F., Uduma, O., Lawal, S.A. et al. (2016). Developing a framework for successful research partnerships in global health. *Global Health*, *12*, 17. https://doi.org/10.1186/s12992-016-0152-1

Leventhal, H., Weinman, J., Leventhal, R.A. & Phillips, A. (2008). Health Psychology: The search for pathways between behavior and health. *Annual Review of Psychology*, *59*, 477–505. https://doi.org/10.1146/annurev.psych.59.103006.093643

Lin, C. L., Ye, Y., Lin, P., Lai, X. L., Jin, Y. Q., Wang, X., & Su, Y. S. (2021). Safe sexual behavior intentions among college students: The construction of an extended theory of planned behavior. *International Journal of Environmental Research and Public Health*, *18*(12), 6349. https://doi.org/10.3390/ijerph18126349

Maddux, J.E., Rogers, R.W. (1983). Protection motivation and self-efficacy: A revised theory of fear appeals and attitude change. *Journal of Experimental and Social Psychology*, *19*, 469–479.

Marja, S.L. & Suvi, A. (2021) Cultural competence learning of the health care students using a simulation pedagogy: An integrative review. *Nurse Education in Practice*, 52. https://doi.org/10.1016/j.nepr.2021.103044

Markus, H.R. & Kitayama, S. (2010) Cultures and selves: A cycle of mutual constitutions. *Perspectives on Psychological Science*, 5(4). https://doi.org/10.1177/1745691610375557

McBride, S. & Morgan, A. (2022) Context matters: A systematic review of neonatal care in humanitarian emergencies. *Journal of International Humanitarian Action*, 7(13). https://doi.org/10.1186/s41018-022-00121-2

Merriman, R., Galizia, I., Tanaka, S., Sheffel, A., Buse, K., & Hawkes, S. (2021). The gender and geography of publishing: A review of sex/gender reporting and author representation in leading general medical and global health journals. *BMJ Global Health*, *6*(5), e005672. https://doi.org/10.1136/bmjgh-2021-005672

Michie, S., Van Stralen, M.M. & West, R. (2011) The behaviour change wheel: A new method for characterising and designing behaviour change interventions. *Implementation Science*, *6*(42). https://doi.org/10.1186/1748-5908-6-42

Miles, J., & Gilbert, P. (Eds.). (2005). *A handbook of research methods for clinical and health psychology*. Oxford University Press. https://doi.org/10.1093/med:psych/9780198527565.001.0001

Morgan, B., Naidoo, A. V., Henn, C., & Rabie, S. (2019). Using interests and Holland's model of vocational personality types in career counselling: Some thoughts and research findings. In J. G. Maree (Ed.), *Handbook of innovative career counselling* (pp. 485–504). Springer.

Morgan, B., Teye-Kwadjo, E., Asumeng, M., Rabie, S., Naidoo, A. V., & de Bruin, G. P. (2021). Psychometric properties of the African Career Interest Inventory in Ghana. *International Journal for Educational and Vocational Guidance*. Advanced online publication. https://doi.org/10.1007/s10775-021-09499-8.

Nafade, V., Sen, P., & Pai, M. (2019). Global health journals need to address equity, diversity and inclusion. *BMJ Global Health*, *4*(5), e002018. https://doi.org/10.1136/bmjgh-2019-002018

Naslund, J.A., Aschbrenner, K.A., Araya, R., Marsch, L.A., Unützer, J. Patel, V. & Bartels, S.J. (2017) Digital technology for treating and preventing mental disorders in low-income and middle-income countries: a narrative review of the literature. *The Lancet Psychiatry*, *4*(6): 486–500. https://doi.org/10.1016/S2215-0366(17)30096-2

Nature (2022). Nature addresses helicopter research and ethics dumping. Nature 606 2 June 2022 pg7.

Nilsen, P. & Bernhardsson, S. (2019) Context matters in implementation science: a scoping review of determinant frameworks that describe contextual determinants for implementation outcomes. *BMC Health Services Research*, *19*(189). https://doi.org/10.1186/s12913-019-4015-3

OECD (2011), Busan Partnership for Effective Development Co-operation: Fourth High Level Forum on Aid Effectiveness, Busan, Republic of Korea, 29 November - 1 December 2011, OECD Publishing, Paris, https://doi.org/10.1787/54de7baa-en.

Ojedokun, O., Henschel, N., Arant, R., & Boehnke, K. (2022). Applying the theory of planned behaviour to littering prevention behaviour in a developing country (Nigeria). *Waste Management*, *142*, 19–28. https://doi.org/10.1016/j.wasman.2022.02.006

Osazuwa, S. & Moodley, R. (2023) "Will there be a willingness to actually engage with it?": Exploring attitudes towards culturally integrative psychotherapy among Canada's African community. *Journal of Psychotherapy Integration*, *33*(1), 68–85. https://doi.org/10.1037/int0000289

Palser, E. R., Lazerwitz, M., & Fotopoulou, A. (2021). *Gender and geographical disparity in editorial boards of journals in psychology and neuroscience* (S. 2021.02.15.431321). bioRxiv. https://doi.org/10.1101/2021.02.15.431321

Pierce, J.L., Kostova, T. & Dirks, K.T. (2001) Toward a theory of psychological ownership in organisations. *The Academy of Management Review*, *26*(2), 298–310.

Posada, A., & Chen, G. (2018, June 15). Inequality in knowledge production: The integration of academic infrastructure by big publishers. *22nd International Conference on Electronic Publishing*. https://doi.org/10.4000/proceedings.elpub.2018.30

Prestwich, A., Webb, T.L. & Connor, M. (2015) Using theory to develop and test interventions to promote changes in health behaviour: evidence, issues and recommendations. *Current Opinion in Psychology*, *5*, 1–5. https://doi.org/10.1016/j.copsyc.2015.02.011

Prochaska, J. O., & DiClemente, C. C. (1983). Stages and processes of self-change of smoking: Toward an integrative model of change. *Journal of Consulting and Clinical Psychology*, *51*(3), 390. https://doi.org/10.1037/0022-006X.51.3.390

Raj, A. (2022). Gender and the COVID-19 pandemic: Multinational research indicates that we must support and compensate LMIC women's leadership in crises. *eClinicalMedicine*, *53*. https://doi.org/10.1016/j.eclinm.2022.101748

Ransing, R., Koh, E. B. Y., Ramalho, R., De Filippis, R., Pinto Da Costa, M., Pereira-Sanchez, V., Noor, I. M., & Shalbafan, M. (2023). Collaborative research on mental health in the post-COVID-19 era: An early career psychiatrists' perspective. *Frontiers in Psychiatry*, *14*, 1230059. https://doi.org/10.3389/fpsyt.2023.1230059

Rosenstock, I. M. (1974). The health belief model and preventive health behavior. *Health Education Monographs*, *2*(4), 354–386. https://doi.org/10.1177/109019817400200405

Saal, W., & Kagee, A. (2012). The applicability of the Theory of Planned Behaviour in predicting adherence to ART among a South African sample. *Journal of Health Psychology*, *17*(3), 362–370. https://doi.org/10.1177/1359105311416875

Schertenleib, A., Sigrist, J., Friedrich, M.N.D., Ebi, C., Hammes, F. & Marks, S.J. (2019) Construction of a low-cost mobile incubator for field and laboratory use. *Journal of Visualized Experiments*, *145*, 58443. https://doi.org/10.3791/58443

Schwarzer, R. (1992). Self-efficacy in the adoption and maintenance of health behaviors: Theoretical approaches and a new model. In R. Schwarzer (Ed.), *Self-efficacy: Thought control of action* (pp. 217–243). Hemisphere

Schwarzer, R. (2016). Health Action Process Approach (HAPA) as a Theoretical Framework to Understand Behavior Change. *Actualidades En Psicología*. *30*(121), 119–130. https://doi.org/10.15517/ap.v30i121.23458

Schwarzer, Ralf (2011). 'Health Behavior Change', In Howard S. Friedman (ed.), The Oxford Handbook of Health Psychology, Oxford Library of Psychology; online edn, Oxford Academic, 18 Sept. 2012), https://doi.org/10.1093/oxfordhb/9780195342819.013.0024, accessed 16 Nov. 2023.

Sharma, S. Palanchoke, J., Reed, D. & Abbott, J.H. (2017) Translation, cross-cultrual adaptation and psychometric properties of the Nepali versions of numerical pain rating scale and global rating of change. *Health and Quality of Life Outcomes*, *15*(236). https://doi.org/10.1186/s12955-017-0812-8

Skevington, S. & Tucker, C. (1999) Designing response scales for cross-cultural use in health care: Data from the development of the UK WHOQOL. *British Journal of Medical Psychology*, *72*(1), 51–61. https://doi.org/10.1348/000711299159817

Smith, E., Hunt, M., & Master, Z. (2014). Authorship ethics in global health research partnerships between researchers from low or middle income countries and high income countries. *BMC Medical Ethics*, *15*(1), 42. https://doi.org/10.1186/1472-6939-15-42

Sniehotta, FF., Presseau, J. & Araújo-Soares, V. (2014) Time to retire the theory of planned behaviour. *Health Psychology Review*, *8*(1): 1–7. 10.1080/17437199.2013.869710

Sumarmi, S., Hsu, Y. Y., Cheng, Y. M., & Lee, S. H. (2021). Factors associated with the intention to undergo Pap smear testing in the rural areas of Indonesia: a health belief model. *Reproductive Health*, *18*(1), 1–10. https://doi.org/10.1186/s12978-021-01188-7

Sumathipala, A., Siribaddana, S., & Patel, V. (2004). Under-representation of developing countries in the research literature: Ethical issues arising from a survey of five leading medical journals. *BMC Medical Ethics*, *5*(5). https://doi.org/10.1186/1472-6939-5-5

Teye-Kwadjo, E. (2021). The job-search self-efficacy (jsse) scale: An item response theory investigation. *International Journal of Applied Positive Psychology*, *6*(3), 301–314.

Teye-Kwadjo, E., Kagee, A., & Swart, H. (2017). Determinants of condom use among heterosexual young men and women in southeastern Ghana: A mediation analysis. *Psychology & Sexuality*, *8*(4), 291–305. https://doi.org/10.1080/19419899.2017.1391870

Teye-Kwadjo, E., Salia, S., Mensah, G. O., & Ofori, R. (2020). Exploring Ghanaian commercial drivers' intentions to wear a seat belt. *Case Studies on Transport Policy*, *8*, 453–459. https://doi.org/10.1016/j.cstp.2019.10.009

THET (n.d.). Principles of Partnership. https://www.thet.org/principles-of-partnership/ Last accessed 30 October 2023.

Tomberge, V. M. J., Harter, M., & Inauen, J. (2022). The importance of collective and individual psychological ownership for safe sanitation: A multilevel analysis in rural Ghana. *Global Public Health*, *17*(7), 1314–1329.

Velin, L., Lartigue, J.-W., Johnson, S. A., Zorigtbaatar, A., Kanmounye, U. S., Truche, P., & Joseph, M. N. (2021). Conference equity in global health: A systematic review of factors impacting LMIC representation at global health conferences. *BMJ Global Health*, *6*(1), e003455. https://doi.org/10.1136/bmjgh-2020-003455

Voller, S., Schellenberg, J., Chi, P., Thorogood, N. (2022) What makes working together work? A scoping review of the guidance on North–South research partnerships. *Health Policy and Planning*, *37*(4), 523–534. https://doi.org/10.1093/heapol/czac008

World Bank. (2022). *Science & Technology Indicators*.

Zingerli, C. A Sociology of International Research Partnerships for Sustainable Development. *The European Journal of Development Research*, *22*, 217–233 (2010). https://doi.org/10.1057/ejdr.2010.1

34

COMMUNITY-BASED PARTICIPATORY ACTION RESEARCH (CBPAR)

A Research Methodology for Impactful, Culturally Sensitive, and Contextually Appropriate Health Psychology

Benjamin Ambuehl, Richard Appiah, Asma Bibi, and Irene A. Kretchy

Introduction

Community development projects using traditional approaches can function effectively to improve health outcomes in situations where the needs of communities are explicit and unambiguous and at the level of basic need provision (Abbott, 1995). However, as described in the previous chapter, traditional community development methodologies have inherent limitations. An alternative methodology is community participation, for example, community-based participatory action research (CBPAR), which is central to impactfully empowering members across cultures and contexts (Vivona & Wolfgram, 2021) and improving health outcomes for communities (Page-Reeves, 2019). CBPAR is a partnership approach to research involving all stakeholders and aiming for their active participation throughout the research process (Israel et al., 1998). CBPAR aims to learn about one's needs and integrate one's resources (Cooke & Kothari, 2007), as well as to support collaboration among stakeholders and enhance action that can lead to community transformation and social change (Wallerstein, Duran, Oetzel, & Minkler, 2017; Weiner & McDonald, 2013).

In this chapter, we focus on the application of CBPAR in health psychology in underserved communities, e.g., in low-and middle-income countries (LMICs), where research projects take on greater complexity and require in-depth

 DOI: 10.4324/9781003318026-41

collaboration between researchers and local communities (Kretchy et al., 2022). We first review published guidelines on how to apply CBPAR as a research methodology. Second, we discuss the benefits and challenges when applying CBPAR in practice. Third, we present three case studies on different psychological health topics, highlighting the success of this research method in different contexts.

Methodology of CBPAR

CBPAR is an ecological approach and a framework for research endeavours that focus on equitable community participation to achieve social change for the community (Collins et al., 2018). The goals of using CBPAR are always threefold: (1) to develop relationships of solidarity between the community and researchers, (2) to learn relevant knowledge and skills from the community, and (3) to engage the results of research in action and to build self-sufficiency for the communities (Stoecker, 2005). This means that CBPAR projects demand extensive capacity development, for example, in developing a common language among and aligning expectations of project implementors and communities (PACT, 2023) in an iterative process (RTI International, 2004; Minkler & Wallerstein, 2008). The core of every iteration is the collaboration research between communities and researchers based on the resources and strengths of the community (Figure 34.1).

When implementing CBPAR, the process of research happens in six phases (Hacker, 2013):

Phase 1 – Assessment of Context and Building Relationships

In the first phase, researchers start working together with the communities rather than in the communities. The main goal is to find out about the difficulties, needs, strengths, and diversity of the communities (Weiner & McDonald, 2013). This demands nurturing collaborations in an ongoing process of exchange by establishing and maintaining equality between parties. Such collaborations require reciprocity (Collins et al., 2018) and respect for community decision-making processes. Reciprocity in the context of CBPAR is an attitude that emerges from reflexive reasoning, becoming aware of and critically examining and owning one's privilege, power, and patterns of intentional and unintentional classism and racism (Muhammad et al., 2015). The collaboration also requires transparent communication and consultation with each other to maintain trustworthy relationships between the community and research staff and to distribute roles and responsibilities based on both parties' wishes (Dyer et al., 2014). In a CBPAR project team, adequate representation of all stakeholders and ongoing discussions help in thinking critically about issues of power, social location, and perspective and are particularly important for assessing the needs of disadvantaged stakeholder groups (O'Mara-Eves et al., 2015).

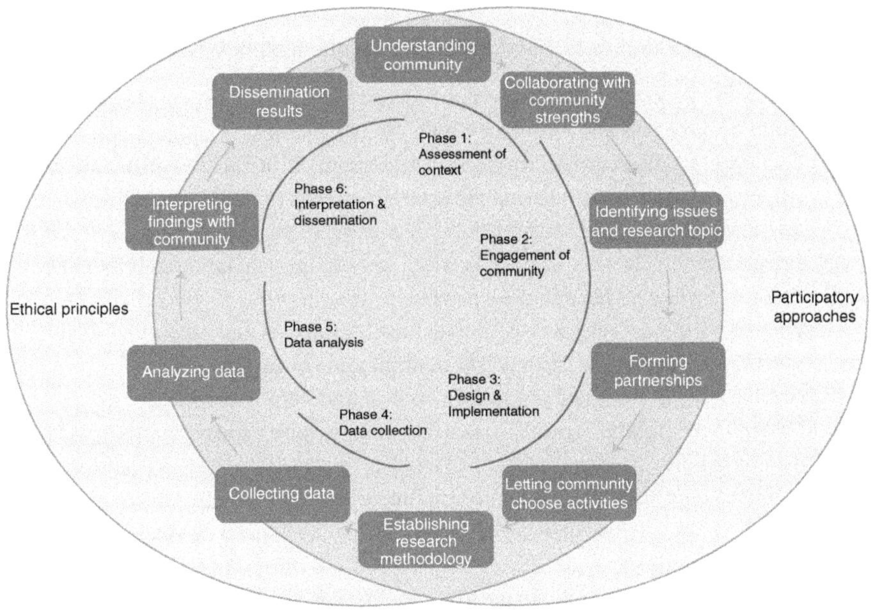

Figure 34.1 CBPAR as an iterative research methodology and its foundations (adapted from Vivona & Wolfgram, 2021).

Phase 2 – Engagement of Community

In the second phase, the focus is to deepen the relationship between research staff and communities and to start discussing the research process and power sharing between researchers and communities (Wallerstein et al., 2019). The aim is to define the scope of the research project upon consultation of researchers and community stakeholders, with meaningful participation of the community to develop common goals (Chess & Purcell, 1999). In this phase, community engagement should be as broad as possible and go beyond the members who already have a strong sense of community (e.g., local leaders; Talo et al., 2014). This phase requires openness from research partners to accept the right of people to be involved in the decision-making process (Abbott, 1995). A very simple example is that the timing and location of meetings can affect whether those with childcare responsibilities can participate. Consultation should therefore be tailored to the community's needs to optimally facilitate communication and decision-making and to create a more equitable distribution of power (e.g., break-out groups, anonymous voting, group discussion, one-on-one meetings), contributing to further strengthen collaborative relations and partnerships (Woolf et al., 2016). Involving the people directly affected by CBPAR encourages community engagement and facilitates learning about the community's needs and possibilities for interventions (Minkler and Wallerstein, 2008). Israel et al.

Box 34.1 Approaches to Participatory Partnerships in CBPAR

1. Recognise the community as a unit of identity.
2. Build on strengths and resources within the community.
3. Facilitate a collaborative, equitable partnership in all phases, involving an empowering and power-sharing process that attends to social inequalities.
4. Foster co-learning and capacity building among all partners.
5. Integrate and achieve a balance between knowledge generation and intervention for the mutual benefit of all partners.
6. Focus on the local relevance of public health problems and on ecological perspectives that attend to the multiple determinants of health.
7. Involve systems development using a cyclical and iterative process.
8. Disseminate results to all partners and involve them in the wider dissemination.
9. Involve a long-term process and commitment to sustainability.
10. Openly address issues of race, ethnicity, racism, and social class and embody 'cultural humility'.
11. Work to ensure research rigour and validity but also seek to "broaden the bandwidth of validity" with respect to research relevance.

(1998 and 2005) suggest 11 approaches to participatory partnerships when conducting research in CBPAR projects (see Box 34.1).

Only through consensus decision-making and co-creation of knowledge in a collaborative and empowering process (ICPHR, 2013) are the scope and activities of research also accepted in the community, and a climate of trust guarantees that people are willing to share personally sensitive information in this project (Etchegary et al., 2013).

Phase 3 – Design and Implementation

In the third phase, intervention activities are developed and tailored specifically to the social and cultural context (Burns et al., 2011). The goal is to divide responsibilities for implementation in an equitable—not necessarily equal—way between researchers and communities. This builds on the strengths and needs of researchers and communities: some communities may have the interest and resources (e.g., time, training) to implement certain aspects of the research project (e.g., participant interviews, qualitative coding, writing), whereas other communities may ask researchers to take on tasks that would otherwise be burdensome (e.g., accessing research grant funding to support the work). These decisions should be made jointly with a focus on capacity building and sustainability (Collins et al., 2018). Generally, greater community involvement leads to more productive partnerships, better research programmes, and stronger implementation of interventions (Minkler et al., 2009) through a collaborative process (Appiah, 2022; Ambuehl et al., 2022).

Phase 4 – Data Collection

In the fourth phase, when collecting data, it is important to follow cultural protocols that resonate with ethical interview style (Ball, 2005) and a variety of methods (Jason & Glenwick, 2016). Pilot-testing of questionnaires and citizen science approaches to data collection (adapted to the culture and context by community participation; Odetola et al., 2021) help to respect the integrity of respondents and increase the quality of data. For data collection, instruments are chosen according to the needs of what data to collect and the skills of the participants. For example, when using questionnaires, though computer-assisted personal interviews (CAPI) or pen-paper instruments are available, some materials to support the respondents in providing adequate data can be introduced (e.g., visual Likert scale, Harter et al. 2020).

Phase 5 – Data Analysis and Interpretation

The first part of phase 5 is the only phase that can happen without the community and may be done by researchers alone or statisticians. But it can also be used for collaboration and capacity building between stakeholders: first, data analysis can be used to develop capacity among community members. For example, community members can be trained in qualitative and quantitative data analysis. In the second part, community members are involved in the interpretation of results by performing member checks – reporting the findings to the community and gathering their input for accurate and valid interpretation (Israel et al., 2010).

Phase 6 – Dissemination of Results and Transfer into Action

In the sixth phase, results from phase five are disseminated using simple numbers and explanations of the statistical models using simple language. The goal is that results dissemination happens as a collaborative effort between the research staff and the community, reporting locally in the communities first and then reporting jointly to a wider audience (i.e., through co-authorships of articles and opportunities of co-presenting). Also, results are translated to and used for impactful actions to improve the reality of livelihood in the communities, e.g., by finding effective community development programmes and impact policymaking (Israel et al., 2010).

Benefits of CBPAR Approaches

Using CBPAR approaches can ensure that underserved communities and underrepresented populations benefit from research projects (Webler and Tuler, 2006;

Twyman et al., 2001). CBPAR also empowers communities and individuals beyond the research project by initiating social change through more equal partnerships (Wallerstein et al., 2019) and by creating community ownership (Dyer et al., 2014). Capacity building within the community through joint learning and skill sharing (Burns et al., 2011) contributes to more equality too. In the following, we explain the selected benefits of using CBPAR in more detail.

Equitable collaborations among research stakeholders and communities through cyclical and iterative processes (Burns et al., 2011) allow to optimise feasibility and relevance of possible interventions and produce realistic visions of what can be done through co-designed, detailed project plans (Dias & Gama, 2014). By using participatory approaches in a person-centred, contextually informed, and ethical way (Butterfoss, 2006), the communities' sense of ownership over the projects is fostered (Ambuehl et al., 2022), which leverages the sustainability of projects. Thus, CBPAR facilitates improving the current situation of the community at the same time as working towards transformative change in the long term (Wallerstein et al., 2020).

Furthermore, CBPAR increases the internal and external validity of the research (Viswanathan et al., 2004) because of improved decision-making: theories that are relevant to the community are selected, research methods are adapted specifically to the context and applied in a culturally sensitive way to solve systemic issues (Rice & McCool, 2022). Measures are adapted specifically to the context, which increases the robustness and ecological validity of findings (Jason & Glenwick, 2016) and presents the opportunity to translate research into practice (Wallerstein & Duran, 2010). Thus, the people affected by the research projects are to be given access to relevant information to support health and well-being through research and innovations. However, to safeguard the integrity of the research process (Kwan & Walsh, 2018), CBPAR is only implemented beneficially if ethical principles are followed (Banks & Manners, 2012). We summarise these as follows:

1 Mutual respect, which is achieved by developing research relationships between stakeholders and participants, based on accepting and embracing different perspectives and listening to the voices of others
2 Equality and inclusion, which are achieved by encouraging and actively enabling people of all backgrounds to lead, design, and take part in research by ensuring formats for meetings are accessible to all while tackling discrimination and oppression
3 Democratic participation, which is achieved by using inclusive methods and communicating in easy language to allow everyone to contribute meaningfully and work towards sharing status and power equally
4 Active learning, which is achieved by sharing responsibilities in the research process and asking for interpretation of research findings and implications for practice
5 Making a difference, which is achieved by creating positive change for communities

6 Collective action, which is achieved by working together with individuals and groups to achieve change for agreed visions
7 Personal integrity, which is achieved by behaving reliably and honestly in a trustworthy manner and being open to challenge and change, including conflict resolution

Additionally, general ethical principles such as the Helsinki Declaration's do no harm principles (Wessells, 2009) and principles of local ethics committees are to be respected as well.

Challenges of CBPAR Approaches

Despite all the benefits, using CBPAR approaches poses several challenges to the research process. The field setting clearly challenges the application of CBPAR. From a methodological point of view, this is a challenge because communities differ substantially from each other, and as a consequence, community participation needs to be defined individually in a process with every community in every research project. For example, in delocalised communities and informal settlements, community engagement has to be different than in urban, wealthier communities with strong institutional structures (i.e., contribution of labour and manpower instead of decision-making on organisational form; Ojha et al., 2016). This challenge can be tackled by ensuring community engagement from early on in project planning and decision-making about the roles and responsibilities of stakeholders.

Another challenge is collaborative community participation in all six phases of a CBPAR project because participants may not be representative of the wider community because of self-assessment (Israel et al., 2005). Researchers must mitigate this challenge by preventing time compression so that intensive sessions over a short time period do not exclude people who cannot commit the time and are busy with other labour. Because if community involvement is in the hands of a small group, the already well-connected get better connected, and there is no guarantee that the wider community will feel the benefits from the CBPAR approach (Webler & Tuler, 2006). Researchers need to be aware of socio-political interactions within a community and who holds power. This is typically the case for formal governance structures, which are often not embedded in the informal everyday spaces of community life.

Also, logistics and resources are a challenge: planning happens in collaboration with researchers and communities. Methodologically rigorous research requires high-skilled capacities (Shadowen et al., 2020) and resources. Involvement of diverse people (e.g., training of enumerators and trainers) over a short time period requires skilled community and academic co-facilitators, too, ensuring participation is not dominated by experts. Thus there are potentially conflicting demands on time, money, administrative resources, and engagement to use the CBPAR methodology in a meaningful way. To cope with these difficulties, the project management can support stakeholders and communities by providing more space for projects to build the right systems to enable successful community leadership, such as through longer start-up stages or by providing more support for locally led development (PACT, 2023).

Finally, CBPAR poses a challenge in not creating false expectations: CBPAR is a research approach which has the goal that the community and researchers collaboratively achieve a result to change the livelihood of a community. However, it does not replace professional developmental and cooperation work to increase the quality of life and basic services infrastructure in a community. Transparent communication is necessary to prevent differing priorities across communities and academic partners and differing priorities between community advisory boards and research funders to ensure that community involvement is not abused and over-demanded (PACT, 2023).

Case Studies

We will now share three case studies to illustrate how CBPAR can be successfully applied in health psychology.

CBPAR and Mental Health Intervention Programmes in Rural Ghana

In most LMICs, including Ghana, mental health is chronically neglected, underfunded, and heavily stigmatised, especially in rural and remote community settings where access to health care is limited (Patel et al., 2018). A proposed solution to mitigate the health treatment gap in LMICs is to scale up evidence-based, context-tailored, community-delivered health promotion programmes (Jordans & Kohrt, 2020). However, in health psychology, a large number of empirically tested behaviour change intervention programmes have been theoretically and fundamentally developed in accordance with Western social value systems (Martín-Martín et al., 2021), but only a few studies have evaluated the effect of context-applicable health behaviour change intervention programmes in Africa (Guse, 2022). In the following, we demonstrate how CBPAR can successfully be used to develop intervention programmes based on psychological theory and adapt them to the local context:

Collaborating with community stakeholders, a new complex intervention was developed by researchers within a seven-step iterative process – the Inspired Life Programme (ILP) (Appiah, Wilson Fadiji et al., 2022). The ILP is constituted by sessions that draw on the principles and constructs of positive psychology and cognitive-behavioural intervention and aim to bolster mental health, foster psychosocial skills, and increase vocational productivity in poor rural adults through group discussions and activity sessions. The ILP has demonstrated effectiveness in improving positive mental health (i.e., well-being, resilience, and strengths use), in reducing symptoms of depression and negative affect, and in increasing vocational productivity in a sample of socioeconomically disadvantaged poor rural adults in Ghana, as evidenced by larger increases in the proportion of flourishers in the programme participants compared to the control group, immediately and three months post-intervention (Appiah, Wilson Fadiji, et al., 2020).

The ILP sessions were developed using CBPAR principles: the overarching method to ensure community participation was to conduct focus group discussions (FGDs) with participating individuals from the target population. Participation during the development was crucial to assess the alignment of the proposed content, session structure, and implementation strategy of the ILP with the needs of the participants. The FGDs were organised for consenting individuals to gather their perspectives on the proposed content, as well as assess the comprehensibility, relevance, and applicability of the themes and lessons to participants. Additionally, researchers sought their input on the structure and implementation strategy. Feedback from these discussions was thoroughly evaluated and incorporated into the programme sessions. Some sessions aimed to practically test and identify potential challenges in delivering the programme and to evaluate implementation strategy. Participants were asked to critique each session's content and contribute to enhancing the draft programme. The simulation sessions also aimed to determine the most effective way to present the content for maximum impact on the target population.

Firstly, although the programme manual may be in English, the sessions needed to be delivered in the native language of participants and by trained facilitators who were native speakers or fluent in the native language. This was important to effectively communicate messages of the sessions, facilitating participants' understanding of the lessons and skills therein. Thus, the research team translated and validated all six mental health and well-being outcome measures into Twi (Appiah, Schutte, et al., 2020), the most widely spoken participant language, before they were administered. Facilitators who were native speakers of participants' dialects were also more likely to understand and adhere to the local cultural norms and values of the people. For instance, some local Ghanaian cultural norms forbid a person to point to another with the left hand or finger, or to interrupt an elderly person who is speaking, or to shake, hug, or establish physical contact with a female Muslim participant, or to take photographs of chiefs and elders at a gathering without their prior consent (Appiah, 2020).

Secondly, because most participants were unable to take notes at the sessions (due to low literacy), it was essential that the session goals and key themes of the sessions were written on a flip chart in the native language and clearly displayed at the sessions. The co-facilitator wrote down keywords from participants' contributions on the flip chart during plenary sessions, as necessary, to demonstrate to participants that their contributions were important and to encourage them to remain attentive and participatory. Another important consideration was to identify and pair up individuals who demonstrated a high level of understanding and performance with those who were slower. Facilitators closely observed participants' level of understanding and strengths in the first session and carefully used this information to pair participants up.

The progress and overall success of this community-based health behaviour change intervention programme depended primarily on the level of group cohesion and interactivity demonstrated by participants at the programme sessions (Appiah, 2020; Appiah, 2023). Important considerations in the project were the FGD meetings: they may be the first of their kind for some participants in the rural African context, but it was important that the facilitators expended effort to build positive group dynamics from the start of the programme. An important strategy to inspire group cohesion and interactivity was to inquire about participants' preferred names that they wish to be called at sessions – and have group members and facilitators call them by those names. Psychologically speaking, calling participants by their right names symbolised respect and indicated to participants that the facilitators and group members recognised their presence and contributions (Agyekum, 2006). Instilling a sense of belongingness and responsibility in participants was not usually arduous since, generally, the communal orientation of most African communities, which was more pronounced in the remote rural context (Appiah, 2020; Gyekye, 2014), fostered a high sense of 'we-ness' (i.e., togetherness, interconnectedness) in participants of FGDs and members of the community.

Health Behaviour Change and Shared Technologies: Participatory Action for Long-Term Arsenic-Safe Water Consumption (PACT)

As important as the Sustainable Development Goals (SDGs) are, their specific means of implementation (MoI) are often neglected in the public discourse (Bartram et al., 2018). For example, to ensure the availability and sustainable management of water and sanitation for all (SDG 6), expanding international cooperation and capacity-building support to developing countries and supporting and strengthening the participation of local communities is crucial (MoI 6a & 6b).

In the project PACT (Participatory Action for Long-Term Arsenic-Safe Water Infrastructure), researchers investigated two key concepts and their impact on the adoption and use of new safe water infrastructure: psychological ownership (the feeling that something is "mine" or "ours") and habit (to automatically associate water-collection with safe water infrastructure). They conducted a Cluster-Randomised Control Trial (C-RCT) in Bihar, India, and used the CBPAR framework to ensure the context specificity of interventions (Ambuehl et al., 2023). By actively involving the community, which meant respecting and acknowledging the difficulties communities were faced with, finding out about what the community needs were, aligning community interests with local government policies, collaborating on decisions for how communities could contribute to achieving their needs, and deciding on processes and protocols in the project, the researchers ensured that the scope and content of the research project were shaped by the communities priorities. This, and the broad collaboration with local stakeholders (e.g., public health and engineering department of the local government, local civil society organisations, and academia), enhanced the uptake of our research findings in the local policymaking and education of government engineers. Similar to other findings, when community participation was meaningful (Shadowen et al., 2020; O'Mara-Eves et al., 2015), PACT identified two key drivers for the success of a participatory approach in research projects: community interests and feedback. PACT communities developed a sense of ownership over the project when inequalities were addressed through the balancing of power, which led to better outcomes through building trust, developing partnerships, mutual respect, and community empowerment. For example, during the preliminary qualitative study, researchers identified relevant insights into the psychological aspects of community-based shared water infrastructure. The research question was collectively defined by the community. Informal local knowledge collection methods (mapping, photo, GPS) were used to foster community knowledge about the research topic by assigning a team of facilitators to certain communities who then accompanied the same community over the entire lifespan of the research project and led community visits by the research team. In workshops, interventions were developed to align community interests and needs and international standards (World Health Organisation quality of water supply infrastructure). Communities also proposed useful activities for every participating household as interventions and helped to refine psychological-theory-based interventions proposed by the researchers. This collaborative process aimed at fostering the communities' sense of ownership and involved offering choices; communities could decide how to implement and what to contribute to interventions and state where they depended on external support. The results were shared in street dramas developed together with the communities and through leaflets comprising simple language and graphics.

It was not easy to conduct his type of intervention research, however, because it demanded more resources from the researchers (time, discussions, compromises on work ethics, etc.) compared to traditional approaches. There was also the tension between scientific rigour and community-based flexibility, which required constant balancing of interests and iterative decision-making. Yet, because it was successfully implemented, this CBPAR approach resulted in more relevant and specific, impactful project outcomes for the communities (Ambuehl et al., 2023). Through CBPAR, researchers and the communities fostered a collaborative and equitable research endeavour that placed community knowledge and needs at the forefront. CBPAR, thus, contributed to an effective implementation of a global research agenda of sustainable development by focusing on the priorities of and empowering the most vulnerable population of our common planet.

As the research representative of the local civil society organisation said,

> Community participation is recognised as an old tradition at many levels in the communities, for example, through Mahatma Gandhi's use of Gram Swaraj in Indian society. But, at present, many communities are found to be divided and community participation is missing a lot. After our intervention, people were found remembering the sense of community ownership similar to as in the old social system.

Environmental Emergencies

The tradition of health psychology follows approaches to changing behaviour with the goal of primary prevention of serious diseases and secondary prevention of mental health issues. From 2010 to 2022, Pakistan saw four major and minor destructive floods. In the flooded areas, there were medical issues and difficult health conditions that were directly affecting women and children. To effectively implement behaviour change approaches, communities had to be empowered and motivated to address their own problems. Collaboration with local participants and an assessment of present health-care facilities and mental health services helped to collect relevant information and address key persons who could help with the matter at hand. The first target was to create an atmosphere of trust with the landlords, town councillors, municipal administration, landowners, and religious leaders in the village where the project was to be implemented to ensure the community's trust and full participation. When these people agreed, it was not a problem for the researcher to implement the project at the grassroots level. In this way, the trust of every person, big and small, in the area was gained, and the benefit proved to help achieve the desired results.

1 Identification of issues: By actively interacting with people, the researcher obtained critical insights, created trust, and generated more sustainable solutions. Listening was an important ability while working in CBPAR because it developed inclusivity and variety in individuals via mutual respect in relationships. It helped the researchers to identify the desired beneficial transformation. However, it was a time-consuming and laborious process.
2 Education of communities helped to convey knowledge about primary prevention.
3 Collaboration and cooperation among diverse stakeholders: Once the researcher established relationships with key individuals in the community, they began conducting sessions on mental health and well-being, physical, psychological, social, or sexual abuse, and educating on the laws that prohibit violence against women, girls, and boys, all embedded in an explanation of the actors and institutions in the social network.
4 Through CBPAR, the researcher promoted multidisciplinary cooperation among existing stakeholders through health education, access to basic amenities, socioeconomic determinants of health, social support networks, and community empowerment: before entering the community for the first time, the researcher sought contact with relevant local authorities to establish a trustworthy relationship and build a reputation. The researcher did this by following the CBPAR approach. However, building trust with communities was a long, tiring, and sometimes boring task. It required patience, commitment, and the passion to sacrifice. Sometimes, putting in too much effort did not necessarily provide the desired results in a given or calculated project's designated time; however, in the long run, those efforts were always not going in vain.

Conclusion

Contrasting traditional non-participatory research methods that have often resulted in findings that cannot be implemented, CBPAR takes into account diverse research representation and collaboration with populations of different cultures and social classes (Rodriguez Espinosa & Verney, 2021). Authentic community engagement is based on ethical principles and happens over all six phases of a CBPAR project to enhance capacity building and impact of the project in the communities (Duea et al., 2022; Vaughn & Jacquez, 2020). Engagement of communities can happen through a variety of participatory activities, increasing acceptability, participation, and feasibility of community-based projects (Ambuehl et al., 2022; Kretchy et al., 2022). CBPAR thus ensures that the community is involved in all stages of the research process and research is conducted jointly with members of the community in a culturally sensitive and context-specific way and not just within the community (Wallerstein et al., 2019). Successful CBPAR involves forming trusting relationships with members of the targeted community and collaborating with them to achieve the desired outcome (Weiner & McDonald, 2013). CBPAR thus makes the research more relevant, impactful, and sustainable (Page-Reeves, 2019; Wallerstein et al., 2018).

Further Reading

CHAT tool (WHO/Unicef) (2022): Community Engagement in Humanitarian Action
ENACT tool (PACT) (2023): Engaged Communities Accountability Commitment Tool

References

Abbott, J. (1995). Community participation and its relationship to community development. *Community Development Journal*, 30(2), 158–168.

Agyekum, K. (2006). The sociolinguistic of Akan personal names. *Nordic Journal of African Studies*, 15(2), 206–235.

Ambuehl, B., Kunwar, B. M., Schertenleib, A., Marks, S. J., & Inauen, J. (2022). Can participation promote psychological ownership of a shared resource? An intervention study of community-based safe water infrastructure. *Journal of Environmental Psychology*, 81, 101818.

Ambuehl, B., Singh, B. K., Kumar, M., Ghosh, A. K., Marks, S., & Inauen, J. (2023). Community Based Participatory Action Research: An Indo-Swiss Project. *Sandec News*, (24), 46–47.

Appiah, R. (2020). Community-based participatory research in rural African contexts: Ethico-cultural considerations and lessons from Ghana. *Public Health Reviews*, 41(1), 27.

Appiah, R. (2022). Context matters: Sociocultural considerations in the design and implementation of community-based positive psychology interventions in sub-Saharan Africa. *Culture & Psychology*, 28(4), 613–639.

Appiah, R. (2023). Facilitating change processes in group-based behaviour change interventions in rural African contexts: practical lessons from Ghana. *International Journal of Mental Health Systems*, 17(1), 3.

Appiah, R., Schutte, L., Wilson Fadiji, A., Wissing, M. P., & Cromhout, A. (2020). Factorial validity of the Twi versions of five measures of mental health and well-being in Ghana. *PLoS One*, 15(8), e0236707.

Appiah, R., Wilson Fadiji, A., Wissing, M. P., & Schutte, L. (2022). The inspired life program: development of a multicomponent positive psychology intervention for rural adults in Ghana. *Journal of Community Psychology*, 50(1), 302–328.

Appiah, R., Wilson-Fadiji, A., Schutte, L., & Wissing, M. P. (2020). Effects of a community-based multicomponent positive psychology intervention on mental health of rural adults in Ghana. *Applied Psychology: Health and Well-Being*, 12(3), 828–862.

Ball, J. (2005). Restorative research partnerships in Indigenous communities. In A. Farrell (Ed.), *Ethical research with children* (pp. 81–96). Maidenhead, UK: Open University Press.

Banks & Manners, (2012). Community-based participatory research: A guide to ethical principles and practice; https://www.fosteropenscience.eu/content/community-based-participatory-research-guide-ethical-principles-and-practice

Bartram, J., Brocklehurst, C., Bradley, D., Muller, M., & Evans, B. (2018). Policy review of the means of implementation targets and indicators for the sustainable development goal for water and sanitation. *NPJ Clean Water*, 1(1), 3.

Burns et al., (2011). A short guide to community based participatory action research. https://www.google.com/url?sa=t&rct=j&q=&esrc=s&source=web&cd=&cad=rja&uact=8&ved=2ahUKEwiA45qfpLWCAxUDxQIHHRc0DUYQFnoECB4QAQ&url=https%3A%2F%2Fhc-v6-static.s3.amazonaws.com%2Fmedia%2Fresources%2Ftmp%2Fcbpar.pdf&usg=AOvVaw0gOey16gB7rlivNpK-t3Dg&opi=89978449

Butterfoss, F. D. (2006). Process evaluation for community participation. *Annu. Rev. Public Health*, 27, 323–340.

CHAT tool (WHO/Unicef) (2022). Community Engagement in Humanitarian Action. https://www.corecommitments.unicef.org/kp/community-engagement-in-humanitarian-action-(chat)-toolkit%3A-updated-version

Chess, C., & Purcell, K. (1999). Public Participation and the Environment: Do We Know What Works? *Environmental Science & Technology*, 33(16), 2685–2692. DOI: 10.1021/es980500g

Collins, S. E., Clifasefi, S. L., Stanton, J., Straits, K. J., Gil-Kashiwabara, E., Rodriguez Espinosa, P., … Wallerstein, N. (2018). Community-based participatory research (CBPR): Towards equitable involvement of community in psychology research. *American Psychologist*, 73(7), 884.

Cooke B, Kothari U. *Participation: the new tyranny?* New York, NY: Zed Books, 2007.

Dias, S., & Gama, A. (2014). Community-based participatory research in public health: potentials and challenges/Investigacao participativa baseada na comunidade em saude publica: potencialidades e desafios. *Revista Panamericana de Salud Pública*, 35(2), 150–155.

Duea, S. R., Zimmerman, E. B., Vaughn, L. M., Dias, S., & Harris, J. (2022). A guide to selecting participatory research methods based on project and partnership goals. *Journal of Participatory Research Methods*, 3(1). https://doi.org/10.35844/001c.32605

Dyer, J., Stringer, L. C., Dougill, A. J., Leventon, J., Nshimbi, M., Chama, F., … Syampungani, S. (2014). Assessing participatory practices in community-based natural resource management: Experiences in community engagement from southern Africa. *Journal of Environmental Management*, 137, 137–145.

ENACT tool (PACT) (2023). Engaged Communities Accountability Commitment Tool. https://www.pactworld.org/library/promise-and-accountability-locally-led-development-lessons-and-recommendations-pact%E2%80%99s-global

Etchegary, H., Green, J., Dicks, E., Pullman, D., Street, C., & Parfrey, P. (2013). Consulting the community: Public expectations and attitudes about genetics research. *European Journal of Human Genetics*, 21(12), 1338–1343.

Guse, T. (2022). Positive psychological interventions in African contexts: A scoping review. In L. Schutte, T. Guse, & M. P. Wissing (Eds.), *Embracing well-being in diverse African contexts: Research perspectives* (pp. 375–397). Springer Nature Switzerland AG. https://doi.org/10.1007/978-3-030-85924-4_16

Gyekye, K. (2014). *Philosophy culture and vision: African perspectives: Selected essays.* Sub-Saharan Publishers.

Hacker, K. (2013). *Community-based participatory research*, Thousand Oaks, CA: Sage Publications.

Harter, M., Inauen, J., & Mosler, H. J. (2020). How does Community-Led Total Sanitation (CLTS) promote latrine construction, and can it be improved? A cluster-randomized controlled trial in Ghana. *Social Science & Medicine*, 245, 112705.

ICPHR – International Collaboration for Participarory Health Research (2013) Position Paper 1: What is Participatory Health Research? Version: Mai 2013. Berlin. Im Internet: www.icphr.org/position-papers/position-paper-no-1 (Stand: 04.09.2014)

Israel, B. A., Coombe, C. M., Cheezum, R. R., Schulz, A. J., McGranaghan, R. J., Lichtenstein, R., … Burris, A. (2010). Community-based participatory research: a capacity-building approach for policy advocacy aimed at eliminating health disparities. *American Journal of Public Health*, 100(11), 2094–2102.

Israel, B. A., Eng, E., Schulz, A. J., & Parker, E. A. (2005). Introduction to methods in community-based participatory research for health. *Methods in Community-Based Participatory Research for Health*, 3, 26.

Israel, B. A., Schulz, A. J., Parker, E. A. & Becker, A. B. (1998) Review of community based research: assessing partnership approaches to improve public health. *Annu. Rev. Public Health* 19, 173–202.

Jason, L., & Glenwick, D. (Eds.). (2016). *Handbook of methodological approaches to community-based research: Qualitative, quantitative, and mixed methods.* Oxford University Press.

Jordans, M. J., & Kohrt, B. A. (2020). Scaling up mental health care and psychosocial support in low-resource settings: a roadmap to impact. *Epidemiology and Psychiatric Sciences*, 29, e189.

Kretchy, I. A., Okoibhole, L. O., Sanuade, O. A., Jennings, H., Strachan, D. L., Blandford, A., … de-Graft Aikins, A. (2022). Scoping review of community health participatory research projects in Ghana. *Global Health Action*, 15(1), 2122304.

Kwan, C., & Walsh, C. A. (2018). Ethical Issues in Conducting Community-Based Participatory Research: A Narrative Review of the Literature. *Qualitative Report*, 23(2), 369–386.

Martín-Martín, J., Roldán-Jiménez, C., De-Torres, I., Muro-Culebras, A., Escriche-Escuder, A., Gonzalez-Sanchez, M., … Cuesta-Vargas, A. I. (2021). Behavior change techniques and the effects associated with Digital behavior change interventions in sedentary behavior in the clinical population: A systematic review. *Frontiers in Digital Health*, 3, 620383.

Minkler, M., Breckwich, V. V., Chang, C., Miller, J. PolicyLink, & University of California Berkley. Promoting healthy public policy through community-based participatory research: Ten case studies. 2009. Retrieved from http://www.policylink.org/sites/default/files/CBPR_PromotingHealthyPublicPolicy_final.pdf

Minkler, M. , & Wallerstein, N. (Eds.) (2008). *Community - based participatory research for health: From process to outcomes* (2nd ed.). San Francisco, CA: Jossey - Bass.

Muhammad, M., Wallerstein, N., Sussman, A. L., Avila, M., Belone, L., & Duran, B. (2015). Reflections on researcher identity and power: The impact of positionality on community based participatory research (CBPR) processes and outcomes. *Critical Sociology*, 41(7–8), 1045–1063.

O'Mara-Eves, A., Brunton, G., Oliver, S., Kavanagh, J., Jamal, F., & Thomas, J. (2015). The effectiveness of community engagement in public health interventions for disadvantaged groups: A meta-analysis. *BMC Public Health*, 15, 1–23.

Odetola, L., Sills, S., & Morrison, S. (2021). A pilot study on the feasibility of testing residential tap water in North Carolina: Implications for environmental justice and health. *Journal of Exposure Science & Environmental Epidemiology*, 31(6), 972–978.

Ojha, H. R., Ford, R., Keenan, R. J., Race, D., Vega, D. C., Baral, H., & Sapkota, P. (2016). Delocalizing communities: Changing forms of community engagement in natural resources governance. *World Development*, 87, 274–290.

Pact. 2023. Promise and Accountability for Locally Led Development: Lessons and Recommendations from Pact's Global Engaged Communities Assessment.

Page-Reeves, J. (2019). Community-Based Participatory Research for Health. *Health Promotion Practice* 20(1), 15–17. doi:10.1177/1524839918809007

Patel, V., Saxena, S., Lund, C., Thornicroft, G., Baingana, F., Bolton, P., … Unützer, J. (2018). The Lancet Commission on global mental health and sustainable development. *The Lancet*, 392(10157), 1553–1598.

Rice, M. L., & McCool, D. (2022). Collaboration and the criteria for success: A case study and a proposed framework for analysis. *Administration & Society*, 54(4), 714–740.

Rodriguez Espinosa, P., & Verney, S. P. (2021). The underutilization of community-based participatory research in psychology: A systematic review. *American Journal of Community Psychology*, 67(3–4), 312–326.

RTI International. (2004, July). Community - based participatory research: Assessing the evidence. Evidence Report/Technology Assessment No. 99, University of North Carolina, Durham.

Shadowen, N. L., Guerra, N. G., Beveridge, R., & McCoy, E. K. (2020). A resilient research approach: Using community-based participatory action research in a rural area of India. *Journal of Community Psychology*, 48(8), 2491–2503.

Stoecker, R. *Research Methods for Community Change: A project-based approach.* Thousand Oaks, CA: Sage; 2005.

Talò, C., Mannarini, T., & Rochira, A. (2014). Sense of community and community participation: A meta-analytic review. *Social Indicators Research*, 117, 1–28.

Twyman, C., Dougill, A., Sporton, D., & Thomas, D. (2001). Community fencing in open rangelands: self-empowerment in Eastern Namibia. *Review of African Political Economy*, 28(87), 9–26.

Vaughn, L. M., & Jacquez, F. (2020). Participatory research methods–Choice points in the research process. *Journal of Participatory Research Methods*, 1(1). doi:10.35844/001c.32605

Viswanathan, M., Ammerman, A., Eng, E., Gattlehner, G., Lohr, K.N., Griffith, D., et al. Whitener L. Community-based participatory research: Assessing the evidence. 2004 Retrieved from Rockville, MD.

Vivona, B. D., & Wolfgram, M. S. (2021). Conducting community based participatory action research. *Human Resource Development Review*, 20(4), 512–521.

Wallerstein, N., & Duran, B. (2010). Community-based participatory research contributions to intervention research: The intersection of science and practice to improve health equity. *American Journal of Public Health*, 100(S1), S40–S46.

Wallerstein, N., Duran, B., Oetzel, J. and Minkler, M. (2018). *Community Based Participatory Research for Health: Advancing Social and Health Equity*, San Francisco, Jossey-Bass.

Wallerstein, N., Duran, B., Oetzel, J. G., & Minkler, M. (Eds.). (2017). *Community-based participatory research for health: Advancing social and health equity*. John Wiley & Sons.

Wallerstein, N., Muhammad, M., Sanchez-Youngman, S., Rodriguez Espinosa, P., Avila, M., Baker, E. A., … Duran, B. (2019). Power dynamics in community-based participatory research: A multiple–case study analysis of partnering contexts, histories, and practices. *Health Education & Behavior*, 46(1_suppl), 19S–32S.

Wallerstein, N., Oetzel, J. G., Sanchez-Youngman, S., Boursaw, B., Dickson, E., Kastelic, S., … Duran, B. (2020). Engage for equity: A long-term study of community-based participatory research and community-engaged research practices and outcomes. *Health Education & Behavior*, 47(3), 380–390.

Webler, T., & Tuler, S. (2006). Four perspectives on public participation process in environmental assessment and decision making: Combined results from 10 case studies. *Policy Studies Journal*, 34(4), 699–722.
Weiner J, McDonald JA (2013) Special issue: Three models of community-based participatory research. *LDI Issue Brief*, 18, 1–8.
Wessells, M. (2009). Do no harm: Toward contextually appropriate psychosocial support in international emergencies. *American Psychologist*, 64, 839–854.
Woolf, S. H., Zimmerman, E., Haley, A., & Krist, A. H. (2016). Authentic engagement of patients and communities can transform research, practice, and policy. *Health Affairs*, 35(4), 590–594.

35

COLLABORATION AND RESEARCH ETHICS IN HEALTH PSYCHOLOGY

Katherine Sorsdahl, Ifeanyichukwu Anthony Ogueji, and Ashraf Kagee

The Need for Collaborative Health Partnerships in Health Psychology

We take our cue from the spirit and ethos of critical health psychology, with its emphasis on research aimed at transformation and change (Fox et al., 2009). Critical health psychology seeks to analyse the sociostructural processes and power relations that sustain disadvantage. To this extent, collaborative health partnerships should seek to dismantle hierarchy and power differentials in the research community.

Scientific progress in today's research environment is increasingly driven by collaboration, a factor well-discussed in the literature (Bozeman & Boardman, 2014). Collaboration can be defined as the "social process whereby human beings pool their human capital for the objective of producing knowledge" (Bozeman & Boardman, 2014, pp. 1–66). Collaboration is a prominent component in the calls to scientific action proposed in the 2019 Global Sustainable Development Report, and its purpose is to contribute to "better-aligning progress and innovation trajectories" for the United Nations 2030 Agenda for Sustainable Development (Messerli et al., 2019). Sustainable Development Goals (SDGs) focus on a range of interrelated goals, comprising 169 targets and 232 indicators, from the eradication of poverty and inequality to taking action on climate change. The COVID-19 pandemic, which is expected to impact SDG 8 (economic growth) and SDG 3 (good health and well-being; see, e.g., United Nations, 2020), has demonstrated the need for research collaboration so as to accelerate new knowledge creation on new interventions and treatment, and to share data and research results worldwide (Addo-Atuah et al., 2020).

Bozeman has identified two kinds of collaborations, namely, knowledge-focused collaborations that are aimed chiefly at expanding the base of knowledge

DOI: 10.4324/9781003318026-42

and property-focused collaborations that emphasise producing economic value and wealth (Bozeman et al., 2013). As has been argued, collaboration is likely to yield an increase in productivity as measured by research articles that are published, cited, or used by policymakers (Hodge, 2019). Economic value, on the other hand, is usually measured in terms of patents, new technology, and new business start-ups. In health psychology, these may take the form of cell phone applications such as health and nutrition guides, fitness calculators and trackers, medication adherence reminders, and mood monitors. However, the overarching goal is an increase in economic good and also an increase in health and well-being in the population that may accrue as a consequence of both knowledge-focused and property-focused collaborations. Collaboration can occur at various levels: intradisciplinary, interdisciplinary, multidisciplinary, transdisciplinary, or national vs international. Increasingly, for many large health psychology projects, team members from a range of fields are required. These include epidemiology, statistics, data science, anthropology, psychiatry, and nursing, in addition to the traditional fields of health psychology and behavioural medicine.

Although not specific to health psychology collaborations, a substantial amount of research has been conducted on the benefits of collaboration in global health. On its website, Springer Nature states that the benefits of collaboration accrue by means of 'maximising outputs' and impact, attracting grant funding, and expanding networks (Hodge, 2019). Health psychology formally emerged in the 1970s (Friedman & Adler, 2007). At present, the field plays a significant role in achieving the SDGs; research collaboration between scientists from low- and middle-income countries (LMICs) and high-income countries (HICs) has become increasingly important. International collaborations have the potential to reduce local and global health inequalities as new knowledge is generated and provides opportunities for researchers from LMICs to be involved in multinational interdisciplinary projects. In the era of big data and machine learning, collaboration between health psychologists, epidemiologists, data scientists, and computer scientists is likely to become increasingly salient (Airhihenbuwa et al., 2011; Godoy-Ruiz et al., 2016; Hanney & González Block, 2006; van den Broucke et al., 2010; Ward et al., 2018).

In many disciplines, including health psychology, one of the reasons for under-representation of research from LMICs, especially in non-Anglophone countries, is English academic writing ability. Limitations in terms of manuscript preparation, especially in terms of language, and uneven access to the scientific literature create conditions under which health psychology research remains unequal between HICs and LMICs. To this extent, grantsmanship, networking, collaboration, and mentoring are necessary. Building research capacity in LMICs, providing more opportunities for LMIC researchers to contribute to research, and expanding the possibility of LMIC researchers to secure grant funding are promising means to bring balance to these relationships. Several initiatives for capacity building in LMICs have been established over the years to increase capacity in mental health research. For example, the establishment of collaborative hubs in mental health research (Pilowsky et al., 2016) and the African Mental

Health Research Initiative (AMARI) (Chibanda et al., 2016) have been fundamental in training the next generation of global mental health researchers. Similar initiatives and programmes could advance the field of health psychology. Furthermore, the requirement of English academic writing could fuel linguistic racism (the discrimination of people on the basis of language resources) (De Costa, 2020). As the requirement of English academic writing can be exclusionary, this requirement must be challenged. At the very least, collaboration to support people with less experience in academic writing is necessary. The specific focus on 'academic English' may also be challenged as it can exclude exclusionary people with good English language skills. It is necessary to challenge linguistic racism in academic writing while at the same time maintaining high standards of scholarship.

The available research on collaborations in health research has found that collaborative projects can have several benefits (Lucas, 2005). Collaborative projects can benefit individual members of research teams in terms of personal growth and development. For instance, collaborative projects offer younger and early career researchers opportunities for mentorship by senior members. These benefits are especially pertinent in a discipline such as health psychology, thus requiring the formalisation of mentoring programmes. An expanded network of collaborators can create opportunities for researchers to learn new skills, develop new perspectives, and embrace alternative paradigms to approach their research. At most research institutions around the world, including universities, academic staff are appointed or considered for promotion in part because of their research output, often in terms of the number of publications. However, increasingly, impact is taken into account, as measured by the number of citations, including the Hirsch index (h-index). The h-index provides an estimate of a researcher's impact on the field by combining the total number of publications (a proxy for productivity) and the number of citations (a proxy for the quality of the publications) (Dinis-Oliveira, 2019). Research articles that result from large international research projects, usually with large samples, are much more likely to be highly cited and thus make a significant impact on the field than those that are single authored.

Collaborative projects can be beneficial by maximising the output and impact of a project and also capacity building. Collaborations allow the sharing of expertise and resources so that complex scientific questions can be addressed. Large teams also allow data collection from several sites and the recruitment of higher numbers of research participants. The impact on the field is usually measured in the impact factor of journals in which research is published and the citation indices of individual researchers. With stronger data, evidence from collaborative projects has the potential to lead to the advancement of knowledge to improve health outcomes. Research outputs that influence policy and practice and have an impact on the public good increase the chances of researchers receiving further funding (Hodge, 2019), for example, from funders such as the European Union's Horizon programme, the National Institutes of Health, and the Wellcome Trust.

Current Challenges in Achieving Equitable and Fair Health Partnerships in Global Health Research

Despite research collaborations being a critical component of global health research (Hook & Vera, 2020), the literature on collaborative health research globally suggests they reproduce relationships and conditions which disproportionately favour HICs and institutions. Concerns regarding whether these collaborations promote equality and fairness are often debated (Munung et al., 2017).

First, at a structural level, funding for research is usually more available in HICs than in LMICs, as many LMICs have modest funds to support research. Commenting on LMICs as opposed to HICs, South Africa, as a high middle-income country (DAC List, 2023), has the National Research Foundation and the Medical Research Council which are key funders of research, including health psychology research. In Nigeria, an LMIC, the Federal Ministry of Health (FMoH), and its research agency, the Nigerian Institute of Medical Research (NIMR), are among the key funders of research, including health psychology-related research. However, Nigeria lacks a professional body for the field health psychology that can advocate on its behalf to the government. States with strong economies, such as those within the Organisation for Economic Cooperation and Development (OECD), are able to direct large resources to funding for health research in ways that LMICs are not able to do. States with smaller economies, such as Mozambique, Malawi, Afghanistan, and Yemen, have far fewer resources to direct to research.

This imbalance of resources creates conditions where global partnerships are necessary. If researchers from LMICs wish to access funds from HICs such as the Wellcome Trust and the British Academy in the United Kingdom, the National Institutes of Health in the United States, or the European Union's Horizon, they usually must partner with researchers from these countries. However, an implication of research funding primarily originating from HICs is that power is often located with these partners and in some instances can impact equity. A few studies conducted in LMICs have highlighted the need for fairness, equity, transparency, and control over the budget and how decisions are made in terms of spending (Matenga et al., 2019; Parker & Kingori, 2016; Walsh et al., 2016).

Second, in an equitable and fair health partnership in global health research, it is imperative that LMIC researchers participate meaningfully in the science as well as the decision-making regarding implementing research projects (London, 2005). Unfortunately, a study conducted by Boshoff (2009) examined publications from global health research collaborations and reported that the most frequent role identified by participants from African countries was conducting fieldwork rather than contributing meaningfully to the research process (Boshoff, 2009; London, 2005; Pratt & Hyder, 2015).

Third, studies in global health research have suggested that researchers in LMICs do not always receive recognition for their contributions. A number of bibliometric studies have found that researchers from LMICs are often not included as authors or are not listed as first or senior authors despite leading the research (Hedt-Gauthier et al., 2019; Jentsch & Pilley, 2003; Pingray et al., 2020; Rees et al., 2017).

There may be various reasons for under-representation of authors from LMICs, especially in non-Anglophone countries, where English academic writing ability may be limited. However, this barrier can be overcome through re-thinking authorship guidance in collaborative global health research (Smith et al., 2014). The ethical principles of beneficence and justice can also be applied to authorship inclusion. Beneficence would require senior authors to avoid taking advantage of junior researchers and instead make decisions that in fact benefit junior researchers, such as creating opportunities for authorship (Washburn, 2008). Yet, including undeserving authors is not appropriate, as it may ultimately be detrimental to their careers (Fine & Kurdek, 1993) and may not be an honest reflection of their efforts. The principle of justice suggests that authorship credit should be decided on in a fair manner. For example, Fine and Kurdek (1993) have suggested that authors at different levels of ability, presumably based on their seniority, should contribute to a research output based on their level of competence. By this logic, more should be expected from authors with greater competence and less from those with less competence.

An overarching principle however is integrity, which requires authors to accurately and honestly report on their contribution to a publication. One way of ensuring justice in this regard is the Contributor Roles Taxonomy (CRediT) (Elsevier, 2022). CRediT was developed to recognise individual author contributions, reduce or eliminate disputes among authors, and facilitate collaboration. It offers authors the opportunity to indicate their relative contributions to the publication. Most health psychology journals have subscribed to the CRediT system, which if properly applied, is intended to ensure authorship credit and that order be based on each author's actual contribution.

As a way to manage authorship under conditions of unequal relationships, the journal *Nature* has suggested a disclosure statement that can be included in the published paper (Nature, 2022). Such a statement would include whether the research design and execution included local scientists, whether the research is locally relevant, and whether there are plans to share the benefits of the research with the communities where the data were collected. The Global Code of Conduct for research in resource-constrained settings provides specific guidelines that are based on principles of fairness, respect, care, and honesty for research partnerships between scholars from high-income and lower-income settings so that they can be advantageous for both parties. Similarly, in a move to counteract exploitative collaborative practices, the *Lancet* recently announced a decision to reject submissions that contain data from Africa if these do not acknowledge African colleagues (Waruru, 2022).

Despite these challenges, as we move towards achieving equitable and fair health partnerships in global health research, understanding how researchers working in this area view equity and strategies for improved collaborations can be useful.

Available Frameworks for Good Collaborative Research Practice

The literature highlighting the inequity in collaborative health research has led to the development of guidelines, policies, and actions for the promotion of equity during collaborative research practice. For instance, Ward et al. (2018) noted that the implementation of the guidance of the International Ethical Guidelines for Health-related Research Involving Humans by the Council for International Organizations of Medical Sciences (CIOMS) (2016) has contributed to reducing inequity in collaborative health research, particularly in resource-limited settings. The authors made several recommendations to enhance good collaborative research practice (Ward et al., 2018). The first is to increase awareness among global actors, funders, institutions, researchers, and ethical review boards of the challenges with collaboration between HICs and LMICs. Second is the need for a memorandum of understanding (MoU) to operationalise the terms of collaboration. The MoU should include contents such as establishing equitable partner inclusion in the area of collaborative research protocol design, project implementation, standards of care, data handling, scientific analysis, authorship, intellectual property rights, and access to novel health research and innovation. The third is to coordinate, strengthen, and implement local laws requiring equitable research partnerships. The last recommendation is to secure good collaborative practice through ethical partnership governance and capacity-strengthening requirements. Beyond these, the International Academy Council (IAC) and the Global Network of Science Academies (Council InterAcademy, 2012), in a bid to provide clarity and advice on international consensus for responsible conduct of global research, recommend that researchers should agree on standards that can be fairly observed during collaborative research. They further recommend that research institutions must have clear and well-communicated rules that define responsible practices and ensure that researchers, research staff, and students are trained in the application of these rules to research. Also, they recommend that funding agencies avoid policies that may lead to inequity. The IAC and the GNSA state that these recommendations can foster international dialogue and action to promote the integrity of the global research enterprise. Further, the Canadian Coalition for Global Health Research, a not-for-profit organisation, adds to this topic through its dedication to ensuring fair research collaborations between Canada and LMICs (Neufeld & Spiegel, 2006). The coalition is committed to nurturing the next generation of global health researchers in Canada and LMICs. It seeks to achieve this through training, mentoring, and providing equitable research collaborations.

The Council on Health Research Development's (COHRED) Fairness Index for international collaborative partnership suggests that collaborative research has not been completely free from inequities and unfair practices (Musolino et al., 2015). For this reason, the council recommends that during collaborative research, indicators, a measurement process, and a reporting system that is unique, transparent, and that can mitigate the key problems of collaborative research must be in place. Ultimately, this will maximise the integrity of research outputs and minimise inequity during collaborative research. This also has benefits for LMICs during research collaborations. Finally, collaborative research offers a valuable opportunity to understand a problem from various perspectives and paves the way for a successful impact in the research community if ethical principles are respected (O'Sullivan et al., 2010). This indeed echoes the need to adopt appropriate frameworks for good collaborative research practice during research collaborations.

Collaborations between Researchers and Communities

One form of collaboration in health psychology research that is, to some extent, implicit is collaboration between researchers and the communities they study and partner with. Research agendas are often determined by the decisions of funders, institutional priorities, and the interests of the researchers themselves. Yet, the research participants and the communities they represent form part of the matrix of players in research collaboration. It has become increasingly important for researchers to engage with community members even prior to planning a study to obtain their buy-in and agreement that the study is needed, is important, and has the potential to positively influence the lives of people. Community-based participatory research (CBPR) offers a means for researchers to create partnerships with communities by sharing decision-making and power in research projects. The assumption of CBPR is that all participants are active collaborators at the various stages of the research process and will thus contribute to shaping the research question and method of inquiry (McQuiston et al., 2005). There is a need to ensure that health measures, interventions, theories, and concepts that are researched and applied in communities are indeed likely to fit in these contexts and that the people for whom they are intended are likely to accept them. For this reason, it is necessary that people with first-hand knowledge of the local terrain, including community members themselves, contribute to the development of interventions. For the past few decades, community advisory boards have become useful mechanisms for researchers to engage communities in health research. Indeed, they are widely used and accepted in global health research (Mlambo et al., 2019). Adopting a CBPR approach where appropriate can assist health researchers in blurring the distinction between themselves as researchers and the population they are studying. CBPR also has the potential to facilitate the effective dissemination and implementation of study findings.

Summary

In summary, collaborative global health research, including health psychology, has significantly increased in scale and scope. Increasingly, for many large health psychology projects, various bodies, including community, policy stakeholders, and team members from a range of fields, are required to collaborate. These collaborations and partnerships are imperative to ensure that complex research questions are well-conceptualised and properly executed. However, collaborative health research globally, in many instances, paves the way for relationships and conditions which disproportionately favour HICs and institutions. Thus, in this chapter, we have highlighted the importance of health partnerships for the improvement of health, via health psychology. We then highlighted the current challenges in achieving equitable and fair health partnerships in global health research that apply to the field of health psychology. We finally reflected on best practices on how researchers and health-care workers (both locally and internationally), community stakeholders, policy, and other decision-makers can form health partnerships for the improvement of health via health psychology. This chapter contributes to reducing relationships and conditions which disproportionately favour HICs and institutions during collaborative global health research and paves the way for future work on this topic, especially in LMICs where the burden of such disproportionate relationships and conditions is often experienced.

Further Reading

Lyons, A.C., Chamberlain, K. (2017). *Critical Health Psychology*. In: Gough, B. (eds) *The Palgrave Handbook of Critical Social Psychology*. Palgrave Macmillan, London. https://doi.org/10.1057/978-1-137-51018-1_26

Nature. (2022). Nature addresses helicopter research and ethics dumping. *Nature*. https://www.nature.com/articles/d41586-022-01423-6

Walsh, A., Brugha, R., & Byrne, E. (2016). "The way the country has been carved up by researchers": ethics and power in north–south public health research. *International Journal for Equity in Health*, *15*(1), 1–11.

References

Addo-Atuah, J., Senhaji-Tomza, B., Ray, D., Basu, P., Loh, F.-H. E., & Owusu-Daaku, F. (2020). Global health research partnerships in the context of the Sustainable Development Goals (SDGs). *Research in Social and Administrative Pharmacy*, 16(11), 1614–1618.

Airhihenbuwa, C. O., Shisana, O., Zungu, N., BeLue, R., Makofani, D. M., Shefer, T., Smith, E., & Simbayi, L. (2011). Research capacity building: A US-South African partnership. *Global Health Promotion*, 18(2), 27–35.

Boshoff, N. (2009). Neo-colonialism and research collaboration in Central Africa. *Scientometrics*, 81(2), 413–434.

Bozeman, B., & Boardman, C. (2014). *Research collaboration and team science: A state-of-the-art review and agenda* (Vol. 17). Springer.

Bozeman, B., Fay, D., & Slade, C. P. (2013). Research collaboration in universities and academic entrepreneurship: The-state-of-the-art. In *Journal of Technology Transfer* (Vol. 38, Issue 1). https://doi.org/10.1007/s10961-012-9281-8

van den Broucke, S., Jooste, H., Tlali, M., Moodley, V., van Zyl, G., Nyamwaya, D., & Tang, K.-C. (2010). Strengthening the capacity for health promotion in South Africa through international collaboration. *Global Health Promotion*, 17(2_suppl), 6–16.

Chibanda, D., Weiss, H. A., Verhey, R., Simms, V., Munjoma, R., Rusakaniko, S., Chingono, A., Munetsi, E., Bere, T., Manda, E., & others. (2016). Effect of a primary care--based psychological intervention on symptoms of common mental disorders in Zimbabwe: a randomized clinical trial. *Jama*, 316(24), 2618–2626.

Council InterAcademy (2012). *Responsible conduct in the global research enterprise. A Policy Report*. Amsterdam: InterAcademy Council.

DAC List (2023). DAC list of ODA recipients. https://www.oecd.org/dac/financing-sustainable-development/development-finance-standards/DAC-List-of-ODA-Recipients-for-reporting-2022-23-flows.pdf

De Costa, P. I. (2020). Linguistic racism: Its negative effects and why we need to contest it. *International Journal of Bilingual Education and Bilingualism*, *23*(7), 833–837.

Dinis-Oliveira, R. J. (2019). The H-index in life and health sciences: advantages, drawbacks and challenging opportunities. *Current Drug Research Reviews Formerly: Current Drug Abuse Reviews*, 11(2), 82–84.

Elsevier. (2022). *Credit author statement*. Elsevier. https://www.elsevier.com/authors/policies-and-guidelines/credit-author-statement

Fine, M. A., & Kurdek, L. A. (1993). Reflections on determining authorship credit and authorship order on faculty-student collaborations. *American Psychologist*, 48(11), 1141.

Fox, D. R., Austin, S., & Prilleltensky, I. (2009). Critical psychology: An introduction. *Critical Psychology*, 1–496.

Friedman, H. S., & Adler, N. E. (2007). The History and Background of Health Psychology. In H. S. Friedman & R. C. Silver (Eds.), *Foundations of health psychology* (pp. 3–18). Oxford University Press.

Godoy-Ruiz, P., Cole, D. C., Lenters, L., & McKenzie, K. (2016). Developing collaborative approaches to international research: Perspectives of new global health researchers. *Global Public Health*, 11(3), 253–275.

Hanney, S. R., & González Block, M. A. (2006). Building health research systems to achieve better health. In *Health Research Policy and Systems* (Vol. 4, Issue 1, pp. 1–6). Springer.

Hedt-Gauthier, B. L., Jeufack, H. M., Neufeld, N. H., Alem, A., Sauer, S., Odhiambo, J., Boum, Y., Shuchman, M., & Volmink, J. (2019). Stuck in the middle: A systematic review of authorship in collaborative health research in Africa, 2014–2016. *BMJ Global Health*, 4(5), e001853.

Hodge, C. (2019). *5 ways that collaboration can further your research and your career*. Springer Nature. https://www.springernature.com/gp/researchers/the-source/blog/blogposts-life-in-research/benefits-of-research-collaboration/17360752

Hook, K., & Vera, E. (2020). Best practices in global mental health: An exploratory study of recommendations for psychologists. *International Perspectives in Psychology*, 9(2), 67–83.

Jentsch, B., & Pilley, C. (2003). Research relationships between the South and the North: Cinderella and the ugly sisters? *Social Science & Medicine*, 57(10), 1957–1967.

London, A. J. (2005). Justice and the human development approach to international research. *Hastings Center Report*, 35(1), 24–37.

Lucas, A. O. (2005). International collaboration in health research. *Bulletin of the World Health Organization*, *83*, 482–482.

Matenga, T. F. L., Zulu, J. M., Corbin, J. H., & Mweemba, O. (2019). Contemporary issues in north–south health research partnerships: perspectives of health research stakeholders in Zambia. *Health Research Policy and Systems*, 17(1), 1–13.

McQuiston, C., Parrado, E. A., Olmos-Muñiz, J. C., & Bustillo Martinez, A. M. (2005). Community-based participatory research and ethnography. *Methods in Community-Based Participatory Research for Health*, 210–229.

Messerli, P., Murniningtyas, E., Eloundou-Enyegue, P., Foli, E. G., Furman, E., Glassman, A., Hernández Licona, G., Kim, E. M., Lutz, W., & Moatti, J.-P. (2019). *Global sustainable development report 2019: the future is now–science for achieving sustainable development*.

Mlambo, C. K., Vernooij, E., Geut, R., Vrolings, E., Shongwe, B., Jiwan, S., Fleming, Y., & Khumalo, G. (2019). Experiences from a community advisory Board in the Implementation of early access to ART for all in Eswatini: A qualitative study. *BMC Medical Ethics*, 20(1), 1–11.

Munung, N. S., Mayosi, B. M., & de Vries, J. (2017). Equity in international health research collaborations in Africa: perceptions and expectations of African researchers. *PloS One*, 12(10), e0186237.
Musolino, N., Lazdins, J., Toohey, J., & IJsselmuiden, C. (2015). COHRED Fairness Index for international collaborative partnerships. *The Lancet*, 385(9975), 1293–1294.
Nature. (2022). Nature addresses helicopter research and ethics dumping. *Nature*. https://www.nature.com/articles/d41586-022-01423-6
Neufeld, V. R., & Spiegel, J. (2006). Canada and global health research: 2005 update. *Canadian Journal of Public Health*, 97(1), 39–41.
O'Sullivan, P. S., Stoddard, H. A., & Kalishman, S. (2010). Collaborative research in medical education: a discussion of theory and practice. *Medical Education*, 44(12), 1175–1184.
Parker, M., & Kingori, P. (2016). Good and bad research collaborations: researchers' views on science and ethics in global health research. *PloS One*, 11(10), e0163579.
Pilowsky, D. J., Rojas, G., Price, L. N., Appiah-Poku, J., Razzaque, B., Sharma, M., Schneider, M., Seedat, S., Bonini, B. B., & Gureje, O. (2016). Building research capacity across and within low-and middle-income countries: The Collaborative Hubs for International Research on Mental Health. *Academic Psychiatry*, 40, 686–691.
Pingray, V., Ortega, V., Yaya, S., & Belizán, J. M. (2020). Authorship in studies conducted in low-and-middle income countries and published by Reproductive Health: advancing equitable global health research collaborations. In *Reproductive health* (Vol. 17, Issue 1, pp. 1–4). Springer.
Pratt, B., & Hyder, A. A. (2015). Global justice and health systems research in low-and middle-income countries. *The Journal of Law, Medicine & Ethics*, 43(1), 143–161.
Rees, C. A., Lukolyo, H., Keating, E. M., Dearden, K. A., Luboga, S. A., Schutze, G. E., & Kazembe, P. N. (2017). Authorship in paediatric research conducted in low-and middle-income countries: parity or parasitism? *Tropical Medicine & International Health*, 22(11), 1362–1370.
Smith, E., Hunt, M., & Master, Z. (2014). Authorship ethics in global health research partnerships between researchers from low or middle income countries and high income countries. *BMC Medical Ethics*, *15*, 1–8. https://doi.org/10.1186/1472-6939-15-42
The Council for International Organizations of Medical Sciences (CIOMS). 2016. *International ethical guidelines*. Geneva: CIOMS. Available at: http://www.cioms.ch/ethical-guidelines-2016/
United Nations. (2020). Sustainable development goals: about the sustainable development goals. https://www.un.org/sustainabledevelopment/sustainable-development-goals
Walsh, A., Brugha, R., & Byrne, E. (2016). "The way the country has been carved up by researchers": ethics and power in north–south public health research. *International Journal for Equity in Health*, 15(1), 1–11.
Ward, C. L., Shaw, D., Anane-Sarpong, E., Sankoh, O., Tanner, M., & Elger, B. (2018). Defining Health Research for Development: The perspective of stakeholders from an international health research partnership in Ghana and Tanzania. *Developing World Bioethics*, 18(4), 331–340.
Waruru, M. (2022). *Renowned journal rejects papers that exclude African researchers*.
Washburn, J. J. (2008). Encouraging research collaboration through ethical and fair authorship: A model policy. *Ethics and Behavior*, 18(1), 44–58. https://doi.org/10.1080/10508420701712917

SECTION 8

Current Challenges and Opportunities

The Future of Health Psychology

36

THE FUTURE OF HEALTH PSYCHOLOGY

Challenges and Opportunities in the Next Decades

Dominika Kwasnicka and Olga Perski

Introduction

In this book section, we highlight key challenges facing the world today in the coming decades and articulate suggestions for how the health psychology community can help tackle these challenges. We are directly experiencing (and will continue to live through) the dire consequences of human activities which have disrupted ecological systems and rigged social structures, including climate change, viral pandemics, a shift in population age structures without adequate support for healthy ageing, and increasing levels of physical and mental health issues faced by the most vulnerable people in our society. This book section reflects on the role health psychologists can play in mitigating these consequences and preventing further decline through, for example, drawing on theory and practical know-how. We propose a set of suggestions for how to more rapidly achieve equitable population-level health impact through the redirection of our research activities towards climate change–related topics, striving for increased interdisciplinarity within our teams, and making a conscious shift towards the use of Open Science practices.

At the time of writing, the global population has already exceeded eight billion people (Ngo, 2023). To enable health, well-being and quality of life for all, people need to be supported to maintain health behaviours, such as physical activity and healthy eating long term and avoiding unhealthy, unsustainable, and environmentally harmful and hazardous behaviours that are often (falsely) equated with economic growth (Cao et al., 2022).

In this chapter, we set the scene for the individual chapters in this book section (Chapters 37–40). First, we provide an overview of some of the most pressing challenges facing society today and in the coming decades, including climate change, viral pandemics, changing population age structures (Hooten et al., 2022), and increasing levels of physical and mental health issues faced by the

 DOI: 10.4324/9781003318026-44

most vulnerable people in our society (Diderichsen et al., 2019). Second, we consider how health psychology can contribute to much-needed improvements in how theory and evidence are considered in the design and implementation of interventions at different system levels, including but not limited to social and health policy. To foster sustainable and equitable living conditions, we need to ensure that health psychology knowledge and practice are effectively considered at different systems levels by key decision-makers in local and national governments and beyond (Hallsworth, 2023).

Finally, challenging the *status quo* in health psychology and signposting to the individual chapters in this section, we discuss ways in which health psychology research and practice can be redirected to allow us to face these challenges and effectively and equitably make a dent in population-level health and well-being. With regard to challenging the *status quo*, we discuss the need to direct some of our research and clinical efforts towards addressing the negative consequences of climate change and elaborate on the need for the popularisation and scaling up of evidence-informed digital health tools (Arigo et al., 2019; Kwasnicka et al., 2022); the investment in interdisciplinary and intersectoral collaboration and communication, with an emphasis on greater involvement of health psychologists in policy discussions (Adhanom Ghebreyesus, 2021); and the move towards Open Science practices (Hesse et al., 2021). Arguably, none of these perspectives or approaches are currently part and parcel of health psychology research and practice – hence the need to challenge the *status quo*.

Key Challenges Facing Our Communities in the 21st Century

An Ageing Population

Thanks largely to improved nutrition and more widespread access to evidence-based health care, the global population is growing. People live longer than ever before; our life expectancy is higher, and quality of life is, on average, better sustained compared with previous decades. By 2030, it is predicted that the number of people aged 60 years and older globally will outnumber youth and be double the number of children under 5 (WHO, 2023). However, the benefits of people living longer notwithstanding, changes in the global population age structures have started to expose substantial vulnerabilities in our social and health systems. For instance, we are ill-prepared to manage the increased resources needed for supporting people with chronic physical and mental health conditions across the lifespan.

Chapter 37, written by Anne Tiedemann and Cathie Sherrington, provides a discussion of the challenges and opportunities related to an ageing population. They discuss common chronic physical and mental health conditions associated with older age (e.g., dementia, cancer, depression, anxiety) and elaborate on how health psychology can contribute to disease prevention and health promotion throughout the life course. Chapter 37 touches on the increased pressures on people acting as formal and informal caregivers and the need for support. It also discusses the issue of accessibility to mobility support for frail people, emphasising that not all older people are frail, and not all frail people are old(er). The authors also emphasise the role of physical activity in promoting well-being and preventing health conditions, providing examples from their own work with interventions designed and implemented at scale. This chapter also signposts practical solutions for how to stay healthy and happy throughout the life course.

The Digitisation of Health Psychology to Increase Access for All

Chapter 38, written by Bradford Hesse, Jessica Lipschitz, David K. Ahern, and Dominika Kwasnicka, provides an overview of the digitisation of health psychology. This chapter provides a brief history of the growth of digital health over the past few decades and highlights specific applications with astounding impact (e.g., personal connected health devices, telemedicine, diagnostics, imaging, pharmaceuticals, implantable devices, surgical innovations, personalised therapeutics, and geospatial and environmental advances in digital health). The authors discuss opportunities uniquely afforded by digital health tools, including improved knowledge generation and integration, in addition to the ability to provide tailored support at much greater volumes than ever before. However, to realise the potential of digital health within and beyond health psychology, the authors argue that we need to embrace the ethos of Open Science, expand access to behavioural and mental health services, and address social determinants of health to ensure that the most vulnerable groups in society are not left behind. However, as discussed further in this chapter (and covered in more detail in Chapter 38), several challenges remain with regard to the rapid scaling of effective digital health solutions and the enablement of researchers and practitioners to build on each other's work through more widespread adoption of Open Science practices.

Climate Change and Viral Pandemics

Human activities over the past two centuries have led to increased emissions of toxic greenhouse gases, which have, in turn, led to the rapid warming of our planet. Anthropogenic climate change – i.e., climate change caused by mankind – leads to rising temperatures, the increased occurrence and intensity of extreme weather events, air pollution, and rising sea levels (The Intergovernmental Panel on Climate Change, IPCC, 2023). Increased land use change and disruptions to ecosystems led to the outbreak of COVID-19 in 2020, which very vividly demonstrated that we, as a global society, are now inevitably connected.

As outlined in the chapter by Guillaume Chevance and Paquito Bernard (Chapter 39), there is an urgent need for behavioural adaptation to the climate crisis. We are already seeing the direct effects of climate change on health behaviours through, for example, the impact of heat extremes on physical activity and sleep behaviours across different continents and countries. As temperatures continue to rise, human behaviour will directly determine the continued course of the climate crisis. We have reached an opportunistic point in time when several individual behaviours can jointly have a population-level effect on the slowing down of the devastation of the environment that has occurred to date. Chapter 39 highlights the urgent need to move rapidly from observation to intervention. We already know that human activity is having a devastating impact on the environment, causing irreversible damage. The authors emphasise that we have conducted enough observational studies and that now is the time to act. We need to start designing and implementing evidence-informed behavioural and environmental interventions. This chapter also highlights the need to improve access to mental health interventions, with a focus on interventions to help manage the trauma of climate-related displacement and forced migration.

Incorporating Health Psychology into Policy and Professional Practice

Specifically (but not exclusively) during the early stages of the COVID-19 pandemic – during which pharmacological interventions (e.g., vaccines) were not yet widely available – governments and policymakers turned to health psychologists to better understand how to encourage the uptake and sustained enactment of health behaviours that limit viral virus spread (e.g., physical distancing, hand-washing, mask-wearing). As outlined in the chapter by Gill A. ten Hoor and Robert A. C. Ruiter (Chapter 40), health psychologists are strongly encouraged to play a more active role in day-to-day decision-making processes at the international, national, or local policy level. Past success stories of health promotion and health psychology treatment programmes have enabled our science to be recognised as important by and embedded within policy and professional practice (Marks, 1996).

Notable progress has been made in getting policymakers, regulators, and health-care professionals (e.g., nurses, physicians, dentists, physiotherapists) to incorporate knowledge and techniques from health psychology in their day-to-day work; however, the progress has been relatively slow and somewhat underwhelming. Although the increased investments in behavioural science by governments are notable, especially in recent years, this has largely been driven by high-income countries' research priorities and needs. For example, only recently – when facing a global pandemic – did the World Health Organization (WHO) formally recognise the importance of behavioural science and announced the forming of its *Behavioural Science Insights Unit*. In the announcement statement, the WHO Secretary wrote,

> [B]ehavioural science is not yet an integral part of daily practice for most public health work and it remains an underutilized resource. Barriers to the adoption of behavioural theories and approaches include practical ones such as lack of capacity, funds and time. Moreover, policymakers and technical managers still lack confidence in the impact of these interventions or in the sustainability and replicability of insights and changes obtained.
>
> *(Adhanom Ghebreyesus, 2021)*

Chapter 40 discusses practical strategies for how health psychologists can effectively influence both policy and practice. The authors provide examples of how health psychology theory and know-how were applied during the COVID-19 pandemic in the Netherlands, advising national and local governments. The authors discuss how we must sometimes adapt available theory to develop timely interventions and rapidly identify evidence-based practices across similar contexts that can positively impact population-level health. The chapter also includes lessons learnt in relation to health psychology, policy, and practice during uncertain times, including the description of how the Intervention Mapping Approach (Bartholomew et al., 1998) was applied to rapidly develop an intervention to promote the enactment of health-protective behaviours during COVID-19.

How Health Psychologists Can Bring Us Safely into the Next Century – Challenging the *Status Quo*

As raised within the individual chapters in this book section, it is time for health psychologists to step up to the challenge of tackling these deeply concerning and pressing issues facing society today. Here, we elaborate further on a set of suggestions for how to more rapidly achieve equitable population-level health impact in times of uncertainty.

First, health psychologists are encouraged to redirect at least some of our research activities towards climate change–related topics. As highlighted in Chapter 39, we cannot wait for numerous observational studies to demonstrate exactly in what ways human activities are speeding up climate change. Instead, the implementation of interventions at multiple systems levels is urgently needed. We encourage health psychologists to draw on our strong theoretical foundations and available frameworks to guide the systematic development of behaviour change interventions to rapidly develop, optimise, and evaluate interventions at different systems levels (e.g., at the individual, community, and population levels) to change climate-related behaviours, such as car use, energy, and meat consumption. We have many success stories to draw on within the health psychology field that can be meaningfully shifted and adapted to tackle climate change–related behaviours and practices. For example, we can apply a wealth of useful frameworks that support the systematic development and evaluation of behaviour change interventions at multiple systems levels (e.g., individual, policy, etc.), such as Intervention Mapping (Bartholomew et al., 1998), the Theoretical Domains Framework (Cane et al., 2012), or the Behaviour Change Wheel (Michie et al., 2011). Health psychology interventions delivered within community or health-care settings have had huge success, including primary and secondary prevention of disease (Lindacher et al., 2018). Additionally, frameworks have been developed that promote evaluating the public health impact of health promotion interventions, including the RE-AIM Framework (Glasgow et al., 1999), evaluating reach, efficacy, adoption, implementation, and maintenance, demonstrating how and why health psychology interventions have a positive impact on population health improvements (Riley et al., 2013).

Second, the aforementioned challenges are – due to systemic marginalisation of minorities and certain subgroups within our societies – hitting the most vulnerable members of our society the hardest. Both mental and physical health conditions are more highly prevalent among underprivileged groups, and trajectories of healthy ageing are less likely among marginalised groups. In addition, most of the evidence generated within the health psychology domain thus far has been produced through recruiting as participants people from so-called WEIRD societies (i.e., Western, Educated, Industrialised, Rich, and Democratic) (Bartusevičius et al., 2020). Similar to the earlier call for action to tackle climate change, we strongly suggest that health psychologists move beyond conducting observational studies to uncover relationships between social determinants of health and health outcomes and use our scientific findings and know-how to communicate to policymakers that systemic change (e.g., to health services) is needed to undo the harm inflicted on marginalised communities over the past centuries.

Third, health psychologists are encouraged to strive for increased interdisciplinary within our teams, in addition to fostering cross-sectoral collaborations. To tackle the aforementioned barriers to the implementation of health psychology know-how, it is vital for health psychologists to learn to communicate our science clearly and effectively. Smarter investments (Kwasnicka et al., 2021) and stronger collaborations with professionals across sectors are needed, in addition to training in science communication and public engagement offered to health psychology professionals at all career stages. In addition to being better able to communicate what health psychologists can bring to the table, we also need to foster curiosity to learn about adjacent scientific disciplines and how we can collaborate with climate scientists, computer scientists, and other researchers and professionals (including, but not limited to, policymakers), to best tackle the aforementioned complex challenges.

Fourth, health psychologists should make a conscious shift towards embracing Open Science practices. Chapter 38 emphasises the need for the increased sharing of intervention materials, data, and analytic and algorithmic code. Limited sharing and cross-disciplinary collaborations mean we are not building on each other's successes as much as we could, thus stifling progress towards population-level health impact. Many health psychology tools require a lot of resources (e.g., interventions are designed to be delivered face-to-face by trained health-care professionals). As health psychology experts, it is imperative for us to help build the science underpinning policy and clinical practice decisions as to when digitisation/hybrid/face-to-face is most effective and for whom – this also relates to interventions targeting climate-related behaviours. However, to build knowledge of what works for whom rapidly yet robustly, we need increased networking and sharing of efforts and resources across different stakeholders, including academic researchers, intervention developers (including programmers), health-care professionals, policymakers, and others.

Conclusions

In this chapter, we have presented an overview of what the future of health psychology is likely to look like in the coming decades. Bringing together theory, evidence, and examples of past interventions, we have suggested what the key upcoming challenges are and highlighted opportunities for health psychologists to get meaningfully involved. The chapters in this book section outline how health psychology knowledge and practice can contribute across the lifespan and how our science can contribute to increased quality of life, and the slowing down of the climate crisis. We have also emphasised how health psychology is playing an active role in shaping the future of health policy and practice, and how policymakers can and should continue to turn to behavioural scientists to help inform policies that meaningfully impact population health. In this book section, we also emphasise the successes, concerns, and future directions of digital health in terms of health self-management and health promotion and prevention. As we take you on a journey of visualising what the future decades of health psychology are likely to bring, we hope we can encourage you to plan for how your own future contributions can continue to impact and improve health. We hope you enjoyed reading this section!

Further Reading

Kwasnicka, D., Keller, J., Perski, O., Potthoff, S., Ten Hoor, G. A., Ainsworth, B., Crutzen, R., Dohle, S., van Dongen, A., & Heino, M. (2022a). White Paper: Open Digital Health–accelerating transparent and scalable health promotion and treatment. White Paper: Open Digital Health. *Health Psychology Review, just-accepted*, 1–37.

Kuehnhanss, C. R. (2019). The challenges of behavioural insights for effective policy design. *Policy and Society*, *38*(1), 14–40.

Lepenies, R., Mackay, K., & Quigley, M. (2018). Three challenges for behavioural science and policy: the empirical, the normative and the political. *Behavioural Public Policy*, *2*(2), 174–182.

References

Adhanom Ghebreyesus, T. (2021). Using behavioural science for better health. *Bulletin of the World Health Organization*, *99*(11), 755–755. https://doi.org/10.2471/BLT.21.287387

Arigo, D., Jake-Schoffman, D. E., Wolin, K., Beckjord, E., Hekler, E. B., & Pagoto, S. L. (2019). The history and future of digital health in the field of behavioral medicine. *Journal of Behavioral Medicine*, *42*(1), 67–83.

Bartholomew, L. K., Parcel, G. S., & Kok, G. (1998). Intervention mapping: A process for developing theory and evidence-based health education programs. *Health Education & Behavior*, *25*(5), 545–563.

Bartusevičius, H., van Leeuwen, F., & Petersen, M. B. (2020). Dominance-driven autocratic political orientations predict political violence in Western, educated, industrialized, rich, and democratic (WEIRD) and non-WEIRD samples. *Psychological Science*, *31*(12), 1511–1530.

Cane, J., O'Connor, D., & Michie, S. (2012). Validation of the theoretical domains framework for use in behaviour change and implementation research. *Implementation Science*, *7*, 1–17.

Cao, X., Kannaiah, D., Ye, L., Khan, J., Shabbir, M. S., Bilal, K., & Tabash, M. I. (2022). Does sustainable environmental agenda matter in the era of globalization? The relationship among financial development, energy consumption, and sustainable environmental-economic growth. *Environmental Science and Pollution Research, 29*(21), 30808–30818.

Diderichsen, F., Hallqvist, J., & Whitehead, M. (2019). Differential vulnerability and susceptibility: How to make use of recent development in our understanding of mediation and interaction to tackle health inequalities. *International Journal of Epidemiology, 48*(1), 268–274.

Glasgow, R. E., Vogt, T. M., & Boles, S. M. (1999). Evaluating the public health impact of health promotion interventions: The RE-AIM framework. *American Journal of Public Health, 89*(9), 1322–1327.

Hallsworth, M. (2023). A manifesto for applying behavioural science. *Nature Human Behaviour, 7*, 1–13.

Hesse, B. W., Conroy, D. E., Kwaśnicka, D., Waring, M. E., Hekler, E., Andrus, S., Tercyak, K. P., King, A. C., & Diefenbach, M. A. (2021). We're all in this together: Recommendations from the Society of Behavioral Medicine's Open Science Working Group. *Translational Behavioral Medicine*, ibaa126. https://doi.org/10.1093/tbm/ibaa126

Hooten, N. N., Pacheco, N. L., Smith, J. T., & Evans, M. K. (2022). The accelerated aging phenotype: The role of race and social determinants of health on aging. *Ageing Research Reviews, 73*, 101536.

Kwasnicka, D., Keller, J., Perski, O., Potthoff, S., Ten Hoor, G. A., Ainsworth, B., Crutzen, R., Dohle, S., van Dongen, A., & Heino, M. (2022). White Paper: Open Digital Health–accelerating transparent and scalable health promotion and treatment. White Paper: Open Digital Health. *Health Psychology Review, just-accepted*, 1–37.

Kwasnicka, D., Ten Hoor, G. A., Hekler, E., Hagger, M. S., & Kok, G. (2021). Proposing a new approach to funding behavioural interventions using iterative methods. *Psychology & Health*, 1–5.

Lindacher, V., Curbach, J., Warrelmann, B., Brandstetter, S., & Loss, J. (2018). Evaluation of empowerment in health promotion interventions: A systematic review. *Evaluation & the Health Professions, 41*(3), 351–392.

Marks, D. F. (1996). Health Psychology in Context. *Journal of Health Psychology, 1*(1), 7–21. https://doi.org/10.1177/135910539600100102

Michie, S., Van Stralen, M. M., & West, R. (2011). The behaviour change wheel: A new method for characterising and designing behaviour change interventions. *Implementation Science, 6*(1), 1–12.

Ngo, T. D. (2023). Demographic trends and population health: Tackling inequality in a world of eight billion people. *BMJ Global Health, 8*(4), e012137.

Riley, W. T., Glasgow, R. E., Etheredge, L., & Abernethy, A. P. (2013). Rapid, responsive, relevant (R3) research: A call for a rapid learning health research enterprise. *Clinical and Translational Medicine, 2*(1), 1–6.

The Intergovernmental Panel on Climate Change (IPCC) (2023). *Special Report: Global Warming of 1.5 °C*. https://www.ipcc.ch/sr15/

WHO. (2023). *Ageing and health*. https://www.who.int/news-room/fact-sheets/detail/ageing-and-health

37

WELL-BEING ACROSS THE LIFESPAN

Healthy and Happy Ageing

Anne Tiedemann and Catherine Sherrington

Introduction

We are currently living in a time of unprecedented and dramatic demographic change. People across the world are living longer than ever before, and today most people can expect to live into their '60s and beyond. By 2030, it is predicted that the number of people aged 60 years and older globally will outnumber youth and be double the number of children under 5 (United Nations, 2017). Population ageing, brought about by increased life expectancy, reduced mortality, and lower fertility rates, creates an even greater need to ensure additional years of life are lived with good health and well-being so that longevity brings opportunity rather than disability. Many chronic conditions that emerge in older age are preventable, and the risk factors that lead to chronic disease can be reduced at any age. This points to a need for targeted action to enhance healthy lifestyle behaviours across the lifespan so that healthy ageing is realised.

Healthy ageing is defined by the World Health Organization as "the process of developing and maintaining the functional ability that enables well-being in older age" (World Health Organization, 2015). Healthy ageing encompasses the capacity to meet basic needs; learn, grow, and make decisions; be mobile; build and maintain relationships; and contribute to society. Importantly, it should be noted that health is not merely the absence of disease but encompasses physical, mental, and social well-being.

The United Nations Decade of Healthy Ageing (2021–2030) shines a spotlight on the needs of our ageing society and prompts ten years of dedicated, collaborative action to improve the lives of older people, their families, and their communities (World Health Organization, 2020). To foster healthy ageing, we need specific targeted actions, such as creating age-friendly cities and communities, and better access to appropriate and effective services and care. We also need to combat ageism by shifting the ways we think, feel, and act towards people on

 DOI: 10.4324/9781003318026-45

the basis of age. Health psychologists are well placed to support people to adopt positive lifestyle behaviours, such as regular physical activity, and to avoid harmful behaviours, such as smoking and excessive alcohol consumption, that can reduce the risk of poor health and promote well-being throughout the lifespan. This chapter highlights how health psychology can contribute towards supporting healthy, happy ageing and how to promote health at any age, with a particular focus on physical activity.

Population Ageing Brings Both Challenges and Opportunities

Across the world, the population is ageing. Between 2015 and 2050, the proportion of the world's population aged over 60 years will nearly double from 12% to 22% (World Health Organization, 2020). This demographic shift is brought about by medical advances in treating chronic conditions of older age that lead to increases in life expectancy and reduced mortality, and by a drop in the birth rate in many countries – as a society, we are living longer and having fewer babies. For example, in 1968, across the world, on average, there were 5 births per woman, falling to a rate of 2.3 births per woman in 2021. In that same time period, life expectancy at birth increased from 57 in 1968 to 71 in 2021 (The World Bank, 2023).

Population ageing brings challenges but also opportunities. Older people have knowledge and experience to share and can make important contributions to their families and communities; however, the ability to participate meaningfully depends on health in older age. Combating age-related chronic disease and associated disability is essential for ensuring additional years of life can be lived with good health and happiness and that older people can continue to flourish and contribute to society in ways that they value. Prevention of health decline across the life course is the best approach for supporting healthy ageing. Many other health conditions can be effectively managed, especially with early detection and treatment (World Health Organization, 2017b).

Prevention of chronic disease and implementation of strategies to support healthy ageing also support ongoing independence in older age. Most older people wish to remain living independently in their own homes for as long as possible, and this is certainly the preference from a social and economic efficiency perspective. To achieve this aim, older people may require support to continue to access health care and social opportunities and to master the use of technology to enhance access (see Chapter 38 in this volume).

In addition to looking after their own health and well-being, many older people will also assume the role of carer for their spouse or other family members. Among Europeans aged 50 years and over, population surveys indicate that between 10% and 35% of people are informal carers (Tur-Sinai et al., 2020). Caring roles present additional challenges and may result in carers' own health and well-being taking a lower priority in the face of competing demands and responsibilities (Mohanty & Niyonsenga, 2019). Informal or unpaid care, however, reduces the burden on the already stretched health-care workforce and therefore should be recognised for its importance and supported appropriately.

One challenge, though, is that not all older people have access to the financial and personal resources required to age independently and in their place of choice. Unfortunately, there is evidence of socio-economic discrepancies in healthy ageing (Wilkinson & Marmot, 2003). This is likely to have complex causes, including access to health services, type of work, education, and nutrition. Equity is a key consideration in the planning of services and supports to promote happy and healthy ageing.

Preparing for older age should include a focus on preventive health, healthy lifestyle habits, and social connection. Starting to focus on these things early in life is also preferred. Encouraging uptake and adherence to health promoting habits in middle age is associated with a greater likelihood of better functional capacity and reduced disability into older age, representing a good long-term investment for individuals and societies. Health psychologists can play a pivotal role in supporting people across the lifespan to achieve these goals. Effective approaches include health coaching, which is demonstrated to promote the uptake of physical activity in older age (Oliveira et al., 2017), and cognitive behavioural therapy, which is effective in supporting people to quit smoking (Vinci, 2020; Krishnamoorthy et al., 2023).

Common Health Conditions Associated with Older Age

With advanced age comes a greater likelihood of developing chronic conditions. The most common chronic conditions experienced by people in older age are cardiovascular disease, chronic obstructive pulmonary disease, diabetes, depression, dementia, osteoarthritis, and other musculoskeletal conditions (Jaul & Barron, 2017). Falls are also common in older age and can lead to significant disability (Lord et al., 2021). Apart from the immediate symptoms associated with the specific conditions, these health conditions can lead to reduced independence, reduced capacity to take part in physical activity, greater risk of social isolation, and reduced well-being.

A focus on the prevention of these chronic conditions and falls should be the priority of policymakers, health professionals, and consumers. Prevention of many of these conditions is possible through lifestyle behaviour change, including eating a balanced diet, engaging in regular physical activity, and avoiding smoking (World Health Organization, 2019). Health psychologists can play a crucial role in supporting behaviour change in middle and older age to promote healthy and happy ageing through engagement and long-term adherence to these crucial health-promoting behaviours, as illustrated in the case study of Ms Smith in Box 37.1. Empowering people to take responsibility for their health and take control of their future well-being should be the focus.

Dementia is a common health condition that is associated with advanced age for which there is currently no treatment. It is estimated that currently, more than 55 million people have dementia worldwide, and it is recognised as the seventh leading cause of death and a leading cause of disability and dependency among older people globally (World Health Organization, 2017a).

Dementia is associated with stigmatisation and barriers to diagnosis and care, often due to a lack of awareness and understanding of dementia. Health psychologists could play a role in improving the lives of people living with dementia by working with the individual and family to develop strategies to enhance quality of life and manage emotions related to the dementia diagnosis (Logsdon et al., 2007).

Efforts to reduce the progression of these health conditions or manage their care and treatment depends on access to evidence-based information to guide care, effective and accessible medications, and healthy lifestyle choices, as mentioned earlier. With support, people can be equipped with the skills and knowledge to maximise their quality of life whilst living with chronic conditions. Messaging around the effectiveness of prevention strategies that target chronic conditions, that investment in health in early adulthood pays dividends in older age (Nagata et al., 2022), and that it is never too late to make lifestyle changes that have significant benefits for health and well-being are important for mobilising an individual's capacity and motivation to take positive steps to build their capacity for healthy ageing.

Support for People Acting as Carers

Playing the role of carer can also provide additional challenges. In 2019, on average across countries in the Organisation for Economic Co-operation and Development (OECD) for which data are available (OECD, 2021), around 13% of people aged 50 years and over report providing informal care on at least a weekly basis to a family member or friend who has a disability, mental illness, chronic condition, terminal illness or who is aged and frail. Carers aged 65 years and over are more likely to be caring for a spouse, which is more likely to require daily care, and men and women are equally likely to take on this role.

Many older people do not consider themselves to be a carer when supporting a spouse, a sibling, or a friend. Being a carer can be personally rewarding; however, there are well-documented costs that include negative impacts on physical and mental health, financial disadvantage, and negative consequences for career and social and emotional well-being. Supporting carers through the provision of paid or unpaid carers leave by employers, financial support from governments, and counselling and training can also assist.

Health psychologists are ideally placed to assist carers in coping with the stress and challenges of being a caregiver. They can also support carers to consider and plan for opportunities to look after their own physical, mental, and emotional health and well-being. The carer can be guided to think about how things are going, how they would like things to be, and what steps they could take towards making that happen. Multidimensional interventions that address the broad range of stressors faced by carers are most effective (Woods & McCormick, 2018). Considering the significant contribution carers make to the health and well-being of people of all ages, it is imperative that they receive the care they themselves need to be healthy and happy into older age.

Accessibility and Mobility Support for Frail Older People

Chronological age is a poor indicator of the physical and mental capacity of an individual. Our capacity in older age is a product of the influence of our environment and our behaviours, and the development of chronic health conditions is not an inevitable consequence of ageing (Khaw, 1997).

Frailty refers to an accumulation of physical and cognitive deficits that are associated with a vulnerability to adverse events (Fried et al., 2004). Around 20% of community-dwelling people aged over 65 years are frail. People who are frail have an increased risk for poor health outcomes, including falls, disability, hospitalisation, and mortality. Frailty is more important in understanding access and mobility requirements than chronological age. Not all older people are frail, and not all frail people are old. Mobility training has been demonstrated to be effective in improving mobility and function among older people with frailty (Treacy et al., 2022).

The concepts of intrinsic capacity and functional ability are used in the *WHO World Report on Ageing and Health* (World Health Organization, 2015), and, like frailty, these concepts emphasise diversity among older adults and ensure a focus on functioning rather than chronological age. 'Intrinsic capacity' is defined as the composite of all the physical and mental capacities of an individual. 'Functional ability' comprises the health-related attributes that enable people to be and to do what they have reason to value. It is made up of the intrinsic capacity of the individual, relevant environmental characteristics, and the interactions between the individual and these characteristics.

Appropriate environmental design can enable safe universal accessibility of public spaces and homes for older people with limited intrinsic capacity and will also benefit younger people with disabilities, infants, and their carers. Supports such as walking aids and wheelchairs can allow someone with impaired intrinsic capacity to participate fully in society by maintaining functional ability. Health psychologists can play a role in encouraging the uptake of such supports by emphasising the improvement in safe mobility and independence that mobility supports can bring and assisting older people to overcome their hesitancy, which is often due to stigma and embarrassment (Lee & Tak, 2023).

Role of Physical Activity in Promoting Well-Being and Preventing Health Conditions

Regular participation in physical activity has significant benefits for the health and well-being of people of all ages. Physical activity is known to reduce the risk of developing the common non-communicable diseases (NCDs) mentioned earlier and also plays an important role in their management and control (Lee et al., 2012). Physical activity can slow the decline in mobility and cognition in older age (Littbrand et al., 2009), is key to maintaining physical capacity to avoid falls (Sherrington et al., 2019), and promotes independent living into older age (Peeters et al., 2013). A large, robust review of the evidence identified which physical activity types are most effective in different populations and settings (Pinheiro et al., 2022).

Physical activity and healthy ageing are critically linked due to the role of physical activity in the treatment and prevention of chronic NCDs, the large NCD disease burden experienced by older people, and the increase of physical inactivity with age (Prince et al., 2015). Chronic NCDs, such as cardiovascular disease, cancer, chronic respiratory, and musculoskeletal, mental, and neurological disorders, account for most of this burden. As the prevalence of chronic conditions and disabilities is greater in older than younger adults, it is important to consider functional ability when catering for older adults but equally important not to assume that all older adults will have impaired intrinsic capacity or functional ability.

The World Health Organization (WHO) Global Guidelines on Physical Activity and Sedentary Behaviour recommend that all children and adults, of all abilities and ages, should undertake regular physical activity (Bull et al., 2020). A summary of the specific amount and type of physical activity recommended is described next.

Young People Aged 5–17 Years

Children and adolescents should do at least an average of 60 min/day of moderate-to-vigorous intensity, mostly aerobic, physical activity, across the week. Vigorous intensity aerobic activities (e.g., running), as well as activities that strengthen muscle and bone (e.g., jumping, lifting weights) should be incorporated at least three days a week. Time spent being sedentary should be limited, particularly the amount of recreational screen time such as social media and video gaming.

Adults and Older Adults, including People Living with Chronic Conditions and Disabilities

Overall, the research evidence shows that every move counts for promoting health, and all adults should do regular physical activity of any intensity or type. Examples of aerobic activities include brisk walking, stair climbing, cycling, swimming, running, or carrying shopping. For substantial health benefits, the guidelines recommend that adults should take part in 150–300 minutes of moderate-intensity aerobic physical activity (e.g., brisk walking) or 75–150 minutes of vigorous activity (e.g., running) throughout the week, or equivalent combinations of both. Provided that there are no contraindications resulting from severe chronic conditions, additional health benefits can be gained by taking part in more activity than the recommended amounts.

In addition to aerobic physical activity, adults should also do muscle-strengthening activities that involve large muscle groups at least two days per week. This is important to combat the age-related decline in muscle mass that starts in middle age and can ultimately lead to an inability to carry out activities of daily living in older years and subsequent relocation to residential aged care. Falls in older age are also a common event that can result in serious injury, threaten independent living, and reduce participation in regular physical activity. For this reason, to reduce the risk of falls, in addition to the previous recommendations, the WHO guidelines recommend that adults aged 65 years and older should engage in 'multicomponent' physical activity that particularly targets functional balance training and muscle strengthening at moderate or greater intensity, on three or more days a week. There is now clear guidance about the types of programmes that are effective in preventing falls and that should be promoted to older adults (World Health Organization, 2021; Montero-Odasso et al., 2022). Importantly, the focus should be on improving capacity early in older age to avoid falls rather than addressing the risk once a fall has occurred.

Role of Health Psychology in Managing Well-Being across the Lifespan

Despite the clear evidence of the importance of physical activity for supporting physical and mental health (Lee et al., 2012; Schuch et al., 2016), population estimates of inactivity range from 28% of adults (Guthold et al., 2018) to 80% of adolescents (Guthold et al., 2020). This illustrates the complexity of physical activity behaviour change and identifies a role for health psychologists in supporting change. The benefits of active lifestyles are generally well acknowledged, yet people often require tailored support to achieve lasting behaviour change. Helping people to identify the factors that could motivate them to change and tapping into their internal strengths that can be drawn upon to make that change can be a starting point.

Health psychologists are well placed to support people to adopt positive behaviours, such as regular physical activity, that can reduce risk factors for poor health and promote well-being. This could occur through physical activity coaching, which has been found to be effective for older people (Oliveira et al., 2017). It is important to recognise the diversity of older adults, tailor interventions to people's circumstances, and adopt a genuinely person-centred approach that starts with listening to the person. This is illustrated in the case study of Ms Smith in Box 37.1, who displays several health-related and structural barriers to lifestyle change. Paying attention to the way support to adopt an intervention is delivered, not just to the components of the intervention, will ensure greater uptake and adherence from the individual. Therapeutic alliance, the interaction between the health psychologist and the patient, enhances intervention uptake and adherence and can improve treatment outcomes (Haynes et al., 2021). Factors that enhance therapeutic alliance, including collaborative decision-making and the development of trusting, person-centred relationships, should be prioritised in the delivery of health promotion strategies.

In terms of supporting people to manage their chronic conditions, health psychologists can assist with promoting adherence to regular physical activity participation and addressing the complex influence of many barriers and enablers to

Box 37.1 Case Study of Health Coaching Approach for an Older Person

Case study: Ms Smith, 65 years old

Session 1

Six-month goals

Take part in moderate-intensity walking for 20 minutes, 3 times/week

Lose weight, aim to reduce weight by 3 kg

Two-week goals

Undertake home exercise programme provided by physiotherapist three to five times/week

Five minutes of walking three times/week

Wear Fitbit daily to monitor progress with being more active

Synchronise Fitbit with iPad every two to three days

Call health coach in two weeks

Session 2

Loves using the activity tracker to monitor herself and motivate to do more.

Has been to the gym two times/week but finds it to be a bit expensive. Will try to find a cheaper option.

Taking the stairs instead of the lift at work. Feels that it is getting easier to go up the stairs. Goes straight up the stairs at the train station and feels less out of breath.

Was sick last week, so she has not been as active as she would like. Feels much better now. Weather was bad in the first week, so this was also a barrier to progress.

Barriers during the Six-Month Intervention

Ms Smith experienced some health-related issues, including bronchitis, low back pain, foot pain, trigeminal neuralgia, and another bad cold that were barriers to activity. Other issues that arose and made it difficult to be active included her dog dying, cold weather, working 28 days straight so she had no time, helping her daughter move house, and her brother became very ill, so she was occupied with him.

Change in Status since Beginning

Balance exercises embedded in day – tandem walking along corridor at work, etc.

Joined gym. Given programme but doesn't get supervision whilst there. Different from last gym with exercise physiologists. Spends approximately 40 minutes at gym using bike, treadmill, weights. Does own balance exercises, sit to stand, etc.

Participant Comments

"You can understand how running becomes addictive.... I'm enjoying the feeling of being more fit."

"I feel a remarkable improvement in my breathing and ability to do things. I walked to the Opera House and felt fine walking up the stairs!"

"I really feel the benefits of being in the study. I can walk anywhere now!"

this behaviour. Reassuring older people about the safety of physical activity in the context of comorbidities is important, and harnessing the support of the individual's primary care physician may enhance participation. Health psychologists can also assist people in avoiding other harmful behaviours, such as smoking and excessive alcohol consumption, and support people in adopting recommendations around medication regimens for the treatment of some conditions. Evidence-based behaviour change techniques such as goal setting, habit formation, and self-monitoring may be particularly important here (Samdal et al., 2017; Janols et al., 2022). These techniques form part of the foundations of health coaching and can be used to maximise an individual's success in initiating and maintaining regular physical activity. The use of motivational interviewing can lead to a discussion clarifying reasons for change – being independent and able to live at home, continuing with social activities and hobbies, being able to travel, caring for family. Rather than being active to follow advice on meeting physical activity guidelines, awareness of the bigger picture can increase motivation. Setting realistic goals that are meaningful and achievable is vital. Confidence in achieving the goal and the level of importance is key and can be measured on a scale from 1 to 10. Other factors to consider in integrating physical activity into a routine are when, where, and with whom. Normalising the possibility of setbacks (due to, for example, illness, caring for others, lack of motivation, bad weather) and how to navigate these improves motivation to continue on the journey of increasing and improving physical activity. The case study of Ms Smith in Box 37.1 provides an example of the approach that could be used to encourage the uptake of physical activity for an older person.

Well-designed physical activity programmes can enhance intrinsic capability (both physical and mental) and can lessen frailty and the risk of falls. Such programmes need to be undertaken regularly and over the long term, as benefits are lost if activity is ceased. Exercises that target mobility, balance, and muscle strength are particularly effective (Fairhall et al., 2011). Health psychologists are ideally placed to advocate for environments and physical activity programmes that maximise intrinsic capacity and functional ability and to assist older adults and their allies in advocating in this way. Regarding falls in older age, health psychologists can play a role in encouraging older people to participate in evidence-based interventions such as health checks and home safety interventions, as well as physical activity interventions. Actions such as having cataracts removed where indicated, taking part in regular exercise that aims to improve balance and leg strength, and having a medication review by a medical practitioner all have the potential to decrease a person's risk of falling (Gillespie et al., 2009; Sherrington et al., 2019).

Conclusion

Our global ageing population brings both challenges and opportunities. Ill health and poor well-being are not inevitable with increased age. Health psychologists can play an important role in supporting people to make healthy choices throughout their lifespans and advocating for designs and services that maximise safe participation for older adults in society regardless of their physical and mental capacity. By harnessing the opportunities provided by adopting healthy lifestyle behaviours, society can reap the benefits of longevity and the potential contributions made by older adults. In turn, older adults can expect to have more years lived in good health and continue to be active members of society.

Further Reading

National programmes for age-friendly cities and communities: a guide. Geneva: World Health Organization; 2023. Licence: CC BY-NC-SA 3.0 IGO.

Progress report on the United Nations Decade of Healthy Ageing, 2021–2023. Geneva: World Health Organization; 2023. Licence: CC BY-NC-SA 3.0 IGO.

References

Bull, F. C., Al-Ansari, S. S., Biddle, S., Borodulin, K., Buman, M. P., Cardon, G., Carty, C., Chaput, J.-P., Chastin, S., Chou, R., Dempsey, P. C., DiPietro, L., Ekelund, U., Firth, J., Friedenreich, C. M., Garcia, L., Gichu, M., Jago, R., Katzmarzyk, P. T., Lambert, E., Leitzmann, M., Milton, K., Ortega, F. B., Ranasinghe, C., Stamatakis, E., Tiedemann, A.,Troiano, R. P., van der Ploeg, H. P., Wari, V., and Willumsen, J. F. (2020). "World Health Organization 2020 guidelines on physical activity and sedentary behaviour." *British Journal of Sports Medicine 54*(24): 1451–1462.

Fairhall, N., Langron, C., Sherrington, C., Lord, S.R., Kurrle, S.E., Lockwood, K., Monaghan, N., Aggar, C., Gill, L., and Cameron, I.D. (2011). "Treating frailty-a practical guide." *BMC Medicine 9*(1): 83.

Fried, L. P., Ferrucci, J., Darer, J., Williamson, J. D., and Anderson, G. (2004). "Untangling the Concepts of Disability, Frailty, and Comorbidity: Implications for Improved Targeting and Care." *The Journals of Gerontology: Series A 59*(3): M255–M263.

Gillespie, L. D., Robertson, M. C., Gillespie, W. J., Lamb, S. E., Gates, S., Cumming, R. G., and Rowe, B. H. (2009). "Interventions for preventing falls in older people living in the community." *Cochrane Database of Systematic Reviews 2*: CD007146.

Guthold, R., Stevens, G. A., Riley, L. M., and Bull, F. C. (2018). "Worldwide trends in insufficient physical activity from 2001 to 2016: a pooled analysis of 358 population-based surveys with 1.9 million participants." *The Lancet Global Health 6*(10): e1077–e1086.

Guthold, R., Stevens, G. A., Riley, L. M., and Bull, F. C. (2020). "Global trends in insufficient physical activity among adolescents: a pooled analysis of 298 population-based surveys with 1·6 million participants." *Lancet Child Adolesc Health 4*(1): 23–35.

Haynes, A., Sherrington, C., Ramsay, E., Kirkham, C., Manning, S., Wallbank, G., Hassett, L., and Tiedemann, A. (2021). ""Sharing Success with Someone": Building therapeutic alliance in physiotherapist-delivered physical activity coaching for healthy aging." *Physiotherapy Theory and Practice 38*(13): 1–17.

Janols, R., Sandlund, M., Lindgren, H., and Pettersson, B. (2022). "Older adults as designers of behavior change strategies to increase physical activity-Report of a participatory design process." *Front Public Health 10*: 988470.

Jaul, E., and Barronm J. (2017). "Age-Related Diseases and Clinical and Public Health Implications for the 85 Years Old and Over Population." *Front Public Health 5*: 335.

Khaw, K. (1997). "Epidemiological aspects of ageing." *Philosophical Transactions of the Royal Society of London. Series B, Biological Sciences 352*(1363): 1829–1835.

Krishnamoorthy, Y., Elangovan, V., and Rajaa, S. (2023). "Non-pharmacological interventions for tobacco cessation in India: A systematic review and network meta-analysis." *Nicotine & Tobacco Research* ePub ahead of print.

Lee, D., and Tak, S. H. (2023). "Barriers and facilitators of older adults' usage of mobility devices: a scoping review." *Educational Gerontology 49*(2): 96–108.

Lee, I. M., Shiroma, E. J., Lobelo, F., Puska, P., Blair, S. N., Katzmarzyk, P. T., and Lancet Physical Activity Series Working Group. (2012). "Effect of physical inactivity on major non-communicable diseases worldwide: an analysis of burden of disease and life expectancy." *Lancet 380*(9838): 219–229.

Littbrand, H., Lundin-Olsson, L., Gustafson, Y., and Rosendahl, E. (2009). "The Effect of a High-Intensity Functional Exercise Program on Activities of Daily Living: A Randomized Controlled Trial in Residential Care Facilities." *Journal of the American Geriatrics Society 57*(10): 1741–1749.

Logsdon, R. G., McCurry, S. M., and Teri, L. (2007). "Evidence-Based Interventions to Improve Quality of Life for Individuals with Dementia." *Alzheimers Care Today 8*(4): 309–318.

Lord, S. R., Sherrington, C., and Naganathan, V. (2021). *Falls in Older People: Risk Factors, Strategies for Prevention and Implications for Practice*. Cambridge, Cambridge University Press.

Mohanty, I., and Niyonsenga, T. (2019). "A longitudinal analysis of mental and general health status of informal carers in Australia." *BMC Public Health 19*(1): 1436.

Montero-Odasso, M. N., van der Velde, F., Martin, F. C., Petrovic, M., Tan, M. P., Ryg, J., Aguilar-Navarro, S., Alexander, N. B., Becker, C., Blain, H., Bourme, R., Cameron, I. C., Camicioli, R., Clemson, L., Close, J., Delbaere, K., Duan, L., Duque, G., Dyer, S. M., Freiberger, E., Ganz, D. A., Gómez, F., Hausdorff, J. M., Hogan, D. B., Hunter, S. M. W., Jauregui, J. R., Kamkar, N., Rose-Anne, K., Lamb, S. E., Latham, N. K., Lipsitz, L. A., Liu-Ambrose, T., Logan, P., Lord, S. R., Mallet, L., Marsh, D., Milisen, K., Moctezuma-Gallegos, R., Morris, M. E., Nieuwboer, A., Perracini, M. R., Pieruccini-Faria, F., Pighills, A., Said, C., Sejdic, E., Sherrington, C., Skelton, D. A., Dzousa, S., Speechley, M., Stark, S., Todd, C., Troen, B. R., van der Cammen, J., Veghese, J., Vlaeyen, E., Watt, J. A., Masud, T., and the Task Force on Global Guidelines for Falls in Older Adults. (2022). "World guidelines for falls prevention and management for older adults: a global initiative." *Age and Ageing 51*(9): afac205.

Nagata, J. M., Vittinghoff, E., Pettee Gabriel, K., Garber, A. K., Moran, A. E., Rana, J. S., Reis, J. P., Sidney, S., and Bibbins-Domingo, K. (2022). "Moderate-to-vigorous intensity physical activity from young adulthood to middle age and metabolic disease: a 30-year population-based cohort study." *British Journal of Sports Medicine 56*(15): 847–853.

Organisation for Economic Cooperation and Development (2021). *Health at a Glance*.

Oliveira, J. S., Sherrington, C., Amorim, A. B., Dario, A. B., and Tiedemann, A. (2017). "What is the effect of health coaching on physical activity participation in people aged 60 years and over? A systematic review of randomised controlled trials." *British Journal of Sports Medicine 51*(19): 1425–1432.

Peeters, G., Dobson, A. J., Deeg, D. J. H., and Brown, W. J. (2013). "A life-course perspective on physical functioning in women." *Bulletin of the World Health Organization 91*(9): 661–670.

Pinheiro, M. B., Oliveira, J. S., Baldwin, J. N., Hassett, L., Costa, N., Gilchrist, H., Wang, B., Kwok, W., Albuquerque, B. S., Pivotto, L. R., Carvalho-Silva, A. P. M. C., Sharma, S., Gilbert, S., Bauman, A., Bull, F. C., Willumsen, J., Sherrington C., and Tiedemann A. (2022). "Impact of physical activity programs and services for older adults: a rapid review." *International Journal of Behavioral Nutrition and Physical Activity 19*(1): 87.

Prince, M. J., Wu, F., Guo, Y., Gutierrez Robledo, L. M., O'Donnell, M., Sullivan, R., and Yusuf, S. (2015). "The burden of disease in older people and implications for health policy and practice." *Lancet 385*(9967): 549–562.

Samdal, G. B., Eide, G. E., Barth, T., Williams, G., and Meland E. (2017). "Effective behaviour change techniques for physical activity and healthy eating in overweight and obese adults; systematic review and meta-regression analyses." *International Journal of Behavioral Nutrition and Physical Activity 14*(1): 42.

Schuch, F. B., Vancampfort, D., Richards, J., Rosenbaum, S., Ward, P. B., and Stubbs, B. (2016). "Exercise as a treatment for depression: A meta-analysis adjusting for publication bias." *J Psychiatr Res 77*: 42–51.

Sherrington, C., Fairhall, N. J., Wallbank, G. K., Tiedemann, A., Michaleff, Z. A., Howard, K., Clemson, L., Hopewell, S., and Lamb S. E. (2019). "Exercise for preventing falls in older people living in the community." *Cochrane Database of Systematic Reviews 1*(1): CD012424.

The World Bank (2023). "Data bank." Retrieved 22/05/2023, from https://databank.worldbank.org/home.aspx

Treacy, D., Hassett, L., Schurr, K., Fairhall, N. J., Cameron, I. D., and Sherrington, C. (2022). "Mobility training for increasing mobility and functioning in older people with frailty." *Cochrane Database of Systematic Reviews 6*(6): CD010494.

Tur-Sinai, A., Teti, A., Rommel, A., Hlebec, V., and Lamura, G. (2020). "How Many Older Informal Caregivers Are There in Europe? Comparison of Estimates of Their Prevalence from Three European Surveys." *Int J Environ Res Public Health 17*(24): 9531.

United Nations, Department of Economic and Social Affairs, Population Division, (2017). World Population Ageing 2017 - Highlights (ST/ESA/SER.A/397).

Vinci, C. (2020). "Cognitive Behavioral and Mindfulness-Based Interventions for Smoking Cessation: a Review of the Recent Literature." *Curr Oncol Rep 22*(6): 58.

Wilkinson, R., and Marmot, M. (eds) (2003). *Social determinants of health. The solid facts*, 2nd edition. Copenhagen: WHO.

Woods, R., and McCormick, S. (2018). Carer Wellbeing and Supports: A review of the literature and directions for research. Centre for Carers Research, Institute of Public Policy and Governance, University of Technology Sydney.

World Health Organization (2015). *World report on ageing and health*. Geneva.

World Health Organization (2019). *Non-communicable disease prevention and control: A guidance note for investment cases*. Geneva.

World Health Organization (2017a). *Global action plan on the public health response to dementia 2017–2025*. Geneva.

World Health Organization (2017b). *Global strategy and action plan on ageing and health*. Geneva.

World Health Organization (2020). *Decade of Healthy Ageing: Baseline Report*. Geneva.

World Health Organization (2021). *Step safely: strategies for preventing and managing falls across the life-course*. Geneva.

38

HEALTH PSYCHOLOGY IN THE AGE OF DIGITAL HEALTH

Bradford W. Hesse, Jessica M. Lipschitz, David K. Ahern, and Dominika Kwasnicka

Introduction

Professionals who depend on psychological evidence to improve the health of individuals have maintained a close alliance with information technologists for decades. The alliance is not surprising; much of health psychology revolves around the study of how individuals and groups *process information* as a precursor to healthy behavior change. Moreover, creating digital health solutions that are effective in the long run requires a "convergence" (Massachusetts Institute of Technology, 2011) of intersectoral perspectives, especially between engineering and the behavioral sciences. Some of the areas in which this alliance has benefited health psychology include (a) enhancing theory by modeling internal cognitive/affective/behavioral processes (Farrell & Lewandowsky, 2018; Nahum-Shani, Hekler, & Spruijt-Metz, 2015), (b) assessing patient status and outcomes in more ecologically valid ways (Fox et al., 2019; Kwasnicka, Kale, et al., 2021), (c) providing support for health-related decision-making (Hesse, 2016; Johnson & Stead, 2022), (d) facilitating behavior change (Ahern, Braun, Cooley, & Bickmore, 2016; Kwasnicka et al., 2020), (f) encouraging personal health management and protecting patient autonomy (Kwasnicka, Ntoumanis, & Sniehotta, 2021; Willems et al., 2017), (g) extending mental health consultation over geographic divides (Hesse, Ahern, & Ellison, 2020; Lipschitz et al., 2022), and (h) reinforcing standards for team-based care and communication (Alfano et al., 2020; Taplin et al., 2015). In the following chapter, we offer a brief history of the alliance between psychology and digital technologies. We then take a look at where the future may take us, paying particular attention to health psychology's contribution across a full gamut of digital health interventions. We conclude with four overarching issues to bear in mind as new technologies come and go.

DOI: 10.4324/9781003318026-46

A Brief History of Digital Technology in Health Psychology

Historically, the very first instantiations of computing technology revolved around the goal of automating numeric calculations in the service of business, defense, and science. This is not surprising to psychology researchers who have depended for decades on the processing power of computers to perform statistical tests on reams of behavioral data. Computing power gave psychologists the ability to process millions of data points in ways that were simply not feasible in a paper-based world, thus catalyzing discovery and boosting productivity.

There is another twist to the early story of computing, however. To enable these computational efficiencies, engineers needed to evolve mechanisms for representing numeric data symbolically for input, processing, storage, and output. What these engineers quickly recognized is that if the internal states of machines could be designed to represent numbers symbolically, they could also be designed to represent logic values or letters. In fact, Alan Turing – the famous British mathematician credited with ushering in modern computing with his 1936 blueprint for a Universal Turing Machine – believed that anything could be represented symbolically in computers, including abstract mental states. If mental processes could be mimicked symbolically, he reasoned, then machines could ultimately be made to think, thus ushering in studies of expert systems and artificial intelligence (AI) and its inferential referent in the human brain, the study of human cognition (Anyoha, 2017). Health psychologists began using computational platforms to model cognitive processes, to develop and refine theories, and to assist in therapeutic tasks such as diagnosis and decision-making.

The Birth of Personal Computing

In the early days of computing, processing power was expensive. Access to computers up until the mid-1980s was often restricted to those who had institutional subscriptions to mainframe computing environments. In the 1970s and 1980s, a group of innovators began pushing back on this centralized computing model with a concerted effort to engineer stand-alone desktop machines purchased directly by individuals. Thus began the era of *personal computing*, an era with at least two significant influences in the field of health psychology. The first was to democratize computing power so that more psychologists could begin experimenting with digital environments and more patients could begin benefiting from computerized assessments and interventions. By 1988, the second edition of the American Psychology Association's *Directory of Computer Software* listed hundreds of personal computer programs written to educate patients, assess psychological and physiological functioning, assist with behavioral goals in areas such as nutrition and smoking cessation, and even assist as adjuvant support in mental health counseling (Stoloff & Couch, 1988). These early affordances, boosted by the personal computer revolution, continue to serve as the foundation for many of the digital health interventions in place today.

The second big influence came as the personal computing market evolved, and technology designers began depending heavily on the expertise of psychologists to improve interactions between humans and technology (Norman, 1990). During this era, the more intuitive graphical user interface (GUI) – which capitalized on recognition memory as opposed to the generational memory needed to work with text-based operating systems – began cornering greater market share than their command-line predecessors. It was not long before the concept of human-centered computing (Shneiderman, 1987) became the byword of an industry trying to push sales beyond early adopters. In medicine, where patient outcomes depended as much on judgment and human behavior as they did on technological advancement, a sociotechnical approach began dominating as a framework for technology implementation (Coiera, 2004; Hesse & Shneiderman, 2007). Such approaches revolved around the recognition that (a) technical systems have social consequences; (b) social systems have technical consequences; (c) we do not design technologies, we design sociotechnical systems; and (d) designing sociotechnical systems requires an understanding of how people and technologies interact (Coiera, 2004).

Diffusion of the Internet

By the early 1990s, personal computing had begun diffusing broadly into the office and home environments. Whereas the diffusion of these technologies offered personal access to some of the vanguard software programs offered by the technology sector, they were limited in their support for electronic communication and connectivity to shared online resources. On 30 April 1993, British computer scientist Tim Berners Lee addressed this gap by releasing the source code for a graphically oriented network language (Hypertext Markup Language, or HTML) aimed at facilitating information sharing across computer networks. This was the birth of the World Wide Web. When mounted on public-facing servers following standardized internet protocols, the easy-to-use interfaces facilitated by HTML created public onramps to a vast *information superhighway* of resources, products, and services. It did not take long before Web-based search engines began registering health and medical issues as some of the most commonly searched terms on the Web (Rice & Katz, 2001). Research conducted at the National Cancer Institute in the United States revealed that by 2003 internet users reported going to the Web first for health information, well before ever contacting their own personal health-care providers (Hesse et al., 2005).

eHealth and Health e-Technologies

Seeking to capitalize on these newly connected resources, international funding agencies and philanthropies began fostering innovation in an area that would come to be known as *eHealth*. The Robert Wood Johnson Foundation recognized the significant potential for the emerging field of eHealth by establishing the Health e-Technologies Initiative as a national program to stimulate research and evaluation of new technologies for behavior change and chronic disease management (Ahern, Phalen, & Mockenhaupt, 2003). Founding editor of the *Journal of Medical Internet Research*, Gunther Eysenbach, defined eHealth as "an emerging field in the intersection of medical informatics, public health and business, referring to health services and information delivered or enhanced through the Internet and related technologies" (Eysenbach, 2000). The domain of health psychology complemented its existing portfolio of electronic applications to incorporate studies of online social support, just-in-time access to online health information, interpersonal messaging through asynchronous and synchronous channels, and – when available – connectivity to patients' electronic health records.

mHealth and Wearable Technology

In 2007, Apple Computer upped the ante on access to the internet through its introduction of smartphone technology, a move that was quickly matched by other mobile device manufacturers. Mobile connectivity introduced affordances built around an "always on, always with you" model of access and, consequently, prompted funding agencies to invest resources into mobile health, or *mHealth*. Health psychologists responded by modifying their theory base to stay abreast of new opportunities in the mobile world (Riley et al., 2011). Innovations included the ability to study peoples' thoughts and behavior in their daily lives by triggering assessments contiguous to the behavior under study (an approach referred to as 'ecological momentary assessment'); the ability to provide the right amount and type of support for a behavior, at the right time, by adapting to an individual's internal and external context (also known as 'just-in-time adaptive interventions'); the use of geo-sensitive sensors to prevent environmental triggers for maladaptive behaviors; and the use of mobile video capacity to support remote psychological consults (Nahum-Shani et al., 2015). The evolution of wearable technologies, implantable medical technologies, and even the popularization of smart devices for the home led to a further expansion of opportunity as health scientists sought to leverage the affordances offered by the "Internet of (Healthy) Things" (Kvedar, Colman, & Cella, 2015; President's Cancer Panel, 2016).

Anticipating Opportunities

To guide a discussion of opportunities in digital health, the US-based National Academy of Medicine (NAM) recently proposed 12 areas in which digital technologies have intersected with medicine in the past and are likely to continue influencing health production into the future (Abernethy et al., 2022). In Figure 38.1, we have adopted the NAM digital health framework to explore comparable areas of opportunity in health psychology. What follows is an analysis of those opportunities to serve as a guide for researchers and practitioners.

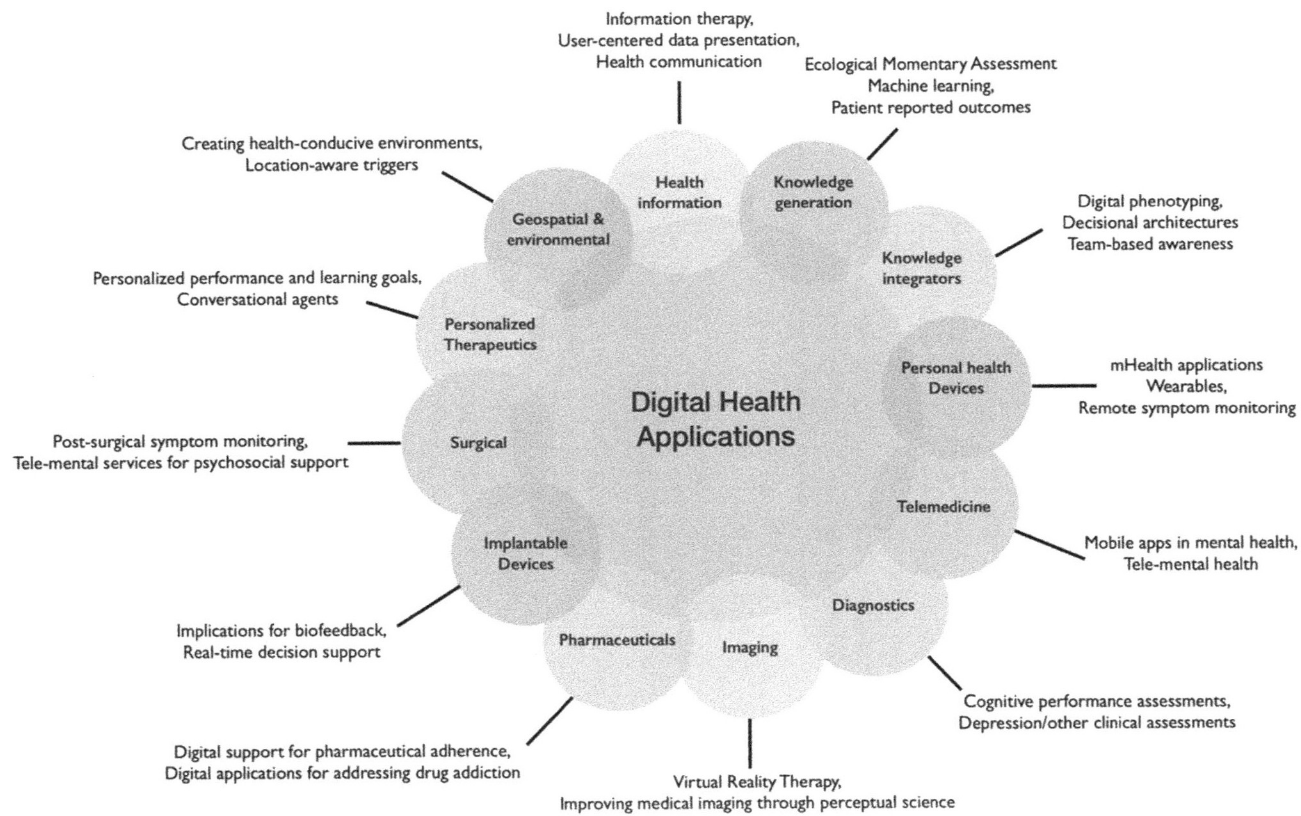

Figure 38.1 Mapping of a digital health framework offered by the NAM (Abernethy et al., 2022) into areas of relevant discovery and practice within health psychology.

Health Information

Health psychologists have worked closely with medical teams and public health specialists to frame health messages that are clear, concise, motivational, and facilitative of action (Cameron & Leventhal, 2003). The effects of media, or channels (e.g., face-to-face, television, radio, print), are routinely factored into the theories underlying these efforts. Digital media have expanded the spectrum of those effects (Hesse, Beckjord, Rutten, Fagerlin, & Cameron, 2015) and will merit ongoing attention as the contours of the media environment change. Health psychologists must continue to be engaged in understanding how the flow of health information across different technology-mediated environments (e.g., bulletin boards, news aggregation services, social media, eCommerce) can be channeled toward health-conducive ends while minimizing the impact of misinformation, disinformation, and social conflict. In another example, the adoption of telemedicine, online patient portals, and encrypted messaging is expanding the palette of communication choices in health care (Barbosa, Zhou, Waddell, Myers, & Dorsey, 2021). Contributions from health psychologists will be needed to mitigate potential cognitive overload in these mediated environments while improving the specificity of health information in an era of personalized medicine (Hesse, Arora, & Klein, 2016).

Knowledge Generation

Digital technologies can inform discovery in health psychology. For instance, we can gather contextually rich information on predictors and outcomes of key health behaviors by using digitally triggered prompts in real time through techniques such as ecological momentary assessment (Perski, Keller, et al., 2022). Based on the data gathered about the individual, we can then gain insight into psychological data patterns, how they impact health behaviors and outcomes over time, and how they can be used to provide personalized, just-in-time adaptive interventions (i.e., JITAI, see Nahum-Shani et al., 2015; Perski, Hebert, et al., 2022). Moreover, wearable devices and remote sensing equipment can obviate the need for self-report (Shum et al., 2022) and, by extension, can create data streams with greater variety, volume, and velocity than was previously possible (Hesse, Moser, & Riley, 2015). This advancement in data collection methodology will allow health psychologists to conduct studies that can provide the abundance of data needed to tailor interventions, fueling a movement coined by some as "precision behavioral medicine" (Stump, Spring, Marchese, Alshurafa, & Robinson, 2019).

We can use technology to learn about the individual, but we can also capitalize on it to learn about populations and to predict data trends through advanced analytic techniques, such as those associated with machine learning (e.g., Hsu, Ahern, & Suzuki, 2020). Machine learning uses pattern-recognition techniques to generate data-informed predictions of future outcomes, to automatically stratify individuals into similarly conditioned categories, and to anticipate who is most likely to be affected by a specific condition or to benefit from a specific (psychological or other) intervention. Here, too, digital technologies can be useful in generating the behavioral data needed to seed newer generations of these machine learning algorithms and to provide the computational power required for processing large swathes of data. Individual data can be contributed with consent through patient-reported outcomes (McMorrow et al., 2021), through mobile sensing devices (California Institute for Telecommunications and Information Technology, 2014), and from designated data fields extracted from a patient's electronic health record (Etheredge, 2007). It is not uncommon to find a sense of "data altruism" among many members of the general public who, in the spirit of true citizen science, wish to contribute data for the betterment of their own communities (Hesse et al., 2021). During the SARS-CoV-2 pandemic, for example, citizens of multiple countries contributed individual-level data on exposure status, screening results, and disease progression in the hopes of enabling more efficient contact tracing while accelerating the pace of scientific discovery. Once volunteered, individual-level data can be melded with other public health datasets to guide population health discovery, policies, and interventions.

Knowledge Integrators

In a timely article published in the *Journal of the American Medical Association*, two thought leaders in medical informatics argued that for medicine to advance in the 21st century, digital infrastructures (e.g., Electronic Health Records) must become both *safer and smarter* in design (Johnson & Stead, 2022). By *smarter*, the authors called for sociotechnical systems that, in essence, would offer greater *cognitive support* for clinicians, patients, and their caregivers and that would *integrate knowledge* ahead of time to inform medical decision-making in more efficient and accurate ways. Health psychologists, who understand how humans process information, are responding by crafting technologies designed to integrate data and evidence into actionable knowledge. These so-called knowledge integrators are crucially needed to support timely and reliable decision-making. Hsu and colleagues offer a glimpse of how efficient knowledge integration might work by using machine learning algorithms to reduce vast amounts of behavioral data from wearable sensors into personalized, just-in-time support for relapse prevention for persons struggling with addiction problems (Hsu et al., 2020). Similarly, health educators have been developing integrative mechanisms to help patients cope with the morass of conflicting information on the open Web by offering up personalized "information prescriptions" to relevant articles and data (Andersen, 2013). Patient portals, serving as a patient's interface to their underlying electronic health record, can work well as knowledge integrators by offering a go-to source for interpreting laboratory results over time, accessing notes from previous office visits, and providing a historical record of vaccinations, therapies, and medications (Ahern, Woods, Lightowler, Finley, & Houston, 2011).

Personal Connected Health Devices

The increased use of personal phones and connected smart devices across both high- and low-income settings allows for wide implementation of mobile phone applications (apps) that are used for self-monitoring (e.g., step counts) and treatment (e.g., mindfulness apps or run tracking). Smartphones and wearables are increasingly used to intervene and improve health behavior and health outcomes. Although an abundance of mobile health apps can be found within the app stores of popular mobile operating systems, only a small fraction of those available programs have undergone formal and systematic evaluation. In 2017, the IQVIA Institute reported that only 0.18% of 325,000 publicly available apps were rigorously evaluated (IQVIA Institute, 2017). To further complicate matters, continued engagement with mobile phone apps can often be an issue. It is estimated that approximately 25% of health apps are only used once, and only 10% of the users continue to engage with health apps that they installed a week after download (Appboy, 2016).

A recent review of mobile health tools and virtual reality therapies (specifically in psychotherapy, clinical rehabilitation, and addiction treatment) has shown that these mobile health tools constantly evolve, but as they evolve, they are finding greater use by health psychologists due to multiple advantages, including relatively low cost and versatility (Caponnetto & Casu, 2022). Smoking cessation apps were reported as the most widespread, followed by apps used for managing alcohol use disorder (Caponnetto & Casu, 2022). Wearable devices have also been gaining in popularity for use in clinical care and in psychological treatment. Factors that predefine the successful implementation of personal devices in health care are described in terms of (a) a clearly defined role and problem that the personal devices are tackling, (b) integration into health-care delivery, (c) technology support provided if and when needed, (d) personalized and tailored experience, (e) alignment with reimbursement models (especially in the fee-for-service health-care settings), and (f) inclusion of clinical advocates who promote and encourage the use of wearables (Passos et al., 2021). Although much progress has been made in aligning personal health devices with standards of care, the devices' full potential has yet to be realized. Future success will depend heavily on designing devices and their applications with their intended users but also in close collaboration with the prescribers and commissioners.

Telemedicine

Unlike other areas covered, telemedicine as a whole is inherently digital. While numerous definitions have been put forth, on the most basic level telemedicine refers to the use of information and communication technologies to deliver care to patients (Sood et al., 2007). It can involve a diverse range of practices, including direct care via telephone or video call, use of remote monitoring devices, and clinical support provided via asynchronous communication such as text message or email (Grady et al., 2011; Hailey, Roine, & Ohinmaa, 2008). Additionally, it can involve care provided by a licensed medical professional or support offered by health coaches or navigators (Gordon et al., 2017).

Telemedicine has evolved notably in the past decade in terms of its evidence base. A number of studies have demonstrated robust clinical outcomes and non-inferiority to in-person clinical care (Bashshur, Shannon, Bashshur, & Yellowlees, 2016; Hilty et al., 2013; Hubley, Lynch, Schneck, Thomas, & Shore, 2016; Varker, Brand, Ward, Terhaag, & Phelps, 2019). A recent meta-analysis of health coaching across multiple domains of behavioral health showed similarly robust effects (An & Song, 2020). Likewise, studies suggest that telemedicine can be met with high patient satisfaction (Kruse et al., 2017). Thus, in the domain of telemedicine, key opportunities lie in the areas of implementation and optimization.

Major leaps have been made in the implementation of telemedicine since the onset of the SARS-CoV-2 pandemic, which necessitated rapid, widespread implementation. In the United States, a national survey found a twelvefold increase in the use of telemedicine by outpatient psychologists (Pierce, Perrin, Tyler, McKee, & Watson, 2021). While this unprecedented public health crisis left clinicians with little choice as to whether to adopt telemedicine, experiences during the pandemic likely shaped attitudes and confidence in ways that may have an enduring impact even when as face-to-face treatment becomes feasible again. Indeed, recent studies of provider attitudes (previously considered a key driver of low uptake; Wade, Eliott, & Hiller, 2014) suggest a shift toward positive attitudes related to telemedicine both among patients and providers (De Simone, Franco, Servillo, & Vargas, 2022; Lipschitz et al., 2022; Taha et al., 2022).

One area of interest is how to maintain and optimize the use of telemedicine and telehealth moving forward. Current wisdom in this area points to the importance of systems-level factors such as reimbursement and integration into routine care in determining the viability of telemedicine across future contexts (Barbosa et al., 2021; Lipschitz et al., 2022). Similarly, significant work has been done to address potential disparities in access to telemedicine (Chunara et al., 2021; Nouri, Khoong, Lyles, & Karliner, 2020), which limit clinical impact. Additionally, interest has mounted in building insight into how to effectively build virtual provider-patient relationships (Modic, Neuendorf, & Windover, 2020), with special attention given to understanding which patients may be most appropriate for remote care (Lipschitz et al., 2022). Addressing these factors is essential for improving the viability and utility of this telemedicine moving forward.

Diagnostics

One emerging area in digital health is the opportunity for digital technologies to play a role in diagnostics via digital phenotyping. Digital phenotyping refers to the moment-to-moment quantification of the individual-level human phenotype, in situ, using data from personal digital devices (Onnela & Rauch, 2016). Personal digital devices, such as smartphones (e.g., iPhones, Androids) and smartwatches (e.g., Fitbits), convert physiological and psychosocial information from patients' day-to-day lives into an electrical signal, which, in turn, can produce objective data on a variety of indicators particularly important for identifying onset or worsening of a variety of health conditions. These methods carry tremendous potential to facilitate more effective diagnostics across many areas of psychology and medicine, and despite this being a nascent field, studies have already generated some evidence that digital phenotyping methods can be useful in areas ranging from cardiovascular disease risk (Teo et al., 2019) to asthma (Jaimini et al., 2018) to mood disorders (Jacobson, Weingarden, & Wilhelm, 2019). While digital phenotyping focuses on a wide array of data, health behavior measures such as daily activity, sleep efficiency, social activity, and self-reported emotional health are key pieces of the digital phenotyping picture.

Similarly, learning health systems that utilize digital phenotyping or high-frequency digital self-reports, among other data collected in routine care, have shown significant promise for improving the accuracy and efficiency of diagnostic practices. Such systems may involve integration of data from wearables or digitally administered ecological momentary assessments to improve prediction of diagnosis and treatment responses. One example of such a system, the Epilepsy Learning Healthcare System (Donahue et al., 2021), illustrates the promise of this approach, as well as the integral role health psychology will play in developing and implementing such systems. In the next decade, we expect that such systems will be applied much more broadly across other areas of disease with opportunities to better understand how health behaviors contribute to disease onset and progression and to deliver just-in-time adaptive interventions.

Imaging

There are at least three ways in which imaging technologies have interfaced with the psychological sciences thus far, with more opportunities certain to develop as imaging technologies advance. On the *discovery* side, functional magnetic resonance imaging has already contributed substantively to our understanding of how the brain functions. Discoveries should accelerate as laboratories share brain scan imaging through collaborative projects such as the Brain Research through Advancing Innovative Neurotechnologies (BRAIN) initiative (Tardif et al., 2016). On the *medical practice* side, the perceptual and sensory sciences routinely contribute to the development of procedures and interfaces that allow diagnosticians to make full use of digital imaging technologies. Feature detection principles drawn from AI research laboratories make it possible to identify a significant portion of potential tumors in an automated reading of, say, a digital mammogram. Perceptual scientists can then work with interface designers and radiologic specialists to design a sociotechnical system that will support an accurate assignment of "hits" into true and false positives while also helping to minimize the risk of false negatives (Horowitz & Rensink, 2016). On the *therapeutic* side, health psychologists have made early use of virtual reality imaging to help place veterans into a peaceful state for coping with post-traumatic stress symptoms (Katz et al., 2020), to provide therapeutic desensitization of anxiety-inducing stimuli (Arnfred et al., 2021), and to provide teens with the psychosocial tools they need to resist addictive impulses (Baumann & Sayette, 2006).

An emerging area of imaging science with promise to health psychology may be in the area of augmented reality (AR). In essence, AR refers to the integration of digital information with the user's environment in real time. Using AR technology, images have been successfully superimposed onto heads-up displays in automobiles, onto specially designed glasses, onto walls and other physical spaces, and through the digital cameras embedded in smartphones. As AR imaging gains broader acceptance, it is possible to envision a world in which multilingual patients gain assistance in navigating complex health-care systems through real-time translations of signage or medical instructions. Similarly, it is possible to envision a practice in which wayfinding and safety cues can be built into the navigational displays of automobiles or smartphones to prevent exposure to toxic environments, to encourage physical activity, or to guide individuals toward healthy resources in stores or neighborhoods. Indeed, studies of players engaged in the AR game *Pokémon Go* have repeatedly demonstrated a statistically significant (albeit clinically modest) effect on the number of daily steps taken by game players engaged in the physical activity of hunting down virtual avatars in their augmented physical world (Khamzina, Parab, An, Bullard, & Grigsby-Toussaint, 2020).

Pharmaceuticals

One type of behavioral target that has attracted considerable attention from health psychologists is adherence to therapeutic regimens or pharmaceutical prescriptions. In 2012, estimates suggested that up to 75% of patients struggle with taking medications according to prescription, while 33% to 69% of medication-related hospital admissions were tied back to pharmaceutical nonadherence (Benjamin, 2012). Memory aids, caregiver communications, and other types of scaffolding have been offered to alleviate the problem. Digital technologies extend that capacity (Karekla et al., 2019). Mobile devices can replace or supplement at-home pill dispensers, with the added advantage of offering electronic prompts through cell phones or electronic watches (Rollman, Muldoon, & Magnani, 2022). Error-trapping routines within the programming modules can ensure that a patient does not erroneously miss a day, as may occur with at-home dispensers. Communication capabilities can invoke additional monitoring by care teams or family members as a further safeguard (Donovan, Hall, Ling, Smith, & Wilkes, 2022).

Pharmaceutical companies have been aggressively experimenting with Electronic Medical Packaging (EMP), which relies on embedded sensors (e.g., in the caps of pill bottles) to detect medication consumption and then offer digital prompts and summaries for patient use and/or for use as part of an integrated medication event monitoring protocol. Early data suggest little to no improvement for the patient-only interfaces but moderate to high improvements for integrated solutions (Checchi, Huybrechts, Avorn, & Kesselheim, 2014). Remote monitoring systems used to track patient-reported outcomes on adverse events have demonstrated statistically significant improvements on patients' medical outcomes and quality of life (Basch et al., 2022) and, in theory, could also serve as a source of post-marketing data on pharmaceutical side effects. Electronic monitoring and error-trapping on the clinical side may have contributed to a ten-year decline in medication errors and adverse events in hospitals, as reported by the Medicare Patient Safety Monitoring System in the United States (Eldridge et al., 2022).

Implantable Devices

In a frequently viewed TEDx Talk, cardiac patient Hugo Campos described the uphill battle he faced in requesting personal access to data recorded from a cardiac defibrillator implanted in his own chest. What Campos wanted to do, explained patient rights activist Dave deBronkart (*ePatient Dave*), was "use his heart's data to save his own life." More broadly, Campos was helping to catalyze a movement in which patients would be allowed to move "from being mere passengers to responsible drivers of their health" (deBronkart, 2012). Campos's case contributed to legal rulings around the world aimed at preventing "data blocking," which in turn contributed to new opportunities for health psychologists to utilize previously inaccessible data from implanted medical devices to bolster patients' capacity for self-determination. The case also became a rallying point for individuals in the "Quantified Self" movement, a movement driven toward the prospects of improving self-knowledge and health through biosensing measurements (Feng, Mantymaki, Dhir, & Salmela, 2021).

Although the adoption of patient-facing interfaces to provide access to these data has been slow thus far, ethical and legal frameworks do offer a path forward in providing patients with the data they need to govern their own health care in the future (Cohen, Gerke, & Kramer, 2020). As health psychologists tackle the problem in the future, we anticipate that they will be able to follow principles derived from self-determination theory (Ryan & Deci, 2017) to (a) preserve patients' sense of autonomy, even when considering the implications of implanted devices; (b) build skills/competence when interpreting biofeedback from implanted devices; and (c) nurture a better sense of relatedness, or connectedness, to their care teams and caregivers. In the not-too-distant future, work on brain-machine interfaces will suggest the feasibility of enhancing afferent (carrying signals from sensory receptors) and even efferent (sending signals to muscles and glands) capacity through neural implantation (Musk & Neuralink, 2019). Needless to say, expertise in neurophysiology, cognition, human factors, and health psychology combined will be needed to ensure that these implantable devices are deployed in ways that are conducive to patients' ethical protection and psychological well-being.

Surgical

Digital sensor monitoring applications for perioperative preparation and post-operative outcome evaluation have emerged across multiple chronic conditions (Memon et al., 2021). Digital applications hold promise in enhancing long-term follow-up and evaluation of functional results following robot-assisted radical prostatectomy for prostate cancer (Leandro et al., 2020). Although at an early stage, existing evidence suggests that harnessing mobile health technology can reduce secondary cardiovascular disease incidence and can improve health outcomes and quality of life (Schorr et al., 2021). Patient-reported outcomes (PROs) collected using digital technologies such as patient portals and tailored apps have been shown to assess long-term outcomes postoperatively and by making those assessments actionable to improve outcomes over time (Basch et al., 2022), including reduced mortality rates (Basch et al., 2017). In another example, digital technologies can help engage patients in understanding the risks and benefits of total joint replacement and provide education support for managing their post-surgical recovery (Lane-Carlson & Kumar, 2012). In sum, the role of measurement-based care, enabled by digital technologies, can "provide a picture of real-world patient functioning" and support postsurgical monitoring and feedback (Chiauzzi & Wicks, 2021).

Personalized Therapeutics

Our research has shown that goals are more likely to be enacted if they are specific, personally relevant, and pursued for autonomous motives (Kwasnicka, Ntoumanis, et al., 2021). These principles apply to the use of technology that needs to be tailored and suitable to users. Health goals are easier to meet if they are flexible and adjustable. Technologies that adjust to accommodate personalized goals flexibly do a better job at maintaining user engagement over time, where engagement and disengagement with a health goal are related to what is currently relevant and important to the given person (Kwasnicka, Ntoumanis, et al., 2021). These are issues worth considering when we encourage users to interact with technology and use it to improve health outcomes.

Moreover, innovations in the modalities through which users interact with health-related technologies show promise in helping to personalize behavioral support and therapeutic care. Richer visual displays can be tailored to offer a more culturally relevant experience with images, symbols, and a language that is in greater harmony with a user's background and self-image (Kreuter & Wray, 2003). Advances in conversational agent technologies, such as those that power 'Siri' or 'Alexa', can be leveraged to provide a more personalized and responsive environment for care (Dingler, Kwasnicka, Wei, Gong, & Oldenburg, 2021). Conversational agents can function as 'digital companions' that sit in a person's home; they are voice activated, and they can serve several health-related functions – they can book medical appointments, give reminders about medications, proactively 'check in' to gather information about the individual, and provide condition relevant information to supplement learning about, e.g., health behavior change, condition management. They can also 'memorize' the users (based on voice recognition), and they can 'speak' several languages, allowing them to be scaled easily across different countries. Together with an unobtrusive and continuous data collection, conversational agents can provide novel and deeply personalized access to digital health care and are likely to become an important part of future health-care delivery.

Geospatial and Environmental

The proliferation of smartphones in health applications brought with it increased access to the geolocation capabilities available through global positioning systems (GPS), along with expanded access to geographical data through map-based geographic information systems (GIS). This expanded capacity has allowed intervention designers to create just-in-time prompts based on locality. In one illustrative application, an intervention designed for individuals struggling with alcoholism allowed users to identify location-specific trigger points, such as bars and after-hours lounges. The system could then send fortifying alerts to the user, warning them when they have entered one of their triggering environments (Gustafson et al., 2011). In another example, users with respiratory issues were recruited into a 'participatory sensing' study in which individuals were encouraged to post measurements of air quality accompanied by GPS tags from their mobile devices. The results of those collection efforts were posted daily on a community-accessible map, giving others with breathing difficulties intelligence on what parts of the community to avoid in their own daily exercise or travel (Burke et al., 2006). The reciprocal nature of giving data back to the community while benefiting from the data contributions of others reflects what some experts have referred to as the "me side" (using GPS/GIS data for personal interventions) and the "we side" (using data for community benefit) of these technologies (King, Glanz, & Patrick, 2015). There should be ample opportunity for health psychologists to explore both sides of the equation in the years to come.

Another way to conceptualize opportunities in the geospatial and environmental space is to take the perspective of environmental psychology. Environmental psychology seeks to understand how the natural and built environments exert influence on behavior. Interventionists seek to create environments that are conducive to better health, say in lobbying for bike paths or healthier food options for children in school environments. As one of the founders of environmental psychology, Dan Stokols, has pointed out, the contemporary built environment is infused with digital technology. These technologies can, and should, be used as a source of contextual data to enrich our understanding of how to create environments that are conducive to healthy behaviors. For that matter, digital environments also exert influence on behavior, as we have seen with the influence of social media on the flow of both beneficent and malevolent information. Creating environments that are healthy, both in the built and digital spaces, will continue to be a priority for health psychologists in the years to come (Stokols, 2018).

Conclusion

The trajectory of health psychology in the digital age has been one of expansive evolution. What started as an augmented analytic capacity held primarily within research institutions has moved into the mainstream of public health and medicine. As digital technologies come and go, we recommend keeping the following four principles in mind.

1 *Embrace an ethos of 'Open Science'*. The work ahead is too expansive to tackle alone; it requires an ethos of transparency and collaboration embodied by an 'open science' philosophy. Open science approaches – defined as a range of scientific activities that aim to increase transparency, reproducibility, and discoverability of data, tools, code, and design features – are gaining popularity in health psychology (Norris & O'Connor, 2019). As a case in point, the Open Digital Health (ODH) organization was established to promote and accelerate health promotion, self-management, and treatment (Kwasnicka et al., 2022). Founding members of the ODH recognized that in order to benefit from recent technological advancements in a manner that would elevate health psychology globally, researchers needed to learn from each other and build upon each other's successes. The old model, in which teams of scientists worked on digital solutions independently and in isolation from each other, offered a limited set of opportunities for replicating and testing digital health interventions across contexts and settings. A new model based on transparency and collaboration should accelerate progress toward global health goals by improving access to effective interventions, encouraging interoperability between solutions, crowdsourcing solutions to common problems, and decreasing health disparities within and between countries (Shneiderman, 2022).
2 *Expand access to behavioral and mental health services*. Much of the enthusiasm behind digital health is driven by the opportunity to expand access to behavioral and mental health services. Behavioral health has for decades been riddled with the issue of inaccessibility. In plain language, traditional modes of service delivery cannot accommodate the demand for services—there are not enough trained providers, weekly transportation and daytime appointments are often not feasible, and the cost is often too high. Digitalization of the diagnosis, treatment, and monitoring processes can go a long way to address these backlog problems. Digital tools for psychological treatment can be widely disseminated at minimal marginal cost, and they do not require transportation or daytime appointments. As an added benefit, they promote patient autonomy (Knowles et al., 2014). The promise of expanding access via digitalization of psychological diagnosis and treatments, however, will require careful implementation and an eye toward optimization. Implementation in this context refers to how these tools are woven into the broader fabric of care provided to patients. Optimization here refers to how and when to use digital versus more standard in-person services. We must keep in mind that the goal is to provide broader access so that patients and the public can thrive and not limit the availability of tried-and-true services (Lipschitz et al. 2022).
3 *Address social determinants, ensure health equity*. The SARS-CoV-2 pandemic put a spotlight on the ever-present health inequities in the United States and globally (Callison & Ward, 2021). Emerging digital technologies offer the

opportunity to address long-standing disparities in health-care access, quality, and improved health outcomes by enabling underserved communities to receive timely, high-quality treatment and support services that defy the boundaries of geography and income (Hesse, Ahern, Ellison, et al., 2020). The social determinants of health (e.g., access to adequate housing, nutrition, transportation) are recognized as critical factors in ensuring adequate access to health care and improved health status. Broadband connectivity increasingly is also recognized as a social determinant of health in that it can enable traditionally underserved communities to benefit from the best treatments and health-care services by overcoming the obstacles of distance and other transportation barriers (Benda, Veinot, Sieck, & Ancker, 2020). As noted previously in this chapter, telemedicine and telehealth became essential during the pandemic for individuals to receive necessary health-care services. But digital access is not distributed equally, and therefore gaps in health equity have become more apparent. The key takeaway from the experience of the pandemic is that it is imperative that all populations have affordable access to broadband connectivity in order to ensure equal access to optimal health and health care (Zelmer, Sheikh, Zimlichman, & Bates, 2022).

4 *Target the 'quadruple aim' in health and health care.* When considering the behavioral affordances offered by digital technologies, it is easy to lose track of the bigger picture of how systems come together to produce health. Current thinking emphasizes a 'quadruple aim' for system improvement: (a) to optimize the patient experience; (b) to improve population health, with a particular focus on reducing inequities; (c) to reduce costs, both economically and in terms of human suffering; and (d) to protect the well-being and productivity of health-care workers. Keeping this quadruple aim in mind when engaging in digital health research should help orient researchers to the overall consequences of individual interventions across systems. The scientific literature is replete with examples of digital health technologies that failed to scale because their designers could not make an argument for overall cost savings or that led to an increase in burden on the shoulders of well-meaning clinical staff precipitating clinical 'burnout' (Wachter, 2017). In a similar vein, digital health technologies will fail at the population level if they end up contributing to, rather than reducing, health disparities.

A Final Caveat

The renowned British physician Sir Cyril Chantler once observed that medicine "used to be *simple*, *ineffective*, and relatively *safe*. Now it is *complex*, *effective*, and potentially *dangerous*" (Chantler, 1999; italics added). In many respects, the same could be said about the role of health psychology in the digital age. As we demonstrated throughout this chapter, the work ahead may be complex and intricate, but it aligns directly with the World Health Organization's strategic plans for improving health and health care worldwide. It has the potential to improve health and well-being at unprecedented scales. The stakes are high though. We know from recent history that if applied incorrectly, these same technologies carry the danger of derailing social systems, disrupting evidence-based practice, proliferating misinformation, and compounding disparities. Health psychology must serve as a stabilizing force to accentuate the positive while minimizing the negative consequences of evolutionary change in digital health.

Further Reading

Abernethy, A. P., Adams, L., Barrett, M., Bechtel, C., Brennan, P., Butte, A., … Valdes, K. (2022b). *The Promise of Digital Health: Then, Now, and the Future*. Washington, DC: National Academies Press. https://nam.edu/the-promise-of-digital-health-then-now-and-the-future/

Kwasnicka, D., Keller, J., Perski, O., Potthoff, S., Ten Hoor, G. A., Ainsworth, B., … Sanderman, R. (2022a). White Paper: Open Digital Health – accelerating transparent and scalable health promotion and treatment. *Health Psychol Rev*, 1–17. doi:10.1080/17437199.2022.2046482

World Health Organization (2021). *Global strategy on digital health 2020-2025*. Geneva, Switzerland: World Health Organization. License: CC BY-NC-SA 3.0 IGO.

References

Abernethy, A. P., Adams, L., Barrett, M., Bechtel, C., Brennan, P., Butte, A., … Valdes, K. (2022). *The Promise of Digital Health: Then, Now, and the Future*. Retrieved from Washington, DC: https://nam.edu/the-promise-of-digital-health-then-now-and-the-future/

Ahern, D. K., Braun, I. M., Cooley, M. E., & Bickmore, T. (2016). Oncology Informatics: Behavioral and Psychological Sciences. In B. W. Hesse, D. K. Ahern, & E. Beckjord (Eds.), *Oncology Informatics: Using Health Information Technology to Improve Processes and Outcomes in Cancer Care* (pp. 231–251). Boston, MA: Elsevier.

Ahern, D. K., Phalen, J. M., & Mockenhaupt, R. E. (2003). Science and the advancement of eHealth: a call to action. *Am J Prev Med*, *24*(1), 108–109. doi:10.1016/s0749-3797(02)00565-2

Ahern, D. K., Woods, S. S., Lightowler, M. C., Finley, S. W., & Houston, T. K. (2011). Promise of and potential for patient-facing technologies to enable meaningful use. *Am J Prev Med*, *40*(5 Suppl 2), S162–172. doi:10.1016/j.amepre.2011.01.005

Alfano, C. M., Mayer, D. K., Beckjord, E., Ahern, D. K., Galioto, M., Sheldon, L. K., … Hesse, B. W. (2020). Mending Disconnects in Cancer Care: Setting an Agenda for Research, Practice, and Policy. *JCO Clin Cancer Inform*, *4*, 539–546. doi:10.1200/CCI.20.00046

An, S., & Song, R. (2020). Effects of health coaching on behavioral modification among adults with cardiovascular risk factors: Systematic review and meta-analysis. *Patient Educ Couns*, *103*(10), 2029–2038. doi:10.1016/j.pec.2020.04.029

Andersen, C. M. (2013). Information therapy: a prescription for the digital era. *Health Care Manag (Frederick)*, *32*(3), 242–245. doi:10.1097/HCM.0b013e31829d766b

Anyoha, R. (2017). The History of Artificial Intelligence. Retrieved from https://sitn.hms.harvard.edu/flash/2017/history-artificial-intelligence/

Appboy. (2016). *Mobile customer retention report: An analysis of retention by day*. Retrieved from New York, NY.

Arnfred, B. T., Bang, P., Winther Davy, J., Larsen, L. Q., Hjorthøj, C., & Christensen, A. B. (2021). Virtual reality exposure in cognitive behavioral group therapy for social anxiety disorder: A qualitative evaluation based on patients' and therapists' experiences. *Translational Issues in Psychological Science*, *7*(3), 229–247. doi:10.1037/tps0000291

Barbosa, W., Zhou, K., Waddell, E., Myers, T., & Dorsey, E. R. (2021). Improving Access to Care: Telemedicine Across Medical Domains. *Annu Rev Public Health*, *42*, 463–481. doi:10.1146/annurev-publhealth-090519-093711

Basch, E., Deal, A. M., Dueck, A. C., Scher, H. I., Kris, M. G., Hudis, C., & Schrag, D. (2017). Overall Survival Results of a Trial Assessing Patient-Reported Outcomes for Symptom Monitoring During Routine Cancer Treatment. *JAMA*, *318*(2), 197–198. doi:10.1001/jama.2017.7156

Basch, E., Schrag, D., Henson, S., Jansen, J., Ginos, B., Stover, A. M., … Dueck, A. C. (2022). Effect of Electronic Symptom Monitoring on Patient-Reported Outcomes Among Patients With Metastatic Cancer: A Randomized Clinical Trial. *JAMA*, *327*(24), 2413–2422. doi:10.1001/jama.2022.9265

Bashshur, R. L., Shannon, G. W., Bashshur, N., & Yellowlees, P. M. (2016). The Empirical Evidence for Telemedicine Interventions in Mental Disorders. *Telemed J E Health*, *22*(2), 87–113. doi:10.1089/tmj.2015.0206

Baumann, S. B., & Sayette, M. A. (2006). Smoking cues in a virtual world provoke craving in cigarette smokers. *Psychol Addict Behav*, *20*(4), 484–489. doi:10.1037/0893-164X.20.4.484

Benda, N. C., Veinot, T. C., Sieck, C. J., & Ancker, J. S. (2020). Broadband Internet Access Is a Social Determinant of Health! *Am J Public Health*, *110*(8), 1123–1125. doi:10.2105/AJPH.2020.305784

Benjamin, R. M. (2012). Medication adherence: helping patients take their medicines as directed. *Public Health Rep*, *127*(1), 2–3. doi:10.1177/003335491212700102

Burke, J., Estrin, D., Hansen, M., Parker, A., Ramanathan, N., Reddy, S., & Srivastava, M. B. (2006). *Participatory Sensing*. Paper presented at the Workshop on World-Sensor Web (WSW '06): Mobile Device Centric Sensor Networks and Applications. https://citeseer.ist.psu.edu/viewdoc/summary?doi=10.1.1.122.3024

California Institute for Telecommunications and Information Technology. (2014). *Personal Data for the Public Good: New Opportunities to Enrich Understanding of Individual and Population Health*. Retrieved from Princeton, NJ.

Callison, K., & Ward, J. (2021). Associations Between Individual Demographic Characteristics And Involuntary Health Care Delays As A Result Of COVID-19. *Health Aff (Millwood)*, *40*(5), 837–843. doi:10.1377/hlthaff.2021.00101

Cameron, L. D., & Leventhal, H. (2003). *The self-regulation of health and illness behaviour*. London; New York: Routledge.

Caponnetto, P., & Casu, M. (2022). Update on Cyber Health Psychology: Virtual Reality and Mobile Health Tools in Psychotherapy, Clinical Rehabilitation, and Addiction Treatment. *Int J Environ Res Public Health*, *19*(6). doi:10.3390/ijerph19063516

Chantler, C. (1999). The role and education of doctors in the delivery of health care. *Lancet*, *353*(9159), 1178–1181. doi:10.1016/S0140-6736(99)01075-2

Checchi, K. D., Huybrechts, K. F., Avorn, J., & Kesselheim, A. S. (2014). Electronic medication packaging devices and medication adherence: a systematic review. *JAMA*, *312*(12), 1237–1247. doi:10.1001/jama.2014.10059

Chiauzzi, E., & Wicks, P. (2021). Beyond the Therapist's Office: Merging Measurement-Based Care and Digital Medicine in the Real World. *Digit Biomark*, *5*(2), 176–182. doi:10.1159/000517748

Chunara, R., Zhao, Y., Chen, J., Lawrence, K., Testa, P. A., Nov, O., & Mann, D. M. (2021). Telemedicine and healthcare disparities: a cohort study in a large healthcare system in New York City during COVID-19. *J Am Med Inform Assoc*, *28*(1), 33–41. doi:10.1093/jamia/ocaa217

Cohen, I. G., Gerke, S., & Kramer, D. B. (2020). Ethical and Legal Implications of Remote Monitoring of Medical Devices. *Milbank Q*, *98*(4), 1257–1289. doi:10.1111/1468-0009.12481

Coiera, E. (2004). Four rules for the reinvention of health care. *BMJ*, *328*(7449), 1197–1199. doi:10.1136/bmj.328.7449.1197

De Simone, S., Franco, M., Servillo, G., & Vargas, M. (2022). Implementations and strategies of telehealth during COVID-19 outbreak: a systematic review. *BMC Health Serv Res*, *22*(1), 833. doi:10.1186/s12913-022-08235-4

deBronkart, D. (2012). Hugo Campos at TEDx Cambridge: "Gimme My Damn Data," Defibrillator Edition. Retrieved from https://participatorymedicine.org/epatients/2012/01/hugo-campos-at-tedx-cambridge-gimme-my-damn-data-defibrillator-edition.html

Dingler, T., Kwasnicka, D., Wei, J., Gong, E., & Oldenburg, B. (2021). The Use and Promise of Conversational Agents in Digital Health. *Yearb Med Inform*, *30*(1), 191–199. doi:10.1055/s-0041-1726510

Donahue, M. A., Herman, S. T., Dass, D., Farrell, K., Kukla, A., Abend, N. S., ... Fureman, B. E. (2021). Establishing a learning healthcare system to improve health outcomes for people with epilepsy. *Epilepsy Behav*, *117*, 107805. doi:10.1016/j.yebeh.2021.107805

Donovan, G., Hall, N., Ling, J., Smith, F., & Wilkes, S. (2022). Influencing medication taking behaviors using automated two-way digital communication: A narrative synthesis systematic review informed by the Behavior Change Wheel. *Br J Health Psychol*, *27*(3), 861–890. doi:10.1111/bjhp.12580

Eldridge, N., Wang, Y., Metersky, M., Eckenrode, S., Mathew, J., Sonnenfeld, N., ... Krumholz, H. M. (2022). Trends in Adverse Event Rates in Hospitalized Patients, 2010–2019. *JAMA*, *328*(2), 173–183. doi:10.1001/jama.2022.9600

Etheredge, L. M. (2007). A rapid-learning health system. *Health Aff (Millwood)*, *26*(2), w107–118. doi:10.1377/hlthaff.26.2.w107

Eysenbach, G. (2000). Towards ethical guidelines for e-health: JMIR theme issue on eHealth ethics. *J Med Internet Res*, *2*(1), E7. doi:10.2196/jmir.2.1.e7

Farrell, S., & Lewandowsky, S. (2018). *Computational modeling of cognition and behavior*. New York, NY: Cambridge University Press.

Feng, S., Mantymaki, M., Dhir, A., & Salmela, H. (2021). How Self-tracking and the Quantified Self Promote Health and Well-being: Systematic Review. *J Med Internet Res*, *23*(9), e25171. doi:10.2196/25171

Fox, R. S., Moreno, P. I., Yanez, B., Estabrook, R., Thomas, J., Bouchard, L. C., ... Penedo, F. J. (2019). Integrating PROMIS(R) computerized adaptive tests into a web-based intervention for prostate cancer. *Health Psychol*, *38*(5), 403–409. doi:10.1037/hea0000672

Gordon, N. F., Salmon, R. D., Wright, B. S., Faircloth, G. C., Reid, K. S., & Gordon, T. L. (2017). Clinical Effectiveness of Lifestyle Health Coaching: Case Study of an Evidence-Based Program. *Am J Lifestyle Med*, *11*(2), 153–166. doi:10.1177/1559827615592351

Grady, B., Myers, K. M., Nelson, E. L., Belz, N., Bennett, L., Carnahan, L., ... Guidelines Working, G. (2011). Evidence-based practice for telemental health. *Telemed J E Health*, *17*(2), 131–148. doi:10.1089/tmj.2010.0158

Gustafson, D. H., Boyle, M. G., Shaw, B. R., Isham, A., McTavish, F., Richards, S., ... Johnson, K. (2011). An e-health solution for people with alcohol problems. *Alcohol Res Health*, *33*(4), 327–337. Retrieved from https://www.ncbi.nlm.nih.gov/pubmed/23293549

Hailey, D., Roine, R., & Ohinmaa, A. (2008). The effectiveness of telemental health applications: a review. *Can J Psychiatry*, *53*(11), 769–778. doi:10.1177/070674370805301109

Hesse, B. W. (2016). Decision Architectures. In M. A. Dieffenbach, S. M. Miller, & D. Bowen (Eds.), *Handbook of Health Decision Science* (pp. 15–28). New York, NY: Springer Verlag.

Hesse, B. W., Ahern, D. K., & Ellison, M. (2020). Barn-raising on the digital frontier: The L.A.U.N.C.H. Collaborative. *Journal of Appalachian Health*, *2*(1), 6–20. doi:https://doi.org/10.13023/jah.0201.02.

Hesse, B. W., Ahern, D. K., Ellison, M., Aronoff-Spencer, E., Vanderpool, R. C., Onyeije, K., ... Norman, D. A. (2020). Barn-Raising on the Digital Frontier: The L.A.U.N.C.H. Collaborative. *J Appalachian Health*, *2*(1), 6–20. doi:10.13023/jah.0201.02

Hesse, B. W., Arora, N. K., & Klein, W. M. (2016). Communication Science: Connecting Systems for Health. In *Oncology Informatics: Using Health Information Technology to Improve Processes and Outcomes in Cancer Care* (pp. 253–276). Boston, MA: Elsevier.
Hesse, B. W., Beckjord, E., Rutten, L. J., Fagerlin, A., & Cameron, L. D. (2015). Cancer communication and informatics research across the cancer continuum. *Am Psychol, 70*(2), 198–210. doi:10.1037/a0036852
Hesse, B. W., Conroy, D. E., Kwasnicka, D., Waring, M. E., Hekler, E., Andrus, S., … Diefenbach, M. A. (2021). We're all in this together: recommendations from the Society of Behavioral Medicine's Open Science Working Group. *Transl Behav Med, 11*(3), 693–698. doi:10.1093/tbm/ibaa126
Hesse, B. W., Moser, R. P., & Riley, W. T. (2015). From Big Data to Knowledge in the Social Sciences. *The Annals of the American Academy of Political and Social Science, 659*(May), 16–32.
Hesse, B. W., Nelson, D. E., Kreps, G. L., Croyle, R. T., Arora, N. K., Rimer, B. K., & Viswanath, K. (2005). Trust and sources of health information: the impact of the Internet and its implications for health care providers: findings from the first Health Information National Trends Survey. *Arch Intern Med, 165*(22), 2618–2624. Retrieved from http://www.ncbi.nlm.nih.gov/entrez/query.fcgi?cmd=Retrieve&db=PubMed&dopt=Citation&list_uids=16344419
Hesse, B. W., & Shneiderman, B. (2007). eHealth research from the user's perspective. *Am J Prev Med, 32*(5 Suppl), S97–103. Retrieved from http://www.ncbi.nlm.nih.gov/entrez/query.fcgi?cmd=Retrieve&db=PubMed&dopt=Citation&list_uids=17466825
Hilty, D. M., Ferrer, D. C., Parish, M. B., Johnston, B., Callahan, E. J., & Yellowlees, P. M. (2013). The effectiveness of telemental health: a 2013 review. *Telemed J E Health, 19*(6), 444–454. doi:10.1089/tmj.2013.0075
Horowitz, T. S., & Rensink, R. A. (2016). Extended Vision for Oncology: A Perceptual Science Perspective on Data Visualization and Medical Imaging. In B. W. Hesse, D. K. Ahern, & E. Beckjord (Eds.), *Oncology Informatics: Using Health Information Technology to Improve Processes and Outcomes in Cancer Care* (pp. 287–303). Boston, MA: Elsevier.
Hsu, M., Ahern, D. K., & Suzuki, J. (2020). Digital Phenotyping to Enhance Substance Use Treatment During the COVID-19 Pandemic. *JMIR Ment Health, 7*(10), e21814. doi:10.2196/21814
Hubley, S., Lynch, S. B., Schneck, C., Thomas, M., & Shore, J. (2016). Review of key telepsychiatry outcomes. *World J Psychiatry, 6*(2), 269–282. doi:10.5498/wjp.v6.i2.269
IQVIA Institute. (2017). *The Growing Value of Digital Health: Evidence and Impact on Human Health and the Healthcare System.* Retrieved from Parsippany, NJ: https://www.iqvia.com/-/media/iqvia/pdfs/institute-reports/the-growing-value-of-digital-health.pdf?_=1668712199256
Jacobson, N. C., Weingarden, H., & Wilhelm, S. (2019). Digital biomarkers of mood disorders and symptom change. *NPJ Digit Med, 2*, 3. doi:10.1038/s41746-019-0078-0
Jaimini, U., Thirunarayan, K., Kalra, M., Venkataraman, R., Kadariya, D., & Sheth, A. (2018). "How Is My Child's Asthma?" Digital Phenotype and Actionable Insights for Pediatric Asthma. *JMIR Pediatr Parent, 1*(2), e11988. doi:10.2196/11988
Johnson, K. B., & Stead, W. W. (2022). Making Electronic Health Records Both SAFER and SMARTER. *JAMA, 328*(6), 523–524. doi:10.1001/jama.2022.12243
Karekla, M., Kasinopoulos, O., Neto, D. D., Ebert, D. D., Van Daele, T., Nordgreen, T., … Jensen, K. L. (2019). Best practices and recommendations for digital interventions to improve engagement and adherence in chronic illness sufferers. *European Psychologist, 24*(1), 49–67. doi:10.1027/1016-9040/a000349
Katz, A. C., Norr, A. M., Buck, B., Fantelli, E., Edwards-Stewart, A., Koenen-Woods, P., … Andrasik, F. (2020). Changes in physiological reactivity in response to the trauma memory during prolonged exposure and virtual reality exposure therapy for posttraumatic stress disorder. *Psychol Trauma, 12*(7), 756–764. doi:10.1037/tra0000567

Khamzina, M., Parab, K. V., An, R., Bullard, T., & Grigsby-Toussaint, D. S. (2020). Impact of Pokemon Go on Physical Activity: A Systematic Review and Meta-Analysis. *Am J Prev Med, 58*(2), 270–282. doi:10.1016/j.amepre.2019.09.005

King, A. C., Glanz, K., & Patrick, K. (2015). Technologies to measure and modify physical activity and eating environments. *Am J Prev Med, 48*(5), 630–638. doi:10.1016/j.amepre.2014.10.005

Knowles, S. E., Toms, G., Sanders, C., Bee, P., Lovell, K., Rennick-Egglestone, S., … Bower, P. (2014). Qualitative meta-synthesis of user experience of computerised therapy for depression and anxiety. *PLoS One, 9*(1), e84323. doi:10.1371/journal.pone.0084323

Kreuter, M. W., & Wray, R. J. (2003). Tailored and targeted health communication: strategies for enhancing information relevance. *Am J Health Behav, 27 Suppl 3*, S227–232. doi:10.5993/ajhb.27.1.s3.6

Kruse, C. S., Krowski, N., Rodriguez, B., Tran, L., Vela, J., & Brooks, M. (2017). Telehealth and patient satisfaction: a systematic review and narrative analysis. *BMJ Open, 7*(8), e016242. doi:10.1136/bmjopen-2017-016242

Kvedar, J. C., Colman, C., & Cella, G. (2015). *The Internet of Healthy Things*. Boston, MA: Partners HealthCare Connected Health.

Kwasnicka, D., Kale, D., Schneider, V., Keller, J., Yeboah-Asiamah Asare, B., Powell, D., … Perski, O. (2021). Systematic review of ecological momentary assessment (EMA) studies of five public health-related behaviours: review protocol. *BMJ Open, 11*(7), e046435. doi:10.1136/bmjopen-2020-046435

Kwasnicka, D., Keller, J., Perski, O., Potthoff, S., Ten Hoor, G. A., Ainsworth, B., … Sanderman, R. (2022). White Paper: Open Digital Health – accelerating transparent and scalable health promotion and treatment. *Health Psychol Rev*, 1–17. doi:10.1080/17437199.2022.2046482

Kwasnicka, D., Luszczynska, A., Hagger, M. S., Quested, E., Pagoto, S. L., Verboon, P., … Naughton, F. (2020). Theory-based digital intervention to promote weight loss and weight loss maintenance (Choosing Health): protocol for a randomised controlled trial. *BMJ Open, 10*(11), e040183. doi:10.1136/bmjopen-2020-040183

Kwasnicka, D., Ntoumanis, N., & Sniehotta, F. F. (2021). Setting performance and learning goals is useful for active and inactive individuals, if goals are personalized and flexible: commentary on Swann et al. (2020). *Health Psychol Rev, 15*(1), 51–55. doi:10.1080/17437199.2020.1762107

Lane-Carlson, M. L., & Kumar, J. (2012). Engaging patients in managing their health care: patient perceptions of the effect of a total joint replacement presurgical class. *Perm J, 16*(3), 42–47. doi:10.7812/TPP/11-143

Leandro, F., Reis, S., Leite, K., Arnaldo Shiomi da Cruz, J., Pimenta, R., Viana, N., … Passerotti, C. (2020). Digital application developed to evaluate functional results following robot-assisted radical prostatectomy: App for prostate cancer. *Computer Methods and Programs in Biomedicine, 197*(105683). doi:https://doi.org/10.1016/j.cmpb.2020.105683

Lipschitz, J. M., Connolly, S. L., Van Boxtel, R., Potter, J. R., Nixon, N., & Bidargaddi, N. (2022). Provider perspectives on telemental health implementation: Lessons learned during the COVID-19 pandemic and paths forward. *Psychol Serv*. doi:10.1037/ser0000625

Masachusetts Institute of Technology. (2011). *The third revolution: The convergence of life sciences, physical sciences, and engineering*. Retrieved from Washington, DC.

McMorrow, R., Hunter, B., Hendrieckx, C., Kwasnicka, D., Cussen, L., Ho, F. C. S., … Manski-Nankervis, J. A. (2021). Effect of routinely assessing and addressing depression and diabetes distress using patient-reported outcome measures in improving outcomes among adults with type 2 diabetes: a systematic review protocol. *BMJ Open, 11*(3), e044888. doi:10.1136/bmjopen-2020-044888

Memon, A., Lec, P., Lenis, A., Sharma, V., Wood, E., Schade, G., & Brisbane, W. (2021). Relationship between mobile digital sensor monitoring and perioperative outcomes: Systematic review. *JMIR Perioper Med*, *4*(1), e21571. doi:10.2196/21571

Modic, M. B., Neuendorf, K., & Windover, A. K. (2020). Enhancing your webside manner: Optimizing opportunities for relationship-centered care in virtual visits. *J Patient Exp*, *7*(6), 869–877. doi:10.1177/2374373520968975

Musk, E., & Neuralink. (2019). An integrated brain-machine interface platform with thousands of channels. *J Med Internet Res*, *21*(10), e16194. doi:10.2196/16194

Nahum-Shani, I., Hekler, E. B., & Spruijt-Metz, D. (2015). Building health behavior models to guide the development of just-in-time adaptive interventions: A pragmatic framework. *Health Psychology*, *34*(Suppl), 1209–1219. doi:10.1037/hea0000306

Norman, D. A. (1990). *The design of everyday things* (1st Doubleday/Currency ed.). New York: Doubleday.

Norris, E., & O'Connor, D. B. (2019). Science as behaviour: Using a behaviour change approach to increase uptake of open science. *Psychology and Health*, *34*(12), 1397–1406.

Nouri, S., Khoong, E. C., Lyles, C. R., & Karliner, L. (2020). Addressing Equity in Telemedicine for Chronic Disease Management During the Covid-19 Pandemic. *NEJM Catalyst, May 4, 2020*, 1–13. doi:10.1056/CAT.20.0123

Onnela, J. P., & Rauch, S. L. (2016). Harnessing smartphone-based digital phenotyping to enhance behavioral and mental health. *Neuropsychopharmacology*, *41*(7), 1691–1696. doi:10.1038/npp.2016.7

Passos, J., Lopes, S. I., Clemente, F. M., Moreira, P. M., Rico-Gonzalez, M., Bezerra, P., & Rodrigues, L. P. (2021). Wearables and Internet of Things (IoT) Technologies for Fitness Assessment: A Systematic Review. *Sensors (Basel)*, *21*(16). doi:10.3390/s21165418

Perski, O., Hebert, E. T., Naughton, F., Hekler, E. B., Brown, J., & Businelle, M. S. (2022). Technology-mediated just-in-time adaptive interventions (JITAIs) to reduce harmful substance use: A systematic review. *Addiction*, *117*(5), 1220–1241. doi:10.1111/add.15687

Perski, O., Keller, J., Kale, D., Asare, B. Y., Schneider, V., Powell, D., … Kwasnicka, D. (2022). Understanding health behaviours in context: A systematic review and meta-analysis of ecological momentary assessment studies of five key health behaviours. *Health Psychol Rev*, *16*(4), 576–601. doi:10.1080/17437199.2022.2112258

Pierce, B. S., Perrin, P. B., Tyler, C. M., McKee, G. B., & Watson, J. D. (2021). The COVID-19 telepsychology revolution: A national study of pandemic-based changes in U.S. mental health care delivery. *Am Psychol*, *76*(1), 14–25. doi:10.1037/amp0000722

President's Cancer Panel. (2016). *Improving Cancer-Related Outcomes with Connected Health*. Retrieved from Washington, DC.

Rice, R. E., & Katz, J. E. (2001). *The Internet and health communication: experiences and expectations*. Thousand Oaks, CA: Sage Publications.

Riley, W. T., Rivera, D. E., Atienza, A. A., Nilsen, W., Allison, S. M., & Mermelstein, R. (2011). Health behavior models in the age of mobile interventions: Are our theories up to the task? *Transl Behav Med*, *1*(1), 53–71. doi:10.1007/s13142-011-0021-7

Rollman, B. L., Muldoon, M. F., & Magnani, J. W. (2022). Four "E"s to speed adoption of mHealth and promote cardiovascular behavioral medicine. *Health Psychol*. doi:10.1037/hea0001171

Ryan, R. M., & Deci, E. L. (2017). *Self-determination theory: Basic psychological needs in motivation, development, and wellness*. New York, NY: The Guilford Press.

Schorr, E. N., Gepner, A. D., Dolansky, M. A., Forman, D. E., Park, L. G., Petersen, K. S., … Cardiometabolic, H. (2021). Harnessing mobile health technology for secondary cardiovascular disease prevention in older adults: A scientific statement from the American Heart Association. *Circ Cardiovasc Qual Outcomes*, *14*(5), e000103. doi:10.1161/HCQ.0000000000000103

Shneiderman, B. (1987). *Designing the user interface: strategies for effective human-computer interaction*. Reading, MA: Addison-Wesley.
Shneiderman, B. (2022). *Human-Centered AI*. Oxford, UK: Oxford University Press.
Shum, L. C., Faieghi, R., Borsook, T., Faruk, T., Kassam, S., Nabavi, H., … Iaboni, A. (2022). Indoor Location Data for Tracking Human Behaviours: A Scoping Review. *Sensors (Basel)*, *22*(3). doi:10.3390/s22031220
Sood, S., Mbarika, V., Jugoo, S., Dookhy, R., Doarn, C. R., Prakash, N., & Merrell, R. C. (2007). What is telemedicine? A collection of 104 peer-reviewed perspectives and theoretical underpinnings. *Telemed J E Health*, *13*(5), 573–590. doi:https://doi.org/10.1089/tmj.2006.0073
Stokols, D. (2018). *Social ecology in the digital age: Solving complex problems in a globalized world*. London; Cambridge, MA: Academic Press, an imprint of Elsevier.
Stoloff, M. L., & Couch, J. V. (1988). *Computer use in psychology: A directory of software, 2nd ed*. Washington, DC: American Psychological Association.
Stump, T. K., Spring, B., Marchese, S. H., Alshurafa, N., & Robinson, J. K. (2019). Toward a precision behavioral medicine approach to addressing high-risk sun exposure: a qualitative analysis. *JAMIA Open*, *2*(4), 547–553. doi:10.1093/jamiaopen/ooz034
Taha, A. R., Shehadeh, M., Alshehhi, A., Altamimi, T., Housser, E., Simsekler, M. C. E., … Alhajri, N. (2022). The integration of mHealth technologies in telemedicine during the COVID-19 era: A cross-sectional study. *PLoS One*, *17*(2), e0264436. doi:10.1371/journal.pone.0264436
Taplin, S. H., Weaver, S., Salas, E., Chollette, V., Edwards, H. M., Bruinooge, S. S., & Kosty, M. P. (2015). Reviewing cancer care team effectiveness. *J Oncol Pract*, *11*(3), 239–246. doi:10.1200/JOP.2014.003350
Tardif, C. L., Schafer, A., Trampel, R., Villringer, A., Turner, R., & Bazin, P. L. (2016). Open science CBS neuroimaging repository: Sharing ultra-high-field MR images of the brain. *Neuroimage*, *124*(Pt B), 1143–1148. doi:10.1016/j.neuroimage.2015.08.042
Teo, J. X., Davila, S., Yang, C., Hii, A. A., Pua, C. J., Yap, J., … Lim, W. K. (2019). Digital phenotyping by consumer wearables identifies sleep-associated markers of cardiovascular disease risk and biological aging. *Commun Biol*, *2*, 361. doi:10.1038/s42003-019-0605-1
Varker, T., Brand, R. M., Ward, J., Terhaag, S., & Phelps, A. (2019). Efficacy of synchronous telepsychology interventions for people with anxiety, depression, posttraumatic stress disorder, and adjustment disorder: A rapid evidence assessment. *Psychol Serv*, *16*(4), 621–635. doi:10.1037/ser0000239
Wachter, R. M. (2017). *The digital doctor: hope, hype, and harm at the dawn of medicine's computer age*. New York: McGraw-Hill Education.
Wade, V. A., Eliott, J. A., & Hiller, J. E. (2014). Clinician acceptance is the key factor for sustainable telehealth services. *Qual Health Res*, *24*(5), 682–694. doi:10.1177/1049732314528809
Willems, R. A., Lechner, L., Verboon, P., Mesters, I., Kanera, I. M., & Bolman, C. A. (2017). Working mechanisms of a web-based self-management intervention for cancer survivors: A randomised controlled trial. *Psychol Health*, *32*(5), 605–625. doi:10.1080/08870446.2017.1293054
Zelmer, J., Sheikh, A., Zimlichman, E., & Bates, D. W. (2022). Transforming care and outcomes with digital health through and beyond the pandemic. *NEJM Catalyst*, *3*(5), 1–14. doi:10.1056/CAT.22.0053

39

SIX WAYS HEALTH PSYCHOLOGY CAN CONTRIBUTE TO CLIMATE CHANGE MITIGATION AND ADAPTATION

Guillaume Chevance and Paquito Bernard

Introduction

Human activities over the last two centuries have resulted in increased greenhouse gases (GHG) emissions and ultimately the sharp warming of our planet (Steffen et al., 2015). Global surface temperature has increased by 1.09°C compared to the preindustrial period (1850–1900; Intergovernmental Panel on Climate Change, IPCC, 2018). Although many governments have considered climate change as a national safety and security threat, a few have initiated some of the necessary transformations required to mitigate its impacts and adapt to it; even the most ambitious actions taken to date are insufficient to slow down global emissions. For any near-term GHG emissions scenario possible under current structural, political, and economic conditions, global surface temperatures are expected to continue to increase until at least mid-century (IPCC, 2018). Current policies and actions are estimated to be taking us to +2.7 °C global warming by 2100 compared to the 1850–1900 baseline temperature (Climate Analytics and New Climate Institute, 2022).

The aforementioned scenario leads to dangerous Earth system trajectories and potential catastrophic consequences, including mass mortality related to food and water shortages, state fragility and international and local conflicts (Kemp et al., 2022). Temperatures of more than 2°C above preindustrial values have not been sustained on Earth's surface since before the Pleistocene Epoch, more than 2.6 million years ago. This is profoundly important because human civilisation did not develop under the conditions that prevailed three million years ago, and

DOI: 10.4324/9781003318026-47

whether our current civilisations can live and thrive in such a climate is unknown. Limiting the worst consequences of climate change requires quick radical behavioural, economic, and societal transformation simultaneously. We believe that health psychology can contribute to this challenge beyond what has been done in other related disciplines, such as environmental psychology.

Through this chapter, our aim is to motivate health psychology researchers and practitioners to redirect some of their research activities towards climate change–related topics. Climate change is defined in the present chapter according to the IPCC definition: "[A] change in the state of the climate that can be identified by changes in the mean and/or the variability of its properties and that persists for an extended period, typically decades or longer". The present chapter notably focuses on the problems caused by anthropogenic climate change, such as rising temperatures, increasing occurrence and intensity of extreme weather events, air pollution, or, again, rising sea levels. The COVID-19 pandemic shows that our scientific community can quickly generate vast amounts of new practical knowledge in record time on topics that are only partially familiar to us. Imagine what could be achieved in one year if, similar to COVID-19, our scientific community shifted to focus on climate mitigation and adaptation. To accelerate this transition, and as a starting point, this chapter proposes six research topics that the field of health psychology and behavioural medicine could take on: (1) behavioural adaptation to climate change; (2) the behavioural aspects of climate change mitigation; (3) health equity; (4) rebound effects in behavioural science; (5) the interplay between behaviours, well-being and energy consumption; and (6) mental health in context of climate change.

Fostering Behavioural Adaptation to Climate Change

We have summarised the impact of climate change on health behaviours in a previous literature review (Chevance et al., 2022). Here, we proposed that climate change is associated with health behaviours through at least two different pathways: (*i*) direct and indirect (or mediated) effects and (*ii*) in the form of behavioural shocks and secular trends. An example of direct effects includes the impact of heat extremes on human physiology and subsequent consequences in terms of physical activity, while indirect effects include, for instance, the impact of hurricanes on sleep via mental health issues such as post-traumatic stress disorders. Behavioural shocks and secular trends refer to the time scales at which climate change can impact behaviours, with extreme weather events leading to situations of emergency in the short term (i.e., behavioural shocks) and slower secular changes in the climate impacting our behaviours in the long run, such as progressive temperature increases and their behavioural effects over several years/decades (see Chevance et al., 2022 for a literature review).

Although relatively few studies have documented the effects of climate-related outcomes on health behaviours (Berrang-Ford et al., 2021), we argue here that it is too late to conduct more observational studies on this topic. In our opinion, the evidence of the disruptive effects of climate change on health and health behaviours is strong, or 'good enough', to avoid wasting time on the (re)estimation of these effects. Instead, the urgent situation requires us to directly invest time and energy in scalable quasi-experimental or interventional studies that could help individuals and communities cope with the negative consequences of climate change (Brown et al., 2022). To our knowledge, very few health behaviour change interventions have been (*i*) specifically designed to help individuals cope with climate outcomes (e.g., how should we promote active transportation in the context of high levels of air pollution) or (*ii*) simply implemented in the context of environmental threats (e.g., how to prevent sleep disorders or dehydration in the context of extreme heat).

Health psychologists are potential key actors in the design, implementation, and evaluation of such interventions. Using our traditional toolboxes, such as the experimental medicine approach to health behaviour change (Sheeran et al., 2017), interventions could focus on individuals, as we are used to, but also on communities (Okvat & Zautra, 2011), or even at larger scales by evaluating and refining the impact of national plans on behavioural outcomes in the context of climate change (Chaloupka et al., 2012). To foster this transition, seeking new collaborations with colleagues skilled in climate and health sciences, planetary health or environmental health and epidemiology will be key. Our experience is that many researchers with a background in these disciplines are keen to transition to more human-centred and interventional initiatives and have few skills compared with us health psychologists when it comes to conducting this type of interventional research. Behavioural and mental adaptation to climate change is in its infancy, and people with a background in health psychology could have a key impact in this domain.

Accelerating Mitigation Efforts

The Intergovernmental Panel on Climate Change suggests the classification of human behaviours into two categories: adaptation and mitigation behaviours (IPCC, 2018). The latter is defined as proactive efforts "*to reduce emissions or enhance the sinks* of *greenhouse gasses*". However, in a consequentialist perspective, all mitigation behaviours are not equal in terms of carbon footprint reduction. For instance, recycling and less frequent car use are considered low and high-impact behaviours, respectively. Unfortunately, a large part of previous research, notably in environmental psychology, has focused on low-impact behaviours, such as recycling (Nielsen et al., 2021), instead of highly impactful ones, such as eating fewer animal products, reducing car use, lowering residential energy use, having fewer children, and decreasing flying frequency (Akenji et al., 2019).

Three main behaviours can be considered as high win-win behaviours for health psychologists interested in health and environmental co-benefits (Bernard, 2019; see also Inauen et al., 2021). First, a meat- and fish-free diet is associated with an individual carbon footprint reduction of 35% and a reduced total and cause-specific mortality (Fresán & Sabaté, 2019). Second, car driving is a major determinant of GHG emissions and local air pollution, and, in parallel, high frequency of car use is related to a higher risk of cardiovascular disease (Patterson et al., 2020). Shifting from car to active transport is also a protective factor of depressive disorders and enhanced well-being. Third, housing energy use is the second-largest carbon footprint source of households behind motorised transports (see Akenji et al., 2019) and is increasingly vital for maintaining good health via adequate temperatures and humidity management, particularly for individuals with scarce economic resources (Jessel et al., 2019). For instance, improved home insulation has been shown to be associated with reduced hospital admissions, incidence and severity of chronic respiratory disease, and improved quality of life (Fyfe et al., 2020).

Mitigation efforts could also be designed to reorganise health systems practices. Indeed, the international health-care sector had a climate footprint equivalent to almost 5% of global net emissions (Health Care Without Harm, 2019). In other words, if health systems were treated as a country, it would be the fifth-largest emitter on the planet. Health-care carbon footprint represents a sizeable percentage of high-income countries' footprints (7.6% United States, 6.7% Switzerland, 6.4% Japan, 6% United Kingdom; Health Care Without Harm, 2019). Thus, the health-care supply chain, infrastructure, and health-care delivery have to be decarbonised. It implies major cultural changes for health care by focusing more on prevention of non-communicable diseases than carbon-intensive care and hospitalisation (Hensher & Zywert, 2020). In practice, health psychologists could contribute to decreasing patients' emissions related to transportation – for example, via tele-consultations or health monitoring at home – and strengthen their efforts to prevent unplanned hospitalisations or complications among patients with chronic diseases via primary prevention. By doing this, the community would contribute to health-care decarbonisation.

Finally, evidence-based psychological and behavioural interventions should be re-designed with regard to their carbon footprints and not only their clinical effectiveness. Traditionally, clinical outcomes and cost-effectiveness are the key indicators to develop guidelines and organise health-care practices. We argue here that carbon effectiveness, the carbon emissions per health gain produced, should also now be considered before scaling up an intervention. For instance, a study showed that smoking cessation delivery modes have different carbon footprints (Smith et al., 2013). They range from high for group or individual counselling (>16 tonnes of CO_2 for 1,000 smokers) to low for short messages or phone calls (<8 tonnes of CO_2 for 1,000 smokers – here the text message support was the most carbon-effective strategy; Smith et al., 2013). From a planetary health perspective, text message support or telemedicine could be more frequently implemented, while less carbon-effective strategies like individual counselling could be delivered to non-responsive smokers only via, for example, Sequential Multiple Assignment Randomised Trials (Collins, Murphy & Strecher, 2007). Health psychologists should now balance clinical effectiveness and carbon effectiveness before scaling up interventions.

Putting Health Equity at the Heart of Any Initiatives

The current climate situation is unfair: (*i*) our current generation and the previous one are responsible for the high emissions, but the worst effects of climate change will be experienced by today's children who do not have control over those situations; (*ii*) the bottom 50% of low-income countries are responsible for only 15% of global emissions but are also those that are already suffering more from climate change and have fewer resources to cope with it; (*iii*) within-countries, a similar pattern is observed, as a strong correlation exists between income and per capita emissions, the higher emitters are the high-income social groups, and people living in socially disadvantaged areas, or with fewer financial resources, are expected to experience more difficulties coping with the health consequences of climate change because of lower rate of access to air conditioning or effective home insulation (Chevance et al., 2022).

These forms of inequity should be at the heart of any interventions and initiatives led by health psychologists. We argue that mitigation efforts should first target wealthy individuals that have the most resource-intensive lifestyle within- and between- countries. The question of intergenerational inequity is difficult to approach. The most consequential decisions today are almost certainly being influenced by intergenerational delay discounting (i.e., countries' focus on short-term vs long-term gains). The field of health psychology could play a role by developing interventions manipulating this construct of delay discounting, which has been relevant for understanding health behaviours in the past (Daugherty & Brase, 2010). Studying and monitoring adolescents' and children's health in this specific context of climate change is also crucial.

Finally, climate change is also expected to impact the health of women and men differently, particularly in low- and middle-income countries (Chevance et al., 2022). For example, rising temperatures could substantially worsen the health impacts of menopause, notably hot flashes. Men could experience other risks, such as suicide due to extreme weather events impacting their occupational activities, such as droughts, in Indian farmers. In parallel, it has been argued that the promotion of climate-friendly policies was associated with a reduction in gender inequality on a worldwide scale (Andrijevic et al., 2020). Based on this, the field of health psychology should consciously monitor and seek to understand and address any disparities that might manifest in relation to sex or gender when developing projects in the domains of climate change and health.

Accounting for Rebound Effects When Promoting Behaviour Change

The adoption of new behaviours such as meat consumption reduction or technologies like electric car use in health or climatic perspectives can sequentially produce new behaviours in individuals. For example, an increase in electricity consumption has been observed in recent adopters of solar panels. This phenomenon is called rebound (Santarius & Soland, 2018) or spillover effects (Geiger et al.,

2021). It can be positive when the new behaviour comes with the adoption of other healthy or climate-friendly behaviours or negative when the adoption of a new behaviour leads to the adoption of other unhealthy or carbon-intensive behaviours. Indeed, new behaviours or technologies can produce some gains in terms of financial, psychological, and temporal resources. For instance, shifting from car to bike use for daily commuting can be associated with money saving. However, if this money is then spent on long-distance vacations and air travel, a negative rebound effect has occurred from an environmental perspective. Also, shopping in plastic-free grocery stores can improve the shopper's green self-identity. However, this new identity, developed by adopting low-impact behaviours, can licence more carbon-intensive behaviours such as long-distance trips and negatively impact the person's overall environmental footprint. In contrast, as an example of an attempt to encourage positive rebound effects in behavioural interventions through incentivisation, new shared electric bike adopters have been offered a 12-month discount for vegetarian meals (York et al., 2022).

Several individual factors are associated with positive or negative rebound effects in behaviour change interventions (Santarius & Soland, 2018). Improved self-efficacy after the adoption of a first behaviour is associated with a higher occurrence of the positive rebound effect. In contrast, having a low income, moral licencing, and compensatory beliefs phenomena are related to negative rebound effects (Santarius & Soland, 2018). In the longer term, rebound effects are also driven by organisational and economic factors, such as energy price, production processes, ancillary applications, and tax credit or exemption.

Possible negative rebound effects should be anticipated in health behaviour change interventions targeting environmental co-benefits. For instance, shifting from car to active transport for daily commuting can be associated with an increase in individual food-related greenhouse gas emissions due to increased energy expenditure (Mizdrak et al., 2020) or a reduction of leisure-related physical activities (Brondeel et al., 2019). Conversely, health behaviour change interventions can also be designed to foster positive rebound effects. A positive behavioural rebound effect occurs more frequently when interventions are autonomy-supportive, provide a strong rationale, do not use financial (dis)incentives, and address normative and personal gain goals (Geiger et al., 2021). For example, an intervention promoting cycling for daily commuting to work could include booster sessions or a second phase designed to include bicycle travel in other life domains.

Decoupling Energy Use, Health, and Well-Being

Many mainstream "solutions" to climate change emphasise the role of technological innovations for climate change mitigation without really questioning our energy-intensive lifestyles and daily behaviours (Akenji et al., 2019). Although we have seen fantastic improvements in energy efficiency over the last few years, technological promises have enabled rapid, effective, and fair mitigation measures (McLaren & Markusson, 2020). The scale of the issue and the urgency are so important that efficiency improvements alone (i.e., replacing objects, like a car, with less carbon-intensive ones but without changing the pattern of utilisation) will not be sufficient in limiting global warming (IPCC, 2022). Two other options exist: (*i*) modal shift (e.g., using public transport instead of cars) and (*ii*) absolute reduction, what we refer to here as 'sufficiency' (e.g., reducing physical consumption of goods and services, such as travelling less instead of travelling differently). In the following paragraphs, we address the challenge of staying healthy with less energy consumption and how health psychologists could contribute to this challenge, notably in high-income countries where the most efforts with regard to lifestyle changes need to be made.

It is crucial to keep in mind that, at the global scale, 85% of our energy comes from fossil fuels (i.e., oil, coal, and gas; see the following graph: https://ourworldindata.org/global-energy-200-years); other major sources being biomass such as wood, nuclear power and hydro-power, and then other renewables like wind and solar energy representing only a tiny percentage of our global energy mix (i.e., around 5%). Therefore, drastically reducing our utilisation of fossil fuels, and thus limiting global warming, will very likely imply a decrease in the quantity and intensity of our daily activities in the way we travel, eat, and consume; again, especially in high-income countries where wealthy individuals have the most resource-intensive lifestyles. To quantify this, a recent report concluded that current per capita lifestyle carbon footprints – which corresponds to the energy consumed at the scale of an individual via their transport, housing, food, goods, and leisure – in high-income countries need to decrease by around 90% by 2050 (in a scenario where global warming is limited to + 1.5°C by 2100 and without extensive use of carbon removal technologies; Akenji et al., 2019). We are not arguing here that the whole responsibility for achieving this target (i.e.,−90%) is on individuals, and, obviously, major structural and political changes will be needed to live within socio-economic contexts that facilitate such lifestyles. But, still, radical behaviour changes towards more sufficiency are needed if we want to safeguard our climate; in explicit terms, travelling less, buying and consuming less of anything, and in a way accepting that we need to cut back on our energy-intensive lifestyles.

The health psychology community could contribute to this transition notably by addressing the challenge of decoupling energy consumption from health outcomes or, in other words, by studying how to stay healthy in societies where we would consume less of everything (Bernard, 2019; Büchs & Koch, 2019). Indeed, positive correlations between energy consumption, at the scale of an individual or a country, and well-being or life expectancy are well demonstrated in the literature (O'Neill et al., 2018). One emerging challenge is thus this decoupling of energy use and health. Especially in high-income countries, well-being relies extensively on the (over)consumption of goods and services.[1] Consuming and travelling less, for example, could thus be seen as a loss of quality of life. Accompanying this transition and monitoring how a decrease in consumption is associated with health markers could be a new topic of research for health psychologists. To our opinion, preparing our societies towards more sufficiency would be both a mitigation measure (i.e., reducing our lifestyle carbon footprints) and, given the current geo-political context, also an adaptation strategy. As we are writing this chapter, in the autumn of the year 2022, the conflict in Ukraine poses serious threats to some European countries with regard to their energy supply, illustrating the fact that, within the current geo-political context, sufficiency should not only be seen as a democratically planned set of actions but also something that could be imposed by the context.

Designing Mental Health Interventions Relevant to Climate Change

From well-being to severe mental disorders, all mental health indicators are and will be severely worsened by climate change (Lawrance et al., 2021). The direct mental health consequences of climate change are related to extreme events, rising temperature, and air pollution. Exposure to climate-related events results in higher rates of mental disorders (Lawrance et al., 2021). Floods, droughts, and wildfires have been associated with higher risk of anxiety, stress, and mood-related disorders. This is particularly concerning because negative psychological impacts from any form of natural disasters exceed physical injuries by a ratio of 40 to 1 (Lawrance et al., 2021). Heat waves exacerbate suicidal thoughts and suicide attempt rates in the general population and symptoms among people with pre-existing mental health disorders. It also increases demands and disruptions of mental health-care services. Finally, short-term exposure to air pollutants (e.g., fine particulate matter) has been associated with increased daily hospital admissions and emergency visits for mental disorders (Bernardini et al., 2020). Exposure to air pollution during childhood is associated with an increased risk of developing psychotic and depressive disorders (Antonsen et al., 2020).

Indirect effects of climate change can also deteriorate mental health, such as rising eco-anxiety (i.e., the fear of environmental collapse that comes from observing the seemingly irrevocable impact of climate change and the associated concern for one's future and that of next generations) and forced migration due to environmental degradation (e.g., sea rising) or social disruptions (e.g., food supply). Uncertainty about the future and a growing communication about climate change–related risks are major sources of eco-anxiety. Eco-anxiety has increased worldwide during the last decade. Authors of a ten-country study concluded that 45% of included adolescents had major worries about future climate change consequences for their daily lives (Hickman et al., 2021). Medium to strong associations between eco-anxiety, depression, and stress have been previously found (Heeren & Asmundson, 2022). In parallel, a moderate level of eco-anxiety has also been associated with a greater likelihood of adoption of pro-environmental behaviours such as meat consumption reduction, active travel, or natural park visits (Heeren & Asmundson, 2022). Thus, young people or adults with a moderate eco-anxiety level could be more receptive to health behaviour change interventions targeting environmental co-benefits.

With regard to forced migration, the permanent or temporary relocation of people due to progressive environmental changes negatively affects their mental health. Studies carried out in countries with high vulnerability to climate change (e.g., the Philippines) showed that forced migration is a highly stressful experience exacerbated by a lack of social support and limited access to housing, health-care, and education. Forced migration consequences were an increased incidence of psychotic, phobic, and mood disorders and reduced self-esteem (Kelman et al., 2021). The (in)direct effects of climate change on public mental health and disadvantaged groups are well identified (Berry et al., 2018). Climate change disproportionately impacts the mental health of children and youth, women and girls, adults with pre-existing mental disorders, and Indigenous people (Berry et al., 2018). For instance, adults with psychotic disorders have a two- or three-times higher risk of death during heat waves than people without mental disorders (Berry et al., 2018). Health psychologists should construct action plans as a community-policy-research endeavour and produce scalable toolboxes incorporating evidence-based psychological interventions for mental disorders prevention and treatment in contexts relevant to climate change (Bernard, 2019). Their mode of delivery should be adapted to stable and crisis situations, as well as culturally tailored.

Conclusion: Living Well and Healthy in a Drastically Decarbonised World

Health psychology, as a community, has the potential to meaningfully contribute to climate change mitigation and adaptation. However, the principal risk for our community is to act too little and too late (Bernard & Chevance, 2023). On the mitigation side, the challenge is to keep or enhance well-being and health while reducing GHG emissions at all levels, from individuals, to health institutions, to countries. On the adaptation side, we need to accelerate our efforts to help individuals and communities to cope and stay resilient to a changing climate, with a focus on vulnerable populations in the short term. Actions need to be coordinated at all levels simultaneously without opposing individual behaviour changes with more systemic changes, and health psychologists should push to be involved in all types of initiatives, from designing individual behaviour change interventions to refining national plans that could have an impact on behavioural and/or psychological outcomes.

As a summary, the different sections of this chapter invite health psychologists to

- focus on behaviours with high health and environmental co-benefits such as meat reduction, active transportation, and behaviours relative to reducing household energy consumption;
- put health equity at the heart of any initiative, keeping in mind that, most of the time, adaptation efforts should target vulnerable groups, and mitigation efforts should target wealthy individuals;
- invest time and energy in experimental and quasi-experimental research, given the urgency of the situation and the fact that previous evidence is good enough to develop interventional initiatives over observational ones that could be redundant;

- account for potential rebound effects that could override all the results of an intervention because secondary effects have not been well anticipated; and
- seek multidisciplinary collaborations with experts in planetary health, climate science, or environmental epidemiology to develop win-win collaborations and bring together our skills in these fields of research.

We hope that this chapter will help motivate health psychologists to think critically about climate change and quickly reorient a part of their activities to contribute more directly to climate change mitigation and adaptation. In 2024, carbon dioxide emissions continue to rise by about 1% per year worldwide, and the 1.5°C global temperature threshold is expected to be exceeded by 2040 under most scenarios. We, as a community, have little time left to meaningfully contribute to climate change mitigation. We contend that climate change is among the most urgent issues facing all scientists and should become a central priority for the health psychology community.

Note

1 Of note, sufficiency involves intentional reduction of consumption and should not be confused with poverty where a reduction in consumption occurs, therefore most of the efforts here in terms of sufficiency concern wealthy individuals (see Akenji et al., 2019).

Further Reading

Bernard, P. (2019). Health psychology at the age of Anthropocene. *Health Psychology and Behavioral Medicine*, *7*(1), 193–201. https://doi.org/10.1080/21642850.2019.1617150

Chevance, G., Fresán, U., Hekler, E., Edmondson, D., Lloyd, S. J., Ballester, J., Litt, J., Cvijanovic, I., Araújo-Soares, V., & Bernard, P. (2022a). Thinking Health-related Behaviors in a Climate Change Context: A Narrative Review. *Annals of Behavioral Medicine*, kaac039. https://doi.org/10.1093/abm/kaac039

References

Akenji, L., Lettenmeier, M., Koide, R., Toivio, V., & Amellina, A. (2019). *1.5-Degree Lifestyles: Targets and options for reducing lifestyle carbon footprints*.

Andrijevic, M., Crespo Cuaresma, J., Lissner, T., Thomas, A., & Schleussner, C.-F. (2020). Overcoming gender inequality for climate resilient development. *Nature Communications*, *11*(1), Art. 1. https://doi.org/10.1038/s41467-020-19856-w

Antonsen, S., Mok, P. L. H., Webb, R. T., Mortensen, P. B., McGrath, J. J., Agerbo, E., Brandt, J., Geels, C., Christensen, J. H., & Pedersen, C. B. (2020). Exposure to air pollution during childhood and risk of developing schizophrenia: A national cohort study. *The Lancet Planetary Health*, *4*(2), e64–e73. https://doi.org/10.1016/S2542-5196(20)30004-8

Bernard, P. (2019). Health psychology at the age of Anthropocene. *Health Psychology and Behavioral Medicine*, *7*(1), 193–201. https://doi.org/10.1080/21642850.2019.1617150

Bernard, P., & Chevance, G. (2023). Health psychology and climate change: A race against time. *The European Health Psychologist*, *23*(1).

Bernardini, F., Trezzi, R., Quartesan, R., & Attademo, L. (2020). Air Pollutants and Daily Hospital Admissions for Psychiatric Care: A Review. *Psychiatric Services*, *71*(12), 1270–1276. https://doi.org/10.1176/appi.ps.201800565

Berrang-Ford, L., Sietsma, A. J., Callaghan, M., Minx, J. C., Scheelbeek, P. F. D., Haddaway, N. R., Haines, A., & Dangour, A. D. (2021). Systematic mapping of global research on climate and health: A machine learning review. *The Lancet Planetary Health*, *5*(8), e514–e525. https://doi.org/10.1016/S2542-5196(21)00179-0

Berry, H.L., Waite, T.D., Dear, K.B.G., Capon, A.G., & Murray, V. (2018). The case for systems thinking about climate change and mental health. *Nature Climate Change*, 8, 282–290. https://doi.org/10.1038/s41558-018-0102-4

Brondeel, R., Wasfi, R., Perchoux, C., Chaix, B., Gerber, P., Gauvin, L., Richard, L., Gaudreau, P., Thierry, B., Chevrier, M., Hoj, S., & Kestens, Y. (2019). Is older adults' physical activity during transport compensated during other activities? Comparing 4 study cohorts using GPS and accelerometer data. *Journal of Transport & Health*, *12*, 229–236. https://doi.org/10.1016/j.jth.2019.02.006

Brown, H. A., Topham, T. H., Clark, B., Smallcombe, J. W., Flouris, A. D., Ioannou, L. G., Telford, R. D., Jay, O., & Périard, J. D. (2022). Seasonal Heat Acclimatisation in Healthy Adults: A Systematic Review. *Sports Medicine (Auckland, N.Z.)*, *52*(9), 2111–2128. https://doi.org/10.1007/s40279-022-01677-0

Büchs, M. and Koch, M. (2019). Challenges for the degrowth transition: The debate about wellbeing. *Futures*, *105*, 155–165. https://doi.org/10.1016/j.futures.2018.09.002

Chaloupka, F. J., Yurekli, A., & Fong, G. T. (2012). Tobacco taxes as a tobacco control strategy. *Tobacco Control*, *21*(2), 172–180. https://doi.org/10.1136/tobaccocontrol-2011-050417

Chevance, G., Fresán, U., Hekler, E., Edmondson, D., Lloyd, S. J., Ballester, J., Litt, J., Cvijanovic, I., Araújo-Soares, V., & Bernard, P. (2022). Thinking health-related behaviors in a climate change context: A narrative review. *Annals of Behavioral Medicine*, kaac039. https://doi.org/10.1093/abm/kaac039

Climate Analytics and New Climate Institute. (2022). *Climate Action Tracker (2022). The CAT Thermometer*. Available at: https://climateactiontracker.org/global/cat-thermometer/

Collins, L.M., Murphy, S.A., & Strecher V. (2007). The Multiphase Optimization Strategy (MOST) and the Sequential Multiple Assignment Randomized Trial (SMART): New Methods for More Potent eHealth Interventions. *American Journal of Preventive Medicine*, 32(5), 112–118. https://doi.org/10.1016/j.amepre.2007.01.022

Daugherty, J. R., & Brase, G. L. (2010). Taking time to be healthy: Predicting health behaviors with delay discounting and time perspective. *Personality and Individual Differences*, *48*(2), 202–207. https://doi.org/10.1016/j.paid.2009.10.007

Fresán, U., & Sabaté, J. (2019). Vegetarian Diets: Planetary Health and Its Alignment with Human Health. *Advances in Nutrition*, *10*, S380–S388. https://doi.org/10.1093/advances/nmz019

Fyfe, C., Telfar, L., Barnard, Howden-Chapman, & Douwes, J. (2020). Association between home insulation and hospital admission rates: Retrospective cohort study using linked data from a national intervention programme. *BMJ*, m4571. https://doi.org/10.1136/bmj.m4571

Geiger, S. J., Brick, C., Nalborczyk, L., Bosshard, A., & Jostmann, N. B. (2021). More green than gray? Toward a sustainable overview of environmental spillover effects: A Bayesian meta-analysis. *Journal of Environmental Psychology*, *78*, 101694. https://doi.org/10.1016/j.jenvp.2021.101694

Health Care Without Harm. (2019). *Health's care carbon footprint*. https://healthcareclimateaction.org/sites/default/files/2021-05/HealthCaresClimateFootprint_092319.pdf

Heeren, A., & Asmundson, G. J. G. (2022). Understanding climate anxiety: What decision-makers, health care providers, and the mental health community need to know to promote adaptative coping. *Journal of Anxiety Disorders*, 102654. https://doi.org/10.1016/j.janxdis.2022.102654

Hensher, M., & Zywert, K. (2020). Can healthcare adapt to a world of tightening ecological constraints? Challenges on the road to a post-growth future. *BMJ*, m4168. https://doi.org/10.1136/bmj.m4168

Hickman, C., Marks, E., Pihkala, P., Clayton, S., Lewandowski, R. E., Mayall, E. E., Wray, B., Mellor, C., & van Susteren, L. (2021). Climate anxiety in children and young people and their beliefs about government responses to climate change: A global survey. *The Lancet. Planetary Health*, *5*(12), e863–e873. https://doi.org/10.1016/S2542-5196(21)00278-3

Inauen, J., Contzen, N., Frick, V., Kadel, P., Keller, J., Kollmann, J., Mata, J., & van Valkengoed, A. M. (2021). Environmental issues Are health issues: Making a case and setting an agenda for environmental health psychology. *European Psychologist*, *26*(3), 219–229. https://doi.org/10.1027/1016-9040/a000438

IPCC, I. P. on C. (2018). *Global warming of 1.5°C*. http://www.ipcc.ch/report/sr15/

IPCC, I. P. on C. (2022). *Climate Change 2022: Mitigation of Climate Change Contribution of Working Group III to the Sixth Assessment*.

Jessel, S., Sawyer, S., & Hernández, D. (2019). Energy, Poverty, and Health in Climate Change: A Comprehensive Review of an Emerging Literature. *Frontiers in Public Health*, *7*, 357. https://doi.org/10.3389/fpubh.2019.00357

Kelman, I., Ayeb-Karlsson, S., Rose-Clarke, K., Prost, A., Ronneberg, E., Wheeler, N., & Watts, N. (2021). A review of mental health and wellbeing under climate change in small island developing states (SIDS). *Environmental Research Letters*, *16*(3), 033007. https://doi.org/10.1088/1748-9326/abe57d

Kemp, L., Xu, C., Depledge, J., Ebi, K. L., Gibbins, G., Kohler, T. A., Rockström, J., Scheffer, M., Schellnhuber, H. J., Steffen, W., & Lenton, T. M. (2022). Climate Endgame: Exploring catastrophic climate change scenarios. *Proceedings of the National Academy of Sciences*, *119*(34), e2108146119. https://doi.org/10.1073/pnas.2108146119

Lawrance, E., Thompson, R., Fontana, G., & Jennings, N. (2021). *The impact of climate change on mental health and emotional wellbeing: Current evidence and implications for policy and practice*. Imperial College London. https://doi.org/10.25561/88568

McLaren, D., & Markusson, N. (2020). The co-evolution of technological promises, modelling, policies and climate change targets. *Nature Climate Change*, *10*(5), Art. 5. https://doi.org/10.1038/s41558-020-0740-1

Mizdrak, A., Cobiac, L. J., Cleghorn, C. L., Woodward, A., & Blakely, T. (2020). Fuelling walking and cycling: Human powered locomotion is associated with non-negligible greenhouse gas emissions. *Scientific Reports*, *10*(1), Art. 1. https://doi.org/10.1038/s41598-020-66170-y

Nielsen, K. S., Cologna, V., Lange, F., Brick, C., & Stern, P. C. (2021). The case for impact-focused environmental psychology. *Journal of Environmental Psychology*, *74*, 101559. https://doi.org/10.1016/j.jenvp.2021.101559

Okvat, H. A., & Zautra, A. J. (2011). Community gardening: A parsimonious path to individual, community, and environmental resilience. *American Journal of Community Psychology*, *47*(3–4), 374–387. https://doi.org/10.1007/s10464-010-9404-z

O'Neill, D. W., Fanning, A. L., Lamb, W. F., & Steinberger, J. K. (2018). A good life for all within planetary boundaries. *Nature Sustainability*, *1*(2), 88–95.

Patterson, R., Panter, J., Vamos, E. P., Cummins, S., Millett, C., & Laverty, A. A. (2020). Associations between commute mode and cardiovascular disease, cancer, and all-cause mortality, and cancer incidence, using linked Census data over 25 years in England and Wales: A cohort study. *The Lancet Planetary Health*, *4*(5), e186–e194. https://doi.org/10.1016/S2542-5196(20)30079-6

Santarius, T., & Soland, M. (2018). How Technological Efficiency Improvements Change Consumer Preferences: Towards a Psychological Theory of Rebound Effects. *Ecological Economics*, *146*, 414–424. https://doi.org/10.1016/j.ecolecon.2017.12.009

Sheeran, P., Klein, W. M. P., & Rothman, A. J. (2017). Health Behavior Change: Moving from Observation to Intervention. *Annual Review of Psychology*, *68*(1), 573–600. https://doi.org/10.1146/annurev-psych-010416-044007

Smith, A. J. B., Tennison, I., Roberts, I., Cairns, J., & Free, C. (2013). The carbon footprint of behavioural support services for smoking cessation. *Tobacco Control*, *22*(5), 302–307. https://doi.org/10.1136/tobaccocontrol-2012-050672

Steffen, W., Broadgate, W., Deutsch, L., Gaffney, O., & Ludwig, C. (2015). The trajectory of the Anthropocene: The Great Acceleration. *The Anthropocene Review*, *2*(1), 81–98. https://doi.org/10.1177/2053019614564785

York, R., Adua, L., & Clark, B. (2022). The rebound effect and the challenge of moving beyond fossil fuels: A review of empirical and theoretical research. *WIREs Climate Change*, *13*(4), e782. https://doi.org/10.1002/wcc.782

40

POLICY IMPLICATIONS – HEALTH PSYCHOLOGY AND THE CASE OF COVID-19

Gill A. ten Hoor and Robert A. C. Ruiter

How Health Psychology Could Play a Role at the Policy Level

Health psychologists have opportunities to effectively influence policy and practice: they have tools that are important for efficiently communicating health psychology science to policymakers and can eventually support evidence-informed policy and practice decisions. Health psychology, as a form of applied psychology, can contribute to health promotion: "[…] the process of enabling people to increase control over, and to improve their health. **It moves beyond a focus on individual behaviour towards a wide range of social and environmental interventions**" (https://www.who.int/). The definition of 'health psychology' as presented by the World Health Organisation (WHO) is broad but accurate: "[H]ealth psychology is about people's behaviour and about behaviour change". The definition correctly goes beyond the tendency to solve a behavioural problem at the individual level, as the solution to undesired behaviour often lies in a combination of change to both the individual behaviour and behaviours of the decision-makers in the surroundings of the individual.

In this chapter, the main focus is on how health psychology can influence individual behaviours by informing policy and policy changes at the environmental level. For that, we first define the 'agents' or stakeholders in charge of policy. Then, we explain how health psychologists could influence policy and practice effectively and what tools are important for efficiently communicating health psychology science to support evidence-informed policy and practice decisions. Health psychologists are sometimes project leads and sometimes are one of the stakeholders themselves, as part of broader teams that serve governments and organisations. The chapter ends with specific examples of how health psychology expertise actually influenced COVID-19-related policy, highlighting

DOI: 10.4324/9781003318026-48

a discrepancy between potential role versus real-life practice, as well as what lessons we learned from those experiences.

The Socio-ecological Approach

There are different ways to define the policy level. In this chapter, the socio-ecological model, as presented in Figure 40.1 (Ruiter et al., 2020; Bartholomew Eldredge et al., 2016; Fernandez et al., 2019b), is used to explain the interrelationships between individuals and their interpersonal, organisational, community, and policy environments (Kok et al., 2016).

The key assumption of the socio-ecological model is that environments (e.g., social, physical, policy) and settings (e.g., work, school) at higher ecological levels influence and shape behaviour at the individual level, and at the same time, individual behaviours influence and shape those higher socio-ecological levels. Within health psychology, promoting change at an environmental level means focusing on the behaviours and decision-making of environmental *agents* or *stakeholders* (Kok et al., 2016) who are influential at those levels, e.g., peers at the interpersonal level, school boards at the organisational level, local media at the community level, or politicians at the societal level. To change policies, important stakeholders in the policy domain at different ecological levels (including the organisational, community, and/or societal level) have to be identified and involved in the planning, development, and execution of behaviour change programmes at the policy level.

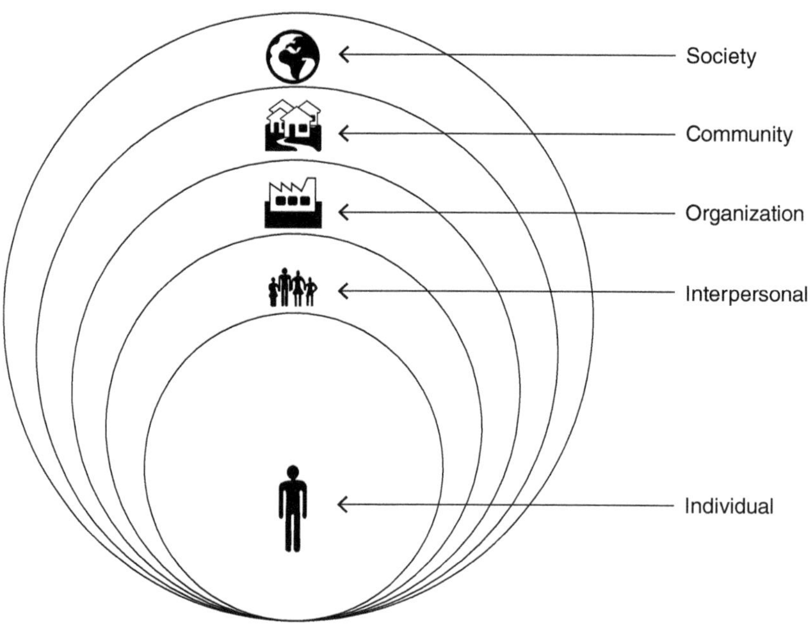

Figure 40.1 Socio-ecological model.

How to Identify and Involve Stakeholders?

Stakeholder Theory (Kok et al., 2015) can be used to identify stakeholders, which in turn may help to make changes at the organisational level. The theory suggests that especially stakeholders' salience (their power, legitimacy, and urgency), interest (support and opposition towards a health problem and their influence), and their position within a network are relevant aspects to consider. To effectively involve stakeholders, health psychologists could use a mix of communicative and compromise strategies (e.g., building a coalition, community involvement, setting new norms, community mobilisation by advocacy, agenda setting, and media usage; see Box 40.1 for an example of how to effectively involve stakeholders). These strategies may be used simultaneously and are likely to change according to the shifting dynamics of the relationships between the focal organisations and health-promoting organisations.

Box 40.1 How to Effectively Involve Stakeholders?

The process consists of

a identifying stakeholders who are knowledgeable about the issue at hand and their "stakes,"
b stakeholder mapping and visualisation in the network,
c identifying stakeholder salience, and
d selecting methods and pathways for change

(Kok et al., 2015).

Step 1: Assessing Stakeholders Who Are Knowledgeable about the Issue at Hand and Their Stakes. The health-promoting organisation first undertakes a stakeholder analysis. Personal experience, existing documents, public consultation, and interviews, starting with obvious stakeholders, are used to identify stakeholders and their interest in the health promotion intervention until no new actors can be identified. Stakes consist of investment in human and financial resources or activities in the programme.

Step 2: Stakeholder Mapping and Visualisation in the Network. The linkages between organisations form the basis for Step 2. Data for this step are answers to questions such as, "Whom do you ask for information related to the health issue", "To whom do you give information?", "Who do you work with?", and "Where do you get resources?"

Step 3: Identifying Stakeholder Salience. Analysing the health-promoting organisation's salience to its stakeholders and to the focal organisation will inform their strategies. Analysing the stakeholders' salience for the focal organisation will help to better anticipate the focal organisation's strategies to cope with the stakeholders' pressure.

> ***Step 4: Selecting Methods and Pathways for Change.*** The final step involves making informed decisions about the methods and pathways the health-promoting organisation will use to influence the focal organisation. Information from earlier analyses forms the basis for these decisions, as the density of the network and the salience and centrality of all stakeholders become visible.

Next to the use of stakeholder theory, *Core Processes* can be used to identify and involve relevant stakeholders (Ruiter en Crutzen, 2020) at different phases/steps of intervention planning following a fixed order of six steps:

In **Step 1**, the initial questions are formulated, for example: who are actually the relevant stakeholders, what role do they play, what is their interest, and what is their position in the broader picture.

In **Step 2**, planning group members will brainstorm an (unedited) list of possible answers to make sure that their current knowledge is ascertained (in this unedited list, also potentially relevant stakeholders can be identified, who – in later steps – are deemed less relevant).

In **Step 3**, additional support for the list of provisional answers is added based on a review of the available empirical findings. The empirical findings can identify potential additional stakeholders (e.g., an implementer who is essential for the execution of a specific policy change) or suggest that the role of some stakeholders is insignificant.

This list is further completed in **Step 4**, where theories (or combinations of theoretical constructs) are consulted (see also Box 40.2 for examples of theories at several ecological levels), first to understand the agents' behaviours and later to make behavioural changes where needed.

Only in **Step 5** is the need for new research identified and addressed by making use of a combination of qualitative and quantitative techniques.

Lastly, in **Step 6**, the provisional list of identified stakeholders can be completed and translated into a working list for which the evidence is sufficient.

Next to the potential use of Core Processes for the identification and involvement of stakeholders, the Core Processes are a practical tool that helps the planner with the complex and time-consuming process of developing an intervention, appropriately based on theory and evidence. Applying theory and evidence is often a challenging task in need of behavioural expertise, and these Core Processes will help the planner to make better choices in all steps of intervention development, at all levels, not just at the individual level but also at the environmental level.

The Essential Role of Planning In Theory- and Evidence-Based Health Psychology

Identifying and involving policy-related stakeholders by using the socio-ecological model, Core Processes, and stakeholder theory is helpful, but not enough. Health psychologists often make use of theories to understand and change stakeholders' behaviour (see Box 40.2 for clear examples of theories that can be used at different ecological levels). Based on those theories, (1) relevant determinants of behaviour and underlying beliefs can be identified, and (2) appropriate behaviour change methods/techniques can be selected that target the determinants of the behaviour (e.g., attitude, self-efficacy, motivation, skills). Note that almost all of the behaviour change methods in psychology (e.g., persuasion, modelling, goal-setting, guided practice) influence behaviour indirectly by influencing the underlying relevant and changeable determinants of behaviour (Crutzen et al., 2017). The behaviour change methods in turn should be translated to intervention applications that fit the characteristics of the target population and intervention context, and are in accordance with the underlying theory that describes the operating mechanism of change (Bartholomew Eldredge et al., 2016; Kok et al., 2016).

Essential for the way behaviour change methods may be applied are the so-called *parameters for effectiveness* that correspond with each method. Translating methods into practical applications demands a sufficient understanding of the theory and empirical evidence behind the method, especially the theoretical conditions (i.e., parameters for use) under which the method is likely to be effective or not. For example, behavioural modelling (providing an appropriate model being reinforced for the desired action) is a strong method, but only when certain parameters are met. For example, environmental decision-makers do not perform behaviour simply because a model demonstrates that behaviour; they do so only when the model exhibits certain characteristics, such as being positively reinforced for that particular behaviour and when they expect to be reinforced in a similar way. All theory-based methods have such parameters, which have to be taken into account when translating a method into practical applications (see Table 40.1. For illustrative examples, see Bartholomew et al., 2016; Kok et al., 2016).

Box 40.2 Example theories at different ecological levels.

There are many individual-level psychological theories, but also theories that specifically focus on the higher ecological levels. For example, at the interpersonal level (e.g., Social Support Theory, Holt-Lunstad & Uchino, 2015, or Stigma Theory, Bos et al., 2013), at the organisational level (e.g., Organisational Development and Change Theories, Cummings & Worley, 2014), the community level (e.g., Social Capital Theory, Jin & Lee, 2013, and Social Norms Theory, Smelser, 1998), the societal level (e.g., Stakeholder Theory, Kok et al., 2015, Agenda-Setting Theory, Clavier & de Leeuw, 2013), and theories and methodologies that can be applied across the various ecological levels that help in understanding the complexity of interacting and mediating and moderating processes that influence behaviour, including feedback loops, e.g., Systems Theories (Mabry et al., 2013), and complexity modelling approaches (Mkhitaryan et al., 2020).

Table 40.1 Methods for changing environmental conditions

Methods	*Method*	*Definition*	*Parameters*	*Application example*
Basic methods for changing the environment	Advocacy and lobbying (Galer-Unti, et al., 2004)	Arguing and mobilising resources on behalf of a particular change; giving aid to a cause; active support for a cause or position	Form of advocacy must match the style and tactics of the people, communities, or organisations represented, and the nature of the issue	Members of the European Health Psychology Society contact their legislators to urge them to vote for pending health-care reform legislation
Methods to change norms, social support, and social networks	Mobilising social networks and social support (Valente et al., 2015)	Encouraging social networks to provide informational, emotional, appraisal, and instrumental support	Availability of social network and potential support givers. Will often include information about others' approval, facilitation, and persuasion	Parents are coached on how to make their negative views about smoking clear to their children as part of tobacco prevention programme
Methods to change organisations	Increasing stakeholder influence (Kok et al., 2015)	Increase stakeholder power, legitimacy, and urgency, often by using community development and social action to change an organisation's policies	The focal organisation perceives that the external organisation or group is one of its stakeholders	A community group uses media advocacy to highlight the groundwater pollution by gas storage tanks located in the community and to demand that the tanks are removed

Methods to change communities	Community development (Wallerstein et al., 2015)	A form of community organisation based on consensus, in which power is shared equally in participatory problem-solving	Starting where the community is; this may be grassroots or professionally driven	A community organiser convenes a task force of the school board, the community, and the city council to address inequities in schools
Methods to change policy	Media advocacy (Dorfman & Krasnow, 2014)	Expose environmental agents' behaviours in the mass media in order to get them to approve health-related conditions; this is a type of advocacy	Requires the media to approve the news value of the message and accept the message without changing its essential content	A public interest group holds a press conference to focus attention on the serving sizes of fat and calories of food served in fast-food restaurants and what they, as responsible community businesses, should do

Selected examples: Bartholomew Eldredge et al. (2016), Kok et al. (2016).

Implementation Mapping

For both the individuals and environmental agents, we explained that the involvement of stakeholders, selecting the most important and changeable determinants and most appropriate methods, and developing the most promising applications are of high importance. To reach the ultimate impact of a health promotion intervention, not only should the programme be effective, but it also should be implemented with high levels of completeness and fidelity. In essence, this means that actions are not only desired with a focus on individuals and agents in the environment related to the problem, but also on agents in the environment who are in charge of implementation. Implementation scientists have developed several frameworks, theories, and models which describe implementation determinants, processes, or outcomes. Unfortunately, there is little guidance about how these can inform the development or selection of implementation strategies (methods or techniques used to improve adoption, implementation, sustainment, and scale-up of interventions).

A practical tool that combines knowledge from both the implementation science field and the health psychology field is *Implementation Mapping* (Fernandez et al., 2019a). Implementation Mapping is a systematic process for planning or selecting implementation strategies and involves five tasks: (1) conduct an implementation needs assessment and identify programme adopters and implementers; (2) state adoption and implementation outcomes and performance objectives, identify determinants, and create matrices of change objectives; (3) choose theoretical methods (mechanisms of change) and select or design implementation strategies; (4) produce implementation protocols and materials; and (5) evaluate implementation outcomes. The tasks are iterative, with the planner circling back to previous steps throughout this process to ensure all adopters and implementers, outcomes, determinants, and objectives are addressed (see, e.g., Markham et al., 2022).

The process of developing a behaviour change intervention can take a long time. However, in times of need, this development process has to be more efficient without losing scientific rigour. COVID-19 confronted health psychologists in such a time of need, causing a dilemma between quality and haste. However, in times of uncertainty, we should not behave like bystanders but be ready to advise and act with what we can contribute. As health psychologists, we were challenged to contribute to solutions from our health psychology expertise. And we can take that challenge; we do have a great amount of insight into understanding human behaviour and changing human behaviour. When needed, in challenging situations, we can apply those insights; we should not hide our light under a bushel. In the following section, examples are given of how health psychologists have worked in the COVID-19 pandemic response, advising national and local governments on how to adapt available theory to devise interventions and rapidly identifying evidence-based practises across similar contexts that can positively impact population-level health. Additionally, based on these health psychology actions, lessons learned are listed.

How Health Psychology Played a Role at Higher Ecological Levels during the COVID-19 Pandemic: Potential Role versus Real-Life Practice

In the Netherlands, the role of health psychologists during the initial months of the COVID-19 pandemic was at the national level somewhat ambiguous. On the one hand, the formal structure for scientific advice supporting the day-to-day political decisions of the government was limited to an advisory team of epidemiologists and medical scientists, with no psychologist present in the Outbreak Management Team (OMT). On the other hand, the Dutch National Institute for Public Health and the Environment, which provided the chair for the OMT, also formed an advisory group of health psychologists who could be asked for advice by the OMT, as well as the Ministry of Health. Additionally, there was a special subgroup for advice on vaccination behaviour. Advice was regularly sought from this group but needed to be given fast and was in practice based on consensus meetings with available expert members. Time-consuming research during this time period was almost impossible. In addition, for all experts involved, the available knowledge was seldom specific enough, while the answers needed to be provided fast. The following case examples illustrate some of these challenges.

Case 1: Risk compensation. Effective policy level interventions should not be made without insights from the health psychology field. A clear example was the implementation of the 1.5m distance rule. In the Netherlands, the behavioural restrictions started with asking people to keep 1.5-metre distance from each other. At some point, that was not considered enough. The question of the OMT to the experts was if making face masks mandatory could lead to the undesirable side effect that people would be less compliant with the 1.5-metre distance rule; in psychological terms, risk compensation.

At that time, Mantzari et al. (2020) had just published an article claiming that risk compensation, increasing risky behaviour after adopting a protective measure, was a non-existent phenomenon. They specifically concluded that wearing masks to prevent COVID-19 infection would not negatively affect keeping one's distance from others. There were also a few Dutch observational studies which supported that claim (Blanken et al., 2021; Liebst et al., 2022). As a result, the majority of the advisory group adopted this same position. Later, ten Hoor et al. (2024) conducted a rapid review of 19 articles on risk compensation in the COVID-19 setting and concluded that risk compensation is "still with us" but is not always strong. Next to the importance of making use of reviews/meta-analyses, a lesson learned – although in hindsight – is that the introduction of the face mask rule should have been accompanied by an intervention to prevent risk compensation.

Case 2: Reactance to vaccination restrictions. In the Netherlands, and many other countries, there was a moment when various interventions to promote COVID-19 vaccination were debated, including vaccination passes, checks, or

> certificates required for entering buildings and public transport. In a review by Brewer et al. (2017) on methods and strategies to increase (general) vaccination, these vaccination certificates can be considered an example of "requirements" (p. 182). Specifically, vaccination requirements make vaccination the default and impose a sanction or penalty on those who want to opt-out, with exemptions for people who are medically contraindicated and, in some cases, also for personal or religious beliefs. Brewer and colleagues conclude that "vaccination requirements are effective in increasing coverage for the targeted vaccines" (p. 183), and they are also effective in preventing vaccine-preventable diseases. They suggested adopting these kinds of requirements when vaccination coverage is very high and other interventions have already been deployed and when confidence in vaccine safety and effectiveness is high.

The downsides were also acknowledged and taken into consideration: people who feel their freedom is curtailed may act with anger, which may also lead to media attention and controversy. Additional issues in these policy discussions were (1) the complex legal issues (making COVID-19-certificates mandatory would require time-consuming changes in the labour laws) and (2) the observation that vaccination certificates seem to be most effective for the people who need them least: the highly educated and high income (Florence et al., 2022; Oliu-Barton et al., 2022). These arguments led to the OMT advice that COVID-19 certificates did not work, ending the debate. However, Albarracin et al. (2021) investigated, with one survey and three experiments, if vaccine requirements, compared to free choice, weaken or strengthen vaccination intentions in the US population. In all four studies, vaccination requirements strengthened vaccination intentions across various ethnic groups, settings, and levels of psychological reactance. These authors conclude that fears of backlash are unfounded and that implementing requirements will promote vaccine uptake (at least in the United States), which is in line with the health psychology insights from the review by Brewer et al. (2017) and later studies by Mills and Rüttenauer (2022), as well as Karaivanov et al. (2022).

Case 3: Supporting prevention with policy: Sanctions for not following preventive guidelines.

Social dilemma situations are not easily solved with communication interventions (van Lange et al., 2013). They often need other types of interventions. An example of how policy was effectively informed by health psychology knowledge is the transition from online to on-campus teaching at the university where we teach. Students work primarily in small tutorial groups with 10 to 15 students under the supervision of a tutor. During COVID-19, those groups were meeting online. In the new academic year (August 2021), tutorial groups started again on-site, but with clear COVID-19-preventive guidelines, at the so-called dark-green level, including a few rules, such as, "*Symptoms of a cold? Stay at home and do a test*", plus information about where to find test facilities. An important rule was that the tutors were instructed to send students home if they did not take this request seriously and were taking part in educational activities while they had symptoms. Tutors were not always happy with this "policing" task, and some expressed doubts about being able to handle those situations effectively. The responsible vice-deans communicated the following guidelines to all tutors to stimulate implementation:

If, during an on-campus teaching activity, a tutor who is in contact with students observes or a student points out that another student has symptoms consistent with COVID-19, the following escalation steps applied:

Step 1: The tutor asks the student to leave the building and get tested. The tutor can say, for example: "*It looks like you have symptoms of a cold. For safety reasons and in line with the current regulations, I have to ask you to leave the session and get tested for COVID-19*".

Step 2: If the student protests, depending on the student's reaction, the tutor can respond, following a number of suggestions, for example: "*There's compulsory attendance for this session – I have to be here*". The lecturer can respond, for example: "*I understand your worries about not complying with the compulsory attendance rule, but symptoms of a cold are a valid reason for absence. Next time, you should report your absence prior to the session. If you do not leave the session, you will be escorted out of the building by the building manager, and we will impose measures in line with the UM safety protocol and internal regulations*" (there were three other examples based on earlier experiences). If the student responds in a different way, the tutor can ask why the student does not want to leave the session and use this to formulate an answer, making sure you refer to the ground rules: stay home if you have symptoms and get tested immediately. Also, warn the students that if they do not leave the building, you will call the building manager and impose a measure in line with the Maastricht University safety protocol and internal regulations.

Step 3: If the student continues to resist, the tutor can call the building manager (or ask a COVID-19 steward to do this) to escort the student from the building. Students will be informed of this measure in writing by the dean/director in accordance with article 3, section 6 of the Maastricht University internal regulations.

What we see here is a mix of health psychology-informed persuasive techniques and power techniques at various levels, which makes sense because this case has all the characteristics of a social dilemma, and social dilemmas cannot simply be solved by persuasive communication. The lecturers needed to feel that they were supported by the university leadership. They had a phone number that would always reach the right person to provide support and, if necessary, someone in charge would come to the venue immediately and provide authority to the lecturer. There was no formal evaluation of this intervention, but there were situations reported where tutors asked students to leave the tutorial sessions. Interestingly, the building managers were never asked to appear, suggesting that tutors felt more support and were therefore more confident in executing the protocol effectively.

Epilogue and Lessons Learned

In this chapter, we discussed how health psychology ideally could play a role at the policy level. Examples were given as to how health psychologists have worked at the forefront during the COVID-19 pandemic, advising national and local governments on how to adapt available theory to devise interventions and rapidly identifying evidence-based practises across diverse contexts. Looking back at the COVID-19 pandemic, we see that behavioural science advisors were mostly asked very limited questions and sometimes gave answers that did not reflect the state of scientific evidence, which is understandable given the complexity of the issues but did not help in convincingly demonstrating the relevant role that health psychologist could and should play in these kinds of crisis situations.

In the Netherlands, for example, the major advisory body for the government on COVID-19 was the OMT, which consisted of only medical experts, especially virologists and public health specialists, none with recognisable expertise in health psychology or health promotion. The argument for this mono-disciplinary constellation was the need to reduce complexity. There was also an advisory group on behaviour change and health communication, with most of the Dutch health psychology experts, but that group responded to specific questions, mostly about practical implementation of the policy measures.

The positive news is that health psychologists were asked for advice at the policy level. Health psychologists were present in the media, while health behaviour change was on the political agenda. There will be moments in the future where health problems, health politics, and policy solutions will again coincide and health psychologists will again be asked for advice. One important development was the instalment of a societal impact team that could provide the Dutch government advice (at any time) on actions that had to be taken based on the consequences of the COVID-19 pandemic.

In this chapter, the main focus was on how health psychology can influence individual behaviours by informing policy and policy changes at the environmental level. We first defined the 'agents' or stakeholders in charge of policy (see Box 40.1). We explained how health psychologists could influence policy and practice effectively and what tools are important for efficiently communicating health psychology science to support evidence-informed policy and practice decisions (see Table 40.1). Health psychologists are sometimes project leads and sometimes are one of the stakeholders themselves, as part of broader teams that serve governments and organisations. We ended with specific examples of how health psychology expertise actually influenced COVID-19-related policy, highlighting a discrepancy between potential role versus real-life practice, as well as what lessons we learned from those experiences (see Box 40.3).

Box 40.3 Lessons Learned from Health Psychology during the COVID-19 Pandemic

ten Hoor et al. (2024) describe the just-in-time, planned development of an online intervention in the field of higher education, promoting COVID-19 vaccination among university students just before these students were eligible to be vaccinated. They showed that, if needed, intervention development can happen fast but still with sufficient empirical and theoretical support. ten Hoor et al. (2024) adapted the following four processes from Hanney et al. (2020): (1) increasing resources (e.g., funding), (2) working in parallel (e.g., starting a next step if there is enough information), (3) starting or working at a certain level of risk (e.g., expert consensus instead of new research), and (4) improving processes (e.g., accelerating procedures). They learned that the whole process is primarily dependent on the trust of those in charge of the quality of the programme developers. Moreover, this type of science is about applying theory, not about theory testing. As there was no COVID-19-related evidence available, evidence from related fields helped to inform decisions, as did theoretical knowledge about change processes, next to having easy access to the target population and getting help from important stakeholders for informed qualitative and quantitative research. This project was executed under time pressure, which made systematic effect evaluation not feasible.

ten Hoor et al. (2024) summarised their experiences in seven health psychology-related lessons:

1. ***Build Mutual Trust between Relevant Stakeholders and Implementers*:** The whole process depends on the trust of those in charge (in this case the leadership of the university) in the competency of the developers. For decision-makers, make sure to include people whose track record you know and who you trust. For implementers: make sure that the people in charge know your expertise in theory- and evidence-based intervention development and implementation.
2. ***Make Use of Theory and Core Processes*:** Theory testing is not part of this process; this is all about applying theory in a real-world and problem-driven context. Especially when time is limited, and therefore elaborate and rigorous research is not always possible, applying theories is the best alternative. One way to systematically apply theories is described in the so-called Core Processes, see page 000.
3. ***Make Use of a Systematic Approach with a Clear Planning Process*:** Existing systematic approaches (see O'Cathain et al., 2019, for an overview of planning frameworks) help with detailed note-taking of the decision-making process in intervention development and design, e.g., what is risky and what is a safe behaviour, what environmental conditions contribute to the problem, who is responsible, what are the determinants of behaviour, how can we change those determinants in the desired direction by an intervention, how can we implement the programme, and how can we measure the final outcomes?

4. ***Make Use of Evidence from Related Fields*:** If there is a lack of evidence around the problem, it can be helpful to rely on evidence from related fields. For example, in Intervention Mapping Step 3, the review of empirical findings was limited to articles on other comparable infectious diseases and vaccination programmes. The careful application of relevant theories in a setting of group discussions with experts formed the basis for 'theory- and evidence-based' programme development.
5. ***Make Use of Evidence from the Past and the Present*:** Several theory-informed methods (and parameters) were identified in the past. Here, the identified outcomes, performance objectives, determinants, and change objectives were based on theory and a survey among the students, providing adequate information about concerns and trust, risk perception, attitudinal, normative, and self-efficacy beliefs. These were linked to the intervention application(s). Given the setting, the target population, and the needs, an online intervention was chosen as the most efficient way to reach the students.
6. ***Identifying and Involving All Relevant Stakeholders*:** It is helpful to identify and involve all stakeholders related to the problem (university students) and solution (experts) throughout the entire process. Students had indicated science-based info as most trustworthy. The intervention consisted of four interviews, each with an expert from our own university, discussing medical aspects: risk for self and others, safety and trust, side effects, and societal aspects: reasons for getting vaccinated and the interaction with others. We had a 'student asking questions of the experts', as a voice of all other students.
7. ***Implementation Can Be More Urgent than Evaluation or Effect Measures*:** When there is no time for a randomised controlled trial to test the intervention, implementation takes precedence. For the timely intervention, the implementation plan was easy, as the university provided all necessary support. The intervention was implemented as soon as it was finished to promote students' responding positively to the vaccination invitations. Intervention Mapping Step 6, the evaluation plan, was not executed, as the focus was on the moment, and even one year later, the situation could have changed to a future where everything could be different.

Further Reading

Fernandez, M. E., ten Hoor, G. A., Van Lieshout, S., Rodriguez, S. A., Beidas, R. S., Parcel, G., Ruiter, R. A. C., Markham, C. M. & Kok, G. (2019). Implementation Mapping: using Intervention Mapping to develop implementation strategies. *Frontiers in Public Health*, *7*, 158.

ten Hoor, G. A., Varol, T., Mesters, I., Schneider, F., Kok, G., & Ruiter, R. A. C. (2023). Just-in-Time, but still planned: Lessons learned from speeding up the development and implementation of an intervention to promote COVID-19 vaccination in university students. *Health Promotion Practice*, 15248399221095077.

Kok, G., Gottlieb, N. H., Peters, G. J. Y., Mullen, P. D., Parcel, G. S., Ruiter, R. A. C., ... & Bartholomew, L. K. (2016). A taxonomy of behaviour change methods: an Intervention Mapping approach. *Health Psychology Review*, *10*(3), 297–312.

Ruiter, R. A. C. & Crutzen, R. (2020). Core Processes: how to use evidence, theories, and research in planning behavior change interventions. *Frontiers in Public Health*, *8*, 247.

Ruiter, R. A. C., Crutzen, R., Leeuw, E. D., Kok, G. (2020). Changing behavior using theories at the interpersonal, organizational, community, and societal levels. In: Hagger, M. S., Cameron, L. D., Hamilton, K., Hankonen, N. & Lintunen, T., *The handbook of behavior change* (pp. 251–266). Cambridge: Cambridge University Press.

References

Albarracin, D., Jung, H., Song, W., Tan, A., & Fishman, J. (2021). Rather than inducing psychological reactance, requiring vaccination strengthens intentions to vaccinate in US populations. *Scientific Reports*, *11*(1), 1–9.

Bartholomew Eldredge, L. K. B., Markham, C. M., Ruiter, R. A. C., Fernández, M. E., Kok, G., & Parcel, G. S. (2016). *Planning health promotion programs: An Intervention Mapping approach*. John Wiley & Sons.

Blanken, T. F., Tanis, C. C., Nauta, F. H., Dablander, F., Zijlstra, B. J., Bouten, R. R., ... Borsboom, D. (2021). Promoting physical distancing during COVID-19: a systematic approach to compare behavioral interventions. *Scientific Reports*, *11*(1), 1–8.

Bos, A. E., Pryor, J. B., Reeder, G. D., & Stutterheim, S. E. (2013). Stigma: Advances in theory and research. *Basic and Applied Social Psychology*, 35(1), 1–9.

Brewer, N. T., Chapman, G. B., Rothman, A. J., Leask, J., & Kempe, A. (2017). Increasing vaccination: putting psychological science into action. *Psychological Science in the Public Interest*, *18*(3), 149–207.

Clavier, C., & de Leeuw, E. (Eds.). (2013). *Health promotion and the policy process*. OUP, Oxford.

Crutzen, R., Peters, G. J. Y., & Noijen, J. (2017). Using confidence interval-based estimation of relevance to select social-cognitive determinants for behavior change interventions. *Frontiers in Public Health*, *5*, 165.

Cummings, T. G., & Worley, C. G. (2014). *Organization development and change*. Cengage learning.

Dorfman, L., & Krasnow, I. D. (2014). Public health and media advocacy. *Annual Review of Public Health*, *35*(1), 293–306.

Fernandez, M. E., ten Hoor, G. A., Van Lieshout, S., Rodriguez, S. A., Beidas, R. S., Parcel, G., Ruiter, R. A. C., Markham, C. M. & Kok, G. (2019a). Implementation Mapping: using Intervention Mapping to develop implementation strategies. *Frontiers in Public Health*, *7*, 158.

Fernandez, M. E., Ruiter, R. A. C., Markham, C. M., & Kok, G. (Eds.). (2019b). Theory- and evidence-based health promotion program planning; Intervention Mapping. *Frontiers in Public Health*, https://doi.org/10.3389/fpubh.2019.00209

Florence, D., Emmanuel, L., Lucie, G., Marie, J., & Anne-Sophie, J. (2022). The French domestic "sanitary pass" did not solve Covid-19 vaccination inequities in France. medRxiv preprint doi: https://doi.org/10.1101/2022.01.03.22268676

Galer-Unti, R. A., Tappe, M. K., & Lachenmayr, S. (2004). Advocacy 101: Getting started in health education advocacy. *Health Promotion Practice*, *5*(3), 280–288.

Hanney, S. R., Wooding, S., Sussex, J., & Grant, J. (2020). From COVID-19 research to vaccine application: Why might it take 17 months not 17 years and what are the wider lessons? *Health Research Policy and Systems*, *18*, 1–10. https://link.springer.com/content/pdf/10.1186/s12961-020-00571-3.pdf

Holt-Lunstad, J., & Uchino, B. N. (2015). Social support and health. In K. Glanz, B. K. Rimer, & K. Viswanath (Eds.), *Health behavior: Theory, research, and practice* (pp. 183–204). Jossey-Bass/Wiley.

Jin, B., & Lee, S. (2013). Enhancing community capacity: Roles of perceived bonding and bridging social capital and public relations in community building. *Public Relations Review*, 39(4), 290–292.

Karaivanov, A., Kim, D., Lu, S. E., & Shigeoka, H. (2022). COVID-19 vaccination mandates and vaccine uptake. *Nature Human Behaviour*, 1–10.

Kok, G., Gottlieb, N. H., Peters, G. J. Y., Mullen, P. D., Parcel, G. S., Ruiter, R. A. C., … Bartholomew, L. K. (2016). A taxonomy of behaviour change methods: An Intervention Mapping approach. *Health Psychology Review*, *10*(3), 297–312.

Kok, G., Gurabardhi, Z., Gottlieb, N. H., & Zijlstra, F. R. (2015). Influencing organizations to promote health: Applying stakeholder theory. *Health Education & Behavior*, *42*(1_suppl), 123S–132S.

van Lange, P. A., Joireman, J., Parks, C. D., & Van Dijk, E. (2013). The psychology of social dilemmas: A review. *Organizational Behavior and Human Decision Processes*, *120*(2), 125–141.

Liebst, L. S., Ejbye-Ernst, P., de Bruin, M., Thomas, J., & Lindegaard, M. R. (2022). No evidence that mask-wearing in public places elicits risk compensation behavior during the COVID-19 pandemic. *Scientific Reports*, *12*(1), 1–7.

Mabry, P. L., Milstein, B., Abraido-Lanza, A. F., Livingood, W. C., & Allegrante, J. P. (2013). Opening a window on systems science research in health promotion and public health. *Health Education & Behavior*, 40(1_suppl), 5S–8S.

Mantzari, E., Rubin, G. J., & Marteau, T. M. (2020). Is risk compensation threatening public health in the covid-19 pandemic? *BMJ*, *370*: m2913

Markham CM, Rushing SC, Manthei J, Singer M, Jessen C, Gorman G, Peskin MF, Hernandez BF, Sacca L, Evans GS, Luna-Meza C, Merritt Z and Shegog R (2022) The Healthy Native Youth Implementation Toolbox: Using Implementation Mapping to adapt an online decision support system to promote culturally-relevant sexual health education for American Indian and Alaska Native youth. *Frontiers Public Health 10*: 889924. doi: 10.3389/fpubh.2022.889924

Mkhitaryan, S., Giabbanelli, P. J., de Vries, N. K., & Crutzen, R. (2020). Dealing with complexity: How to use a hybrid approach to incorporate complexity in health behavior interventions. *Intelligence-Based Medicine*, 3–4, 100008. https://doi.org/10.1016/j.ibmed.2020.100008

Mills, M. C., & Rüttenauer, T. (2022). The effect of mandatory COVID-19 certificates on vaccine uptake: synthetic-control modelling of six countries. *The Lancet Public Health*, 7(1), e15–e22.

O'Cathain, A., Croot, L., Sworn, K., Duncan, E., Rousseau, N., Turner, K., … Hoddinott, P. (2019). Taxonomy of approaches to developing interventions to improve health: a systematic methods overview. *Pilot and Feasibility Studies*, 5(1), 1–27.

Oliu-Barton, M., Pradelski, B. S., Woloszko, N., Guetta-Jeanrenaud, L., Aghion, P., Artus, P., … Wolff, G. B. (2022). The effect of COVID certificates on vaccine uptake, health outcomes, and the economy. *Research Square*, DOI: https://doi.org/10.21203/rs.3.rs-1242919/v2

Ruiter, R. A. C. & Crutzen, R. (2020). Core Processes: how to use evidence, theories, and research in planning behavior change interventions. *Frontiers in Public Health*, *8*, 247.

Ruiter, R. A. C., Crutzen, R., Leeuw, E. D., Kok, G. (2020). Changing behavior using theories at the interpersonal, organizational, community, and societal levels. In: Hagger, M. S., Cameron, L. D., Hamilton, K., Hankonen, N. & Lintunen, T., *The handbook of behavior change* (pp. 251–266). Cambridge: Cambridge University Press.

Smelser, N. J. (1998). Social Structure. In: N.J. Smelser (Ed.), *Handbook of Sociology* (pp. 103–130). Newbury Park, CA: Sage.
ten Hoor, G. A., Ruiter, R. A.C., & Kok, G. (2024). Risk compensation in times of COVID-19: Do people keep distance when wearing a facemask? A rapid review. *Discover Social Science and Health*, *4*(1), 50.
Valente, T. W., Palinkas, L. A., Czaja, S., Chu, K. H., & Brown, C. H. (2015). Social network analysis for program implementation. *PloS one*, *10*(6), e0131712.
Wallerstein, N., Minkler, M., Carter-Edwards, L., Avila, M., & Sánchez, V. (2015). Improving health through community engagement, community organization, and community building. In: Glanz, K. Rimer, B. & Viswanath, K. (Eds.), *Health behavior: Theory, research, and practice* (pp. 277–300). Jossey-Bass/Wiley.

INDEX

Pages in *italics* refer to figures, pages in **bold** refer to tables, and pages followed by "*b*" refer to boxes.

For Product Safety Concerns and Information please contact our EU
representative GPSR@taylorandfrancis.com
Taylor & Francis Verlag GmbH, Kaufingerstraße 24, 80331 München, Germany

www.ingramcontent.com/pod-product-compliance
Ingram Content Group UK Ltd.
Pitfield, Milton Keynes, MK11 3LW, UK
UKHW020156200926
475702UK00016B/2744
* 9 7 8 1 0 3 2 3 3 0 6 6 2 *